Neurobiology of Alzheimer's Disease

(Molecular and Cellular Neurobiology)

Neurobiology of Alzheimer's Disease

(Molecular and Cellular Neurobiology)

David Dawbarn
Reader in Medicine, University of Bristol

Shelley J. Allen
Research Fellow in Medicine, University of Bristol

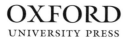
OXFORD
UNIVERSITY PRESS

OXFORD

UNIVERSITY PRESS

Great Clarendon Street, Oxford OX2 6DP

Oxford University Press is a department of the University of Oxford. It
furthers the University's objective of excellence in research, scholarship,
and education by publishing worldwide in

Oxford New York

Athens Auckland Bangkok Bogotá Buenos Aires Calcutta Cape Town
Chennai Dar es Salaam Delhi Florence Hong Kong Istanbul Karachi
Kuala Lumpur Madrid Melbourne Mexico City Mumbai Nairobi
Paris São Paulo Singapore Taipei Tokyo Toronto Warsaw

with associated companies in Berlin Ibadan

Oxford is a registered trade mark of Oxford University Press in the UK
and in certain other countries

Published in the United States by Oxford University Press Inc., New York

British Library Cataloguing in Publication Data Data available

Library of Congress Cataloguing in Publication Data

Neurobiology of alzheimer's disease/David Dawbarn, Shelly J. Allen
[editors].
      p.cm. — (Molecular and cellular neurobiology)
   Includes index.
   1. Alzheimer's disease—Pathophysiology. 2. Molecular neurobiology.
I. Dawbarn, David. II. Allen, Shelly J. III. Molecular and cellular
neurobiology series.

RC523. N417 2000   616.8'3107—dc21   00-045314

ISBN 0-19-852460-9 (hbk.)
ISBN 0-19-852459-5 (Pbk.)

1 3 5 7 9 10 8 6 4 2

Typeset in Minion by Expo Holdings, Malaysia
Printed in Great Britain on acid-free paper
by T. J. International Ltd., Padstow

Preface

Each new year has brought revelations about molecules implicated in Alzheimer's disease (AD), both veteran, such as amyloid and tau, and newly discovered, such as the presenilins and beta-site amyloid precursor protein (APP)-cleaving enzyme (BACE/Asp2). Discovery is speeding up; research papers with Alzheimer in the title have increased five-fold since 1991 compared with the increase in number of papers published, in general, on the brain. At the moment there is a raised level of expectation in both the academic and public domains.

We have come a long way since the discoveries of the cholinergic deficit in the 1970s and the characterization of plaques and tangles in the 1980s when there seemed to be a specialization and separation of various key aspects of the disease. More recent discoveries such as apolipoprotein E4 (apoE4) as a risk factor and the presenilins as causative factors have facilitated a merging and interweaving of various aspects of this disease. It is becoming crucial that researchers working in one field of Alzheimer's research understand the discoveries in the other fields too.

This book aims to present an accessible overview of each of the predominant aspects of this disease. Included are chapters on neuropathology, genetics, inflammation, neurochemical pathology and pharmacology, diagnosis, models of the disease, therapeutics, and of course key molecules such as Aβ, tau, apoE, and the presenilins. Also included are appendices covering the protein sequences and other information on APP, tau, the presenilins, and apoE.

We hope that this approach will provide not only a readable introduction for those new to the subject, but also allow researchers to seek out and appreciate overlap of their areas of expertise with other aspects of the disease.

David Dawbarn
Shelley J. Allen

Contents

List of Contributors

Allen, Shelley J.
Molecular Neurobiology Unit
Research Centre for Neuroendocrinology
University of Bristol
Address for correspondence:
Molecular Neurobiology Unit
URCN
Bristol Royal Infirmary
Bristol BS2 8HW. UK
shelley.allen@bristol.ac.uk

Allsop, David
Department of Biological Sciences
Lancaster University, Lancaster LA1 4YQ. UK
d.allsop@lancaster.ac.uk
http:/bssv01.lancs.ac.uk/bs/home.html

Al-Mohanna, Futwan
Biological & Medical Research
King Faisal Specialist Hospital and Research
  Centre
Riyadh 11211, Saudi Arabia

Arai, Hiroyuki
Department of Geriatric and Respiratory
  Medicine
Tohoku University School of Medicine
Sendai, Miyagi 980, Japan

Burns, Alistair
University Dept of Psychiatry
Withington Hospital
West Didsbury
Manchester M20 8LR U.K
A_Burns@fs1.wph.man.ac.uk

Citron, Martin
Amgen Inc. Dept. of Neurobiology
One Amgen Center Drive
Thousand Oaks
CA 91320–1799 USA
mcitron@amgen.com

Collison, Kate
Biological & Medical Research
King Faisal Specialist Hospital and Research
  Centre
Riyadh 11211, Saudi Arabia

Davies, Peter
Departments of Pathology and Neuroscience
Albert Einstein College of Medicine
1300 Morris Park Ave
Bronx, New York 10461 USA
Davies@mailserver.aecom.yu.edu

Dawbarn, David
Molecular Neurobiology Unit
Research Centre for Neuroendocrinology
University of Bristol
Address for correspondence:
Molecular Neurobiology Unit
URCN
Bristol Royal Infirmary
Bristol BS2 8HW. UK
dave.dawbarn@bristol.ac.uk

Duff, Karen
Nathan Kline Institute for Psychiatric Research
Dementia Research Program
140 Old Orangeburg Road
Orangeburg, New York
10962–2210. USA

Eastley, Rebecca
Avonmead
Mental Health Unit
Southmead Hospital
BS10 5NB U.K

Emmerling, Mark
Parke-Davis Pharmaceutical Research
A Warner-Lambert Company
2800 Plymouth Road
Ann Arbor Michigan, USA

Esiri, Margaret M
Department of Clinical Neurology and
  Neuropathology
University of Oxford and Radcliffe Infirmary
  NHS Trust
Address for correspondence:
Department of Neuropathology
Radcliffe Infirmary
Oxford OX2 6HE. UK
margaret.esiri@clneuro.ox.ac.uk

Fox, Nick
Dementia Research Group
Department of Clinical Neurology
Institute of Neurology, Queen Square
London WC1N 3BG. UK

Gracon, Stephen I
Parke-Davis Pharmaceutical Research
A Warner-Lambert Company
2800 Plymouth Road
Ann Arbor Michigan
MI 48105. USA

Harrington, Charles R.
Department of Mental Health
University Medical Buildings
University of Aberdeen
Foresterhill, Aberdeen.
AB25 2ZD. UK
c.harrington@abdn.ac.uk

Higuchi Makoto
Department of Geriatric and Respiratory
    Medicine
Tohoku University School of Medicine
Sendai, Miyagi 980, Japan

Higuchi, Susumu
Department of Psychiatry
Kurihama National Hospital
National Institute on Alcoholism
Kanagawa 239, Japan

Høgh, Peter
Memory Disorders Research Unit
The Neuroscience Center
Copenhagen University Hospital
Rigshospitalet, Copenhagen, Denmark

Howlett, D. R.
SmithKline Beecham Pharmaceuticals
New Frontiers Science Park
Third Avenue, Harlow, Essex
CM19 5AW. UK
david_howlett-1@sbphrd.com

Iwatsubo, Takeshi
Department of Neuropathology and
    Neuroscience
Faculty of Pharmaceutical sciences
University of Tokyo
Tokyo, 174, Japan

Jeffries, Suzanne
University Dept of Psychiatry
Withington Hospital
West Didsbury, Manchester
M20 8LR. UK

Karran, E. H.
Pfizer Central Research
Ramsgate Road
Sandwich, Kent
CT13 9NJ UK

Morikawa, Yu-ichi
Department of Geriatric and Respiratory
    Medicine
Tohoku University School of Medicine
Sendai 980, Miyagi, Japan

Okamura, Nobuyuki
Department of Geriatric and Respiratory
    Medicine
Tohoku University School of Medicine
Sendai 980, Miyagi, Japan

Roher, Alex
Haldeman Laboratory for Alzheimer's Disease
    Research Laboratory
Sun Health Research Institute
Sun City, Arizona 85372. USA

Rossor, Martin N.
Dementia Research Group
Department of Clinical Neurology
Institute of Neurology
Queen Square
London WC1N 3BG and Imperial College
School of Science
Technology and Medicine
St Mary's Campus, Norfolk Place
London W2 1PG. UK

Saunders, Ann M.
Joseph and Kathleen Bryan Alzheimer's Disease
    Research Center
Division of Neurology
Duke University Medical Center
Durham
NC 27710. USA
saund005@mc.duke.edu

Sasaki, Hidetada
Department of Geriatric and Respiratory
  Medicine
Tohoku University School of Medicine
Sendai 980, Miyagi, Japan

Scahill, Rachael
Dementia Research Group
Department of Clinical Neurology
Institute of Neurology, Queen Square
London WC1N 3BG. UK

Schmidt, Ann Marie
Departments of Pathology
Physiology & Cellular Biophysics
Surgery and Medicine
College of Physicians and Surgeons of Columbia
  University
New York, NY 10032. USA

Soto, Claudio
Department of Pathology
New York University Medical Center
New York, NY 10016. USA

Stern, David
Departments of Pathology
Physiology & Cellular Biophysics
Surgery and Medicine
College of Physicians and Surgeons of Columbia
  University
New York, NY10032. USA

Theuring, Franz
Campus Charité Mitte
Institut für Pharmakologie und Toxikologie
Dorotheenstrasse 94–10117
Berlin, Germany
Theuring@charite.de

Trojanowski, John Q.
Division of Anatomic Pathology
Department of Pathology and Laboratory
  Medicine
University of Pennsylvania
Philadelphia, PA 19104, USA

Vanderstichele, Hugo
Department of Molecular Science
Innogenetics, Ghent, Belgium

Vanmechelen, Eugeen
Department of Molecular Science
Innogenetics, Ghent, Belgium

Wasco, Wilma
Genetics and Aging Unit
Department of Neurology
Massachusetts General Hospital
Harvard Medical School
Building 149, 13th Street
Charlestown, MA 02129–9142. USA
wasco@helix.mgh.harvard.edu

Wilcock, Gordon
Department of Care of the Elderly
Frenchay Hospital
Frenchay, Bristol
BS16 ILE. UK

Wischik, Claude M.
Department of Mental Health
Institute of Medical Sciences
University of Aberdeen
Foresterhill, Aberdeen
AB25 2ZD. UK
c.m.wischik@abdn.ac.uk

Yan, Shi Du
Department of Pathology
Physiology and Cellular Biophysics
Surgery and Medicine
College of Physicians and Surgeons of Columbia
  University
Address for correspondence:
Department of Pathology
P&S 17–401
College of Physicians & Surgeons
Columbia University
630 West 168th Street
New York, NY 10032 USA

List of Abbreviations

α2M	α-2 macroglobulin
Aβ	amyloid beta-protein (e.g. Aβ1–40)
ABAD	amyloid β peptide binding protein alcohol dehydrogenase
ACE	angiotensin-converting enzyme
ACh	acetylcholine
AChE	acetylcholinesterase
ACT	α_1-antichymotrypsin
AD	Alzheimer's disease
ADAM	a disintegrin and metalloprotease like
ADAS	Alzheimer's disease assessment scale
ADFACS	Alzheimer's disease functional assessment and change scale
ADL	activities of daily living
ADRDA	Alzheimer's disease and related disorders association
AGE	advanced glycation endproducts
ALG-3	apoptosis-linked gene 3
AMPA	alpha-amino-3-hydroxy-5-methyl-4-isoxazole propionic acid
AMTS	abbreviated mental test score
APM	affected pedigree member
apoE	apolipoprotein E
APP	amyloid precursor protein (sAPP secreted APP)
ATP9	ATP synthase subunit 9
BACE	β-site APP cleaving enzyme
BDNF	brain-derived neurotrophic factor
CAMDEX	Cambridge examination for mental disorders of the elderly
CBD	corticobasal degeneration
CBF	cerebral blood flow
cdk	cyclin dependant kinase
CEI	cholinesterase inhibitor
CERAD	Consortium to Establish a Registry for Alzheimer's Disease
CIE	Canberra interview for the elderly
ChAT	choline acetyltransferase
CHO	Chinese hamster ovary
CJD	Creutzfeldt-Jakob disease
CNS	central nervous system
COX-2	cyclooxygenase 2
CRF	corticotropin-releasing factor
CSF	cerebrospinal fluid
CT	computerised tomography
CTF	C-terminal fragment (of presenilin)
DAD	disability assessment for dementia
DBB	diagonal band of Broca

DCP1	dipeptidyl carboxypeptidase 1
DDPAC	disinhibition dementia parkinsonism amyotrophy complex
DLB	dementia with Lewy bodies
Dll1	Delta-like ligand 1
DSM	Diagnostic and Statistical Manual
EEG	electroencephalogram
EGF	epidermal growth factor
ELISA	enzyme-linked immunosorbent assay
EPI	echo planar imaging
ER	endoplasmic reticulum
ERAB	ER-associated Aβ binding protein
ERα	oestrogen receptor gene α
ERK	extracellular signal-related kinase
ERT	oestrogen replacement therapy
FBD	familial British dementia
FDG	fluorodeoxyglucose
FENIB	familial encephalopathy with neuroserpin inclusion bodies
FITC	fluorescein isothiocyanate
FTDP	frontotemporal dementia and Parkinsonism
GFAP	glial fibrillary acidic protein
GMSS	geriatric mental state schedule
GS	glutamine synthetase
GSK-3β	glycogen synthase kinase 3β
HCHWA-D	hereditary cerebral haemorrhage with amyloidosis- Dutch type
HMG-coA	3-hydroxy-3-methylglutaryl coenzyme A
ICD	International Classification of Disease
ICE	interleukin-converting enzyme
IDDD	interview for deterioration in daily living activities in dementia
IL-1	interleukin 1
icv	intracerebroventricular
ITT	intention to treat
KPI	Kunitz protease inhibitor domain (on APP)
LDL	low density lipoprotein
LRP	LDL receptor-related protein
MAC	membrane attack complex
MAO	monoamine oxidase
MAP	mitogen activated protein (kinase)
MAP	microtubule-associated protein
MCI	mild cognitive impairment
M-CSF	macrophage-colony stimulating factor
MMSE	mini-mental state examination
MRI	magnetic resonance imaging
MRS	magnetic resonance spectroscopy
NACP	α-synuclein derived non-amyloid component
NBM	nucleus basalis of Meynert
NCAM	neural cell adhesion molecule

NFκβ	nuclear factor κβ
NFT	neurofibrillary tangles
NGF	nerve growth factor
NICD	Notch intracellular domain
NINCDS	National Institute of Neurological and Communicative Disorders and Stroke
NMDA	N-methyl-D-aspartate
NOS	nitric oxide synthase
NPC	Niemann-Pick type C disease
NPI	neuropsychiatric inventory
NSAD	non-steroidal anti-inflammatory drugs
NT-3	neurotrophin-3
NT-4	neurotrophin-4
NTF	N-terminal fragment (of presenilin)
NTP	neural thread protein
PD	Parkinson's disease
PDGF	platelet-derived growth factor
PDPK	proline-directed protein kinase
PET	positron emission tomography
PHF	paired helical filaments
PKC	protein-kinase C
PLC	phospholipase C
PNLD	pallido-nigro-luysian-degeneration
PP	protein phosphatases
PPND	pallido-ponto-nigral-degeneration
PS1 or PS2	presenilin 1 or 2
PSP	progressive supranuclear palsy
QOL	quality of life
RAGE	receptor for advanced glycation end products
RAP	receptor associated protein
ROS	reactive oxygen species
RR	relative risk
SAP	stress-activated protein kinase
SCAP	SREBP cleavage activation protein
SIDAM	structured interview for the diagnosis of dementia of the Alzheimer type multi-infarct dementia and other dementias
SOD	superoxide dismutase
SPECT	single photon emission computed tomography
SPM	statistical parametric mapping
SREBP	sterol regulatory element binding protein
SSRI	selective serotonin reuptake inhibitor
STEM	scanning transmission electron microscopy
TGF	transforming growth factor
TACE	TNFα converting enzyme
THA	tetrahydroaminoacridine, Tacrine
TIMP	tissue inhibitor of matrix metalloproteases

TNF   tumour necrosis factor
TP   temporal-parietal
Trk   tyrosine receptor kinase (neurotrophin receptors)
VLDL   very low density lipoprotein
WMH   white matter hyperintensities

Chapter 1

Alzheimer's disease: past, present and future themes

Shelley J. Allen

Alzheimer's disease (AD) is the most common form of dementia in the elderly, affecting up to twenty million people world-wide. It is estimated that by 2025, that number will have nearly doubled (review Prince 1997). Estimates of prevalence vary, however, the generally accepted chance of developing the disease is <0.05% in those aged below 60, >5% chance for those over 60 years, and >20% in those over 80. Survival in developed countries is currently approximately six years (median value) after diagnosis.

AD is a form of dementia characterized by symptoms of memory loss and confusion, coupled with a distinctive combination of neuropathological changes including neuronal loss, intracellular neurofibrillary tangles (NFT) and extracellular amyloid plaques. Few cases are familial with autosomal dominance, however, those that are, appear similar to sporadic cases, except that the symptoms and pathology can be more severe and present at an earlier age. NFT and amyloid plaques may be found in many normal non-demented elderly, but in reduced numbers, and are classified as 'age-related changes'.

Speculating on the aetiology of the disease from these facts alone might suggest that AD is simply the ageing process speeded up. It seems to be inevitable that if we live long enough we will all succumb to this dementing illness. But is that true?

Clues as to the mechanisms of neurodegeneration can be found in some families where there is evidence of mutations in a protein called amyloid precursor protein (APP). In these families APP is cleaved, more frequently than normal, to form a 4 kDa peptide Aβ, which is then deposited in the core of the senile plaques. A single point mutation in the gene for APP is able to produce the full neuropathological and symptom profile of AD. Mutations in two newly discovered multi-transmembrane proteins, namely presenilin 1 (PS1) and PS2, are also causative of AD, and are involved in cleavage of APP to form Aβ.

Most researchers agree that Aβ plays a major part in the initiation of events which lead to neurodegeneration in AD. However, if we ask by what *means* Aβ is able to cause this neurodegeneration, which results in dementia, we may be less sure of a consensus. A number of factors have been shown to influence the process of degeneration including PS mutations, risk factors such as age, head injury, and the presence of one particular polymorphic protein product of the apolipoprotein E gene, apoE4. Conversely other factors may protect against AD, such as the presence of apoE2, non steroidal anti-inflammatory drugs (NSAID), and hormone replacement therapy, or may ameliorate symptoms, such as cholinesterase inhibitors.

In any hypothetical pathway between APP cleavage and neuronal loss we should be able to account for the effects of these factors at some point along this pathway. We should also be able to explain the pattern of neuropathology and the symptoms of the dementia. Can we explain each of these in *one* model of neurodegeneration? The following overview touches on some of these aspects, and provides a brief introduction to the chapters within this book which then deal with each subject in depth.

1.1 Alzheimer

The official introduction to Alzheimer's disease as a presenile dementia was presented by a German physician, Dr Alois Alzheimer in 1907 (Alzheimer 1907) (Fig. 1.1). He described the post-mortem analysis of the brain of a 51-year-old woman who, in life, had exhibited signs of cognitive impairment, depression, and hallucinations. Neuropathological analysis revealed extensive senile plaque and NFT formation. Although AD-associated neuropathology had been described in the aged brain in the two preceding decades, this study of what is now termed an 'early onset' case led to its naming as 'Alzheimer's disease' by Kraeplin in 1910. However, the term is now used loosely to describe all patients, of whatever age, who present the characteristic symptoms of dementia and neuropathology (see Chapter 2 for a discussion of neuropathology by Margaret Esiri).

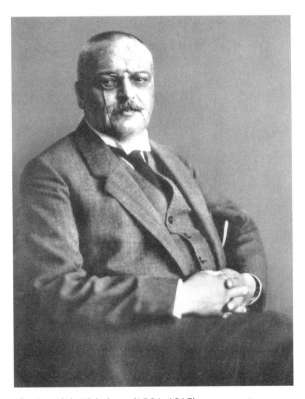

Fig. 1.1 Alois Alzheimer (1864–1915)

The gross neuropathological changes to the brain of both early and late onset cases involves, to a greater or lesser degree, thinning of the cortical gyri, widening of the sulci, and enlarging of the ventricles (see Chapter 2, Fig. 2.1). Microscopically this translates largely as a loss of grey matter. Measurements of cell loss vary but in severe cases it can amount to a greater than 40% loss in certain regions of the neocortex and in some sub-cortical nuclei.

1.2 Amyloid pathology

Plaques are microscopic areas of degeneration which contain deposits of amyloid protein, comprising aggregated Aβ peptides up to 43 amino acids in length. The most common forms present are known as Aβ1–40 and Aβ1–42, and are derived from APP. Plaques may be 'cored', that is with a dense core of amyloid protein aggregated to form beta pleated sheets, or they may be 'diffuse' in nature. Cored plaques may be 'neuritic', that is surrounded and infiltrated by degenerating neurites or 'burned out', with only a dense core of amyloid remaining. Cored plaques can be viewed in a variety of ways, one of which is by staining with Congo Red. Under polarized light this stain produces a green birefringence due to its binding to the beta pleated sheet form of the amyloid. In a similar way, stains such as Thioflavin S will bind to amyloid when it is in a beta pleated sheet formation. Diffuse plaques, which are more abundant, cannot be seen in this way and require staining with antibodies, usually to Aβ, in order to be made visible. About 80% of AD patients also have cerebrovascular amyloid deposited in the small vessels (Masters *et al.* 1985*a*) in the leptomeninges and cortices, resulting in congophilic angiopathy, which can also be seen using stains described above.

Deposited amyloid is uncommonly perverse, biochemically speaking, as it is impervious to degradation, and initially it was extremely difficult to isolate. After much effort it was extracted, purified from brain, and characterized, and the amino acid sequencing of cerebrovascular amyloid was finally achieved by Glenner and Wong in 1984 (Glenner and Wong 1984). The plaque core cerebral amyloid protein was also purified and characterized and found to be similar to that of amyloid of cerebrovascular origin and to amyloid found in the brains of Down patients (Masters *et al.* 1985*b*). In all three cases the protein consisted of multimeric aggregates of a 4kDa polypeptide of about 40 residues. In 1987 this peptide was shown to be derived from a much larger, 695 amino acid, protein precursor APP (Goldgaber *et al.* 1987; Kang *et al.* 1987; Robakis *et al.*1987; Tanzi *et al.*1987), which resembled a cell surface receptor with a single transmembrane domain. The gene for APP was localized to the long arm of chromosome 21. This was in accord with the fact that Down patients, with three copies of chromosome 21 (Trisomy 21), were known to produce cerebral amyloid deposits similar to that of AD, and in fact usually developed AD by their fourth decade.

In 1990 a report was published showing a mutation in the *APP* gene (E693Q) in a family with hereditary cerebral haemorrhage with amyloidosis, Dutch type (HCHWA-D, Levy *et al.* 1990). Following this was a report of an AD kindred with a mutation in the *APP* gene (V717I London mutation; Goate *et al.* 1991). Although, as it turned out, these families with *APP* mutations are rare (roughly 120 families have been discovered world-wide), the discovery showed that a single mutation in the *APP* gene was able to increase Aβ production, and that this was evidently upstream of NFT formation.

1.3 **Amyloid precursor protein**

APP is a member of a superfamily of amyloid precursor-like proteins (APLP) and APP homologues. The Aβ peptide sequence is only conserved in the APP forms. Alternative splice forms of the *APP* gene code for a protein of up to 770 amino acid residues, most commonly APP695, APP751 and APP770. On the Swiss-Prot database the longest form of APP is given (770: primary accession no. P05067) and mutations are usually denoted using this form. David Howlett and co-authors give a detailed account of APP and its processing in Chapter 4. APP sequence and details are given in Appendix I. This form is used throughout this chapter. One of the alternatively transcribed exons encodes a 56 amino acid Kunitz protease inhibitor (KPI) domain and the KPI-containing form of APP, also known as Protease Nexin II, is able to inhibit a number of serine proteases. APP is widely expressed in various neuronal and non-neuronal tissues; the predominant form of APP in neurons does not contain the KPI domain, in general that produced in astrocytes and microglia, and in peripheral tissues does.

The function of APP is still not fully understood, although from its cDNA sequence and from *in vitro* experiments we can see that it is a single transmembrane protein with potential functions which include cell adhesion molecule, aid to neurite outgrowth and synaptogenesis, and promoter of cell survival. It has been suggested that cell death in AD is not so much due to the formation of Aβ, but rather that the beneficial secreted APP, sAPPα, is not formed. Surprisingly then, APP null mice seem to suffer little from its absence (Zheng *et al.* 1995). They are viable, though underweight, with decreased locomotor activity, and some reactive gliosis; however not showing the, perhaps expected, extensive cell death. Similarly, the APLP2 knockout mouse is healthy. However, mice with a double knockout of APP and APLP2 are very different. 80% of these die a week after birth and those that survive have deficits in balance and lack strength (Von Koch *et al.* 1997). The inference is that APP and APLP2 are able normally to compensate for each other in the single knockouts.

Central to the understanding of the importance of APP in the AD neurodegenerative process must be the way in which the molecule is processed to form the Aβ peptide. APP is cleaved predominantly by the enzyme α-secretase, between K16 and L17 of Aβ. This cleavage precludes the production of the Aβ domain and, as noted above, results in the secretion of the N-terminal portion of APP as sAPPα. sAPPα appears to be protective in that it can reduce the excitotoxic effects of various molecules such as Aβ or glutamate. APP is synthesized in the rough endoplasmic reticulum (ER), and transported to the plasma membrane via the secretory pathway through the Golgi and secretory vesicles to the surface. After cleavage at the plasma membrane the C-terminal membrane bound fragment of APP consisting of 83 amino acids (c83) is internalized via clathrin coated vesicles and degraded by lysosomes. A resulting 3kDa fragment known as p3 is formed during this process. Recent papers give evidence to suggest that two members of the ADAMs family of proteases (A member of the Disintegrin And Metalloprotease family), tumour necrosis factor alpha (TNFα) converting enzyme (TACE or ADAM17) (Buxbaum *et al.* 1998) and ADAM10 (Lammich *et al.* 1999) have α-secretase activity. Overexpression of ADAM10 in HEK293 cells resulted in a marked increase in basal and protein kinase C- (PKC) stimulated α-secretase cleavage of APP. The active form of ADAM10 was found to be in the plasma membrane, the proenzyme was mainly in the Golgi. TACE and ADAM10 have only 21% amino acid homology but their catalytic domains are probably structurally similar. They may not be the only enzymes involved in α-secretase cleavage.

In addition, a minor component of the APP is cleaved by β-secretase. This cleavage occurs between M671 and D672 of the APP770 form, resulting in the formation of the N-terminal secreted APPβ (sAPPβ) and a C-terminal peptide, of 99 amino acids, known as c99. This contains, embedded within it, the Aβ fragment. β-secretase has now been cloned independently by four separate groups: at Amgen (BACE: Vassar *et al.* 1999), SmithKline Beecham (Asp2: Hussain *et al.*1999), Pharmacia & Upjohn Inc. (Asp2; Yan *et al.* 1999) and Elan Pharmaceuticals (β-secretase; Sinha *et al.* 1999) (see Appendix VI for more detail). BACE (beta site APP cleaving enzyme) or Asp2 is a novel transmembrane aspartyl protease. Amgen discovered BACE using an expression cloning strategy. The team at SmithKline Beecham searched on the EST database for putative novel aspartyl proteases, and found Asp2, and Yan and colleagues at Pharmacia & Upjohn Inc had a similar strategy and scanned the *C. elegans* genome for the D(S/T)G(S/T) motif which denotes an aspartyl protease. By comparison of sequences on the database they identified human equivalents, membrane bound aspartyl proteases named Asp1 and Asp2. Purification of recombinant Asp2 from Chinese hamster ovary (CHO) cells showed that it was able to act as β-secretase. Sinha and the team at Elan Pharmaceuticals identified β-secretase activity in triton solubilized membranes from a variety of tissues using an assay for sAPPβ. A synthetic peptide resembling the region around the β-secretase site inhibited β-secretase activity and was used in an affinity column in purification of BACE from solubilized human brain extracts. All four versions of this β-secretase were identical.

In order to determine the intracellular localization of 'BACE', C-terminal tagged (haemagglutanin epitope) BACE was stably transfected into HEK293 cells, and cells stained with anti-haemagglutanin (Vassar *et al.* 1999). For the localization of 'Asp2' (Hussain *et al.* 1999) a C-terminal myc epitope tag was added to the cDNA encoding Asp2 and transfected into COS7 cells expressing APP751; anti-myc was used for detection. The groups at Amgen and SmithKline Beecham both agree that BACE/Asp2 and APP seem to co-stain. The actual localization is not clear cut, but both agree a large proportion is present in the Golgi. Vassar and coworkers visualized BACE mRNA mainly in neurons rather than astrocytes, although it is known that astrocytes are able to produce Aβ in culture (LeBlanc *et al.* 1997). From the Amgen study we can see that α- and β-secretase compete for the APP substrate. When BACE is overexpressed, cleavage of APP (with the Swedish double mutation — a form which favours formation of Aβ) to form sAPPβ and c99 is increased, and cleavage by α-secretase to form c83 is decreased.

Subsequent to α- and β-secretase cleavage, c83 or c99 can then be cleaved by γ-secretase to form p3 or Aβ. There is currently some controversy as to whether γ-secretase is presenilin 1 (see below and Appendix VI). Under normal conditions very small amounts of Aβ1–40 and Aβ1–42 are formed in the cell. In both CSF and in cell culture, Aβ1–40 is the major component (50–70%) with Aβ1–42 as the minor component (5–20%) (Murphy *et al.* 1999). Information as to the site of production of Aβ1–40 and Aβ1–42 is clouded by the fact that neuronal and non-neuronal cells process APP differently. However, it seems that, in neuronal cells, most Aβ1–40 is secreted through the trans-Golgi network whereas Aβ1–42 is produced in the ER and nuclear envelope (Hartmann *et al.* 1997). This would mean that if neuronal Aβ1–42 were the basis of amyloid plaques then this could only occur after cell death. In non- neuronal cells both Aβ1–40 and Aβ1–42 may be produced at the cell membrane and secreted.

In Chapter 4 David Howlett and colleagues list comprehensively the factors implicating Aβ in the aetiology of AD, the most obvious of which is the fact that a single mutation in the *APP* gene leads to early onset AD. From the pattern of mutations in the *APP* gene which actually result in AD it seems that they fall around the α-, β- and γ-secretase cleavage sites. The most accessible explanation would be that cleavage by the three enzymes is affected in some way by these mutations. An overview of the genetic aspects of AD is given in Chapter 3 by Wilma Wasco. Briefly, five APP mutations at three amino acid positions have been identified at the γ-site, which appear to be directly causative of AD: the V715M (French), I716V (Florida), V717I (London), and V717G/F mutations. The 716 and 717 mutations cause an increase in the ratio of Aβ1–42:Aβ1–40 (Suzuki *et al.* 1994; Eckman *et al.* 1997). At the β-secretase cleavage site, the Swedish double mutation (KM670/671NL) causes an increase in both Aβ1–40 and Aβ1–42 (Citron *et al.* 1992; Cai *et al.* 1993; Felsenstein *et al.* 1994) and increases plasma Aβ concentration (Jensen *et al.* 1995). In addition there are two mutations near the α-secretase site. These are E693Q, which is the causative mutation linked to hereditary cerebral haemorrhage with amyloidosis, Dutch type (HCHWA-D) and A692G which is linked to the cerebral haemorrhage with amyloidosis (CHWA), Flemish type. Both result in chronic and fatal cerebral haemorrhages associated with the deposition of Aβ in the cerebral blood vessel walls. The Flemish type also has AD pathology. E693Q does not seem to cause an increase in Aβ production whereas A692G does (Haass *et al.* 1994).

Thus the position of the mutations influences whether more c99 or c83 is made available (at the β-site), a differential increase in Aβ1–42 (γ-site) or whether there is predominantly cerebrovascular amyloid (α- secretase site). Since we now know that BACE/Asp2 has about a 100 fold increased activity with an APP-derived substrate containing the Swedish double mutation compared with wild type (Vassar *et al.* 1999) we can see that in this case more c99 is made available for cleavage into Aβ. The 'α-secretase site' mutations result mainly in deposition of Aβ1–40 in the cerebral vessel walls. This species is also deposited in cored plaques along with Aβ1–42, although in general mainly Aβ1–42 is present in diffuse plaques (Fukumoto *et al.* 1994; Iizuka *et al.* 1995; Mann *et al.* 1996), possibly Aβ17–42 (Gowing *et al.* 1994). It is not clear at present why an APP mutation around the 'α-secretase site' results in Aβ1–40 being deposited by non-neuronal cells in the vessel walls in preference to deposition in neuronal senile plaques.

Karen Duff discusses models of AD in Chapter 8. In the case of the mutations I717F or KM670/671NL, some mice do show signs of pathology similar to that of AD (Games *et al.* 1995; Hsiao *et al.* 1996; Sturchler-Pierrat *et al.* 1997). All develop amyloid deposits in the cortex and hippocampus, none develop tangles, although there is a report of some abnormally phosphorylated tau immunoreactivity (Sturchler-Pierrat *et al.*1997). Cognitive impairment is relatively mild. This may be evidence against the toxicity of Aβ *per se* or is it that the mechanisms of Aβ toxicity are different in rodents?

1.4 Toxic amyloid

So let us examine whether or not Aβ is toxic, and if so which form is toxic. The original assumption of the 'amyloid hypothesis' was that the deposition of Aβ is necessary for the cell death observed in AD. This has led to discussion as to whether it is actually the deposited Aβ that causes neuronal death or whether it is the presence of Aβ *before* it aggregates which is toxic. Some would extend the hypothesis to say that it is merely the presence of Aβ, in whatever form, which is required for neurotoxicity. If Aβ is toxic then most researchers seem to agree that it is the fibrillar form that is most toxic. Looking at the NMR structure [NCBI accession code 1AML] of Aβ1–40 it appears mainly in α helix form.

Spontaneously, protomers of four or five molecules are able to form, this initial step is very slow and concentration dependent. During this process the molecules form beta strands, and it seems that Aβ1–42 can do this more readily (Jarrett *et al.* 1993) and that may be why it is more toxic. A combination of factors may conspire to induce fibrilization, including Aβ concentration, pH and elements which may act as 'seeds.' These may be in the form of metal ions, apoE, proteoglycans, or even such molecules as acetylcholinesterase which accelerate the aggregation of Aβ by lowering the concentration required for fibrilization. Shi Du Yan and colleagues (Chapter 9) suggest that the tightly packed deposits in amyloid cores may actually have a *protective* function by sequestering toxic amyloid from cellular elements. He argues that, early on, Aβ fibrils are probably oligomeric and soluble and it is at this stage when their interactions with the cell surface are more likely to be relevant. But if Aβ is more toxic in this form, by what mechanism may this toxicity manifest itself? It may be able to activate a receptor that precipitates cell destruction. In 1996 Shi Du Yan (Yan *et al.* 1996) reported the discovery that the Receptor for Advanced Glycation Endproducts or RAGE, a member of the immunoglobulin superfamily of cell surface molecules, is able to bind Aβ. AGEs form as a result of glycoxidation of free amino groups on proteins and lipids and this modification could be expected to enhance the pathogenicity of Aβ.

In human AD brain, expression of RAGE is increased in neurons, microglia and cells of the vessel wall (Yan *et al.* 1996). Shi Du Yan and colleagues also describe the identification of a polypeptide ER-associated Aβ binding protein (ERAB) using the yeast two-hybrid system (Yan *et al.* 1997*a*). When ERAB was shown to be an alcohol dehydrogenase it was renamed ABAD or amyloid β-peptide binding protein alcohol dehydrogenase (Yan *et al.* 1997*b*). ABAD is a reversible, NAD/NADH-dependent, β-hydroxyacyl coenzyme A dehydrogenase participating in the β-fatty acid oxidation pathway and is a generalized alcohol dehydroge-nase which uses a wide range of substrates (e.g. ethanol, oestradiol). It is widely distributed in normal tissues and resides mainly in the ER and mitochondria. ABAD is increased in both aged and AD brain, binds Aβ in the nanomolar range, and appears to potentiate Aβ toxicity. Interestingly, apoE4 is able to bind to AGEs more readily than apoE3 (Li and Dickson 1997) (see Section 1.7).

Shi Du Yan and co-authors suggest that at higher concentrations of Aβ, the involvement of RAGE and ABAD may well be minimal, as increased levels of Aβ directly destabilize membranes, and that it is probably only at the initial stages of Aβ formation that these mol-ecules exert their influence. The RAGE promoter has sites for nuclear factor κβ (NF-κβ) which are involved in ligand-induced enhancement of RAGE expression. RAGE appears to have properties of a signal transduction receptor for Aβ which results in sustained nuclear translocation of NF-κβ and induction of the expression of proteins such as macrophage-colony stimulating factor (M-CSF). AD brain shows an increased level of M-CSF in neurons and microglia. Microglia will thus be attracted to the vicinity, which sets up a vicious circle by which microglial RAGE promotes further M-CSF expression, increased microglial sur-vival and proliferation. With the release of various molecules such as cytokines, we may expect an escalation of toxic events.

1.5 **Neurofibrillary tangles and tau**

The other pathological hallmark of AD are NFT. A definitive description of NFT is given in Chapter 5 by Claude Wischik and colleagues. Briefly, NFT have been shown to correlate with loss of hippocampal neurons (Bondareff *et al.* 1993) and synapse formation (Terry *et al.* 1991) and to correlate with dementia more strongly than with senile plaques (Wilcock and Esiri 1982). A study of the distribution of tangles showed that tangles, unlike plaques, increase in numbers throughout the disease process in a circumscribed manner. Braak and Braak (1991) showed that this could be defined by a series of six stages correlating pathology and dementia. Early on in the disease process NFT appear in the transentorhinal cortex, and subsequently the CA1 of the hippocampus. In the limbic stages of the disease there are numerous tangles in the transentorhinal and entorhinal cortex, amygdala and CA1, with tangles beginning to appear in temporal cortex. In the final stages they are also present in large numbers in all neocortical association areas.

Tangles form intracellularly, but after cell death, may be dispersed and somewhat degraded by astrocytes. Electron microscope studies show that the main structural constituent of NFT is an abnormal fibre consisting of paired helical filaments (PHF); straight filaments are also present. These filaments also occur in dystrophic neurites which are scattered amongst senile or neuritic plaques. Early immunohistochemical studies revealed a range of associated proteins including ubiquitin, neurofilament proteins, β-amyloid and tau.

Like amyloid, PHF were extremely difficult to work with and were also resistant to most well known methods of protein extraction. In 1988 Claude Wischik and colleagues (Wischik *et al.* 1988*a*) showed that by digesting PHFs with proteases they were able to remove the 'coat' around the PHF and leave the core structure intact. Acid treatment of this core fraction produced a 12 kDa protein, and sequence analysis showed that it contained three of a possible four tandem repeat regions of the microtubule-associated protein tau (Wischik *et al.* 1988*b*; Jakes *et al.* 1991).

cDNA libraries from AD cerebral cortex were screened and the cDNA for tau was isolated. This was shown to encode a 352 amino acid protein, with a sequence homologous to that of the mouse tau (Goedert *et al.* 1988). Tau was then shown to exist in six isoforms (352–441 amino acids, see Appendix V for sequence) formed by alternate splicing (Goedert *et al.* 1988). The gene is located at chromosome 17q21–22. Isoforms contain either 3 or 4 tandem repeats of 31 or 32 amino acids towards the carboxy-terminal, these are the microtubule binding domains. In addition there are two possible inserts of 29 amino acids near the amino terminus. Only the form of tau with three repeats and no amino terminal inserts is present in fetal brain (Goedert *et al.* 1993) whereas all six tau isoforms are expressed in adult human brain.

Depending on the splice variant, tau has 3 or 4 binding domains comprising predominantly basic amino acids, these are able to stabilize microtubules by binding to negatively charged tubulin. As for APP knockouts, tau null mice are healthy with only apparently minor deficiencies in small calibre axons (Harada *et al.* 1994). However, the researchers did note that there was an increase in MAP1A and perhaps, as for APP, there is some compensatory mechanism. Further studies, as discussed in Chapter 5, demonstrate that these mice exhibit behavioural and memory changes reminiscent of frontotemporal dementia patients. Interestingly, double knockouts of tau and MAP1B have severe defects and die prematurely (Takei *et al.* 1999).

Tau is a neuronal phosphoprotein. In 1990 abnormally phosphorylated forms were reported (Bancher *et al.* 1990) and in AD and Down syndrome brains a fraction of tau was found with decreased solubility and increased phosphorylation (Hanger *et al.* 1991). Tau was reported to be both hyperphosphorylated and abnormally phosphorylated in AD

(Morishima-Kawashima *et al.* 1994). Over twenty sites of phosphorylation have been identified on tau; many are threonine or serines, followed by proline, usually localized to the amino- and carboxyl-terminal regions flanking the microtubule binding domain, although serine-262 is within this domain. Preparations of PHFs from the AD and Down brains revealed only three principal bands (corresponding to abnormally phosphorylated tau) on gels. This compared with the six bands seen in normal adults. By dephosphorylation the three abnormal bands were shifted to align with the six nonphosphorylated tau isoforms (Goedert *et al.* 1992).

There is ongoing controversy about the role of phosphorylation in tau and it has been suggested that the abnormal phosphorylation results in conformational change which leads to aggregation into PHF. Arguments supporting the necessity of hyperphosphorylation for tau–tau aggregation however, were disproved when Goedert and co-workers in 1996 showed that phosphorylation of tau was not *necessary* for PHF formation (Goedert *et al.* 1996). Heparan sulphate and other negatively charged sugar-containing glycosaminogly-cans are able to bind with tau and induce aggregation, and thus prevent tau from binding to microtubules. Earlier work had already shown that NFT often contained proteoglycans (Snow *et al.* 1988) and these molecules are able to 'seed' the fibrillization of tau. They are also similarly implicated in enabling amyloid to fibrillise. Further to this it has been argued that phosphorylation at ser262 and ser214 actually protects against tau aggregation (Schneider *et al.* 1999). However, phosphorylation of ser262, within the microtubule binding domain, also results in a reduced ability of tau to bind to microtubules (Drewes *et al.* 1992; Biernat *et al.* 1993). Glycogen synthase kinase 3β (GSK3β) is able to phosphorylate tau which results in destabilization of microtubules (Wagner *et al.* 1996). Since protein kinase C (PKC) is able to activate MAP kinases and thus inhibit GSK3β, its activation may be expected to cause a decrease in tau phosphorylation. Acetylcholine release results in an increase in PKC, and PC12 cells, transfected with M1 receptors, causes a reduction in tau phosphorylation when stimulated with acetylcholine agonists (Sadot *et al.* 1996). GSK3β is also able to phosphorylate APP in its cytoplasmic domain (Aplin *et al.* 1996).

Recently Tsai and colleagues (Patrick *et al.* 1999) have shown that Cyclin-dependent kinase 5 (Cdk5), a kinase able to phosphorylate tau, is abnormally activated in AD brain. Cdk5 is a serine/threonine kinase, important in development and required for neurite growth. Under normal conditions, p35, a regulatory subunit, binds to Cdk5 and anchors it to the plasma membrane. Cdk5 is present in the processes and growth cones of neurons and p35 is found at the plasma membrane. p35 protein is usually tightly regulated, with a very short half-life, but it can be cleaved to form p25 and p10. The p25 fragment maintains the activity of p35 and can still switch on Cdk5 but is unable to anchor it, thus the activity of Cdk5 is not limited to the membrane. p25 has a long half life, is present in the cytosol, and absent from nerve terminals. Tsai and colleagues conclude that the accumulation of p25 in AD may cause mislocation and prolonged action of Cdk5. In cells transfected with p25 or p35, and tau and Cdk5, p25 and Cdk5 were able to hyperphosphorylate tau more efficiently than p35 and Cdk5. Neuronal cells transfected with p25 and Cdk5 showed disruption of the cytoskeleton and cell death. p25 is stable, and found in vastly elevated amounts in AD brain, these high levels are also associated with cells containing NFT. It will be interesting to see which molecule is responsible for the cleavage of p35 and if this forms a link between Aβ formation and phosphorylation of tau. Phosphorylation of tau has also been shown to occur as a result of applying Aβ to primary neuronal cultures. Fibrillar, rather than soluble or amorphous aggregated Aβ, was shown to cause hyperphosphorylation of tau at Ser-202 and Ser- 396/Ser-404 (Busciglio *et al.* 1995), rendering it unable to bind with microtubules. Dephosphorylation of this tau restores its capacity to bind to microtubules.

Transgenic models with *APP* mutations show a relative paucity of tau pathology. Transgenic mice that over-express one of the isoforms of human tau with four microtubule binding repeats, show some hyperphosphorylation but no real sign of neurodegeneration (Gotz *et al.* 1995). However, others which overexpress the smallest tau isoform accumulate intraneuronal filamentous inclusions associated with axonal degeneration (Ishihara *et al.* 1999).

Mutations in the tau gene, on chromosome 17, have not been associated with AD; however, they have been identified as the cause of certain frontal temporal lobe dementias (FTDP-17). Claude Wischik and colleagues deal with this in detail in Chapter 5. These mutations will allow the study of 'pure' tauopathies without the presence of deposited Aβ. The most common mutations result in an increased splicing in of exon 10, which increases production of the 4-repeat isoforms. *In vitro* experiments showed that recombinant tau with exonic mutations G272V, P301L, V337M, and R406W were markedly less able to promote microtubule assembly (Hasegawa *et al.* 1998). However, others, using CHOs and neuroblastoma cells, and *in vitro* conditions, found that these mutants caused only a small reduction in affinity for microtubules or in ability to promote tubulin assembly (DeTure *et al.* 2000). Since, although these mutations clearly result in FTDP-17, the mechanism by which this happens may not be so straightforward.

1.6 **Neurochemical changes**

In terms of neuropathology, not all neurons are affected; there appears to be selective vulnerability. In the mid 1970s, attention was focused on a specific set of neurons affected in AD brain (Davies and Maloney 1976; Bowen *et al.* 1976; Perry *et al.*, 1977) (Chapter 10, Peter Davies). Cortical activity of the enzyme choline acetyltransferase, responsible for the synthesis of the neurotransmitter acetylcholine, was found to be dramatically reduced. This early loss in cholinergic function was thought to be responsible for the first symptom in AD, the short-term memory loss. The majority of the cholinergic neurons innervating the cortex originate from nuclei in the basal forebrain, the medial septal nucleus, the diagonal band of Broca (DBB) and the nucleus basalis of Meynert (NBM) (Mesulam *et al.* 1983, 1986; Mesulam and Geula 1988). Lesions of the innervating cholinergic pathways, or administration of anti-cholinergics such as scopolamine or hemicholinium-3 result in impaired ability to perform certain memory tasks (e.g. Dunnett *et al.* 1987; Ridley *et al.* 1984). The effects of this loss in AD may be compensated for by administration of the acetylcholine precursor, choline, or by the use of acetylcholinesterase inhibitors. Later, other neurotransmitter deficits were reported, for instance glutamatergic, noradrenergic and serotoninergic neurons, somatostatin and corticotropin releasing factor (CRF) (e.g. Davies *et al.* 1980; Benton *et al.* 1982; Bowen *et al.* 1983) were all found to be affected to a greater or lesser degree. However, cholinergic loss has turned out to be one of the better-publicized and indeed most consistent neurochemical changes in AD brain. Over twenty years later, in AD most of the therapies used act on cholinergic function, and anticholinesterase inhibitors are still the only drugs widely available.

Why is the cholinergic system so vulnerable so early (Sims *et al.* 1983) in the disease process? Cholinergic neurons project from the NBM to the hippocampus and neocortex;

80–90% of the neurons in the human/primate NBM are cholinergic, perhaps slightly less so (around 70–80%) in the DBB (Mesulam *et al.* 1983; Mesulam and Geula 1988). However, they are not all affected equally in AD; although the hippocampus receives most of its inner-vation from the medial septal nucleus and the DBB in the primate brain (Mesulam and Geula 1988) these areas are relatively spared in AD brain (Wilcock *et al.* 1988; Mufson *et al.* 1989; Allen *et al.* 1990). By contrast, the NBM provides the main innervation to the cerebral cortex (Mesulam *et al.* 1983, Mesulam and Geula 1988) and it is the posterior part of the NBM which shows marked neuronal loss in AD brain (Wilcock *et al.* 1988; Mufson *et al.* 1989; Allen *et al.* 1990). The loss of cholinergic activity in the cortex seems to far outstrip the neuronal loss in the NBM.

Cholinergic function correlates highly with the level of insoluble phosphorylated tau in the neocortex, hippocampus, and NBM (Arendt *et al.* 1999). Claude Wischik and colleagues reason (Chapter 5) that since PHF content in the neocortex correlates highly with neuritic pathology in the cortex it is likely to be associated with cell bodies rather than from a cholinergic input; but since NBM tau pathology precedes neocortical pathology, loss of cholinergic activity probably results from tau pathology in this nucleus. As mentioned above, in PC12 cells, stimulation with acetylcholine agonists results in decreased tau phos-phorylation (Sadot *et al.* 1996), in addition muscarinic agonists cause a decrease in APP levels and an increase in sAPPα (Lin *et al.* 1999). Loss of cholinergic cells then may result from tau burden but their damage and eventual loss will have a direct effect on their own pathology, and on those cells to which they project. In this way small changes may accelerate their demise, rendering them apparently more vulnerable.

The nature of the cholinergic neuron requires that it is able to synthesize acetylcholine, and for this the substrates acetyl coenzyme A and choline are necessary. Neurons are unable to synthesize choline *de novo* but can obtain this postsynaptically from the breakdown of phosphatidylcholine and presynaptically from reuptake of choline at the synaptic cleft after breakdown of acetylcholine by acetylcholinesterase. Choline is also intrinsic to the choles-terol synthesis/degredation pathway. This dual role may have some bearing on the selective vulnerability of these neurons and which may be enhanced by an *apoE4* ε 4 allele. In the presence of the *apoE* ε 4 allele, cholinergic function is reduced in AD brain (Soinenen *et al.* 1995; Beffert and Poirier 1996; Allen *et al.* 1997) and even in non demented controls (Allen *et al.* 1997). The effect of the presence of apoE4 is discussed in more detail below.

1.7 ApoE

One of the principal areas of discovery in AD research has been in the search for causative genes using early onset families, as exemplified by mutations in *APP* (e.g. Goate *et al.* 1991) giving rise to an autosomal dominant form of AD. However in 1994 a late-onset AD family was shown to be associated with the presence of a polymorphism of apoE (Sequence data is given in Appendix IV).

ApoE is a lipid transport molecule, a constituent of liver-synthesized very low density lipoproteins (VLDL) and a subclass of high density lipoproteins (HDL). ApoE mediates the cellular uptake of lipid complexes mainly through binding to the low density lipoprotein receptor (LDL — the principal cholesterol-ester transporter in plasma (Mahley 1988)) and the LDL receptor-related protein (LRP).

In the CNS, LRP is believed to be a major apoE receptor (Rebeck *et al.* 1993). Brain apoE is not synthesized by the liver, but locally by astrocytes and microglia, although low levels of

APOE mRNA have been seen in some cortical neurons and also human neuronal cell lines. The *APOE* gene has three common alleles on human chromosome 19, these are ε 2 (8%), ε 3 (78%) and ε 4 (14%). Percentages of alleles are given in brackets, although these vary somewhat from population to population. Certainly, in most Caucasian populations ε 3 is the most common allele. The three haplotypes give rise to six genotypes; ε 2ε 2 (1%), ε 2ε 3 (15%) ε 2ε 4 (3%), ε 3ε 3 (55%), ε 3ε 4 (23%), and ε 4ε 4 (3%) (Utermann *et al.* 1980). These code for apoE proteins that differ by one or two amino acids out of 317. ApoE3 has cysteine at position 112 and arginine at 158, apoE2 has cysteine, and apoE4 has arginine residues at both positions. In response to neuronal damage, production of apoE is increased to allow for the redistribution of lipid breakdown products and cholesterol during neuronal regeneration.

Ann Saunders reviews apoE as a risk factor for AD in Chapter 6. Rapidly following its association with late onset familial AD, it was shown that the ε 4 allele was also associated with sporadic AD (Chartier-Harlin *et al.* 1994; Nalbantoglu *et al.* 1994). This appeared to be a risk factor rather than a direct causative factor, in other words, inheritance is not sufficient to cause the disease. In Chapter 6, Ann Saunders cites an increased frequency of the ε 4 allele in late-onset families (~52%) and in sporadic AD (~40%) compared with age-matched normal (~16%) (Saunders *et al.* 1993*a*, *b*). Other events, maybe environmental or genetic, must be present to cause the pathology and symptoms of AD. Others reported that ε 4/4 patients had more senile plaques than ε 3/3 patients (Rebeck *et al.* 1993). In contrast the ε 2 allele has been suggested to have a protective effect on AD, as evidenced by a decreased frequency of this allele (Corder *et al.* 1994). The mean age of onset of individuals with an ε 4/4 genotype is younger than 70 years while the mean age of onset for the ε 2/3 genotype is older than 90 years.

A large number of experiments have been carried out to determine differences between the isoforms of apoE in order to explain the reason for the increased risk of apoE4. *In vitro* studies of complex formation between apoE4 and Aβ are a little confusing since using purified apoE, binding is much faster for apoE4 than apoE3, whereas using unpurified apoE from conditioned media, apoE3 binds Aβ more avidly than apoE4. Whatever the *in vitro* studies show however, there is increased amyloid deposition in AD patients with an ε 4 allele compared with ε 3. Interestingly, *APOE* genotype affects levels of Aβ in the CSF of patients. Aβ1–42 decreases regardless of genotype, but total Aβ levels differentially decrease in those patients with an ε 4 allele (Pirttila *et al.* 1998). ApoE levels also decrease with length of illness.

Since apoE plays a role in lipid redistribution during regeneration, it will affect the way in which neurons are able to cope with insults. Data seem to support the hypothesis that the presence of an ε 4 allele is detrimental to efficient recovery from head trauma. Likewise intracerebral haemorrhage patients with an ε 4 allele have a much higher mortality and recovery rate than ε 3 and dementia pugilistica is more severe with an ε 4 allele present. Head injury alone does not increase risk for AD and so apoE is probably important during recovery from trauma.

Ann Saunders observes, in her appraisal of the subject in Chapter 6, that there is another connection: apoE binds to NFT. One of the effects of apoE in AD may therefore be through its association with tau. ApoE3, but not apoE4, binds to the microtubule-binding repeat regions of tau (Strittmatter *et al.* 1994*a*, *b*). Tau, in turn, binds to the LDL-receptor binding domain of apoE3, but only if unphosphorylated, since phosphorylation of the repeat regions of tau stops it binding to apoE3. *In vitro*, apoE3 has been shown to be more effective than apoE4 in promoting neurite sprouting and extension in neurons and neuronal cell lines (Fagan *et al.* 1996; Narita *et al.* 1997). In fact apoE4 seems to inhibit neurite outgrowth *in vitro* and is associated with microtubule depolymerization. ApoE-null mice have synaptic and dendritic disruption in the neocortex and limbic system due to cytoskeletal abnormalities and it has been suggested that the presence of apoE4 allele in man is, in effect, similar to a reduction in apoE3. Buttini and colleagues (Buttini *et al.* 1999) find age-related differences between apoE (-/-) and wild type mice including lower levels of various neuronal markers (e.g. synaptophysin, MAP-2) in the neocortex. When human apoE3 or apoE4 was reintroduced into the embryos of these null mice, under the neuron-specific enolase promoter, those expressing human apoE3 were similar to wild type whereas those with apoE4 were similar to null mice.

We know that Aβ deposition is virtually eradicated in crosses between apoE (-/-) and the V717F APP mouse (Bales *et al.* 1997, 1999). Thus amyloid deposition is dependent on the presence of apoE. The absence of apoE did not alter the transcription or translation of the *APP*(V717F) transgene or its processing to Aβ so apoE may facilitate the deposition and fibrillization of Aβ, reducing clearance of protease-resistant Aβ/apoE aggregates (Bales *et al.* 1999). The reduction in plaque numbers is startlingly evident, however, since the cognitive deficits of APP mutant mice are quite subtle, and apoE-deficient mice are known to have memory deficits associated with synaptic loss of basal forebrain cholinergic projections, it will be difficult to be sure of the effect of reducing plaque numbers on cognition.

There seems to be no increased risk for apoE4 with Parkinson's disease, with or without dementia. We might therefore assume that, unlike Aβ, the deposition of α-synuclein, the main constituent of Lewy bodies, is not affected by the presence of apoE4. However, there is an increased risk for diffuse Lewy body disease (DLB) with apoE4 (Harrington *et al.* 1994), perhaps due to the presence of Aβ pathology.

The presence of apoE4 does not increase the risk for FTDP-17 (Bird *et al.* 1999; Houlden *et al.* 1999). If the effect of apoE4 is upon recovery, why is there not an effect of apoE4 on all types of neuronal stress? Does it mean that apoE4 is more relevant to amyloid-related damage?

ApoE4 does lower the age of onset of AD patients with *APP* mutations, but has no effect on those with PS1 mutations. It is not obvious why that should be if the result of both the mutations in APP and PS1 is to increase production of Aβ1–42, especially since the effect of APP mutations and PS1 mutations are additive in transgenic models in terms of amyloid burden (Holcomb *et al.* 1998).

1.8 **Presenilins**

In 1995 linkage studies revealed a new gene involved in FAD. This was finally localized to chromosome 14 (Sherrington *et al.* 1995), at the same time five missense mutations in seven AD pedigrees were reported. The gene coded for a previously unknown protein, initially referred to as S182, the name of one of the isolated clones. S182 was predicted as being multi-transmembrane (thought to be seven transmembrane by hydropathy plots). In the same year, another novel gene named *STM2* (second seven transmembrane gene associated with AD) was attributed to the cause of an autosomally dominant form of FAD in a kindred of Volga Germans (Levy-Lehad *et al.* 1995; Li *et al.* 1995; Rogaev *et al.* 1995). This gene was localized to chromosome 1, identified through EST databases due to its homology with S182. Overall the S182 and STM2 proteins are 67% identical and were subsequently renamed presenilin 1 (PS1) and PS2.

PS1 mutations account for 30–50% of all early onset cases of AD (Cruts *et al.* 1996). A comprehensive description of the presenilins is given by Martin Citron in Chapter 7, and Appendices II and III show sequences of PS1 and PS2 and the mutations found to date. The proteins encoded by *PS1* and *PS2* genes are 467 and 448 amino acids long respectively. The number of putative transmembrane domains in both PS1 and PS2 is uncertain and has been suggested to be six, seven, eight, or nine. The most commonly accepted form is that with eight transmembrane domains with the C- and N-terminus both on the cytoplasmic side, although a recent model (Nakai *et al.* 1999) opts for a seven transmembrane structure with one membrane embedded domain. Either way, the large hydrophilic loop and the N-terminus are in the cytosol.

The presenilins are cleaved within the large hydrophilic loop to form an N-terminal and C-terminal fragment (NTF and CTF). Endogenously, little full length PS1 or PS2 is detected, suggesting that the NTF and CTF are the primary form of the protein present in cells. The holoproteins appear to be rapidly degraded, by contrast the fragments are stabilized within large molecular weight complexes.

To date, approximately 50 individual point mutations in PS1 have been identified and found to be responsible for early-onset FAD. There has also been found an intronic mutation which causes the disruption of a splice acceptor site which results in an in-frame deletion of exon 9 (Perez-Tur *et al.* 1995). The pathological effect of this mutation (referred to as delta-9 or ΔE9) is actually due to an additional point mutation (S290C) occurring at the aberrant exon splice junction (Steiner *et al.* 1999). By contrast only three mutations have been found in the PS2 gene. There have been reports of presenilin localization at the cell surface (Dewji and Singer 1997) and at the nuclear membrane (Li *et al.* 1997) but there is some agreement that the primary subcellular localization of both endogenous and transfected presenilin appears to be within the intracellular membranes of the ER (full length PS1 and PS2 in particular) and the Golgi complex (NTF and CTF particularly) (Kovacs *et al.* 1996; De Strooper *et al.* 1997; Zhang *et al.* 1998). *In situ* hybridization shows mRNA for PS1 and PS2 is mainly neuronal in the brain, and is particularly intense in large pyramidal neurons.

Fibroblasts from AD patients with *PS1* mutations show an increase in Aβ (Scheuner *et al.* 1996). Transgenic mice overexpressing mutant PS1 show an increase in Aβ1–42, but not Aβ1–40 (Duff *et al.* 1996; Borchelt *et al.* 1996; Citron *et al.* 1997). There appears however, to be little obvious pathology or cognitive deficits in these mice. By contrast, Karen Duff describes the dramatic neuropathological changes in crosses between *PS1* mutant and *APP* mutant transgenic mice. In a double transgenic PS/APP cross Aβ-containing deposits can be identified in the cortex and hippocampus as early as 12 weeks of age (Holcomb *et al.* 1998), accelerating the deposition seen in single transgenics by many months.

Some indication of normal function of the presenilins may be gleaned from homologous proteins. *C. elegans* proteins SEL-12 and SPE-4 are both believed to be involved in the trafficking and/or sorting of intracellular molecules. A *sel-12* mutant is unable to suppress the constitutive action of *lin-12* (a member of the *lin-12/Notch* family of receptors) and thus has an egg-laying defect. This can be rescued by human PS1 and PS2 (Levitan *et al.* 1996). Using the rescue assay it was shown that the endoproteolytic cleavage is dispensable for presenilin function, because the ΔE9 mutant, which is not cleaved, can rescue (Levitan et al. 1996; Baumeister et al. 1997). In this assay the C-terminal domain of PS1 including trans-membrane 7 is dispensable, but the large loop between transmembrane 6 and 7 is not (Baumeister et al. 1997).

Yeast two hybrid studies using either the main hydrophilic loop or the C-terminus of PS1 or PS2 show many binders. Martin Citron in Chapter 7 gives a table of some confirmed binding proteins most notably GSK 3β, tau, calsenilin, β and δ-catenins. Since recent evidence shows that PS1 is involved in the cleavage of Notch proteins we can see that this is a multifunctional protein. β- catenin interacts with the Wnt signalling pathway. Phosphorylation of β- catenin, by GSK3β results in its destabilization and ubiquination ready for degradation. Wnt signalling inhibits GSK3β, allowing β- catenin to translocate to the nucleus. PS1 is able to bind GSK3β and β- catenin, and also tau, perhaps enabling phosphorylation of β- catenin or tau by GSK3β. Mutations in PS1 may thus alter the balance of phosphorylation. Furthermore, β- catenin may be involved in stabilization of the microtubules by interaction with such molecules as cadherin (Kaufmann et al. 1999).

PS1 knockouts are lethal probably due to the effect on Notch processing (Wong et al. 1997, Shen et al. 1997). In vitro culture of neurons from PS1$^{-/-}$ mice embryos show an 80% reduction in both Aβ1–40 and Aβ1–42 (De Strooper et al. 1998). This γ-secretase activity (or action upon γ-secretase) is not unique for APP and it seems, amongst other proteins, Notch receptor is cleaved in a similar fashion.

Three recent papers in Nature (DeStrooper et al. 1999; Struhl and Greenwald 1999; Ye et al. (1999); Appendix VI) bear witness to the close association between γ-secretase and PS1. They also show that PS1 is required for Notch processing in the same way as for APP processing. DeStrooper and colleagues show that PS1 deficiency reduces the proteolytic release of the Notch intracellular domain (NICD) from a truncated Notch construct. Struhl and Greenwald (1999) show that after ligand-induced processing, in Drosophila the NICD enters the nucleus and is involved in transcriptional control of downstream target genes. Null mutations in the Drosophila presenilin gene abolish Notch signal transduction and prevent its intracellular domain from entering the nucleus. In concurrence Ye et al. 1999 report that presenilin is required for the normal proteolytic production of C-terminal Notch fragments, and that it acts upstream of both the membrane-bound form and the activated nuclear form of Notch.

A fourth paper (Wolfe et al. 1999) reports that mutation of either of two conserved TM aspartate residues in PS1, Asp 257 (in TM6) and Asp 385 (in TM7) to alanines, substantially reduces Aβ production and increases the amounts of the C-terminal fragments of APP in cell lines and in cell-free microsomes. Either mutation prevents the normal endoproteolysis of PS1. In the ΔE9 PS1 variant, which does not undergo cleavage, the Asp385Ala mutation still inhibits γ-secretase activity. The authors suggest that PS1 is either a diaspartyl cofactor for γ- secretase or is itself γ-secretase, an autoactivated intramembranous aspartyl protease. However, although inhibition or knockout of PS1 results in reduction of γ- secretase activity, until purified PS1 is shown to cleave APP in a cell-free system we cannot be sure that PS1 is γ- secretase.

So far all presenilin mutations examined increase Aβ1–42 generation relative to Aβ1–40 and transgenic mice expressing mutant PS1 also show increased Aβ1–42 (Duff et al. 1996). The effects of presenilin mutations and the Swedish APP mutation which enhances β-secretase cleavage are additive, *in vitro*, and so are the effects of combined PS1 mutations and the APP717 mutation at the γ-secretase site (Citron *et al.* 1998).

Increases in β-secretase cleavage do not automatically lead to increases in Aβ as γ- secretase appears to be limiting (Vassar *et al.* 1999). If Aβ is the main reason for neuronal death then the double Swedish mutation, which increases β-secretase cleavage 100 fold, or the London mutation which increases Aβ1–42 production, would presumably have as early, or an earlier age of onset than PS1 mutations. In fact this is not so, generally the age of onset of disease in patients with the PS1 mutations appears to occur earlier (Appendices I and II). The increase in Aβ1–42 is unrelated to the age of disease onset (Citron *et al.* 1998, Mehta *et al.* 1998). Is this because PS1 is able to affect both the Aβ production and the depolymerisation of microtubules by phosphorylation of tau?

There are probably other genes involved in this disease process. However, as we move away from early onset families and autosomal dominant genes, to late onset or sporadic cases of AD, it becomes more difficult to show statistically that any given gene is implicated. Genetic linkage analyses indicate that there is a late-onset AD risk factor locus located on chromosome 12 (Pericak-Vance *et al.* 1998; Rogeava *et al.* 1999; Wu *et al.* 1998; Zubenko *et al.* 1998). Candidate genes include LRP and alpha-2 macroglobulin (A2M). LRP binds and internalizes KPI-containing forms of APP as well as acting as a receptor for apoE, while A2M is present in senile plaques and binds Aβ (Du *et al.* 1997). There is still considerable debate about these proteins.

1.9 Diagnosis

Having looked at the theoretical aspects of AD we must now face the problems involved with the complex reality of this disease: the clinical aspects by which we may determine the type and extent of the dementia in sufferers. Diagnosis is separated into three chapters covering aspects of clinical diagnosis, biochemical tests, and imaging techniques.

Suzanne Jeffries and Alistair Burns (Chapter 11) describe the clinical presentation of dementia and the assessment of contribution of the different elements. These include amnesia and the focal symptoms (e.g. aphasia, apraxia, agnosia), a psychiatric element including depression and aggression, and deficits in activities of daily living (ADL). The authors note that, although we focus on clinical symptoms such as short-term memory loss in AD often a psychiatric presentation may be a greater problem to families than memory impairment. Obviously, correct diagnosis of patients allows us to treat those for whom there is a valid treatment available and there are many treatable causes of dementia-like symptoms. The authors remark that accuracy of diagnosis has advanced such that AD can now be symptomatically diagnosed, rather than being largely a diagnosis of exclusion. Diagnosis of AD can only be guaranteed to be correct at post-mortem neuropathological examination, however, the success rate of diagnosis in life in those patients receiving a full battery of tests is remarkably high (around 85%). As Hiroyuki Arai and colleagues observe in Chapter 12, it is still difficult to detect AD accurately in its presymptomatic stage, that is at a time when it would be most useful (provided we had a therapy to deal with it!). Perhaps biological markers can help in this.

The most likely candidates for assessment as biological markers are Aβ1–42 and tau. Both can be measured using sensitive ELISAs. CSF-tau is significantly increased in CSF in patients with AD compared to patients with other neurological diseases and controls (Arai *et al.* 1995), while Aβ1–42 is decreased (Motter *et al.* 1995). Total Aβ remains the same as in control. The mean values for CSF tau are much higher than for other dementias but the variation is quite large. Aβ1–42 levels decline with increasing dementia but there is, again, overlap with other groups. Used in a simultaneous assay this may prove very useful for patients undergoing clinical trials in which neuropathological confirmation of disease would not be a viable option for five to ten years, or in situations where diagnosis is difficult.

However, it must be decided whether the risks associated with sampling of CSF are outweighed by the additional confirmation by biological tests. As more treatments become available it may well be a valid option. The idea that there may be more genetic markers, perhaps polymorphisms, in the near future, which will assist in the diagnostic procedure may not be realistic. Even though there is a marked enrichment of the ε 4 allele in AD, there are still at least 16% of normal elderly who have this allele and yet do not have the disease, it would be unethical to use APOE genotype as a predictor of AD. Are we likely to find a polymorphism which has a much greater predictive ability than that of APOE, considering the late age of onset of sporadic AD and the likelihood of the multifactorial nature of the disease? If not then such markers may still only be useful after the symptoms of AD have become evident.

There are two other diagnostic tests of interest. One is related to the protein melanotransferrin, or p97 protein, first identified as a surface marker of melanoma cells (Brown *et al.* 1981). This iron-binding protein, resembling serum transferrin, has a role in cellular iron uptake and exists in two forms: either attached to the cell surface by a glycosyl-phosphatidylinositol anchor or secreted. p97 is present on reactive microglial cells specifically associated with senile plaques in AD (Jefferies *et al.* 1996), and is not associated with other degenerative disorders such as Parkinson's disease or with microglial cells not associated with senile plaques (Yamada *et al.* 1991,1994). Increased levels of p97 are seen in CSF and serum in AD (Kennard *et al.* 1996). Serum diagnostic kits are currently being developed and marketed in Japan.

The second test relies on the production of a 41kDa protein known as AD7C-NTP (neuronal thread protein). This is a protein which is expressed in neurons and overexpressed in AD. Originally, increased immunoreactivity of a pancreatic protein was detected in AD pancreas (de la Monte *et al.* 1990). Antibodies to this were used to pull out AD7C-NTP from a human brain library (de la Monte *et al.* 1997). This was not similar to the pancreatic form in sequence, but only in structure as evidenced by its affinity for the same antibody. This was a novel putative seven transmembrane protein, elevated in AD CSF, as measured by ELISA. Further studies show that this is also true of urine samples (Ghanbari *et al.* 1998).

Neuroimaging is already used in the clinical diagnosis of AD. A description and consideration of the role of both structural and functional imaging techniques in diagnosis is given in Chapter 13 by Nick Fox and colleagues. Structural imaging techniques, such as computed tomography (CT) and magnetic resonance imaging (MRI) allow detection of atrophy, ischaemic changes, tumours, hydrocephalus, and subdural haematomata. Functional imaging highlights changes in metabolism, using such techniques as positron emission tomography (PET), single photon emission computed tomography (SPECT) and functional MRI (fMRI). The sensitivity and specificity of diagnosis by structural imaging is generally better than that of functional imaging.

CT scans are widely used as they are relatively cheap and quick to use. MRI has a better resolution but is more expensive. CT requires the use of X-rays whereas MRI uses the resonant frequencies of hydrogen protons. Nick Fox and colleagues give a comprehensive evaluation of these various approaches and their applicability for the identification of structural lesions, differentiation of symptomatic and presymptomatic AD from normal ageing and in differentiation of AD patients from those with other dementias.

As Nick Fox and Martin Rossor observe (Fox and Rossor 2000), the holy grail of non-invasive diagnostic markers would be measurement of plaques and tangles within the brain. By using magnetic resonance microscopy (MRM), which uses the principles of MRI but with strong magnetic field gradients and specialized radio frequency coils, Benveniste and colleagues (1999) were able to visualize neuritic plaques in formalin-fixed hippocampal tissue. Images were T2* -weighted; the presence of metals, such as iron, in the plaques may enhance visibility; scan times were around 18 hours. Neuritic plaques are between approximately 5 and 100 µm in diameter, plaques of around 80 µm could be detected. Scan times are obviously far too long but Benveniste and colleagues suggest that translating this to an *in vivo* situation may be possible using high-temperature superconducting radio frequency coils.

Functional neuroimaging uses measurement of glucose metabolism (CMR-glu) or cerebral blood flow (CBF) as indicators of neural activity under conditions of rest or during specific tasks. PET uses radioactive tracers which emit positrons, which in turn produce gamma rays, which are converted to visible photons and thus an image. Radioactive isotopes are expensive as they require a cyclotron for production. The main advantage is the production of high resolution images and the ability to measure quantitatively such functions as receptor binding. ^{18}F fluorodeoxyglucose (^{18}F-FDG) enables cerebral glucose metabolism to be estimated and $^{15}O_2$ oxygen is used to measure cerebral oxygen metabolism. SPECT also involves the detection of gamma rays produced by radioactive tracers using technetium ^{99m}Tc, these are relatively inexpensive but have poorer resolution than PET tracers. However, they use standard gamma ray detection cameras and so are more available than PET scanners. fMRI uses the magnetic properties of oxygenated and deoxygenated blood to estimate CBF. It can be used to assess abnormalities in resting blood flow as well as during activation by cognitive tasks.

Various studies have shown deficits in AD, in brain regions implicated by neuropathology, but the pattern of hypometabolism in normal ageing is variable, and so differentiating between AD and normal elderly is difficult. Nicotinic (Nordberg 1993) and muscarinic (Yoshida *et al.* 1998) binding has been shown to be decreased in AD using PET and evaluation of drug treatment by this method is potentially valuable. Such studies using tacrine and also NGF, for instance, have shown a drug-related increase in nicotine binding. More therapies are being made available and it will be important to see, in particular, functional changes with these drugs.

1.10 **Therapeutics**

The question of treatment is covered in two chapters dealing with current pharmacological approaches (Rebecca Eastley and colleagues, Chapter 14) and current perspective and future directives (Stephen Gracon and Mark Emmerling, Chapter 15).

Treatments may be grouped according to whether they are symptomatic, modify the disease process, or lower the risk or delay the onset of the disease. Symptomatic treatments generally encompass actions on the neurotransmitter systems, in particular deficits in the cholinergic system in terms of memory loss but also other systems, particularly the monoaminergic system which has effects on the behavioural aspects of AD. Despite the fact that clearly many neuronal systems are involved, the cholinergic hypothesis of AD has produced the first clinically relevant therapeutics. Historically, the earliest of these, physostigmine, showed improvement in memory function but its side effects were problematic. Similar difficulties exist for the more recently produced Tacrine or tetrahydroaminoacridine (THA). However, the work of Summers and colleagues (1986), which showed great improvements in patients using Tacrine, did much to promote cholinesterase inhibitors. Although by comparison, later studies with patients were disappointing, enough trials from large multicentre studies do now show that Tacrine treatment is of some benefit in some AD patients. It is able to improve cognitive function (Arrieata and Artalejo 1998) although the side effects are still cause for concern.

With the advent of the second generation cholinesterase inhibitors Donepezil (Aricept) and Rivastigmine (ENA 713, Exelon), we now have well tolerated drugs, that in over half the patients receiving them are able to provide improvement or stabilization in cognitive function. Rebecca Eastley and colleagues point out that improvements shown in trials with Rivastigmine corresponded to a relative delay in cognitive deterioration of about 6 months over placebo. In addition to these, the organophosphate Metrifonate and also Galanthamine (Reminyl), both with cholinesterase inhibitory actions, are currently undergoing trials. Both seem to be well tolerated and have beneficial effects on cognitive function. Galanthamine is a reversible inhibitor of brain acetylcholinesterase but is also able to modulate nicotinic receptors, improving cognition, global function and behavioural disturbance. Despite the recent evidence to show beneficial effects of M1 agonists on sAPPα production, the results of postsynaptic muscarinic agonists may be less hopeful in the short-term. Xanomeline, seems to have significant positive effects on cognitive and global function and reduced behavioural disturbance has been noted in trial, but side effects, particularly on the gut, are a problem.

The use of nerve growth factor (NGF) as a therapeutic is still an unknown quantity. The theory is that, since it is able selectively to increase cholinergic function and rescue cholinergic neurons after trauma, it will be able to benefit AD sufferers by virtue of support of surviving cholinergic neurons. NGF is produced in the cerebral cortex and hippocampus and retrogradely transported to the basal forebrain cholinergic cells (Seiler and Schwab 1984). Administration of NGF to basal forebrain cholinergic neurons *in vitro* results in increased survival and up regulation of ChAT, and intracerebroventricular administration of NGF abolishes degeneration and cognitive deficits caused by fimbria fornix lesions (e.g. Hefti 1986). Perhaps most convincing is the work of Walter Fischer and colleagues showing that a sub-population of aged rats that perform poorly in the Morris water maze are able to perform normally after infusion of NGF (Fischer *et al.* 1987, 1994). Although we discuss acetylcholine therapy as if all it does is ameliorate symptoms, since, it appears that it also has an effect on sAPPα and Aβ this may actually also be modifying the disease process.

Other neurotransmitter-based therapies include those that act on the monoaminergic systems including monoamine oxidase A (MAOA) which deaminates noradrenaline and serotonin (5HT) (e.g. moclobemide) and MAOB which deaminates dopamine, and additionally selective serotonin reuptake inhibitors (SSRI) (e.g.citalopram). In general these work effectively to reduce symptoms such as depression but also improve cognitive function.

Oestrogen has been associated with beneficial effects on cognition in post menopausal women and has been suggested as a therapeutic alternative in AD. The reasoning behind this, apart from empirical data from hormone replacement studies, may be rationalized by evidence of the association between oestrogen, cholesterol metabolism, apoE and amyloid production. For instance, reducing the cholesterol/protein ratio in membranes inhibits the production of Aβ (Simons *et al.* 1998; Frears *et al.* 1999) and physiological levels of 17 beta-oestradiol also reduce the generation of Aβ, in primary cultures of cerebrocortical neurons (Xu *et al.* 1998) and protect neurons from oxidative stress (Behl *et al.* 1995). Increased cholesterol reduces α-secretase cleavage (Bodowitz and Klein 1996). Oestradiol is also able to increase dendritic spine and synapse formation in cultured hippocampal neurons (Murphy and Segal 1996). Furthermore, 17 beta-oestradiol has been shown to increase apoE mRNA levels in mixed cultures of astrocytes and microglia (Stone *et al.* 1997) and some strains of mice respond to injections of oestradiol by raising their apoE levels 2.5-fold (Srivastava *et al.* 1997). Therapeutic trials have been controversial but two in particular strongly suggest that oestrogen reduces onset of AD (Tang *et al.* 1996; Kawas *et al.* 1997) although this is by no means universally accepted. There is some evidence that the protective effect of oestrogen appears strongest in those with the *APOE* ε4 allele (Van Duijn *et al.* 1996; Tang *et al.* 1996).

It has been known for some time that rheumatoid arthritis sufferers are less likely to develop AD. This may be related to the fact that many sufferers take non-steroidal anti-inflammatory drugs (NSAID). Trials of NSAID have mixed results but in general confer some benefit in reducing risk of AD. Pilot studies of prednisone and indomethacin are being carried out. One drug to have caught the imagination of the public, particularly since it can be bought over the counter, is Ginkgo biloba. This plant extract seems to have beneficial effects on cognition in clinical trials but has side effects due to its inhibition of platelet-activating factor. Positive effects on cognitive and global function have also been found with such drugs as Idebenone, which may act as a free radical scavenger and protect cell membranes against lipid peroxidation.

In terms of modifying the disease process we must cover tau–tau aggregation. If the destabilization of tau–microtubule interactions could be prevented it might be possible to preserve cellular structure and reduce the pathology and symptoms of AD. Whether prevention of tau–tau aggregation will be important, any more than Aβ de-aggregation would help, is unclear. However, Claude Wischik and colleagues (Chapter 5) discuss the possibility of differentiating between tau–microtubule binding domains and tau–tau binding domains. They look at the feasibility of using the tau–tau binding assay as a screening tool for identifying inhibitors of aggregation without destabilizing tau–tubulin interactions.

Since the importance of Aβ production and/or deposition is a central tenet of AD, then it is not unreasonable to argue that if this were hindered then all events downstream of this would be moderated and the neuropathology and symptoms associated with AD would be reduced. We may consider some of the approaches to this: to remove amyloid deposits already laid down, to prevent the Aβ formed from acting as a toxin or to prevent the production of Aβ altogether.

With regards to the first of these approaches: Dale Schenk and colleagues at Elan Pharmaceuticals reported the immunization of a transgenic mouse model of AD (over-expressing mutant human APP (V717F; Games *et al.* 1995) with a synthetic form of Aβ (1–42) called AN-1792 (Schenk *et al.* 1999). Animals were immunized either before the onset of AD-type neuropathology (at 6 weeks) or later, (11 months) when amyloid deposition and neuropathology was well established. Immunization prevented β-amyloid-plaque formation, neuritic dystrophy, and astrogliosis in the young animals and reduced the extent and progression of the neuropathology in the older animals. However, the problem with models used so far lies in the relative lack of synaptic and neuronal loss and cognitive deficits. AD-like neurofibrillary pathology is particularly difficult to emulate, and although, in particular the Novartis Pharma mouse (Sturchler-Pierrat *et al.* 1997; with human APP751 with Swedish and London mutations), does show hyperphosphorylated tau present in distorted neurites associated with congophilic plaques, this does not in reality constitute a perfect model of AD. However, currently AN-1792 is in Phase I clinical trials and we await the outcome with interest.

The second approach, reducing toxicity of Aβ may involve blocking pathways, such as those which are RAGE dependant, or preventing the formation of fibrils of Aβ which may be the toxic substrate leading to cell death. There has been a suggestion that Aβ fibrils may be prevented from forming by using small molecules which bind to Aβ, but there is no sign of clinically applicable treatments yet.

The third approach, prevention of formation of Aβ seems much more likely given the cloning of β-secretase. BACE/Asp2 is an aspartyl protease. A lot of work has been carried out on aspartyl proteases (e.g. pepsin, cathepsin D, HIV protease). The category to which BACE belongs is that with an active site of D[s/t]G[s/t]×2, such as for pepsin, renin, and cathepsin D. Other aspartyl proteases such as HIV I protease are homodimers with each monomer contributing to the active site. Inhibitors already exist to these proteases and so by a combination of rational design from crystal structure and screening from databases it should be possible to produce an inhibitor to BACE. Specificity may be more of an issue but we await the results of the BACE knockout.

Figure 1.2 tries to provide a starting point for looking at a hypothetical pathway between APP and cell death. For convenience it separates Aβ formation (Fig. 1.2a) and tau interactions (Fig. 1.2b) into two pathways. However, part of the uniqueness of AD is that it requires both features. Furthermore we know that in some way aberrant cleavage of APP results in neurofibrillary pathology, whereas tau mutations do not lead to amyloid deposition. So far, no causative or risk factor has been shown to act independently of amyloid formation or deposition. Although PHF are a defining feature of AD, and may even be the ultimate reason for cell dysfunction and destruction, mutations in tau lead to FTDP-17 not AD. Connecting factors may not yet be known but glycosaminoglycans appear in both 'pathways' — along with other 'seeding' agents including apoE. Direct or indirect phosphorylation of tau may also be a common feature. There is some evidence of direct Aβ-induced phosphorylation of tau (Busciglio *et al.* 1995) and perhaps presenilins may play a part in hyperphosphorylation of tau, although probably not directly (Irving and Miller 1997; Julliams *et al.* 1999). Certainly, the importance of mutations in PS1 is evidenced by the very low age of onset seen in these FAD cases. We don't know whether there is still a large clue missing or whether we now have all the pieces and merely need to put them together, and we also don't know how many 'red herrings' there are amongst the pieces.

This book tries to make these pieces of evidence more accessible in the hope that it will help in their assembly into a clear picture.

A recent study in Toronto (Yu *et al.* 2000) shows that the presence of a Type 1 transmembrane glycoprotein (110kDa, 709 amino acids) named nicastrin, coprecipitates with PS1

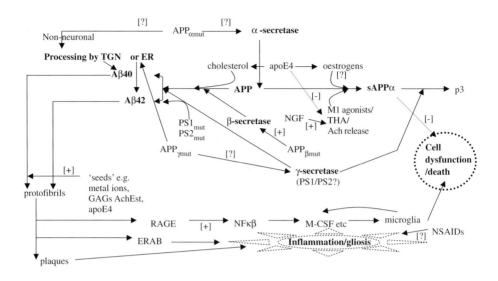

Fig. 1.2 Interaction of key molecules in the Alzheimer's disease process of neurodegeneration.
(a) Aβ: formation of, in particular, Aβ1–42 from APP may depend on many influencing factors.
A mutation in APP at the β-secretase cleavage site (APPβ_mut) will cause an increased production in both Aβ1–40 and Aβ1–42. This may build up inside the neuronal cell at the ER. By producing oligomers or protofibrils it may then be toxic to the neuron. Glycosaminoglycans
(GAGs) will 'seed' fibrillization of Aβ as may other proteins such as apoE4. ApoE3 does not
bind so avidly to Aβ. Cleavage of APP to sAPPα may be encouraged by oestrogen and discouraged by higher cholesterol content. These may be influenced by apoE4, or lack of apoE3.
Mutations in PS1 or PS2 will increase production of Aβ1–42, either by acting directly on
γ-secretase (or *is* γ-secretase) or by affecting localization of APP and products in the cell (arrow
not shown). Mutations in APP at the α-secretase site (APPα_mut) may act on α-secretase
directly, but if so must act also in some way to increase Aβ1–40 deposition in blood vessels,
e.g. affecting only non-neuronal cells by their secretory pathway, which is different from neuronal cells. Mutations in APP at the γ-secretase site (APPγ_mut) cause an increase in Aβ1–42,
either by affecting the binding of γ-secretase or on processing (via PS?). As Aβ forms it may
interact with RAGE and ERAB resulting in NFkβ activation. Resulting inflammation will fuel the
situation causing influx of reactive astrocytes and microglia into the vicinity. This may also
cause increased apoE production. If apoE4 is produced it may result in increased deposition of
Aβ and the local deposition of Aβ from astrocytes. Acetylcholine release or M1 agonists or
maybe acetylcholinesterase inhibitors such as THA may result in an increase in protective
sAPPα.

and PS2 in human brain. A sequence, DIYGS, on the N-terminal side of the transmembrane
region, is required for interaction with PS; deletion of this region results in loss of association
with PS and subsequent reduction in γ-secretase activity; mutation to AAIGS results in
an increase in Aβ1–40 and Aβ1–42 production. Furthermore, PS FAD mutations increase
nicastrin binding to C99 and C83 and increase Aβ secretion, whereas PS aspartate mutants
(D257 or D385) decrease nicastrin binding and Aβ secretion. It seems likely that nicastrin
will turn out to be key protein in processing of *APP*, and may also pay a part in the pathological mechanism of AD.

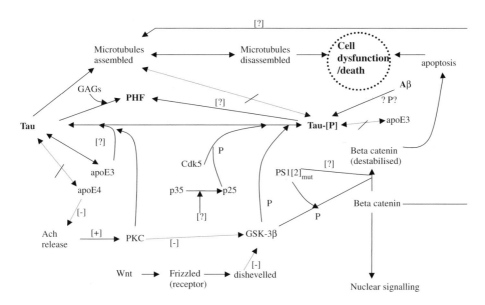

Fig. 1.2 (b) Tau: Tau is able to bind to microtubules and thus stabilize them. Self aggregation of tau to form PHF leads to microtubule destabilization. GAGs may promote this destabilization by providing a 'seed' by which tau may self aggregate. PHF contain some hyperphosphorylated tau. Phosphorylated tau is less likely to bind to microtubules and so may lead to destabilization, but is also less likely to self aggregate. ApoE3 may protect tau from self aggregation, or phosphorylation, by binding to the microtubule binding domain, or may be able in some way to 'pass on' the tau to tubulin. ApoE4 may contribute to destabilization of microtubules by not protecting these sites, also after trauma it is less useful in synapse re-formation. Phosphorylation of tau may occur by means of various kinases, one candidate is GSK3β. Presenilins are able to bind this and tau, mutations may encourage aberrant phosphorylation. Another candidate is Cdk5 which is regulated by anchorage to the membrane by p35. If p35 is degraded, by an unknown factor, to p25, this is able to phosphorylate in an unregulated fashion. Cholinergic function causes an increase in PKC, which in turn leads to dephosphorylation of tau. ApoE4 appears to result in a decrease in cholinergic function, which will then be less able to activate PKC and inhibit the constitutively active GSK3β. β-catenin may be involved in stabilization of microtubules. Phosphorylation of β-catenin will lead to degredation of catenin. Aβ may directly phosphorylate tau. P is phosphorylation. Dotted lines denote negative influence.

References

Allen, S. J., Dawbarn, D., MacGowan, S. H., *et al.* (1990). A quantitative morphometric analysis of basal forebrain neurons expressing β-NGF receptors in normal and Alzheimer's disease brains. *Dementia*, **1**, 125–37.

Allen, S. J., MacGowan, S. H., Tyler, S., *et al.* (1997). Reduced cholinergic function in normal and Alzheimer's disease brain is associated with apolipoprotein ε4 Genotype. *Neuroscience Letters*, **239**, 33–6.

Alzheimer, A. (1907). Über eine eigenartige Erkrankung der Hirnrinde (Concerning a novel disease of the cortex). *Allgemeine Zeitschrift für Psychiatrie Psychisch-Gerichtlich Medizine*, **64**, 146–8.

Aplin, A. E., Gibb, G. M., Jacobsen, J. S., *et al.* (1996). *In vitro* phosphorylation of the cytoplasmic domain of the amyloid precursor protein by glycogen synthase kinase-3 beta. *Journal of Neurochemistry*, **67**, 699–707.

Arai, H., Terajima, M., Miura, M., *et al.* (1995). Tau in cerebrospinal fluid. A potential diagnostic marker in Alzheimer's disease. *Annals of Neurology*, **38**, 649–52.

Arrieata, J. L. and Artalejo, F. R. (1998). Methodology, results, and quality of clinical trials of tacrine in the treatment of Alzheimer's disease: a systematic review of the literature. *Age and Ageing*, **27**, 161–79.

Arendt, T., Holzer, M., Gertz, H. J., and Bruckner, M. K. (1999). Cortical load of PHF-tau in Alzheimer's disease is correlated to cholinergic dysfunction. *Journal of Neural Transmission*, **106**, 513–23.

Bales, K. R., Verina, T., Dodel, R. C., *et al.* (1997). Lack of apolipoprotein E dramatically reduces amyloid beta-peptide deposition. *Nature Genetics*, **17**, 263–4.

Bales, K. R, Verina, T., Cummins, D. J., *et al.* (1999). Apolipoprotein E is essential for amyloid deposition in the APP(V717F) transgenic mouse model of Alzheimer's disease. *Proceedings of the National Academy of Sciences (USA)*, **96**, 15233–8.

Bancher, C., Grundkeiqbal, I., Iqbal, K., *et al.* (1990). Abnormal phosphorylation of tau precedes ubiquitination in neurofibrillary pathology of Alzheimer-disease. *Neurobiology of Ageing*, **11**, 281.

Baumeister, R., Leimer, U., Zweckbronner, I., *et al.* (1997). Human presenilin-1, but not familial Alzheimer's disease (FAD) mutants, facilitate *Caenorhabditis elegans* Notch signalling independently of proteolytic processing. *Gene Function*, **1**, 149–59.

Beffert, U., and Poirier, J. (1996). Apolipoprotein E plaques, tangles and cholinergic dysfunction in Alzheimer's disease. *Annals of New York Academy of Science*, **777**, 166–74.

Behl, C., Widmann, M., Trapp, T., and Holsboer, F. (1995). 17-beta estradiol protects neurons from oxidative stress-induced cell-death in vitro. *Biochemical and Biophysical Research Communications*, **216**, 473–82.

Benton, J. S, Bowen, D. M. Allen, S. J., *et al.* (1982). Alzheimer's disease as a disorder of isodendritic core. *The Lancet*, (i), 456.

Benveniste, H., Einstein, G., Kim, K. R., *et al.* (1999). Detection of neuritic plaques in Alzheimer's disease by magnetic resonance microscopy. *Proceedings of the National Academy of Sciences (USA)*, **96**, 14079–84.

Biernat, J., Gustke, N., Drewes, G., *et al.* (1993). Phosphorylation of Ser262 strongly reduces binding of tau to microtubules, distinction between PHF-like immunoreactivity and microtubule binding. *Neuron*, **11**, 153–63.

Bird, T. D., Nochlin, D., Poorkaj, P., *et al.* (1999). A clinical pathological comparison of three families with frontotemporal dementia and identical mutations in the tau gene (P301L). *Brain*, **122**, 741–56.

Bodovitz, S. and Klein, W. L. (1996). Cholesterol modulates alpha-secretase cleavage of amyloid precursor protein, *Journal of Biological Chemistry*, **271**, 4436–40.

Bondareff, W., Mountjoy, C. Q., Wischik, C. M., *et al.* (1993). Evidence for subtypes of Alzheimer's disease and implications for etiology. *Archives of General Psychiatry*, **50**, 350–6.

Borchelt, D. R., Thinakaran, G., Eckman, C. B., *et al.* (1996). Familial Alzheimer's disease-linked presenilin 1 variants elevate Abeta1–42/1–40 ratio *in vitro* and *in vivo*. *Neuron*, **5**, 1005–13.

Bowen, D. M., Smith, C. B., White, P., and Davison, A. N. (1976). Neurotransmitter-related enzymes and indices of hypoxia in senile dementia and other abiotrophies. *Brain*, **99**, 459–96.

Bowen, D. M. Allen, S. J., Benton, J. S., *et al.* (1983). Biochemical assessment of serotonergic and cholinergic dysfunction and cerebral atrophy in Alzheimer's disease. *Journal of Neurochemistry*, **41**, 266–72.

Braak, H. and Braak, E. (1991). Neuropathological stageing of Alzheimer-related changes. *Acta Neuropathology*, **82**, 239–59.

Brown, P., Woodbury, R. C., Hart, C. E., *et al.*(1981). Quantitative analysis of melanoma-associated antigen p97 in normal and neoplastic tissues. *Proceedings of the National Academy of Science (USA)*, **78**, 539-43.

Busciglio, J., Lorenzo, A., Yeh, J., and Yankner, B. A. (1995). Beta-amyloid fibrils induce tau-phosphorylation and loss of microtubule-binding. *Neuron*, **14**, 879–88.

Buttini, M., Orth, M., Bellosta, S., *et al.* (1999). Expression of human apolipoprotein E3 or E4 in the brains of Apoe (-/-) mice: Isoform-specific effects on neurodegeneration. *Journal of Neuroscience*, **19**, 4867–80.

Buxbaum, J. D., Liu, K. N., Luo, Y. X., *et al.* (1998). Evidence that tumor necrosis factor alpha converting enzyme is involved in regulated alpha-secretase cleavage of the Alzheimer amyloid protein precursor. *Journal of Biological Chemistry*, **273**, 27765–7.

Cai, X. D., Golde, T. E., and Younkin, S. G. (1993). Excess amyloid β production is released from a mutant amyloid β protein precursor linked to familiar Alzheimer's disease. *Science*, **259**, 514–16.

Chartier-Harlin, M. C., Parfitt, M., Legrain, S., *et al.* (1994). Apolipoprotein E, epsilon4 allele as a major risk factor for sporadic early and late-onset forms of Alzheimer's disease: Analysis of the 19q13. 2 chromosome. *Human Molecular Genetics*, **3**, 569–74.

Citron, M., Oltersdorf, T., Haass, C., *et al.* (1992). Mutation of the β-amyloid precursor protein in familial Alzheimer's disease increases β-protein production. *Nature*, **360**, 672–4.

Citron, M., Westaway, D., Xia, W., *et al.* (1997). Mutant presenilins of Alzheimer's disease increase production of 42-residue amyloid beta-protein in both transfected cells and transgenic mice. *Nature Medicine*, **3**, 67–72.

Citron, M., Eckman, C. B., Diehl, T. S., *et al.* (1998). Additive effects of PS1 and APP mutations on secretion of the 42-residue amyloid ß-protein. *Neurobiology of Disease*, **5**, 107–16.

Corder, E. H., Saunders, A. M., Risch, N. J., *et al.* (1994). Protective effect of apolipoprotein E type 2 allele for late onset Alzheimer disease. *Nature Genetics*, **7**, 180–4.

Cruts, M., Hendriks, L., and Van Broeckhoven, C. (1996). The presenilin genes: a new gene family involved in Alzheimer's disease pathology. *Human Molecular Genetics*, **5**, 1449–55.

Davies, P. and Maloney, A. J. F. (1976). Selective loss of central cholinergic neurons in Alzheimer's disease. *Lancet;* II, l403.

Davies, P., Katzman, R., and Terry, R. D. (l980). Reduced somatostatin- like immunoreactivity in cerebral cortex from cases of Alzheimer disease and Alzheimer senile dementia. *Nature*, **288**, 279–80.

de la Monte, S. M., Ozturk, M., and Wands, J. R. (1990). Enhanced expression of an exocrine pancreatic protein in Alzheimer's disease and the developing human brain. *Journal of Clinical Investigation*, **86**, 1004–13.

de la Monte, S. M., Garner,W., and Wands, J. R. (1997). Neuronal thread protein gene modulation with cerebral infarction. *Journal of Cerebral Blood Flow and Metabolism*, **17**, 623–35.

De Strooper, B., Beullens, M., Contreras, B., *et al.* (1997). Phosphorylation, subcellular localization and membrane orientation of the Alzheimer's disease associated presenilins. *Journal of Biological Chemistry*, **272**, 3590–8.

DeStrooper, B., Saftig, P., Craessaerts, K., *et al.* (1998). Deficiency of presenilin-1 inhibits the normal cleavage of amyloid precursor protein. *Nature*, **391**, 387–90.

DeStrooper, B., Annaert, W., Cupers, P., *et al.* (1999). A presenilin-1-dependent gamma-secretase-like protease mediates release of Notch intracellular domain. *Nature*, **398**, 518–22.

DeTure, M., Ko, L. W., Yen, S., *et al.* (2000). Missense tau mutations identified in FTDP-17 have a small effect on tau–microtubule interactions. *Brain Research*, **853**, 5–14.

Dewji, N., and Singer, S. J. (1997). Cell surface expression of the Alzheimer's disease-related presenilin proteins. *Proceedings of the National Academy of Sciences (USA)*, **94**, 9926–31.

Drewes, G., Lichtenberg-Kraag, B., Döring, F., *et al*. (1992). Mitogen activated protein (MAP) kinase transforms tau protein into an Alzheimer-like state. *EMBO Journal*, **11**, 2131–8.

Du, Y. S., Ni, B. H., Glinn, M., *et al*. (1997) Alpha(2)-macroglobulin as a beta-amyloid peptide-binding plasma protein. *Journal of Neurochemistry*, **69**, 299–305.

Duff, K., Eckman, C., Zehr, C., *et al*. (1996). Increased amyloid-beta 42(43) in brains of mice express-ing mutant presenilin 1. *Nature*, **383**, 710–3.

Dunnett, S. B., Whishaw, I. Q., Jones, G. H., and Bunch, S. T. (1987). Behavioural, biochemical and histochemical effects of different neurotoxic amino acids injected into nucleus basalis magnocellu-laris of rats. *Neuroscience*, **20**, 653–69.

Eckman, C. B., Mehta, N. D., Crook, R., *et al*. (1997). A new pathogenic mutation in the APP gene (I716V) increases the relative proportion of A-beta 42(43). *Human Molecular Genetics*, **12**, 2087–9.

Fagan, A. M., Bu, G., Sun, Y., *et al*. (1996). Apolipoprotein E-containing high density lipoprotein pro-motes neurite outgrowth and is a ligand for the low density lipoprotein receptor-related protein. *Journal of Biological Chemistry*, **271**, 30121–5.

Felsenstein, K. M., Hunihan, L. W., and Roberts, S. B. (1994). Altered cleavage and secretion of a recombinant beta-APP bearing the Swedish familial Alzheimer's-disease mutation. *Nature Genetics*, **6**, 251–6.

Fischer, W., Wictorin, K., Bjorklund, A., *et al*. (1987). Amelioration of cholinergic neuron atrophy and spatial memory impairment in aged rats by nerve growth factor. *Nature*, **328**, 65–8.

Fischer, W., Sirevaag, A., Wiegand, S. J., *et al*. (1994). Reversal of spatial memory impairments in aged rats by nerve growth factor and neurotrophins 3 and 4/5 but not by brain-derived neurotrophic factor. *Proceedings of the National Academy of Sciences (USA)*, **91**, 8607–11.

Fox, N. C. and Rossor, M. N. (2000). Seeing what Alzheimer saw- with magnetic resonance microscopy. *Nature Medicine*, **6**, 20–1.

Frears, E. R., Stephens, D. J., Walters, C. E., *et al*.(1999). The role of cholesterol in the biosynthesis of beta-amyloid. *Neuroreport*, **10**, 1699–705.

Fukumoto, H., Asami-Odaka, A., Suzuki, N., *et al*.(1994). Amyloid β protein deposition in normal ageing has the same characteristics as that in Alzheimer's disease: predominance of Aβ42(3) and association of Aβ40 with cored plaques. *American Journal of Pathology*, **148**, 259–65.

Games, D., Adams, D., Alessandrini, R., *et al*. (1995). Alzheimer-type neuropathology in transgenic mice over-expressing the V717F β-amyloid precursor protein. *Nature*, **373**, 523–7.

Ghanbari, H. A., Ghanbari, K., Beheshti, I., *et al*. (1998). Biochemical assay for AD7C-NTP in urine as an Alzheimer's disease marker. *Journal of Clinical Laboratory Analysis*, **12**, 285–8.

Glenner, G. G. and Wong, C. W. (1984). Alzheimer's disease: initial report of the purification and characterisation of a novel cerebrovascular amyloid protein. Biochemical Biophysical Research Communication, **120**, 885–90.

Goate, A., Chartier-Harlin, M. C., Mullan, M., *et al*. (1991). Segregation of a missense mutation in the amyloid precursor protein gene with familial Alzheimer's disease. Nature, **349**, 704–6.

Goedert, M. (1993). Tau protein and the neurofibrillary pathology of Alzheimer's disease. *Trends in Neuroscience*, **16**, 460–5.

Goedert, M., Wischik, C. M., Crowther, R. A., *et al*. (1988). Cloning and sequencing of the cDNA encoding a core protein of the paired helical filament of Alzheimer's disease: identification as the microtubule-associated protein. *Proceedings of the National Academy of Science (USA)*, **85**, 4051–5.

Goedert, M., Spillantini, M. G., Cairns N. J., and Crowther, R. A. (1992). Tau proteins of Alzheimer paired helical filaments: Abnormal phosphorylation of all six brain isoforms. *Neuron*, **8**, 159–68.

Goedert, M., Jakes, R., Crowther, R. A., *et al.* (1993). The abnormal phosphorylation of tau-protein at ser-202 in Alzheimer-disease recapitulates phosphorylation during development. *Proceedings of The National Academy of Sciences (USA)*, **90**, 5066–70.

Goedert, M., Jakes, R., Spillantini, M. G., *et al.* (1996). Assembly of microtubule-associated protein tau into Alzheimer-lke filaments induced by sulphated glycosaminoglycans. *Nature*, **383**, 550–3.

Goldgaber, D., Lerman, M. I., McBride, O. W., *et al.* (1987). Characterization and chromosomal localization of a cDNA encoding brain amyloid of Alzheimer's disease. *Science*, 235, 877–80.

Gotz, J., Probst, A., Spillantini, M. G., *et al.* (1995). Somatodendritic localization and hyperphosphorylation of tau protein in transgenic mice expressing the longest human brain tau isoform. *European Molecular Organisation Journal*, 14, 1304–313.

Gowing, E., Roher, A. E., Woods, A. S., *et al.* (1994). Chemical characterization of A beta 17–42 peptide, a component of diffuse amyloid deposits of Alzheimer disease. *Journal of Biological Chemistry*, 269, 10987–90.

Haass, C., Hung, A. Y., Selkoe, D., and Teplow, D. B. (1994). Mutations associated with a locus for familial Alzheimer's disease result in alternative processing of amyloid beta-protein precursor. *Journal of Biological Chemistry*, **269**, 17741–8.

Hanger, D. P., Brion, J. P., Gallo, J. M., *et al.* (1991). Tau in Alzheimers-disease and Downs-syndrome is insoluble and abnormally phosphorylated. *The Biochemical Journal*, 275, 99–104.

Harada, A., Oguchi, K., Okabe, S., *et al.* (1994). Altered microtubule organization in small-calibre axons of mice lacking tau protein. *Nature*, **369**, 488–91.

Harrington, C. R., Louwagie, J., Rossau, R., *et al.* (1994). Influence of apolipoprotein E genotype on senile dementia of the Alzheimer and Lewy body types. Significance for etiological theories of Alzheimer's disease. *American Journal of Pathology*, **145**, 1472–84.

Hartmann, T., Bieger, S. C., Bruhl, B., *et al.* (1997). Distinct sites of intracellular production for Alzheimer's disease A beta40/42 amyloid peptides. *Nature Medicine*, **3**, 1016–20.

Hasegawa, M., Smith, M. J., and Goedert, M. (1998). Tau proteins with FTDP-17 mutations have a reduced ability to promote microtubule assembly. *FEBS Letters*, 437, 207–10

Hefti, F. (1986). Nerve growth factor promotes survival of septal cholinergic neurons after fimbrial transections. *Journal of Neuroscience*, 6, 2155–62.

Holcomb, L., Gordon, M. N., McGowan, E., *et al.* (1998). Accelerated Alzheimer-type phenotype in transgenic mice carrying both mutant amyloid precursor protein and presenilin 1 transgenes. *Nature Medicine*, 4, 97–100.

Houlden, H., Rizzu, P., Stevens, M., *et al.* (1999). Apolipoprotein E genotype does not affect the age of onset of dementia in families with defined tau mutations. *Neuroscience Letters*, 260, 193–5.

Hsiao, K., Chapman, P., Nilsen, S., *et al.* (1996). Correlative memory deficits, Aβ elevation, and amyloid plaques in transgenic mice. *Science*, 274, 99–102.

Hussain, I., Powell, D., Howlett, D. R., *et al.* (1999). Identification of a Novel Aspartic Protease (Asp 2) as β–Secretase. *Molecular and Cellular Neuroscience*, 14, 419–27.

Iizuka, T., Shoji, M., Harigaya, Y., *et al.* (1995). Amyloid beta-protein ending at thr43 is a minor component of some diffuse plaques in the Alzheimers-disease brain, but is not found in cerebrovascular amyloid. *Brain Research*, **702**, 275–8.

Irving, N. G. and Miller, C. C. J. (1997). Tau phosphorylation in cells transfected with wild-type or an Alzheimer's disease mutant Presenilin 1 *Neuroscience Letters*, 222, 71–4.

Ishihara, T., Hong, M., Zhang, B., *et al.* (1999). Age-dependent emergence and progression of a tauopathy in transgenic mice overexpressing the shortest human tau isoform. *Neuron*, 24, 751–62

Jakes, R., Novak, M., Davison, M., and Wischik, C. M. (1991). Identification of 3- and 4-repeat tau isoforms within the PHF in Alzheimer's disease. *EMBO Journal*, 10, 2725–9.

Jarrett, J. T., Berger, E. P., and Lansbury, P. T., Jr. (1993). The carboxy terminus of the beta amyloid protein is critical for the seeding of amyloid formation: implications for the pathogenesis of Alzheimer's disease. *Biochemistry*, 32, 4693–7.

Jefferies, W. A. Food, M. R. Gabathuler, R. *et al.* (1996). Reactive microglia specifically associated with amyloid plaques in Alzheimer's disease brain tissue express melanotransferrin. *Brain Research*, 712, 122-6.

Jensen, M., Song, X. H., Suzuki, N., *et al.* (1995). The delta-NL Alzheimer mutation (Swedish) increases plasma amyloid-beta protein-concentration. *Journal of Neurochemistry*, 65, S136.

Julliams, A., Vanderhoeven, I., Kuhn, S., *et al.* (1999). No influence of presenilin 1 I143T and G384A mutations on endogenous tau phosphorylation in human and mouse neuroblastoma cells, *Neuroscience Letters*, 269, 83–6.

Kang, J., Lemaire, H., Unterbeck, A., *et al.* (1987). The precursor of Alzheimer's disease amyloid A4 protein resembles a cell-surface receptor. *Nature*, 325, 733–6.

Kaufmann, U., Kirsch, J., Irintchev, A., *et al.* (1999). The M-cadherin catenin complex interacts with microtubules in skeletal muscle cells: implications for the fusion of myoblasts. *Journal of Cell Science*, 112, 55–67.

Kawas, C., Resnick, S., Morrison A., *et al.* (1997). A prospective study of estrogen replacement therapy and the risk of developing Alzheimer's disease: the Baltimore longitudinal study of ageing. *Neurology*, 48, 1517-21.

Kennard, M. L. Feldman, H. Yamada T., and Jefferies, W. A. (1996). Serum levels of the iron binding protein p97 are elevated in Alzheimer's disease. Increased levels of p97 are seen in CSF and serum in AD. *Nature Medicine*, 2, 1230-5.

Kovacs, D. M., Fausett, H. J., Page, K. J., *et al.* (1996). Alzheimer associated presenilins 1 and 2, Neuronal expression in brain and localization to intracellular membranes in mammalian cells. *Nature Medicine*, 2, 224–229.

Lammich, S., Kojro, E., Postina, R., *et al.* (1999). Constitutive and regulated alpha-secretase cleavage of Alzheimer's amyloid precursor protein by a disintegrin metalloprotease. *Proceedings of the National Academy of Sciences (USA)*, 96, 3922–7.

LeBlanc, A. C., Papadopoulos, M., Belair, C., *et al.* (1997). Processing of amyloid precursor protein in human primary neuron and astrocyte cultures. *Journal of Neurochemistry*, 68, 1183–90.

Levitan, D., Doyle, T. G., Brousseau, D., *et al.* (1996). Assessment of normal and mutant human pre-senilin function in *Caenorhabditis elegans*. *Proceedings of the National Academy of Sciences (USA)*, 93, 14940–4.

Levy, E., Carman, M. D., Fernandez-Madrid, I. J., Power, M. D., Lieberburg, I., Van Duinen, S. G.,*et al.* (1990). Mutation of the Alzheimer's disease amyloid gene in hereditary cerebral hemorrhage, Dutch type. *Science*, 248, 1124–6.

Levy-Lahad, E., Wasco, W., Poorkaj, P., *et al.* (1995). Candidate gene for the chromosome 1 familial Alzheimer's disease locus. *Science*, 269, 973–7.

Li, J., Ma, J., and Potter H (1995). Identification and expression analysis of a potential familial Alzheimer disease gene on chromosome 1 related to AD3. *Proceedings of the National Academy of Sciences (USA)*, 92, 12180–4.

Li, Y. M. and Dickson, D. W. (1997). Enhanced binding of advanced glycation end products (AGE) by the ApoE4 isoform links the mechanism of plaque deposition in Alzheimer's disease. *Neuroscience Letters*, 226, 155–8.

Li, J., Xu, M., Zhou, H., *et al.* (1997). Alzheimer presenilins in the nuclear membrane, interphase kine-tochores, and centrosomes suggest a role in chromosome segregation. *Cell*, 90, 917–27.

Lin, L., Georgievska, B., Mattsson, A., and Isacson, O. (1999). Cognitive changes and modified processing of amyloid precursor protein in the cortical and hippocampal system after cholinergic synapse loss and muscarinic receptor activation. *Proceedings of the National Academy of Sciences (USA)*, 96, 12108–13.

Mahley, R. W. (1988). Apolipoprotein E, cholesterol transport protein with expanding role in cell biology. *Science*, **240**, 622–30.

Mann, D. M. A., Iwatsubo, T., and Snowden, J. S. (1996). Atypical amyloid (A beta) deposition in the cerebellum in Alzheimer's disease: An immunohistochemical study using end-specific A beta monoclonal antibodies. *Acta Neuropathologica*, **91**, 647–653.

Masters, C. L., Multhaup, G., Simms, G., *et al.* (1985*a*). Neuronal origin of a cerebral amyloid—neurofibrillary tangles of Alzheimers-disease contain the same protein as the amyloid of plaque cores and blood-vessels. *EMBO Journal*, **4**, 2757–63.

Masters, C. L., Simms, G., Weinman, N. A., *et al.* (1985*b*). Amyloid plaque core protein in Alzheimer's disease and Down syndrome. *Proceedings of the National Academy of Science (USA)*, **82**, 4245–9.

Mehta, N. D., Refolo, L. M., Eckman, C., *et al.* (1998). Increased Aβ42(43) from cell lines expressing presenilin 1 mutations. *Annals of Neurology*, **43**, 256–8.

Mesulam, M. M. and Geula, C. (1988). Nucleus basalis (CH4) and cortical cholinergic innervation in the human brain: observations based on the distribution of acetylcholinesterase and choline acetyltransferase. *Journal of Comparative Neurology*, **275**, 216–40.

Mesulam, M. M., Mufson, E. J., Levey, A. I., and Wainer, B. H. (1983). Cytochemistry and cortical connections of the septal area, diagonal band, nucleus basalis (substantia innominata), and hypothalamus in the rheusus monkey. *Journal of Comparative Neurology*, **214**, 170–97.

Mesulam, M. M., Mufson, E. J., and Wainer, B. H. (1986). Three-dimensional representation and cortical projection topography of the nucleus basalis (Ch4) in the macaque: Concurrent demonstration of choline acetylttransferase and retrograde transport with a stabilized tetramethybenzidine method for horseradish peroxidase. *Brain Research*, **367**, 301–8.

Morishima-Kawashima, M, Hasegawa, M, Takio, K, *et al.* (1994). Proline-directed and non-proline-directed phosphorylation of PHF-tau. *Journal of Biological Chemistry*, **270**, 823–9.

Motter, R., Vigo-Pelfrey, C., Kholodenko, D., *et al.* (1995). Reduction of β-amyloid42 in the cerebrospinal fluid of patients with Alzheimer's disease. *Annals of Neurology*, **36**, 903–11.

Mufson, E. J., Bothwell, M., and Kordower, J. H. (1989). Loss of nerve growth factor receptor-containing neurons in Alzheimer's disease: a quantitative analysis across sub-regions of the basal forebrain. *Experimental Neurology*, **105**, 221–32.

Murphy, D. D. and Segal, M. (1996). Regulation of dendritic spine density in cultured rat hippocampal neurons by steroid hormones. *Journal of Neuroscience*, **16**, 4059–68.

Murphy, M. P., Hickman, L. J., Eckman, C. B., *et al.* (1999). Gamma secretase, evidence for multiple proteolytic activities and influence of membrane positioning of substrate on generation of amyloid beta peptides of varying length. *Journal of Biological Chemistry*, **274**, 11914–23.

Nakai, T., Yamasaki, A., Sakaguchi, M., *et al.* (1999). Membrane topology of Alzheimer's disease-related presenilin 1—Evidence for the existence of a molecular species with a seven membrane-spanning and one membrane-embedded structure. *Journal of Biological Chemistry*, **274**, 23647–58.

Nalbantoglu, J., Gilfix, B. M., Bertrand, P., *et al.* (1994). Predictive value of apolipoprotein E genotyping in Alzheimer's disease: results of an autopsy series and an analysis of several combined studies. *Annals of Neurology*, **36**, 889–95.

Narita, M., Bu G., Holtzman, D. M., and Schwartz, A. L. (1997). The low-density lipoprotein receptor-related protein, a multifunctional apolipoprotein E receptor, modulates hippocampal neurite development. *Journal of Neurochemistry*, **68**, 587–95.

Nordberg, A. (1993). In-vivo detection of neurotransmitter changes in Alzheimers- disease. *Annals of New York Academy of Science (USA)*, **695**, 27–33.

Patrick, G. N., Zukerberg, L., Nikolic, M., *et al.* (1999). Conversion of p35 to p25 deregulates Cdk5 activity and promotes neurodegeneration. *Nature*, **402**, 615–22.

Perez-Tur, J., Froelich, S., Prihar, G., *et al.* (1995). A mutation in Alzheimer's disease destroying a splice acceptor site in the presenilin-1 gene. *Neuroreport*, **7**, 297–301.

Pericak-Vance, M. A., Bass, M. L., Yamaoka, L. H., *et al.* (1998). Complete genomic screen in late-onset familial Alzheimer's disease. *Neurobiology of Ageing*, 19, S39–42.

Perry, E. K., Gibson, P. H., Blessed, G., *et al.* (1977). Neurotransmitter enzyme abnormalities in senile dementia. Choline acetyltransferase and glutamic acid decarboxylase activities in necropsy brain tissue. *Journal of Neurological Science*, 34, 247–65.

Prince, M. (1997). The need for research on dementia in developing countries. *Tropical Medicine and International Health*, 2, 993–1000.

Rebeck, G. W., Reiter, J. S., Strickland, D. K., and Hyman, B. T. (1993). Apolipoprotein E in sporadic Alzheimer's disease, allelic variation and receptor interactions. *Neuron*, 11, 575–80.

Ridley, R. M., Barratt, N. G., and Baker, H. F. (1984). Cholinergic learning deficits in the marmoset produced by scopolamine and ICV hemicholinium. *Psychopharmacology*, 83, 340–5.

Robakis, N. K., Ramakrishna, N., Wolfe, G., and Wisniewski, H. M. (1987). Molecular cloning and characterization of a cDNA encoding the cerebrovascular and neuritic plaque amyloid peptides. *Proceedings of the National Academy of Sciences (USA)*, 84, 4190–4.

Rogaev, E. I., Sherrington, R., Rogaeva, E. A., *et al.* (1995). Familial Alzheimer's disease in kindreds with missense mutations in a gene on chromosome 1 related to the Alzheimer's disease type 3 gene. *Nature*, 376, 775–8.

Rogaeva E; Premkumar S; Song y *et al.* (1998). Evidence for an Alzheimer disease susceptibility locus on chromosome 12 and for further locus heterogeneity. *Journal of the American Medical Association*, 280, 614–8.

Sadot, E., Gurwitz, D., Barg, J., *et al.* (1996). Activation of M1 muscarinic acetylcholine receptor regulates tau phosphorylation in transfected PC12 cells. *Journal of Neurochemistry*, 66, 877–80.

Saunders, A. M., Schmader, K., Breitner, J. C., *et al.* (1993a). Apolipoprotein E epsilon4 allele distributions in late-onset Alzheimer's disease and in other amyloid-forming disease. *Lancet*, 342, 710–11.

Saunders, A. M., Strittmatter, W. J., Schmechel, D., *et al.* (1993b). Association of apolipoprotein E allele epsilon4 with late-onset familial and sporadic Alzheimer's disease. *Neurology*, 43, 1467–72.

Schenk, D., Barbour, R., Dunn, W., *et al.* (1999). Immunization with amyloid-β attenuates Alzheimer-disease-like pathology in the PDAPP mouse. *Nature*, 400, 173–177.

Scheuner, D., Eckman, C., Jensen, M., *et al.* (1996). The amyloid β-protein deposited in the senile plaques of Alzheimer's disease is increased in vivo by the presenilin 1 and 2 and APP mutations linked to familial Alzheimer's disease. *Nature Medicine*, 2, 864–70.

Schneider, A., Biernat, J., von Bergen, M., *et al.* (1999). Phosphorylation that detaches tau protein from microtubules (Ser262, Ser214). also protects it against aggregation into Alzheimer paired helical filaments. *Biochemistry*, 38, 3549–58.

Seiler, M. and Schwab, M. E. (1984). Specific retrograde transport of nerve growth factor (NGF) from neocortex to nucleus basalis in the rat. *Brain Research*, 300, 33–9.

Shen, J., Bronson, R. T., Chen, D. F., *et al.* (1997). Skeletal and CNS defects in presenilin-1-deficient mice. *Cell*, 89, 629–39.

Sherrington, R., Rogaev, E. I., Liang, Y., *et al.* (1995). Cloning of a novel gene bearing missense mutations in early onset familial Alzheimer disease. *Nature*, 375, 754–60.

Simons, M, Keller, P, De Strooper, B, *et al.* (1998). Cholesterol depletion inhibits the generation of β-amyloid in the hippocampal neurons. *Proceedings of the National Academy of Science (USA)*, 95, 6460–4.

Sims, N. R., Bowen, D. M. Allen, S. J., *et al.* (1983). Presynaptic cholinergic dysfunction in patients with dementia. *Journal of Neurochemistry*, 40 503–9.

Sinha, S., Anderson, J. P., Barbour, R., *et al.* (1999). Purification and cloning of amyloid precursor protein β-secretase from human brain. *Nature*, 402, 537–40.

Snow, A. D., Mar, H., Nochlin, D., *et al.* (1988). The presence of heparan sulphate proteoglycans in the neuritic plques and congophilic angiopathy in Alzheimer's disease. *American Journal of Pathology*, 133, 456–63.

Soinenen, H., Kosunen, O., Helisalmi, S., *et al.* (1995). A severe loss of choline acetyltransferase in the frontal cortex of Alzheimer patients carrying Apolipoprotein-epsilon4 allele. *Neuroscience Letters*, 187, 79–82.

Srivastava R. A. K., Srivastava N., Averna M., *et al.* (1997). Estrogen up-regulates apolipoprotein E (ApoE) gene expression by increasing ApoE mRNA in the translating pool via the estrogen receptor alpha-mediated pathway. *Biological Chemistry*, 272, 33360–6.

Steiner, H., Romig H., Grim, M. G., *et al.* (1999). The biological and pathological function of the presenilin-1 Delta exon 9 mutation is independent of its defect to undergo proteolytic processing. *Journal of Biological Chemistry*, 27, 7615–8.

Stone D. J., Rozovsky I., Morgan T. E., *et al.* (1997). Astrocytes and microglia respond to estrogen with increased apoE mRNA in vivo and in vitro. *Experimental Neurology*, 143, 313–18.

Strittmatter, W. J., Saunders, A. M., Goedert, M., *et al.* (1994a). Isoform-specific interactions of apolipoprotein E with microtubule- associated protein tau: implications for Alzheimer disease. *Proceedings of the National Academy of Science (USA)*, 91, 11183–6.

Strittmatter, W. J., Weisgraber, K. H., Goedert, M., *et al.* (1994b). Hypothesis: microtubule instability and paired helical filament formation in the Alzheimer disease brain are related to apolipoprotein E genotype. *Experimental Neurology*, 125, 163–71.

Struhl, G. and Greenwald, I. (1999). Presenilin is required for activity and nuclear access of Notch in Drosophila. *Nature*, 398, 522–5.

Sturchler-Pierrat, C., Abramowski, D., Duke, M., *et al.* (1997). Two amyloid precursor protein transgenic mouse models with Alzheimer disease-like pathology. *Proceedings of the National Academy of Science (USA)*, 94, 13287–92.

Summers, W. K., Majovski, L. V., Marsh, G. M., *et al.* (1986). Oral tetrahydroaminoacridine in long-term treatment of senile dementia, Alzheimer type. *New England Journal of Medicine*, 315, 1241–5.

Suzuki, N., Cheung, T. T., Cai, X. -D., *et al.* (1994). An increased percentage of long amyloid β protein secreted by familial amyloid β protein precursor (βAPP717) mutants. *Science*, 264, 1336–40.

Takei, Y, Teng, J. L., Harada, A., *et al.* (1999). Defects in neuronal morphogenesis in mutant mice lacking microtubule-associated proteins, tau and MAP1B. *Molecular Biology of The Cell*, 10, No. SS, 2159.

Tang, M. X. Jacobs, D. Stern Y., *et al.* (1996). Effect of oestrogen during menopause on risk and age at onset of Alzheimer's disease. *Lancet*, 348, 429-432

Tanzi R. E., Gusella J. F., Watkins P. C., *et al.* (1987). Amyloid β protein gene: cDNA, mRNA distribution, and genetic linkage near the Alzheimer locus. *Science*, 235, 880–4.

Terry, R. D., Masliah, E., Salmon, D. P., *et al.* (1991). Physical basis of cognitive alterations in Alzheimer's disease, synapse loss is the major correlate of cognitive impairment. *Annals of Neurology*, 30, 572–80.

Uterman, G., Langenbeck, U., Beisiegel, U., and Weber, W. (1980). Genetics of the apolipoprotein E system in man. *American Journal of Human Genetics*, 32, 339–47.

Van Duijn, C. M. Meijer, H. Witteman J. C. M., *et al.* (1996). Estrogen, apolipoprotein E and the risk of Alzheimer's disease. *Neurobiology of Ageing*, 17, 79.

Vassar, R., Bennett, B. D., BabuKhan, S., *et al.* (1999). Beta-secretase cleavage of Alzheimer's amyloid precursor protein by the transmembrane aspartic protease BACE. *Science*, 286, 735–41.

Von Koch, C. S., Zheng, H., Chen, H., *et al.* (1997). Generation of APLP2 KO mice and early postnatal lethality in APLP2/APP double KO mice. *Neurobiology of Ageing*, 18, 661–9.

Wagner, U., Utton, M., Gallo, J-M., and Miller, C. C. J. (1996). Cellular phosphorylation of tau by GSK-3β influences tau binding to microtubules and microtubule organisation. *Journal of Cell Science*, 109, 1537–43.

Wilcock, G. K. and Esiri, M. M. (1982). Plaques, tangles and dementia: a quantitative study. *Journal of Neurological Science*, 56, 407–17.

Wilcock, G. K., Esiri, M. M., Bowen, D. M., and Hughes, A. O. (1988). The differential involvement of subcortical nuclei in senile dementia of the Alzheimer type. *Journal of Neurology, Neurosurgery and Psychiatry*, 51, 842–9.

Wischik C. M., Novak M., Thogersen H. C., *et al.* (1988*a*). Isolation of a fragment of tau derived from the core of the paired helical filament of Alzheimer's disease. *Proceedings of the National Academy of Science (USA)*, 85, 4506–4510.

Wischik C. M., Novak M., Edwards P. C., *et al.* (1988*b*) Structural characterization of the core of the paired helical filament of Alzheimer disease. *Proceedings of the National Academy of Science (USA)*, 85, 4884–8.

Wolfe, M. S., Xia, W. M., Ostaszewski, B. L., *et al.* (1999). Two transmembrane aspartates in prese-nilin-1 required for presenilin endoproteolysis and gamma-secretase activity. *Nature*, 398, 513–17.

Wong, P. C., Zheng, H., Chen, H., *et al.* (1997). Presenilin 1 is required for Notch1 and DII1 expres-sion in the paraxial mesoderm. *Nature*, 387, 288–92.

Wu, W. S., Holmans, P., WavrantDevrieze, F., *et al.* (1998). Genetic studies on chromosome 12 in late-onset Alzheimer disease. *Journal of The American Medical Association*, 280, 619–22.

Xu, H. X., Gouras, G. K., Greenfield, J. P., *et al.* (1998). Estrogen reduces neuronal generation of Alzheimer beta-amyloid peptides. *Nature Medicine*, 4, 447–51.

Yamada, T., McGeer P. L., and McGeer, E. G. (1991). Relationship of complement-activated oligoden-drocytes to reactive microglia and neuropathology in neurodegenerative disease. *Dementia*, 2, 71-7.

Yamada, T. McGeer, P. L. Shigeatsu, K., *et al.* (1994). Immunohistochemical features which distinguish pallido-nigro-lysial atrophy from progressive supranuclear palsy. *Japanese Journal of Psychiatric Neurology*, 48, 855–63.

Yan, S. D., Chen, X., Fu, J., *et al.* (1996). RAGE and amyloid-beta peptide neurotoxicity in Alzheimer's disease. *Nature*, 382, 685–91.

Yan, S. D., Zhu, H., and Fu J. (1997*a*). Amyloid-β peptide-receptor for advanced glycation end product interaction elicits neuronal expression of macrophage-colony stimulating factor. A pro-inflammatory pathway in Alzheimer's disease. *Proceedings of the National Academy of Science (USA)*, 94, 5296–301.

Yan, S. D., Fu, J., Soto, C., *et al.* (1997*b*). An intracellular protein that binds amyloid-beta peptide and mediates neurotoxicity in alzheimers-disease. *Nature*, 389, 689–95.

Yan, R., Bienkowsi, M. J., Shuck, M. E., *et al.* (1999). Membrane-anchored aspartyl protease with Alzheimer's disease β-secretase activity. *Nature*, 402, 533–7.

Ye, Y. H., Lukinova, N., and Fortini, M. E. (1999). Neurogenic phenotypes and altered Notch process-ing in *Drosophila* Presenilin mutants. *Nature*, 398, 525–9.

Yoshida, T., Kuwabara, Y., Ichiya, Y., *et al.* (1998). Cerebral muscarinic acetylcholinergic receptor mea-surement in Alzheimer's disease patients on 11C-N-methyl-4-piperidyl benzilate — comparison with cerebral blood flow and cerebral glucose metabolism. *Annals of Nuclear Medicine*, 12, 35–42.

Yu, G., Nishimura, M., Arakawa, S., *et al.* (2000). Nicastrin modulates presenilin–mediated *notch/glp–1* signal transduction and APP processing. *Nature*, 407, 48–54.

Zhang, J., Kang, D. E., Xia, W., *et al.* (1998). Subcellular distribution and turnover of presenilins in transfected cells. *Journal of Biological Chemistry*, 273, 12436–42.

Zheng, H., Jiang, M., Trumbauer, M.E., *et al.* (1995). Beta-Amyloid precursor protein-deficient mice show reactive gliosis and decreased locomotor activity. *Cell*, 81, 525–31.

Zubenko, G. S., Hughes, H. B., Stiffler, J. S., *et al.* (1998). A genome survey for novel Alzheimer disease risk loci, results at 10-cM resolution. *Genomics*, 50, 121–8.

Chapter 2

The neuropathology of Alzheimer's disease

Margaret M. Esiri

2.1 Introduction

The neuropathology of Alzheimer's disease (AD) is arguably its most distinguishing feature. Although its clinical features of progressive dementia with prominent and early memory failure are characteristic, there are other dementing disorders from which distinction can be difficult and the definite diagnosis of AD still requires neuropathological examination of the brain. The diagnostic pathological features are microscopic and were first described in the late nineteenth and early twentieth centuries (Beljahow 1889; Alzheimer 1907). Despite long familiarity with this pathology it is only recently that understanding about its development is beginning to be achieved.

2.2 Gross neuropathology

The naked eye appearance of the brain in cases of AD varies from normal to grossly atrophic. Atrophy, when present, affects the cerebral hemispheres in a fairly generalized distribution but in some cases the medial temporal lobes, hippocampus and amygdala are relatively selectively picked out (Fig 2.1). Severe, generalized atrophy is more common in the

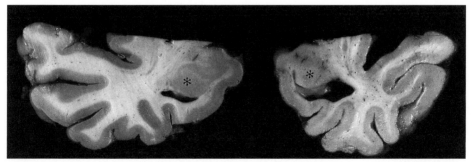

Fig. 2.1 Normal (left) and Alzheimer's disease (right): appearance of a coronal slice through the anterior temporal lobe and amygdala (*). Note reduction in size of both temporal lobe and amygdala in Alzheimer's disease with compensatory dilation of the inferior horn of the lateral ventricle.

minority of cases of early onset than in cases of AD developing very late in life. The early and selective medial temporal lobe atrophy has been detected and found to be diagnostically useful using neuroimageing during life. Some genetically affected members of families with a mutation that causes AD have had neuroimageing performed serially, commencing when they were asymptomatic. These studies have shown that in such cases cerebral atrophy can be detected before the onset of unequivocal psychological or clinical deterioration (Fox *et al.* 1996 see also chapter 13).

Externally the brain usually shows some evidence of gyral narrowing and sulcal widening though this may be no more obvious than is normally seen with increasing age. In slices through the cerebrum there may be increased ventricular size ranging from well within the limits seen with normal ageing to very severe, involving lateral and third ventricles but not the aqueduct and fourth ventricle. Cerebral white matter participates in the atrophic process as well as cortex (de la Monte 1989). The striatum may also show some atrophy. In the brain stem the only noteworthy feature is that the locus coeruleus is characteristically lacking some pigment. In contrast, unless Parkinson's disease pathology with Lewy bodies is also present, the substantia nigra appears normally pigmented in AD.

2.3 **Microscopic pathology**

There are several different components to the microscopic pathology of AD, the most distinctive and widespread of which are argyrophilic plaques and neurofibrillary tangles (NFT). The other six components are neuron loss, glial cell reactions, neuropil threads, granulovacuolar degeneration, Hirano bodies, and amyloid angiopathy. These will be considered in turn.

2.3.1 **Argyrophilic plaques**

These are complex, extracellular foci best visualized with a variety of silver stains or with immunocytochemistry using antibodies to the chief protein constituent of plaques, β-amyloid peptide (Aβ) (Fig 2.2). They vary in size from about 5 μm to 200 μm across and can be divided on the basis of their structural appearance into two main types: diffuse and neuritic. Diffuse plaques consist of homogeneous deposits of fibrillary material unaccompanied by any local reactive glial cells or abnormal neuritic processes. They do not take up the Congo red stain for amyloid and ultrastructurally contain no more than a few amyloid fibrils. In contrast, neuritic plaques have a more heterogeneous, sculpted, appearance with a central dense core which reacts with the Congo red stain. Around this core is clustered a peripheral more or less circular halo of similarly stained material. The halo contains additional elements in the form of glial and abnormal swollen, neuritic, processes (Figs 2.2c, d). Between the core and the halo are interposed the processes of microglial cells. Occasionally plaque cores with no discernible halo can be seen in AD, but these make up only a very small proportion of total plaques even when present. Ultra-structurally the core contains a dense mass of extracellular amyloid fibrils and the neuritic processes contain collections of multi-vesicular bodies and mitochondria. Some are filled with abnormal bundles of helically-wound paired filaments ('paired helical filaments', PHF) (Kidd 1964; Terry *et al.* 1964). Some neuritic processes are axonal and others dendritic. They display an abnormal deficiency of microtubules which causes their cytoskeleton to collapse (Gray *et al.* 1987). The glial components consist of the

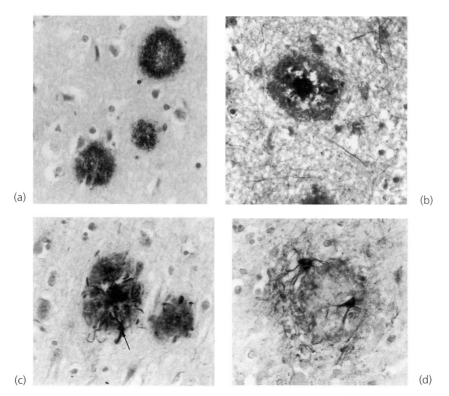

Fig. 2.2 Argyrophilic plaques in cerebral cortex. (a) Diffuse plaques immunostained with an antibody to β amyloid protein; (b) plaque with a central core stained with silver; (c) plaque with a core and neuritic processes (arrow) around it stained with silver; (d) plaque immunostained for glial fibrillary acidic protein and showing two astrocyte cell bodies near the margins of the plaque.

processes of astrocytes and of microglial cells, the latter displaying coated pits in intimate apposition to amyloid filaments.

The relationship between these two main types of plaques — diffuse and neuritic — is not certain. Diffuse plaques are the more abundant and in Down syndrome, in which by late middle age the pathological features of AD have invariably already developed, they appear earlier than neuritic plaques (Lemere *et al.* 1996; Iwatsubo *et al.* 1995; Mann 1997). While both types of plaque contain Aβ, in diffuse plaques this consists of a polypeptide 42–43 amino acids in length (Aβ1–42), while in neuritic plaques much of it lacks the last one or two N-terminal amino acids (Aβ1–40). The two main possible interpretations are that diffuse plaques evolve into neuritic ones with the passage of time and the interaction of the deposited protein with components of the neuropil, or that they have different origins and often occur together, but with a tendency for diffuse plaques to form more readily than neuritic ones. At some sites in the brain, most notably the cerebellum, only diffuse plaques are found in AD, whereas in the other regions of the brain affected by plaque formation both diffuse and neuritic plaques are found (Joachim *et al.* 1989).

The exact nature and development of plaques is the subject of intense interest because it is known that mutations that cause familial AD either involve alterations to the structure of the precursor protein that gives rise to Aβ or they influence the amount of this protein that is produced and skew its metabolism usually in such a way as to increase the amount of Aβ, particularly in its more fibrillogenic 1–42 form that is produced.

Although Aβ is believed to be the main biochemical constituent of plaques a host of other molecules are also found concentrated in them. Many of these are proteins including enzymes such as acetylcholinesterase (Mesulam and Moran 1987) and α1-antichymotrypsin (Abraham et al. 1988); amyloid P component (Kalaria and Perry 1993), complement components (Eikelenboom and Stam 1982; Eikelenboom et al. 1989), apolipoproteins E (apoE) and J (clusterin) (Namba et al. 1991; McGeer and Rogers 1992) and growth factors and their receptors. In addition there are other constituents such as glycosaminoglycans (Snow et al. 1988) and receptor for advanced glycation end-products (RAGE) (Yan et al. 1997). Yet further molecules are found in the cellular processes in neuritic plaques such as the amyloid precursor protein (APP), neuropeptides, lysosomal enzymes, ubiquitin, α-synuclein-derived non-amyloid component (NACP), RNA and markers of apoptosis. The extent to which these components are integral to the plaque and essential for its formation or evolution, or are passively trapped in the fibrillary matrix is unclear. The Congo red reactivity in the cores of neuritic plaques and the amyloid fibrils that can be found ultrastructurally are thought to represent an important difference from diffuse plaques; in neuritic plaques the Aβ adopts the form of a twisted β-pleated sheet that is characteristic of all amyloids. Studies of Aβ *in vitro* indicate that in this form it is neurotoxic whereas in a soluble form and perhaps in diffuse plaques it is non-toxic.

Argyrophilic plaques are not entirely specific for AD but occur also in normal ageing, in Down syndrome, and in some other neurodegenerative conditions (dementia pugilistica, William's disease, progressive supranuclear palsy). The essential difference between normal ageing and AD with respect to plaques is that they are more numerous and include, in particular, more neuritic elements in AD than in normal ageing (see Section 2.7 below). Their occurrence in Down syndrome is considered a forerunner of AD. The most widely used pathological criteria for the diagnosis of AD are based on a semi-quantitative assessment of the density of cortical neuritic plaques (CERAD; Mirra et al. 1991).

2.3.2 Neurofibrillary tangles

NFT are abnormal intraneuronal structures that are formed in the perikarya of neurons in AD. Like plaques, they are well seen with silver stains or using immunocytochemistry with antibodies to their principal biochemical constituent which in this case is hyperphosphorylated tau (Fig 2.3). They also stain well with thioflavine S. They are generally smaller than plaques and their size relates to that of the neuron cell body containing them. Some of the largest are found in subcortical nuclei such as the locus coeruleus and raphe nuclei, where they are sometimes described as 'globose'. They appear as dense skein-like, looped or flame-shaped fibrillary structures occupying the cell body and proximal apical dendrite of affected neurons. In most NFT-bearing neurons a nucleus can still be discerned but in some cells the nucleus and cell outline may not be present and some NFT are clearly extracellular and represent the insoluble contents of a neuron that has died ('ghost' tangle). Under these circumstances NFT take on additional staining properties presumably through accrual of additional molecules such as glial fibrillary acidic protein (GFAP) and Aβ.

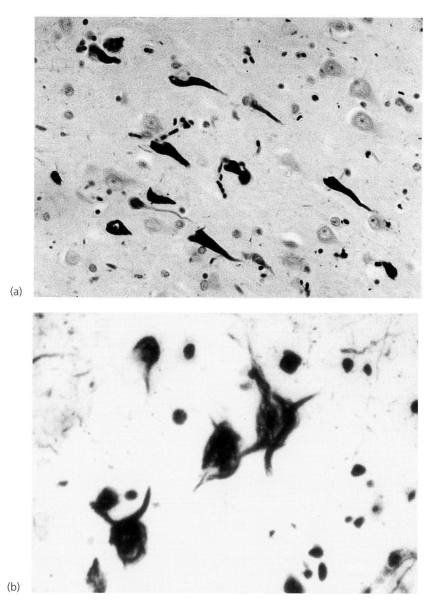

(a)

(b)

Fig. 2.3 Neurofibrillary tangles (a) in the hippocampus, immunostained with an antibody to hyperphosphorylated tau (AT8) and (b) at higher power, in the entorhinal cortex stained with silver. The fibrillary nature of these structures can be appreciated in (b).

The ultrastructure of NFT is revealing (Kidd 1964; Terry 1963; Wisniewski *et al.* 1976). They consist of bundles of distinctive unbranched filaments measuring 20 μm across, pairs of which are wound helically around each other with a periodicity of 80 nm. They do not resemble any normal neuronal ultrastructural constituent. Mixed with these PHF are a few straight, unpaired, filaments 50–20 nm across (Gibson *et al.* 1976; Yagashita *et al.* 1981).

Some neurons containing NFT also contain abnormal tubular or cylindrical cytoplasmic profiles of uncertain significance (Sloper *et al.* 1986; Ghatak 1992).

Despite the lack of resemblance of the PHF forming NFT to any normal neuronal cytoskeletal element, biochemical analysis of NFT has shown that they are formed from a normal cytoskeletal component, a microtubule-associated protein, tau (Grundke-Iqbal *et al.* 1986). However, in comparison to normal tau, the tau found in NFT is abnormally highly phosphorylated.

Whilst being characteristic of AD, NFT have also been described in human brain in a wide range of other diseases including rare, inherited dementia associated with mutations in the tau gene on chromosome 17 (Poorkaj *et al.* 1998), progressive supranuclear palsy, dementia pugilistica, subacute sclerosing pancencephalitis, Guam disease, Niemann-Pick disease, lead poisoning, post encephalitic parkinsonism, myotonic dystrophy, Kuf's disease, Cockayne's syndrome, Hallevorden-Spatz disease and in some varieties of prion disease. They also occur in a restricted distribution in normal ageing (see Section 2.7 below).

2.3.3 **Neuron loss**

Many neurons containing NFT appear healthy despite many of the perikaryal organelles being displaced to the margins of the cell. However, there are indications that NFT-bearing neurons are cells under stress. In particular they express ubiquitin, a protein which is up-regulated in response to various forms of stress including oxidative stress (Mayer *et al.* 1998). As described above, some neurons containing NFT die, leaving behind a 'ghost' tangle. Furthermore, quantitative studies of neuronal populations have shown considerable neuron loss in AD (e.g. West *et al.* 1994). Drop-out of neurons occurs mainly in the types of neurons susceptible to NFT formation. For example, in the neocortex large pyramidal neuron density is reduced by 40%, hippocampal CA1 neurons by 68%, basal nucleus neurons by 40–70% and dorsal raphe and locus coeruleus neurons by 40% and 55% respectively (Terry *et al.* 1981; Arendt *et al.* 1983; Wilcock *et al.* 1988; Aletrino *et al.* 1992; West *et al.* 1994). Some shrinkage of remaining neurons is also seen in AD.

2.3.4 **Glial cell reactions**

As occurs with almost any type of neuropathology in the central nervous system (CNS), the glial cells show evidence of a reaction in AD. This is seen mainly in astrocytes and microglial cells. Astrocytes in grey and subcortical white matter appear enlarged with increased numbers and size of processes, and increased expression of GFAP. Many neuritic plaques are decorated with GFAP-positive astrocytic fibres (Fig 2.2d).

Microglial cells are also increased in regions of grey matter containing neuritic plaques and NFT in AD. The microglial cells are enlarged with increased numbers of processes and increased expression of MHC Class II antigens as well as a moderately increased expression of lysosomal enzymes and complement receptors (McGeer and Rogers 1992; Rogers *et al.* 1992; Itagaki *et al.* 1994). These are features of microglial cells displaying some evidence of activation. A particularly noteworthy involvement of microglial cells with the pathology of AD is an intimate relationship between microglial cells and the cores of neuritic plaques. This has led to the suggestion that microglial cells are either attempting to endocytose the amyloid fibrils or even that they contribute to amyloid formation (Gray *et al.* 1987; Wisniewski 1996). Microglial cells also express RAGE to which Aβ binds on their surface

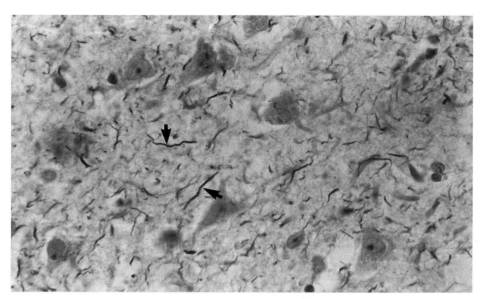

Fig. 2.4 Neuropil threads (arrows) in the neocortex from a case of Alzheimer's disease, stained with silver.

(Yan *et al.* 1997) and it is likely that interactions with these substances in plaques immobilize microglial cells there and expose components of plaques to neurotoxic influences such as nitric oxide and other free radicals as well as to lysosomal enzymes produced by microglial cells.

2.3.5 **Neuropil threads**

Neuropil threads are microscopic argyrophilic (straight or curved) linear structures resembling tiny threads that are present in large numbers in NFT-containing neuropil in AD (Braak *et al.* 1986) (Fig 2.4). They are thought to consist predominantly of dendrites of neurons that contain NFT and they react in similar ways to NFT with antibodies to hyperphosphorylated tau.

2.3.6 **Granulovacuolar degeneration**

Simchowicz (1911) was the first to describe granulovacuolar degeneration in cases of senile dementia. The change is largely confined to hippocampal pyramidal neurons that accumulate one or several cytoplasmic vacuoles in which are located dot-like granules (Fig 2.5). The vacuoles measure 3–5 μm across and the granules 1–2 μm across. Granulovacuolar degeneration is readily visible with routine stains and the granules are also prominently stained by silver. Ultrastructurally they consist of membrane-bound electron-dense granules (Hirano *et al.* 1968). Immunocytochemically the granules react with antibodies to phosphorylated neurofilaments, tubulin, tau, and ubiquitin. Granulovacuolar degeneration is thought to represent autophagic lysosomal degradation of cytoskeletal components. It occurs to a slight extent with normal ageing and can be found in other neurodegenerative conditions as well as in AD.

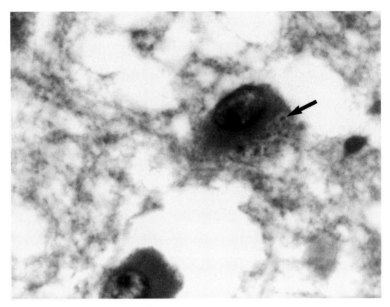

Fig. 2.5 Granulovacuolar degeneration in a hippocampal pyramidal neuron from a case of Alzheimer's disease. One of the granules is arrowed.

2.3.7 **Hirano bodies**

Hirano bodies were first described in cases of dementia-parkinsonism complex of Guam (Hirano *et al.* 1966) but they can be found in many cases of AD and to a much lesser extent with normal ageing. Like granulovacuolar degeneration they are most prominent in the hippocampus. They are strongly eosinophilic rod or carrot-shaped structures 10–30 μm in length and 6–8 μm in width. They are located adjacent to or apparently within pyramidal neurons. Ultrastructurally they consist of tightly aligned parallel filaments and they react immunocytochemically for actin and the actin-associated proteins α-actinin, tropomyosin and vinculin (Goldman 1983; Galloway *et al.* 1987). They are thought to represent an abnormal accumulation of cytoskeletal microfilaments.

2.3.8 **Congophilic angiopathy**

Congophilic angiopathy is a pathological change affecting small blood vessels in the leptomeninges and cerebral and cerebellar cortex in AD. Deep to the cortex, vessels are hardly ever affected. The effect of the change is that the media of small arteries and arterioles is replaced by a homogeneous deposition of Aβ (Fig 2.6). Leptomeningeal vessels provided the original source from which Glenner and Wong (1984) isolated and characterized this protein. Both 1–42 and 1–40 forms of the protein can be found in affected vessel walls, but the shorter 1–40 form predominates, particularly in severe cases (Prelli *et al.* 1988; Roher *et al.* 1993; Alonso *et al.* 1998). Incompletely affected vessels first show deposits of Aβ at the interface between the media and adventitia. The proportion of vessels affected varies greatly from case to case. Within a case there is a less marked variation in severity from one cerebral lobe to another. Most cases show one or a few vessels to be affected in a medium sized microscopic section. The occipital lobe vessels are those most frequently affected, followed

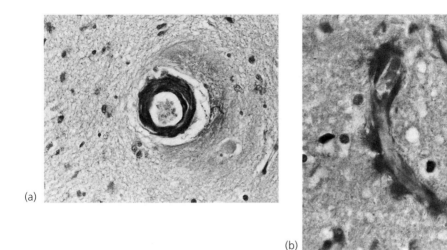

Fig. 2.6 (a) Small cortical arteriole stained with Congo red for amyloid from a case of Alzheimer's disease. The media is replaced by a homogeneous deposit of amyloid; (b) cortical capillary stained with Congo red from a case of Alzheimer's disease. Subendothelial deposits of amyloid have fine spicules extending into the surrounding neuropil.

by the parietal and then frontal and temporal lobes. The hippocampal vessels, in contrast, are rarely affected. Cerebellar leptomeningeal vessels are commonly mildly affected.

The vessels affected are predominantly small branches of leptomeningeal arteries or cortical arterioles. Their walls become converted to featureless, largely acellular tubes of amyloid covered by a thin, sometimes apparently discontinuous, endothelium. Smooth muscle cells eventually disappear. The adventitia is represented by a few collagen fibrils. In severe cases there may be secondary changes consisting of small perivascular haemorrhages, vascular occlusions or reduplications, fibrinoid necrosis or mild perivascular inflammation. Adjacent neuropil may show evidence of haemorrhage or infarction. Not infrequently a massive lobar and subarachnoid haemorrhage may occur from affected vessels and constitute a fatal terminal event. Occasionally the amyloid deposits in cortical vessels involve capillaries as well as arterioles and spicules of amyloid are then seen radiating into the surrounding neuropil where there may be perivascular plaques evident (Fig 2.6b). In such cases a close association between plaques and congophilic angiopathy is clearly shown. More commonly the association is only qualitative with no clear quantitative correlation between the extent of congophilic angiopathy and the density of plaques in a given region of cortex. Some genetically determined cases of AD have particularly severe congophilic angiopathy with much less neuritic pathology than in the typical case (Nochlin *et al.* 1998). Congophilic angiopathy also occurs in normal ageing but it is then usually mild and is associated with some cortical plaque formation, though not necessarily enough to meet pathological criteria for AD. In one study amyloid angiopathy was detected in 30% of brains from elderly undemented subjects (Esiri and Wilcock 1986) and in another study in 36% (Vinters and Gilbert 1983). As with cases of AD with congophilic angiopathy, undemented elderly subjects with amyloid angiopathy may develop major lobar or subarachnoid haemorrhages. Among elderly subjects with such haemorrhages those with the *APOE ε 2* genotype are over-represented (Nicoll *et al.* 1997). In contrast, among cases of AD with severe congophilic angiopathy those with the *APOE* ε *4* genotype are over-represented (Alonso *et al.* 1998). Among subjects with vascular dementia congophilic angiopathy is more common than in age-matched undemented subjects (Esiri *et al.* 1997*a*).

There are other rare genetically determined diseases associated with congophilic angiopathy. One of these, in which recurrent cerebral haemorrhages occur, is due to a mutation in the *APP* gene close to sites at which other mutations cause AD (Levy *et al.* 1990; van Broekhoven *et al.* 1990) and Aβ is deposited, as in AD. There are other forms of inherited cerebral congophilic angiopathy in which the amyloid is not Aβ and combinations of stroke-like symptoms and dementia arise (reviewed in Plant and Esiri 1997).

The source of the Aβ that is deposited in vessel walls is not certain but smooth muscle is one possible source, the extracellular space another and the nerve endings innervating the vessel walls a third.

2.4 Anatomy of plaque and tangle pathology

Having described the microscopic appearance of plaques and tangles we consider the relationships between these two hallmark lesions of AD and their distribution in the brain.

2.4.1 Relationship of plaques to tangles

Neuritic plaques have PHF, as one of their many components, contained in abnormal neuritic processes which are identical ultrastructurally and immunocytochemically in PHF, in NFT, and neuropil threads. Neurons containing NFT probably have axonal processes that contribute to neuritic plaques and dendritic processes that form neuropil threads as well as contributing to neuritic plaques. These structural relationships are difficult to prove but they are supported by the common finding of a distinctive row of plaques in the molecular layer of the dentate gyrus of the hippocampus, at the known site of termination of axonal processes arising from entorhinal pyramidal neurons which are very prone to NFT formation in AD (Hyman *et al.* 1984), and by the location of neuropil threads in regions of the brain that are rich in NFT.

Whether PHF form first in neuronal processes or in the cell body, or at the two sites simultaneously, has not been determined. Evidence from studying Down syndrome brains suggests that plaques make an appearance before NFT and therefore that PHF may form initially in plaques. What does seem clear is that only some of the brain's neurons are prone to NFT formation and that the distribution of plaques is consistent with these forming at sites to which NFT-prone neurons project. Another aspect of the plaque-tangle relationship that is worth bearing in mind is that neuritic processes in plaques display features suggestive of regenerative as well as degenerative activity (Hyman *et al.* 1987).

2.4.2 Distribution of neurons that are prone to neurofibrillary tangle formation in Alzheimer's disease

NFT-prone neurons are to be found in cerebral cortex, hippocampus, and certain subcortical nuclei. In the cortex it is the pyramidal neurons and some large stellate cells that are affected predominantly but their susceptibility to NFT formation varies markedly depending on where in the cortex they are positioned. Those that are most susceptible are situated in transentorhinal cortex occupying the anterior parahippocampal gyrus (Braak and Braak 1991; Arnold *et al.* 1991). Also highly susceptible are the large stellate cells of the adjacent entorhinal cortex followed in turn by the pyramidal neurons of the subiculum and CAI region of the hippocampus, pyramidal neurons of the corticomedial amygdaloid nuclei and periamygdaloid cortex and pyramidal neurons of the inferior and middle temporal gyrus, cingulate gyrus, insula, anterior olfactory nucleus, and association cortex of the frontal, parietal, and occipital lobes. Last in this susceptibility hierarchy of pyramidal neurons are those of the primary motor and sensory cortices which are notably spared from NFT formation (Pearson *et al.* 1985; Esiri *et al.* 1986; Arnold *et al.* 1991). The ordering of this hierarchy shows a striking inverse resemblance to the sequential anatomical connections linking primary sensory cortex via association cortex to entorhinal cortex and hippocampus (van Hoesen 1982). This resemblance has led to the suggestion that NFT pathology may spread from the transentorhinal region both to the hippocampus and to association cortex. In general, cortical brain regions to which the tangle pathology spreads account for the functional impairment in AD (Grabowski and Damasio 1997). Thus, almost universal involvement of transentorhinal, entorhinal, and hippocampal regions underlies the characteristic early and severe memory deficits seen (van Hoesen and Damasio 1987; Hyman *et al.* 1984; Nagy *et al.* 1996), whereas occasional cases with severe and early occipital and occipito-temporal pathology suffer from deficits in associative visual function (Balint's syndrome) (Hof *et al.* 1990).

The consistent hierarchical pattern of involvement of these different regions of cortex with NFT formation forms the basis of a practical stageing scheme that has been developed (Braak and Braak 1991). The first two stages have NFT confined to transentorhinal, entorhinal, and subicular/CAI regions of the hippocampus. At stages III and IV there are increased numbers of NFT in these limbic regions. At stages V and VI isocortical areas are also involved. The first two or three stages are considered as largely subclinical and are exhibited commonly in undemented elderly patients' brains, whereas most cases of pure AD reach stages V and VI. Stages III and IV are commonly found in cases of AD mixed with other pathology such as Parkinson's disease (Nagy *et al.* 1999).

If we accept the suggestion made in Section 2.4.1 that plaques are to be found at the axonal and dendritic terminations of NFT-bearing neurons we can predict from knowledge based on animal, particularly primate, experimentation of cortical connectivity where plaques may be expected to occur: in neuropil that is rich in NFT (because many dendritic endings and some axonal endings project to local cortex) and in neuropil receiving a distant afferent supply from hippocampus and association cortex. This is, in general, the case. Plaques are particularly numerous in the outer three layers of the association cortex and in the molecular layer of the hippocampal dentate gyrus. They are less numerous but nevertheless present in sensory cortex where there is less sparing from plaques than from NFT. If we extend consideration to the subcortical nuclei that are affected in AD, nuclei with rich projections to association cortex and hippocampus, such as the basal nucleus, dorsal raphe, locus coeruleus, some hypothalamic and thalamic nuclei (though not the sensory relay nuclei), and the amygdala develop NFT, whereas those subcortical nuclei to which the cortex projects heavily, such as the striatum, develop plaques (Pearson and Powell 1989; Rogers and Morrison 1985; Lewis *et al.* 1987).

These anatomical projections between tangle-bearing neurons and plaques are liable to suffer from impaired anterograde and retrograde axonal transport as a consequence of NFT formation and depletion of normal tau. This has implications for transport of growth factors which depend on such mechanisms. In particular, delivery of nerve growth factor (NGF), which is synthesized in cortex and hippocampus and delivered to the cholinergic subcortical nuclei by retrograde transport, is likely to be impaired. Sofroniew and Mobley

(1993) have drawn attention to the potential that such impairment might have to provoke a spiralling decline in which deprivation of a growth factor needed to support healthy cholinergic cells could lead to impaired cholinergic stimulation of the cortex and, in turn, to diminished growth factor production there.

2.5 Relationship between the neuropathology of Alzheimer's disease and dementia and behavioural scores

Recent longitudinal follow-up studies to autopsy of people with pathologically confirmed AD generally agree with Wilcock and Esiri (1982) that the severity of dementia correlates best with the density of NFT in the neocortex. Likewise, NFT density in the hippocampus correlates closely and specifically with memory impairment (Nagy *et al.* 1996). In contrast, the total plaque density in neocortex is only weakly related to the severity of dementia (Arriagada *et al.* 1992; Berg *et al.* 1993; Bierer *et al.* 1995; Nagy *et al.* 1995). Neuritic plaque density in neocortex shows an intermediate level of correlation between that of total plaque and NFT densities with dementia severity. Other measures besides NFT density that show good correlations with dementia severity are measures of cortical synapse density (de Kosky and Scheff 1990) or indirect markers of this such as synaptophysin immunoreactivity (Terry *et al.* 1991), cortical neuron density (Neary *et al.* 1986; Hyman *et al.* 1994), and cortical neuritic threads (McKee *et al.* 1991). Biochemical markers that correlate well are the amount of hyperphosphorylated tau (Holzer *et al.* 1995) and markers of cholinergic enzyme activity (Francis *et al.* 1993).

Behavioural symptomatology, in contrast to cognitive decline, has been less studied in relation to neuropathology in AD. However, significant correlates have been found linking behavioural symptoms to subcortical pathology. Thus, depressive symptoms have been linked to loss of neurons in the locus coeruleus (Zweig *et al.* 1988; Zubenko *et al.* 1990) and to loss of serotonergic endings in the cortex (Chen *et al.* 1996). Aggressive behaviour has also been correlated with reduced 5-hydroxytryptamine (5HT) function (Palmer *et al.* 1988) and preserved noradrenergic function (Russo-Neustadt *et al.* 1998) and anxiety to relative preservation of 5HT 2A receptors in cortex (Chen *et al.* 1994). Further work is needed before a full understanding of the clinically important behavioural features of AD is reached. For example, the reason for the apparently beneficial effects of anticholinesterase therapy on the behavioural symptoms of AD is not readily apparent based on current understanding of the contribution of cholinergic deficits (Francis *et al.* 1999). These have been shown to correlate better with cognitive than behavioural scores in AD. However, the greater plasticity that is evident in the serotonergic and noradrenergic systems than in the cholinergic system renders brain functions that are dependent on these subcortical projections more readily supported by anticholinesterase therapy than cognitive function which depends heavily on an intact neocortex and hippocampus.

2.6 The heterogeneity of Alzheimer's disease and its complication of interpretation of clinico-pathological correlations

Clinicopathological studies have shown that although most clinical AD sufferers have exclusively AD pathology at autopsy, a not unsubstantial minority show additional pathology as well. The best correlates between clinical dementia severity and AD pathology are, not surprisingly, obtained when cases of pure AD are considered (e.g. Nagy *et al.* 1995). The two commonest additional pathologies found with AD are cerebrovascular disease and Parkinson's disease. Since these two pathological processes are known to be capable, on their own, of causing symptoms of dementia it is logical to expect that when they are combined with AD the severity of AD pathology for a given severity of cognitive decline will tend to be less because the two types of pathology that are present can have additive effects. This has been shown to be the case in a study of AD combined with vascular disease in which the NFT and plaque density were significantly lower than in a group of cases of pure AD with an equivalent severity of dementia (Nagy *et al.* 1997). In the presence of vascular disease it is of interest that the plaque load showed a more significant correlation with dementia severity than in pure AD. In the presence of Parkinson's disease pathology demented subjects have been described as having an abundance of plaques but little neuritic pathology — a finding that has led to the description of 'plaque only' AD (Hansen *et al.* 1993). This finding is open to a similar interpretation to that suggested above with respect to vascular disease combined with AD; that is, AD pathology when augmented by Parkinson's disease pathology becomes symptomatic at an earlier stage, when plaques are present but few NFT have developed. The finding generally of lower Braak stages in cases of mixed pathology also supports this view (Nagy *et al.* 1999).

Quite apart from the complications in clinicopathological correlation that are posed by cases of mixed pathology there are also some subtypes of AD that are beginning to be discerned. For example, vascular complications occur with some forms of AD, particularly certain familial forms with severe amyloid angiopathy (Poorkaj *et al.* 1998). In such cases NFT are not prominent and dementia may be contributed to more by the vascular complications of the amyloid angiopathy than by neuritic pathology. Clearly such cases do not conform to the usual finding of a close correlation between neuritic pathology and dementia severity.

2.7 The interface between Alzheimer's disease and normal ageing

It was mentioned in Sections 2.2. and 2.3 above that a number of the macroscopic and microscopic features of AD can be found, albeit in a less well developed form or in lower numbers, in the brains of elderly undemented people. Here we take a closer look at the overlap between ageing and AD.

The most conspicuous epidemiological characteristic of AD is its close relationship to ageing (Evans *et al.* 1989; Hofman *et al.* 1991; Ott *et al.* 1995), and some investigators view AD as an exaggerated form of brain ageing. Certainly, changes that occur with ageing present conditions that favour the development of AD. Age-related changes are diverse (reviewed in Esiri 1994) and include slight reductions in the volume and weight of the cerebral hemispheres, enlargement of the ventricles and subarachnoid spaces and mild fibrosis of the leptomeninges. The reduction in hemisphere weight and volume affects white as well as grey matter. At the microscopic level the most prominent changes are an increase in lipofuscin in neurons, the development of corpora amylacea, atrophy of neurons, and loss of neurons among some populations including cerebral cortical and hippocampal neurons, substantia nigra neurons, and cerebellar Purkinje cells. Also noted are a reduction in synaptic density, a change which accompanies reduction in number and length of dendrites and the number of dendritic spines, and a reduction in neuron nucleolar volume, reflecting a reduction of RNA transcription with an accompanying reduction in neuronal cytoplasmic RNA content. These changes do not affect all populations of neurons but many of them affect neurons which are also vulnerable to drop-out or NFT formation in AD.

Added to these universal age-associated changes is the common appearance with ageing of argyrophilic plaques in neocortex and of NFT in transentorhinal, entorhinal, and hippocampal neurons. The dorsal raphe is another site at which NFT in small numbers form, even with normal ageing. Granulovacuolar degeneration and Hirano body formation also develop to a slight extent in the hippocampus and amyloid angiopathy in leptomeningeal and cortical blood vessel walls. All these features tend to be displayed to a lesser extent in normal ageing than in AD, though there can be considerable overlap, particularly in the density of diffuse plaques and the extent of amyloid angiopathy. Neuritic pathology is much less in evidence in normal ageing. What determines its topographic restriction to transentorhinal and adjacent cortex (where it may be related to age-associated benign memory loss) in normal ageing and loss of this restriction in AD is an important unanswered question.

2.8 The interface between Alzheimer's disease and dementia with Lewy bodies

Dementia with Lewy bodies is a relatively recently introduced term to describe a clinico-pathological syndrome in which, on the clinical side, there is fluctuating but progressive dementia, extrapyramidal motor symptoms, and visual hallucinations, and on the pathological side Lewy bodies in the substantia nigra and cerebral cortex usually accompanied by considerable cortical AD pathology as well, particularly plaques (McKeith *et al.* 1996). Lewy bodies in the substantia nigra are of course a hallmark of Parkinson's disease so that what, in pathological terms, is being described here is a combination of features of Parkinson's disease and AD. There may be a tendency for Parkinson's disease and AD pathology to occur together more frequently than would be expected by chance since Lewy bodies in the substantia nigra are found consistently, in large pathological series of AD cases, in about 20% of cases (Gearing *et al.* 1995); whereas they occur in only 1–2% of age matched, undemented controls (Smith *et al.* 1991). The extent of the Lewy body formation and neuron loss in Parkinson's disease is recognized to vary in subcortical nuclei such as the substantia nigra, nucleus basalis, locus coeruleus, hypothalamus, amygdala, and dorsal vagal nucleus, but all these nuclei are commonly affected. Improved methods of detection, using immunocytochemistry with antibodies to ubiquitin and α-synuclein (Lennox *et al.* 1989; Spillantini *et al.* 1998a), show that Lewy bodies invariably also occur in the neocortex, particularly cortex of the parahippocampal gyrus, cingulate gyrus and insula in Parkinson's disease (Hughes *et al.* 1993). The pathological stage would, therefore, seem to be set for the development of dementia with Lewy bodies when Parkinson's disease pathology bears particularly heavily on nuclei such as the nucleus basalis that project to the cortex as well as affecting the cortex itself quite severely, and when the cerebral cortex is simultaneously affected by considerable AD pathology, particularly argyrophilic plaque formation.

Clinical recognition of dementia with Lewy bodies is important because those suffering from it deteriorate significantly if treated with neuroleptic drugs (McShane *et al.* 1997). An explanation for the hallucinations that occur is not readily apparent. The severity of dementia has also been linked to Lewy body density (Lennox *et al.*; 1989 Hortig *et al.* 2000), and neurochemical studies have emphasized the pre-eminence of the severe cholinergic deficit in determining the severity of dementia (Perry *et al.* 1990).

2.9 **A mention of frontal lobe dementia**

Frontal lobe dementia is a clinical term applied to a subset of dementia subjects in whom symptoms of frontal lobe dysfunction such as changes in personality, disinhibited behaviour and impulsivity predominate over those attributable to temporal lobe, parietal lobe, and hippocampal dysfunction such as language disorders, memory deficits, and apraxia (Brun *et al.* 1994). Some cases of frontal lobe dementia show typical (with Pick bodies) or atypical (without Pick bodies) pathology of Pick's disease, but slightly more than half of them show less distinctive pathology with less prominent frontal lobe atrophy than is typically seen in Pick's disease (Esiri *et al.* 1997b). There are also relatively non-specific microscopic changes which are as characteristic for what they lack as for what they include. The features that are lacking are those of AD (in any more than a degree related to age alone), Lewy bodies, and Pick bodies or Pick cells. The features that are present are spongy change confined to lamina 2 of the cortex in frontal and anterior temporal lobes, neuron loss in the same distribution and astrocytosis of affected cortex and subcortical white matter. Another noteworthy feature is the presence of ubiquitin-positive filamentous inclusions in neurons and neuritic processes in affected cortex. The nature of these inclusions is not yet clear as they do not react with antibodies to recognized cytoskeletal components (Jackson and Lowe 1996). Some subcortical sites including the substantia nigra, corpus striatum, and medial thalamus may also show neuron loss and gliosis. Thus, frontal lobe degeneration represents another form of partially selective neurodegeneration which, to judge from the relatively high familial occurrence, probably has important but as yet uncharacterized genetic components to its aetiology. Already rare familial forms of frontotemporal dementia with parkinsonism, associated with NFT (but not plaques), in the brain have been linked to mutations in the gene coding for tau protein (Poorkaj *et al.* 1998; Spillantini *et al.* 2000b)

2.10 **Conclusions and aetiological considerations**

We now have a fairly clear picture of the pathology of AD and of how this relates to symptomatology. There is also a remarkable amount of recently accumulated information about genetic influences. However, we still lack much understanding of pathogenesis and therefore of how best to intervene to slow the process down or prevent it. Other chapters in this volume address aetiology and pathogenesis more directly. The way in which ageing plays such a prominent part in most cases needs clarification. Likewise, the selectivity of the process for particular parts of the brain remains an enigma.

When the interconnectedness of the regions affected was first appreciated the question arose as to whether a virus might be responsible (Esiri 1988). This was based on the known selectivity of some viruses for damageing specific subsets of anatomically connected neurons such as the predilection of herpes simplex virus, when causing acute encephalitis, to damage rather similar limbic regions of the brain to those damaged in AD (Esiri 1982). There has indeed been recent work purporting to implicate herpes simplex virus in the aetiology of AD, although the manner in which this ubiquitous virus might be involved is not at all clear and it will require more evidence to substantiate this suggestion (Lin *et al.* 1998). A more favoured possibility is that age-related free radical damage to neurons has an important role and that apoptotic mechanisms of cell death play an important part . The selectivity of the neuroanatomical distribution of pathology may eventually find an explanation in a particular vulnerability of neurons that retain the long-term plasticity needed to enable life-long learning to be maintained. Understanding the nature of this plasticity is likely to increase understanding of AD.

References

Abraham, C. R., Selkoe, D. J., and Potter, H. (1988). Immunochemical identification of the serine protease inhibitor α-1 antichymotrypsin in the brain amyloid deposits of Alzheimer's disease. *Cell*, 52, 487–501.

Aletrino, M. A, Vogels, D. J. M., and Van Doinburg, P. H. M. F., Ten Donkelaar, H. J. (1992). Cell loss in the nucleus raphe dorsalis in Alzheimer's disease. *Neurobiology of Ageing*, 13, 461–68.

Alonso, N. C., Hyman, B. T, Rebeck, G. W., and Greenberg, S. M. (1998). Progression of cerebral amyloid angiopathy: accumulation of amyloid-beta 40 in affected vessels. *Journal of Neuropathology and Experimental Neurology*, 57, 353–9.

Alzheimer, A. (1907). Über eine eigen artige Erkrankung der Hirnrinde. *Allgemeine Zeitschrift für Psychiatrie Psychisch-Gerichtlich Medizine*, 64, 146–8.

Arendt, T., Bigl ,V., Arendt, A., and Tennstedt, A. (1983). Loss of neurons in the nucleus basalis of Meynert in Alzheimer's disease, paralysis agitans and Korsakoff's disease. *Acta Neuropathologica*, 61, 101–8.

Arnold, S. E., Hyman, B. T., Flory, J., *et al.* (1991). The topographical and neuroanatomical distribution of neurofibrillary tangles and neuritic plaques in cerebral cortex of patients with Alzheimer's disease. *Cerebral Cortex*, 1, 103–16.

Arriagada, P. V., Growdon, J. H., Hedley-Whyte, E. T., and Hyman, B. T. (1992). Neurofibrillary tangles but not senile plaques parallel duration and severity of Alzheimer's disease. *Neurology*, 42, 631–9.

Beljahow, S. (1889). Pathological changes in the brain in dementia senilis. *Journal of Mental Science*, 35, 261–2.

Berg, L., McKeel, D. W., Miller, J. P., *et al.* (1993). Neuropathological indexes of Alzheimer's disease in demented and nondemented persons aged 80 and older. *Archives of Neurology*, 50, 349–58.

Bierer, L., Hof, P., and Purohit, D., *et al.* (1995). Neocortical neurofibrillary tangles correlate with dementia severity in Alzheimer's disease. *Archives of Neurology*, 52, 81–8.

Braak, H. and Braak, E (1991). Neuropathological stageing in Alzheimer-related changes. *Acta Neuropathologica*, 82, 239–59.

Braak, H., Braak, E., Grundke-Iqbal, I., and Iqbal, K. (1986). Occurrence of neuropil threads in the senile human brain and in Alzheimer's disease: a third location of paired helical filaments outside of neurofibrillary tangles and neuritic plaques. *Neuroscience Letters*, 65, 351–5.

Brun, A., Englund, E., Gustafson, L., *et al.* (1994). Clinical and neuropathological criteria for frontotemporal dementia. *Journal of Neurology, Neurosurgery and Psychiatry*, 57, 416–18.

Chen, C. P. L-H, Hope, R. A., Alder, J. T., *et al.* (1994). Loss of $5HT_{2A}$ receptors in Alzheimer's disease neocortex is associated with cognitive decline whilst preservation of $5HT_{2A}$ receptors is associated with anxiety. *Annals of Neurology*, 36, 308–9.

Chen, C. P. L. -H, Alder, J. T., Bowen, D. M., *et al.* (1996). Presynaptic serotonergic markers in community recruited cases of Alzheimer's disease: correlations with depression and neuroleptic medication. *British Journal of Pharmacology*, 66, 1592–8.

De Kosky, S. T. and Scheff, S. W. (1990). Synapse loss in frontal cortex biopsies in Alzheimer's disease: correlation with cognitive severity. *Annals of Neurology*, 27, 457–64.

de la Monte, S. M. (1989). Quantitation of cerebral atrophy in preclinical and end stage Alzheimer's disease. *Annals of Neurology*, 25, 450–9.

Eikelenboom, P. and Stam, F. C. (1982). Immunogobulins and complement factors in senile plaques: an immunoperoxidase study. *Acta Neuropathologica*, 57, 239–42.

Eikelenboom, P., Hack, C. E., Rozemuller, J. M., and Stam, F. C. (1989). Complement activation in amyloid plaques in Alzheimer's dementia. *Virchows Archives B. Cellular Pathololology*, 56, 256–62.

Esiri, M. M. (1982). Herpes simplex encephalitis. An immunohistological study of the distribution of viral antigen within the brain. *Journal of Neurological Science*, 54, 209–26.

Esiri, M. M. (1988). Typical and atypical viruses in the aetiology of senile dementia of the Alzheimer type. In *Histology and histopathology of ageing brain. Interdisciplinary Topics in Gerontolology*, Vol. 25, pp. 119–39. Karger.

Esiri, M. M. (1994). Dementia and normal ageing: neuropathology. In *Dementia and normal ageing* (ed. F. Huppert, C. Brayne, and D. W. O'Connor), pp. 385–436. Cambridge University Press.

Esiri, M. M. (1997). Other neurodegenerative diseases causing dementia. In *The neuropathology of dementia*, (ed. M. M. Esiri., and J. H. Morris), pp. 241–259. Cambridge University Press.

Esiri, M. M., and Wilcock, G. K. (1986). Cerebral amyloid angiopathy in dementia and old age. *Journal of Neurology, Neurosurgy and Psychiatry*, 49, 1221–6.

Esiri, M. M., Pearson, R. C. A., and Powell, T. P. S. (1986). The cortex of the primary auditory area in Alzheimer's disease. *Brain Research*, 366, 385–7.

Esiri M. M., Wilcock G. K., and Morris J. H. (1997*a*). Neuropathological assessment of the lesions of significance in vascular dementia. *Journal of Neurology, Neurosurgery and Psychiatry*, 63, 749–53.

Esiri, M. M., Hyman, B. T., Beyreuther, K., and Masters, C. (1997*b*). Neurodegeneration: ageing and dementia. In *Greenfield's Neuropathology*, 6th edn, Vol II (ed. D. I. Graham and P. L. Lantos), pp. 153–233. Arnold, London.

Evans, D. A., Funkenstein, H. H., Albert, M. S., *et al*. (1989). Prevalence of Alzheimer's disease in a community population of older persons. *Journal of the American Medical Association*, 262, 2551–6.

Fox, N. C., Warrington, E. K., Freeborough, P. A., *et al*. (1996). Presymptomatic hippocampal atrophy in Alzheimer's disease. *Brain*, 119, 2001–7.

Francis, P., Webster, M., Chessell, I., *et al*. (1993). Neurotransmitters and second messengers in ageing and Alzheimer's disease. *Annals New York Academy of Science*, 695, 19–26.

Francis, P., Palmer, A. M., Snape, M., and Wilcock, G. K. (1999). The cholinergic hypothesis of Alzheimer's disease: a review of progress. *Journal of Neurology, Neurosurgery and Psychiatry*, 66, 137–47.

Galloway, P. G., Perry, G., and Gambetti, P. (1987). Hirano body filaments contain actin and actin-associated proteins. *Journal of Neuropathology and Experimental Neurology*, 46, 185–99.

Gearing, M., Mirra, S., Hedreen, J. C., *et al*. (1995). The consortium to establish a registry for Alzheimer's disease (CERAD). Part X. Neuropathology confirmation of the clinical diagnosis of Alzheimer's disease. *Neurology*, 45, 461–6.

Ghatak, N. R. (1992). Intraneuronal cylindrical particles in Alzheimer's disease. *Acta Neuropathologica*, 84, 105–9.

Gibson, P. H., Stones, M., and Tomlinson, B. E. (1976). Senile changes in the human neocortex and hippocampus compared by the use of the electron and light microscopes. *Journal of Neurological Science*, 27, 389–405.

Glenner, G. G. and Wong, C. W. (1984). Alzheimer's disease: initial report of the purification and characterisation of a novel cerebrovascular amyloid protein. *Biochemistry Biophysical Research Communications*, 120, 885–90.

Goldman, J. E. (1983). The association of actin with Hirano bodies. *Journal of Neuropathology and Experimental Neurology*, 42, 146–52.

Grabowski, T. J. and Damasio, A. R. (1997). Definition, clinical features and neuroanatomical basis of dementia. In *The neuropathology of dementia* (ed. M. M. Esiri and J. H. Morris), pp. 1–20. Cambridge University Press.

Gray, E. G., Paula-Barbosa, M., and Roher, A. (1987). Alzheimer's disease: paired helical filaments and cytomembranes. *Neuropathology and Applied Neurobiology*, **13**, 91–110.

Grundke-Iqbal, I., Iqbal, K., Tung, Y. C. H., *et al.* (1986). Abnormal phosphorylation of the micro-tubule-associated protein tau in Alzheimer cytoskeletal pathology. *Proceedings of the National Academy of Science (USA)*, **83**, 4913–17.

Hansen, L., Masliah, E., Galasko, D., and Terry, R. D. (1993). Plaque-only Alzheimer's disease is usually the Lewy body variant and vice versa. *Journal of Neuropathology and Experimental Neurology*, **52**, 648–54.

Hirano, A., Maland, N., Elizan, T. S., and Kurland, L. T. (1966). Amyotrophic lateral sclerosis and Parkinsonism-dementia complex of Guam. *Archives of Neurology*, **15**, 35–51.

Hirano, A., Dembitzer, H. M., Kurland, L. T., and Zimmerman, H. M. (1968). The fine structure of some intraganglionic alterations. *Journal of Neuropathology and Experimental Neurology*, **27**, 167–82.

Hof, P. R., Bouras, C., Constantinidis, J., and Morrison, J. H. (1990). Balint's syndrome in Alzheimer's disease: specific disruption of the occipito-parietal visual pathway. *Brain Research*, **493**, 368–75.

Hofman, A., Rocca ,W. A., Brayne, C., Breteler, M. M. B., Clarke, M., Cooper, B., *et al.* (1991). The prevalence of dementia in Europe: a collaborative study 1980–1990 findings. *International Journal of Epidemiology*, **20**, 736–48.

Holzer, M., Holzapfel, H. P., Zedlick, D., *et al.* (1995). Abnormally phosphorylated tau protein in Alzheimer's disease: heterogeneity of individual regional distribution and relationship to clinical severity. *Neuroscience*, **63**, 499–516.

Hughes, A. J., Daniel, S. E., Blankson, S., and Lees, A. J. (1993). A clinico pathological study of 100 cases of Parkinson's disease. *Archives of Neurology*, **50**, 140–80.

Hurtig, H. I., Trojanowski, J.Q., Galvin, J., *et al.* (2000). Alpha–synuclein cortical Lewy bodies corre-late with dementia in Par kinson's disease. *Neurology*, **54**, 1916–21.

Hyman, B. T., Van Hoesen, G. W., Damasio, A. R., and Barnes, C. L. (1984). Alzheimer's disease: cell specific pathology isolates the hippocampal formation in Alzheimer's disease. *Science*, **225**, 1168–70.

Hyman, B. T., Kromer, L. J., and Van Hoesen, G. W. (1987). Reinnervation of the hippocampal per-forant pathway zone in Alzheimer's disease. *Annals of Neurology*, **21**, 259–67.

Hyman B., West H., Gomez-Isla T., and Mui S. (1994). Quantitative neuropathology in Alzheimer's disease: neuronal loss in high order association cortex parallels dementia. In *Research advances in Alzheimer's disease and related disorders* (ed. K. Iqbal, A. Mortimer, B. Winblad, and H. Wisniewski), pp. 363–70. Wiley and Sons, NY.

Itagaki S., Akiyama H., Saito H., and McGeer P. L. (1994). Ultrastructural localisation of complement membrane attack complex (MAC)-like immunoreactivity in brains of patients with Alzheimer's disease. *Brain Research*, **645**, 78–84.

Iwatsubo, T., Mann, D. M. A., Odaka, A., *et al.* (1995). Amyloid β protein (Aβ) deposition: Aβ42(43) precedes Aβ40 in Down syndrome. *Annals of Neurology*, **37**, 294–9.

Jackson, M. and Lowe, J. (1996). The new neuropathology of degenerative fronto-temporal demen-tias. *Acta Neuropathologica*, **91**, 127–34.

Joachim, C. L., Morris, J. H., and Selkoe, D. J. (1988). Clinically diagnosed Alzheimer's disease: autopsy results in 150 cases. *Annals of Neurology*, **24**, 50–6.

Joachim, C. L., Morris, J. H. N., and Selkoe, D. J. (1989). Diffuse senile plaques occur commonly in the cerebellum in Alzheimer's disease. *American Journal of Pathology*, **135**, 309–19.

Kalaria, R. N. and Perry, G. (1993). Amyloid P component and other acute-phase proteins associated with cerebellar A-beta deposits in Alzheimer's disease. *Brain Research*, **631**, 151–5.

Kidd, M. (1964). Alzheimer's disease: an electron microscopic study. *Brain*, **87**, 307–20.

Lemere, C. A., Blusztajn, J. K., Yamaguchi, H., *et al*. (1996). Sequence of deposition of heterogeneous amyloid β-peptides and ApoE in Down Syndrome: implications for initial events in amyloid plaque formation. *Neurobiology of Disease*, 3, 16–32.

Lennox, G., Lowe, J., Landon, M., *et al*. (1989). Diffuse Lewy body disease: correlative neuropathology using anti-ubiquitin immunocytochemistry. *Journal of Neurology, Neurosurgery and Psychiatry*, 52, 1236–47.

Levy, E., Carman, M. D., Fernandez-Madrid, I. J., *et al*. (1990). Mutation of the Alzheimer's disease gene in hereditary cerebral haemorrhage, Dutch type. *Science*, 248, 1124–6.

Lewis, D. A., Campbell, M. J., Terry, R. D., and Morrison, J. H. (1987). Laminar and regional distributions of neurofibrillary tangles and neuritic plaques in Alzheimer's disease: a quantitative study of visual and auditory cortices. *Journal of Neuroscience*, 7, 1799–808.

Lin, W-R., Graham, J., MacGowan, S. M., *et al*. (1998). Alzheimer's disease, herpes virus in brain, apolipoprotein E_4 and herpes labialis. *Alzheimer's Reports*, 1, 173–8.

McGeer, P. L. and Rogers, J. (1992). Complement proteins and complement inhibitors in Alzheimer's disease. *Research into Immunology*, 143, 621–4.

McKee, A., Kosik, K., and Kowall, N. (1991). Neuritic pathology and dementia in Alzheimer's disease. *Annals of Neurology*, 30, 156–65.

McKeith, I. G., Galasko, D., Kosaka, K., *et al*. (1996). Consensus guidelines for the clinical and pathological diagnosis of dementia with Lewy bodies. *Neurology*, 47, 1113–24.

McShane, R., Keene, J., Gedling, K., *et al*. (1997). Do neuroleptic drugs hasten cognitive decline in dementia? Prospective study with necropsy follow-up. *British Medical Journal*, 314, 266–70.

Mann, D. M. A. (1997). Neuropathological changes of Alzheimer's disease in persons with Down Syndrome. In *The neuropathology of dementia*, (ed. M. M. Esiri and J. H. Morris), pp. 122–136. Cambridge University Press.

Mayer, R. J., Landon, M., and Lowe, J. (1998). Ubiquitin and the molecular pathology of human disease. In *Ubiquitin and the biology of the cell*, (ed. J. -M. Peters, J. R. Harris, and D. Finley), pp. 429–62. Plenum Press, NY

Mesulam, M-M. and Moran, A. M. (1987). Cholinesterases within neurofibrillary tangles related to age and Alzheimer's disease. *Annals of Neurology*, 22, 223–8.

Mirra, S. S., Heyman, A., McKeel, D., *et al*. (1991). The consortium to establish a registry of Alzheimer's disease (CERAD) Part II. Standardisation of the neuropathologic assessment of Alzheimer's disease. *Neurology*, 41, 479–86.

Nagy, Zs., Esiri, M. M., Jobst, K. A., *et al*. (1995). Relative roles of plaques and tangles in the dementia of Alzheimer's disease: correlations using three sets of neuropathological criteria. *Dementia*, 6, 21–31.

Nagy, Zs., Jobst, K. A., Esiri, M. M., *et al*. (1996). Hippocampal pathology reflects memory deficit and brain imageing measurements in Alzheimer's disease: clinicopathologic correlations using three sets of pathologic diagnostic criteria. *Dementia*, 7, 76–81.

Nagy, Zs., Esiri, M. M., Jobst, K. A., *et al*. (1997). The effects of additional pathology on the cognitive deficit in Alzheimer's disease. *Journal of Neuropathol Experimental Neurology*, 56, 165–70.

Nagy, Zs., Hindley, N. J., Braak, H., *et al*. (1999). The progression of Alzheimer's disease from limbic regions to the neocortex: clinical, radiological and pathological relationships. *Dementia and Geriatric Cognitive Disorders*, 10, 115–20.

Namba, Y., Tomonaga, M., Kawaskai, H., *et al*. (1991). Apolipoprotein E immunoreactivity in cerebral amyloid deposits and neurofibrillary tangles in Alzheimer's disease and Kuru plaque amyloid in Creutzfeldt-Jakob disease. *Brain Research*, 541, 163–6.

Neary,D., Snowden, J., Mann, D., *et al*. (1986). Alzheimer's disease — a correlative study. *Journal of Neurology, Neurosurgery and Psychiatry*, 49, 229–37.

Nicoll, J. A., Burnett, C., Love, S., *et al.* (1997). High frequency of apolipoprotein E epsilon 2 allele in haemorrhage due to cerebral amyloid angiopathy. *Annals of Neurology*, **41**, 716–21.

Nochlin, D., Bird, T. D., Nemens, E. J., *et al.* (1998). Amyloid angiopathy in a Volga German family with Alzheimer's disease and a presenilin-2 mutation ($N^{141}I$). *Annals of Neurology*, **43**, 131–5.

Ott, A., Breteler, M. M. B., Van Harskamp, F., *et al.* (1995). Prevalence of Alzheimer's disease and vascular dementia: association with education. The Rotterdam study. *British Medical Journal*, **310**, 970–3.

Palmer, A. M., Stratmann, G. C., Procter, A. W., and Bowen, D. M. (1988). Possible neurotransmitter basis of behavioural changes in Alzheimer's disease. *Annals of Neurology*, **23**, 616–20.

Pearson, R. C. A., and Powell, T. P. S. (1989). The neuroanatomy of Alzheimer's disease. *Reviews in Neuroscience*, 2101–21.

Pearson, R. C. A., Esiri, M. M., Hiorns, R. W., *et al.* (1985). Anatomical correlates of the distribution of the pathological changes in the neocortex in Alzheimer's disease. *Proceedings of the National Academy of Science (USA)*, **82**, 4531–4.

Perry, E. K., Marshall, E., Perry, R. H., *et al.* (1990). Cholinergic and dopaminergic activities in senile dementia of Lewy body type, *Alzheimer Disease Association Disorders*, **4**, 87–95.

Plant, G., and Esiri, M. M. (1997). Familial cerebral amyloid angiopathies. In *The neuropathology of dementia*, (ed. M. M. Esiri and J. H. Morris), pp. 260–76. Cambridge University Press.

Poorkaj, P., Bird, T. D., Wijsman, E., Nemens, E., Garruto, R. M., Anderson, L., *et al.* (1998). Tau is a candidate gene for chromosome 17 frontotemporal dementia. *Annals of Neurology*, **43**, 815–25.

Prelli, F., Castano, E., Glenner, G. G., and Frangione, B. (1988). Differences between vascular and plaque core amyloid in Alzheimer's disease. *Journal of Neurochemistry*, **51**, 648–51.

Rogers, J. and Morrison, J. H. (1985). Quantitative morphology and regional and laminar distributions of senile plaques in Alzheimer's disease. *Journal of Neuroscience*, **5**, 2801–8.

Rogers, J., Cooper, N. R., Webster, S., *et al.* (1992). Complement activation by β amyloid in Alzheimer's disease. *Proceedings of the National Academy of Science (USA)*, **89**, 10016–20.

Roher, A. E., Lowenson, J. D., Clark, S., *et al.* (1993). β amyloid (1–42) is a major component of cerebrovascular amyloid deposits: implications for the pathology of Alzheimer's disease. *Proceedings of the National Academy of Science (USA)*, **90**, 10836–40.

Russo-Neustadt, A., Zomorodian, T. J., and Cotman, C. W. (1998). Preserved cerebellar tyrosine hydroxylase-immunoreactive neuronal fibres in a behaviourally aggressive subgroup of Alzheimer's disease patients. *Neuroscience*, **87**, 55–61.

Simchowicz, T. (1911). Histologische Studien ueber die senile Demenz. *Histol Histopathol Arb Grosshirn*, **4**, 267–444.

Sloper, J. J., Barnard, R. O., Eglin, R. P., and Powell, T. P. S. (1986). Abnormal tubular structures associated with the granular endoplasmic reticulum of the neocortical neurons in a biopsy from a patient with Alzheimer's disease. *Neuropathology and Applied Neurobiology*, **12**, 491–501.

Smith, P. E. M., Irving, D., and Perry, R. H. (1991). Density, distribution and prevalence of Lewy bodies in the elderly. *Neuroscience Research Communications*, **8**, 127–35.

Snow, A. D., Mar, H., Nochlin, D., *et al.* (1988). The presence of heparan sulphate proteoglycans in the neuritic plaques and congophilic angiopathy in Alzheimer's disease. *American Journal of Pathology*, **133**, 456–63.

Sofroniew, M. V. and Mobley, W. C. (1993). On the possibility of positive feedback in trophic interactions between afferent and target neurons. *Journal of Neuroscience*, **5**, 309–12.

Spillantini, M. G., Crowther, R. A., Jakes, R., *et al.* (1998a). Alpha-synuclein in filamentous inclusions of Lewy bodies from Parkinson's disease and dementia with Lewy bodies. *Proceedings of the National Academy of Science (USA)*, **95**, 6469–73.

Spillantini, M. G., Murrell, J. R., Goedert, M., *et al.* (1998b). Mutation in the tau gene in familial multisystem tauopathy with presenile dementia. *Proceedings of the National Academy of Science (USA)*, **95**, 7737–41.

Terry, R. D. (1963). The fine structure of neurofibrillary tangles in Alzheimer's disease. *Journal of Neuropathology and Experimental Neurology*, 22, 629–42

Terry, R. D., Gonatas, N. K., and Weiss, M. (1964). Ultrastructural studies in Alzheimer's presenile dementia. *American Journal of Pathology*, 44, 269–97.

Terry, R. D., Peck, A., DeTeresa, R., *et al.* (1981). Some morphometric aspects of the brain in senile dementia of the Alzheimer type. *Annals of Neurology*, 10, 184–92.

Terry, R. D., Masliah, E., Salmon, D. P., *et al.* (1991). Physical basis of cognitive alterations in Alzheimer's disease: synapse loss is the major correlate of cognitive impairment. *Annals of Neurology*, 30, 572–80.

Van Broeckhoven, C., Haan, J., Bakker, F., *et al.* (1990). Amyloid β protein precursor gene and hereditary cerebral haemorrhage with amyloidosis (Dutch). *Science*, 248, 1120–2.

Van Hoesen, G. W. (1982). The parahippocampal gyrus: new observations regarding its cortical connections in the monkey. *Trends in Neuroscience*, 5, 345–50.

Van Hoesen, G. and Damasio, A. (1987). Neuronal correlates of cognitive impairment in Alzheimer's disease. In *The Handbook of Physiology*, Vol 5, (ed. F. Plum), pp. 871–98. American Physiological Society, Baltimore.

Vinters, H. V. and Gilbert, J. J. (1983). Cerebral amyloid angiopathy: incidence and complications in the ageing brain II. The distribution of amyloid vascular changes. *Stroke*, 14, 924–8.

West, M. J., Coleman, P. D., Flood, D. G., and Troncoso, J. C. (1994). Differences in the pattern of hippocampal neuronal loss in normal ageing and Alzheimer's disease. *Lancet*, 344, 764–72.

Wilcock, G. K., and Esiri, M. M. (1982). Plaques, tangles and dementia: a quantitative study. *Journal of Neurological Science*, 56, 343–56.

Wilcock, G. K., Esiri, M. M., Bowen, D. M., and Hughes, A. O. (1988). The differential involvement of subcortical nuclei in senile dementia of the Alzheimer type. *Journal of Neurology, Neurosurgery and Psychiatry*, 51, 842–9.

Wisniewski, H. M., Narang, H. K., Corsellis, J. A. N., and Terry, R. D. (1976). Ultrastructural studies of the neuropil and neurofibrillary tangles in Alzheimer's disease and post-traumatic dementia. *Journal of Neuropathol Experimental Neurology*, 35, 367.

Wisniewski, H. M., Wegiel, J., and Kotula, L. (1996). Some neuropathological aspects of Alzheimer's disease and its relevance to other disciplines. *Neuropathology and Applied Neurobiology*, 22, 3–11.

Yagashita, S. T., Itoh, T., Nan, W., and Amano, N. (1981). Reappraisal of the fine structure of Alzheimer's neurofibrillary tangles. *Acta Neuropathologica*, 54, 239–46.

Yan, S. D., Zhu, H., and Fu J. (1997). Amyloid-β peptide-receptor for advanced glycation end product interaction elicits neuronal expression of macrophage-colony stimulating factor. A pro-inflammatory pathway in Alzheimer's disease. *Proceedings of the National Academy of Science (USA)*, 94, 5296–301.

Zubenko, G. S., Moossy, J., and Kopp, U. (1990). Major depression in primary dementia: clinical and neuropathologic correlates. *Archives of Neurology*, 45, 1182–86.

Zweig, R. M., Ross, C. A., Hedreen, J. C., *et al.* (1988). The neuropathology of aminergic nuclei in Alzheimer's disease. *Annals of Neurology*, 24, 233–42.

Chapter 3

Molecular genetics of Alzheimer's disease

Wilma Wasco

3.1 Introductions

The aetiologic events that lead to the generation of the intracellular neurofibrillary tangles (NFT) and extracellular deposits of amyloid that are the pathological hallmarks of Alzheimer's disease (AD), as well as to the accompanying synaptic loss and neurodegeneration are not well understood. However, a significant portion of the disease has a genetic basis (for review see Tanzi *et al.* 1994; Schellenberg 1995; Selkoe 1996; Hardy 1997; Blacker and Tanzi 1998). The familial forms of Alzheimer's disease (FAD) can be classified based on both the age-of-onset and the type of gene defect inherited. The majority of early-onset (<60 years) FAD is attributed to 'causative' defects in one of three genes.

   The first of these causative gene defects were identified as mutations in the amyloid β protein precursor (*APP*) gene located on chromosome 21 (Levy *et al.* 1990; Chartier-Harlin *et al.* 1991a; b; Goate *et al.* 1991; Murrell *et al.* 1991; Hendriks *et al.* 1992; Mullen *et al.* 1992). Since this discovery, it has become clear that mutations in APP cause a only a small percentage of early-onset FAD, and that the vast majority of this form of the disease is caused by mutations in the more recently identified gene *PS1*, located on chromosome 14 (Sherrington *et al.* 1995) and coding for the protein presenilin 1. In addition, mutations in a second presenilin gene, *PS2*, located on chromosome 1, result in a small percentage of early onset FAD (Li *et al.* 1995; Levy-Lahad *et al.* 1995; Rogeav *et al.* 1995). An allele of a fourth gene, coding for apolipoprotein E (*APOE*), which is located on chromosome 19, confers increased 'risk' for late-onset FAD (> 60 years) (Pericak-Vance *et al.* 1991; Strittmatter *et al.* 1993; Corder *et al.* 1993; Rebeck *et al.* 1993). Finally, a recent study indicates that polymorphisms in the α-2 macroglobulin gene (*α2M*), which is located on chromosome 12, are genetically associated with AD (Blacker *et al.* 1998, Liao 1998).

3.2 The amyloid precursor protein

The main component of the AD-associated senile plaques, a 39–43 amino acid amyloidogenic peptide termed Aβ, is derived by the proteolytic processing of APP. A series of mutations in the gene coding for APP, were the first FAD gene defects to be described (Levy *et al.* 1990; Chartier-Harlin *et al.* 1991a; b; Goate *et al.* 1991; Murrell *et al.* 1991; Hendriks *et al.* 1992; Mullen *et al.* 1992). APP can exist either as an integral membrane-associated type-1 transmembrane domain protein or, after cleavage at a site near the membrane, as a secreted protein (sAPP). Both versions of the protein can contain a variety of post-translational modifications (Goldgaber *et al.* 1987; Kang *et al.* 1987; Robakis *et al.* 1987; Tanzi *et al.* 1987; Van Nostrand *et al.* 1988; Oltersdorf *et al.* 1989; Weidemann *et al.* 1989; Podlisny *et al.* 1990). The gene for APP is encoded by eighteen exons, three of which can be alternatively transcribed to produce a variety of mRNA species (APP695, APP751, APP770, LAPP). The three alternatively transcribed exons encode a 19 amino acid domain of unknown function that has homology to the MRC Ox-2 antigen, a 56 amino acid Kunitz protease inhibitor (KPI) domain, and a 15 amino acid domain which, when included in APP transcripts, disrupts a consensus site used for heparin sulfate modification of the protein (see Appendix I for structure and sequence of APP).

APP mRNA transcripts appear to be widely, if not ubiquitously expressed, however northern blot analysis does provide evidence for tissue-specific and developmental regulation of APP transcription. The expression of APP mRNA is relatively high in heart, brain, and kidney, and low in lung and liver. All of the major APP transcripts have been localized in brain, however individual alternatively spliced transcripts appear to be expressed with some cellular specificity. The predominant form of APP mRNA in neurons does not contain the KPI domain, while the majority of APP transcripts produced in astrocytes and microglia do, and in peripheral tissues KPI-containing APP transcripts are more abundant. Interestingly, in normal ageing a relative decrease in the production of transcripts lacking the KPI domain as compared to KPI-containing transcripts is observed, perhaps as a result of increased production of APP-KPI forms by reactive astrocytes.

APP is a member of an evolutionarily conserved gene family. To date, two mammalian amyloid precursor-like proteins, APLP1 and APLP2 have been identified and APP-like proteins have also been found in *Drosophila* and *C. elegans*. (Rosen *et al.* 1989; Wasco, *et al.* 1992; Diagle and Li, 1993; Sprecher *et al.* 1993; Slunt *et al.* 1994). The overall structure and the majority of APPs specific structural/functional domains are extremely well conserved in all five of these proteins. In fact, the only region of APP that is not well conserved in either of the mammalian APLPs or in the *Drosophila* or *C. elegans* APP-like genes is the Aβ domain. The conspicuous absence of Aβ in the APLPs indicates that, although it is likely that APP and the APLPs have similar normal physiological roles, only APP can directly give rise to the main component of the amyloid-containing senile plaques.

3.3 **Processing of amyloid precursor protein**

The intracellular trafficking and processing of APP has been intensively investigated (for review, see Gandy and Greengard 1994; Gandy *et al.* 1994; Goate 1998; Selkoe 1998; Mills and Reiner 1999), and specific attention has been given to elucidating the mechanism(s) that are involved in the liberation of Aβ from APP. The two forms of Aβ that have been most extensively examined are the forms that are either 40 or 42 amino acids in length, referred to as Aβ1–40 and Aβ1–42. Aβ1–42 is the more amyloidogenic form of the peptide and is associated with the onset of the disease. APP contains a signal sequence that allows it to be inserted into the plasma membrane after maturation via constitutive secretory pathways (Weidemann *et al.* 1989). The molecule can then be metabolized via one of at least three pathways that produce fragments of APP that do or do not contain 'intact' Aβ. The majority of APP appears to be processed through an 'α-secretase' pathway, where cleavage of full-length APP takes place within the Aβ domain, at the plasma membrane or at an undefined intracellular site. Cleavage at the membrane results in the secretion of the N-terminal portion of APP, termed sAPP (Weidemann *et al.* 1989; Esch *et al.* 1990; Sisodia *et al.* 1990), and the clathrin coated vesicle associated-re-internalization and subsequent lysosomal degradation of the C-terminal membrane bound fragment (Esch *et al.* 1990; Caporaso *et al.* 1992; Golde *et al.* 1992; Haass *et al.* 1992; Nordstedt *et al.* 1993; Ramabhadran *et al.* 1993). Because α-secretase cleavage takes place within the Aβ domain, utilization of this pathway precludes formation of amyloid aggregates.

Recently tumour necrosis factor alpha converting enzyme (TACE), a member of the disintegrin and metalloprotease family of proteases, has been demonstrated to be the enzyme responsible for the α-secretase regulated cleavage of APP (Buxbaum *et al.* 1998). These investigators demonstrated that inhibiting this enzyme affects both APP secretion and Aβ formation in cultured cells. Interestingly, basal secretion of APP was not affected in cultured cells derived from TACE knock out mice, indicating that there may be two classes of α secretase, one involving regulated secretion (TACE) and an as-of-yet identified activity involved in basal secretion.

The ability to detect soluble Aβ in the cerebrospinal fluid (CSF) of individuals unaffected by AD as well as in a variety of APP-transfected cultured cell systems indicates that an alternative APP processing pathway(s) must exist. Indeed, in what has been termed the β-secretase pathway, cleavage of APP at the N-terminal amino acid of Aβ produces a C-terminal fragment that contains an intact Aβ domain, which may then be further cleaved by 'γ-secretase' to produce Aβ (Gandy *et al.* 1992; Golde *et al.* 1992; Knops *et al.* 1992; Nordstedt *et al.* 1993; Seubert *et al.* 1992). A precarious balance between these pathways probably needs to be maintained to keep the amounts of Aβ below pathological levels.

Seven APP mutations have been identified and demonstrated to cause AD in autosomal dominant families with early onset forms of the disease and to alter the ratio of Aβ1–40 to Aβ1–42 production — increasing the relative amounts of Aβ1–42 (for review see Goate 1998; Selkoe 1998; Mills and Reiner 1999). Two other APP mutations that are associated with other amyloid phenotypes have been identified. APP693 (E693Q), is the causative mutation linked to hereditary cerebral haemorrhage with amyloidosis, Dutch type (HCHWA-D) (Levy *et al.* 1990). This rare autosomal dominant disease results in chronic and fatal cerebral haemorrhages that are associated with the deposition of Aβ in the cerebral blood vessel walls and diffuse plaques in the brain parenchyma, two of the pathological hallmarks of AD. A mutation at APP692 (A692G) is linked to cerebral haemorrhage with amyloidosis (CHWA) (Hendriks *et al.* 1992). To date, all of the identified mutations in APP are located within exons 16 or 17 of the gene. Interestingly, these exons encode the Aβ domain, suggesting that the mutations effect the generation of Aβ. Unfortunately, the majority of the APP mutation analyses have focused exclusively on these two exons; thus it is unclear whether there are disease-associated mutations in other regions of the *APP* gene. Although it is now known that mutations in *APP* are responsible for only a small percentage of reported early-onset FAD (Tanzi *et al.* 1992), a clear understanding of the molecular mechanism by which these mutations result in an increase in Aβ and ultimately to the synaptic loss characteristic of FAD, may provide valuable clues regarding the mechanism of Aβ generation in other forms of the disease.

3.4 **Presenilins**

3.4.1 **Presenilin mutations**

The presenilins constitute an evolutionarily conserved family of ubiquitously expressed, multiple transmembrane domain proteins. The genes for two mammalian presenilin proteins, PS1 and PS2, have been identified and localized to human chromosome 14 (Sherrington *et al.* 1995) and chromosome 1 (Levy-Lahad *et al.* 1995; 1996; Li *et al.* 1995; Rogeav *et al.* 1995) respectively. *PS1*, which is the dominant early onset FAD gene, was identified by classical position cloning techniques (Schellenberg 1992; Sherrington *et al.* 1995). *PS2*, which was isolated based on its homology to *PS1* and was then tested as a candidate gene for the non-chromosome 14-linked form of FAD present in pedigrees of Volga German descent (Levy-Lahad *et al.* 1995; 1996; Li *et al.* 1995; Rogeav *et al.* 1995). Pathogenic mutations in both of these genes have been identified and mutations in these two genes, together with those in APP account for most early-onset FAD. Although the proteins encoded by the two presenilin genes are 63% homologous at the amino acid level, (Levy-Lahad *et al.* 1995; Rogeav *et al.* 1995), intensive mutation and epidemiological analyses have revealed some interesting differences between the two proteins. Most evidently, the number of identified mutations in *PS1* is far greater than those in *PS2*. To date, more than 45 individual point mutations in *PS1* have been identified and found to be responsible for the majority of early-onset FAD (for reviews see Kovacs and Tanzi 1998, Hardy 1997; also Appendices II and III). All but one of these alterations are point mutations that result in single amino acid changes in residues that are conserved between the PS1 and PS2 proteins. An additional intronic mutation results in the disruption of a splice acceptor and the in-frame deletion of exon 10 (Perez-Tur *et al.* 1995). It has recently been demonstrated that the pathological activity of this mutation (referred to as ΔE9) is independent of its lack of ability to undergo proteolytic processing, but instead is due to a point mutation (S290C) occurring at the aberrant exon splice junction (Steiner *et al.* 1999). Although the point mutations are distributed throughout the *PS1* gene, more than half of the changes are clustered within two specific regions, exons 6 and 9, which encode transmembrane domain 2 and hydrophilic loop 6, respectively. The clustering of these mutations suggests that the function of the PS1 protein is particularly dependent on these two domains, perhaps by affecting conformation or position within the membrane. Interestingly, the mutations clustered in these regions appear to cause particularly aggressive forms of FAD (Kovacs and Tanzi 1998). The mean age of onset in all *PS1* families is about 45 years old with a range of 28–62 years. The set of individuals with mutations in exon 6 has a mean age of onset of 40, and for those with mutations in exon 9 it is 43.

In contrast to PS1, only two mutations in PS2, both of which are point mutations, have been identified and clearly linked to kindred-specific forms of the disease. The first PS2 mutation to be identified results in an asparagine to isoleucine change at amino acid 141 (N141I) and is responsible for the disease in large Volga German kindred (Li *et al.* 1995; Levy-Lahad *et al.* 1995; Rogeav *et al.* 1995). The second PS2 mutation causes a methionine to valine change at amino acid 239 (M239V) and was identified in an Italian pedigree (Rogeav *et al.* 1995). Whether the preponderance of PS1 versus PS2 mutations is due to the differing genomic environment of the two genes or to factors related to differing biological function of the two molecules remains unclear. Mutation analysis of the two proteins has also led to the identification of a phenotypic difference. Overall, mutations in PS1 result in a relatively early and constant age-of-onset while those in PS2 lead to a somewhat later and more variable age-of-onset (Bird *et al.* 1996). The identification of a PS1 asparagine to isoleucine disease-associated mutation at amino acid 135, a position and alteration that corresponds to the PS2 Volga German mutation, and the finding that the affected members of this pedigree have a relatively constant age-of-onset suggests that the observed variations in age-of-onset are dependent on the molecule itself as opposed to the specific position or nature of the amino acid alteration (Crook *et al.* 1997).

Although the normal function(s) of PS1 and PS2 remain unknown, it is evident that like APP the mammalian presenilins are members of an evolutionarily conserved gene family. Presenilin homologues have been identified in *C. elegans* (L'Hernault and Arduengo 1992; Levitan and Greenwald 1995), *Drosophila* (Boulianne *et al.* 1997; Hong and Koo 1997) and *Xenopus* (Tsujimura *et al.* 1997). Although little is known about the function of the homologues in *Drosophila* or *Xenopus*, the two *C. elegans* proteins, termed SEL-12 and SPE-4, are both believed to be involved in the trafficking and/or sorting of intracellular molecules. Mutation analyses of these proteins indicates that SEL-12 modulates signalling in the LIN-12/Notch mediated pathway and that SPE-4 is involved in intracellular protein sorting and trafficking during spermatogenesis. The ability of the mammalian presenilin proteins to rescue the SEL-12 phenotype in *C. elegans* (Levitan *et al.* 1996; Baumeister *et al.* 1997) indicates that clues to the biological role of the mammalian presenilins, and to the mechanism(s) by which the FAD-associated mutations act, ultimately may come from a clearer understanding of the function of the presenilin homologues in organisms that are easily manipulated at the genetic level.

The gene for PS1 has been localized to a 75 kb region of chromosome 14 and the open reading frame is encoded by 10 exons (Clark *et al.* 1995). PS2 is encoded by a twelve exon gene that spans 24 kb (Levy-Lahad *et al.* 1996, Prihar *et al.* 1996,) and is located on the long arm of chromosome 1 at 1q42 (Levy-Lahad *et al.* 1996; Takano *et al.* 1997). The sequence of the mouse *PS1* gene has been reported (Sherrington *et al.* 1995) and it encodes a protein that is 92% identical to the human gene at the amino acid level. Although the full length *PS2* sequence is unpublished, it is available in Genbank (accession #AF038935) and it is predicted to encode a protein that is 96% identical to the human protein.

There is considerable debate concerning the membrane topology of the presenilins. Although topological analyses have centred on PS1, the extreme similarity of PS2 to PS1 makes it probable that the two proteins take up comparable positions within the membrane and for the purposes of this discussion it will be assumed that the two proteins have similar topologies. The original analysis of hydropathy plots, which indicate that both PS1 and PS2 have ten putative hydrophobic domains, predicted that six to nine of these domains actually spanned the membrane. Originally, the favoured model was a seven transmembrane domain which predicted that the N- and C-termini were on opposite sides of the membrane and that there was a large hydrophilic loop located between transmembrane domains 6 and 7. Subsequently, the analyses from three groups, two of which focus on PS1 (Doan *et al.* 1996; Lehmann *et al.* 1997) and one on SEL 12 (Li and Greenwald 1996), a *C. elegans* presenilin homologue, have refined the original predictions. All three of these groups assume that the presenilins are located in the intracellular membranes of the ER and Golgi and that consequently, the hydrophilic regions of the molecules are either cytoplasmic or lumenal. These studies utilized constructs that produce a series of presenilin or SEL-12 fusion proteins in combination with enzymatic assays and immunochemical analysis to determine the number of the hydrophobic domains that actually span the membrane and which side of the membrane (cytoplasmic or lumenal) specific domains are situated. The results of all three studies indicate that the first six hydrophobic regions span the membrane. This agrees with the original model. The SEL-12 analysis goes on to predict that although the 8th and 9th hydrophobic domains also span the membrane, the 7th and 10th do not (Li and Greenwald 1997). These findings suggest an eight-transmembrane domain model. The results of a similar study of presenilin 1 concluded that there was either a six- or eight-transmembrane domain, but did not allow for differentiation between the two possibilities (Doan et al. 1996). The most recent PS1 topology study predicts that only the first six hydrophobic domains span the membrane and that the last four hydrophobic domains remain on the cytoplasmic side of the membrane to create a relative large C-terminal domain (Lehmann et al. 1997). An important consequence of this model is the loss of the large hydrophilic loop that is a prominent characteristic of the other models. This domain becomes part of a larger C-terminal domain in the six-transmembrane domain model. Notably, each of the studies conclude that the N- and C-termini are on the cytoplasmic side of the membrane, that a ~32 amino acid loop located between transmembrane domain 1 and 2 is on the lumenal side of the membrane, and the remainder of the hydrophilic loops located before transmembrane domain 6 are relatively small, ranging from only 5 to 9 amino acids. Accordingly, proteins that interact with PS2 in the cytoplasm have been predicted to do so by interaction with the N- or C-termini or with the large hydrophilic loop, while interactions with proteins located within the lumen of the ER/Golgi would most likely do so via the smaller transmembrane domain 1/2 hydrophilic loop.

Two specific regions of PS1 and PS2 — the first eighty amino acids and the single large hydrophilic loop — stand out because they are not particularly well conserved either among the two mammalian proteins or in the C. elegans, Xenopus, or Drosophila homologues. The lack of homology raises the possibility that these regions impart specificity of function or localization to the different family members.

Northern blot analysis indicates that the genes encoding PS1 and PS2 both produce two major transcripts. The PS1 messages migrate at approximately 2.7 and 7.5 kb (Sherrington et al. 1995) and the PS2 transcripts at 2.3 and 2.6 kb (Levy-Lahad et al. 1996). While both of the PS1 transcripts are expressed in all tissues examined, it appears that there is clear tissue specific regulation of the production of the two different PS2 transcripts; only the smaller of the two transcripts is detected in brain, placenta, lung, and liver, while both transcripts are detected in heart, skeletal muscle, and pancreas. To date, only the cDNA sequences for the smaller of the two messages from each gene have been reported, therefore whether the differences in size of each genes two main transcripts are the result of alternative splicing or of alternative polyadenylation has not yet been resolved.

In situ hybridization and immunohistochemical studies indicate that, within the brain message for both presenilins are primarily detectable in neurons, and particularly in somal cytoplasm (Boissiere et al. 1996; Deng et al. 1996; Kovacs et al. 1996; Lee et al. 1996; McMillian et al. 1996; Benovic et al. 1997; Berezovska et al. 1997; Blanchard et al. 1997). These studies found that a relatively intense staining signal was most commonly found in large pyramidal neurons, and that moderate or faint staining was usually present in smaller neurons and that the expression of the presenilins is not limited to the neuronal populations that are known to degenerate in AD.

Although there have been reports of presenilin localization at the cell surface (Dewji and Singer 1997) and at the nuclear membrane (Li *et al.* 1997) there is general agreement that the primary subcellular localization of both endogenous and transfected PS2 is within the intracellular membranes of the endoplasmic reticulum (ER) and the Golgi complex (Cook *et al.* 1996; Kovacs *et al.* 1996; Walter *et al.* 1996). In neuronal cell lines PS1 staining has also been observed in dendrites, but not in axons (Cook *et al.* 1996). These findings are supported by the results of an immunoelectron microscopy study of primate brain where PS1 was found to be associated with the cytoplasmic face of the ER/Golgi intermediate compartment as well as in certain coated transport vesicles and dendrites (Lah *et al.* 1997).

3.4.2 Presenilin protein processing

The presenilin proteins both have a tendency to form high molecular weight ubiquitinated aggregates (Kim 1997*a*). In addition, both proteins are endoproteolytically cleaved within the large hydrophilic loop by an unidentified but regulated activity — in transfected cells and transgenic animals the fragments are produced to saturable levels. Endogenously, little full length PS1 or PS2 is detected, suggesting that the N-and C-terminal fragments are the primary form of the protein present in cells (Doan *et al.* 1996; Thinakaran *et al.* 1996; 1997; Kim *et al.* 1997*a*, *b*; Lehman *et al.* 1997; Ratovitski *et al.* 1997).

Studies using cultured cells which have been transiently or stably transfected with wild-type or mutant presenilins indicate that the FAD-associated mutation in the molecule has no obvious effect on the subcellular localization, production or processing of the protein (Kovacs *et al.* 1996; Walter *et al.* 1996; Tomika *et al.* 1997). Interestingly, an analysis of the effects of presenilin mutations in a tetracycline-regulated inducible cell system did reveal mutation-associated alterations in the proteolytic processing of PS2 (Kim *et al.* 1997 *a*, *b*). In this system, a Triton-soluble PS2 25kDa C-terminal fragment (CTF) believed to represent the primary transgene-derived cleavage product, as well as a smaller Triton-insoluble 20kDa alternative CTF were detected). In cells expressing PS2 containing the N141I Volga German FAD mutation, the ratio of alternative to primary-site PS2 cleavage fragments was increased relative to cells expressing wild type PS2. In addition, during apoptosis endogenous PS2 was shown to be cleaved at the alternative site by a caspase-3 family protease. Importantly, this cleavage was increased in molecules containing the FAD-associated mutation as compared to wild type molecules, suggesting a potential mechanism for the mutations. Similar results were found for PS1 (Kim *et al.* 1997*b*). The caspase 3-type cleavage of PS2 was also observed in transiently or stably transfected hamster kidney cells and mouse and human neuroblastoma cells, although in these cells the N141I Volga German mutation did not have a detectable effect on processing (Loetscher *et al.* 1997). In addition, the overexpression of a truncated form of PS2 in a mouse T cell hybridoma study was found to lead to the activation of interleukin converting enzyme (ICE)/Ced-3 cysteine proteases. The caspase 3- family proteases are CPP32-like cysteine proteases. The association of this family of molecules with the processing of the presenilins is particularly interesting in light of a number of studies which indicate that expression of PS2 is pro-apoptotic (Deng *et al.* 1996; Wolozin *et al.* 1996) and that the expression of a C-terminal fragment of PS2 rescues cells from Fas-mediated apoptosis (Vito *et al.* 1996*a*, *b*).

Both the six or eight transmembrane domain models predict that the N- and C-terminal domains and the site for PS2 proteolytic cleave are on the cytoplasmic side of the membrane. Accordingly, both models dictate that the enzymes responsible for the proteolytic cleavage of the presenilins, at either the primary cleavage site or the caspase-3 family cleavage site, would be cytoplasmic in origin.

3.4.3 Clues to the normal biological roles of APP and the presenilins

The normal biological roles of APP and the presenilins remain unclear. The existence of secreted forms of APP in plasma and CSF as well as in growth conditioned media of cultured cells suggests a role for these molecules *in vivo*. APP has been demonstrated to have growth promoting effects on fibroblasts, PC12 cells, cortical and neuronal cells, and a specific amino acid sequence (RERMS) within the N-terminal domain of APP has been shown to be responsible for some of these trophic effects. Studies on hippocampal neurons suggest that secreted APP can protect cells from excitotoxic effects of glutamate by regulating intracellular levels of calcium (Mattson *et al.* 1993). The most clearly defined role for APP so far is that of protease inhibitor. KPI-containing forms of APP have the ability to inhibit a number of serine proteases *in vitro* and these forms of the molecule have been shown to be identical to protease nexin II, a molecule that was previously identified based on its tight association with proteases. In addition KPI-containing forms of APP are also identical to factor XIa inhibitor which is released from the α-granules of platelets and inhibits activated factor XIa at the late stages of the cascade.

There is also evidence for the interaction of APP with the extracellular matrix, where it is believed to be influential in the guidance of neurites in the developing nervous system and during regeneration of neurites after injury. APP preadsorbed to the culture dish clearly promotes cell adhesion to the substratum. It interacts with heparan sulfate proteoglycan (Small *et al.* 1994; Buee *et al.* 1993), collagen, and laminin (Narindarasorasak *et al.* 1992; Kibbey *et al.* 1993), which are all significant protein components of the extracellular matrix that have been localized in amyloid plaques. In addition, APP, APLP1, and APLP2 all bind heparin, a heparan analog, and this binding is promoted by the presence of zinc (Bush *et al.* 1994). In B103 cells, a clonal central nervous system (CNS) neuronal cell line that make little or no endogenous APP, the ability of an APP695 transgene to promote neurite outgrowth has been determined to lie within the 17 amino acids contained between amino acids 319–335 (Jin *et al.* 1994). In this system, the effects of APP do not appear to be mediated by stimulation of cell adhesion. However, the addition of the 17-mer did increase the turnover of inositol polyphosphates, suggesting that in these cells APP may promote neurite extension through cell surface interaction and subsequent activation of inositol phosphate signal transduction systems.

Data that indicates that the low density lipoprotein (LDL) receptor-related protein (LRP) binds secreted APP, and mediates its degradation, provide a biochemical link for APP and apoE in a single metabolic pathway. LRP is a multifunctional, muti-ligand receptor that is a member of the LDL receptor family. Other members of this family include the very low density lipoprotein (VLDL) receptor, megalin or glycoprotein 330 (gp330) and the LDL receptor itself. One function of LRP is to bind and mediate the uptake and degradation of proteins (including tissue factor pathway inhibitor and urokinase plasminogen activator), proteinase-inhibitor complexes, and matrix proteins such as apoE-enriched lipoproteins. In the CNS, LRP is believed to be a major apoE receptor (Rebeck *et al.* 1993). The binding of a 39-kDa protein receptor-associated protein (RAP) blocks the ligand binding ability of LRP and of other members of the family. Kounnas *et al.* (1995) have demonstrated that LRP is responsible for the endocytosis of forms of secreted APP that contain the KPI domain. The degradation of internalized APP is inhibited by RAP and by LRP antibodies, and is significantly diminished in cell lines that are genetically deficient in LRP. Forms of APP that do not contain a KPI domain are poor LRP ligands. Taken together, these data suggest that LRP serves as a receptor for APP and for apoE, two of the four molecules that have been genetically linked to AD. LRP can serve as a receptor for a variety of other molecules including α2M (for review see Rebeck 1998). Interestingly, α2M, which has recently been identified as a risk factor in AD (see below), has also been demonstrated to interact *in vitro* with Aβ (Du *et al.* 1997). Whether there is also a link between this metabolic pathway and the presenilins remains unknown.

The normal physiological roles of both of the presenilins remain unknown however, clues about their function in mammalian cells can be derived from the observation that both PS1 and PS2 share significant amino acid homology with two *C. elegans* proteins, SEL-12 (Levitan and Greenwald 1995) and SPE-4 (L'Hernault and Arduengo 1992) *Sel 12* was isolated during a screen for suppressors of a *lin-12* gain-of-function mutation. The *lin-12* gene is a member of the *lin-12/Notch* family of receptors for intracellular signals that specify cell fate in the nematode (see Greenwald 1994 for review). It produces a protein that has a single membrane-spanning domain. A hypermorphic mutation in the *lin-12* gene results in a multivulva phenotype that is characterized by the production of ectopic pseudovulvae. The fact that this phenotype can be corrected by specific mutations in *sel 12* indicates that there is an interaction between the SEL-12 and LIN-12 proteins, and that the function of SEL-12 may be to facilitate the *lin-12* mediated reception of intracellular signals. The exact details of the interaction remain unclear. The *sel-12* gene product, SEL-12 may be directly involved in the *lin-12* mediated reception of signals by functioning as a co-receptor, or it may act as a downstream effector that is influenced by LIN-12 activation. It has also been proposed that SEL-12 plays a role in receptor trafficking, localization or recycling of LIN-12 (Levitan and Greenwald 1995).

Although the identity of the presenilins with SPE-4 is not quite as striking as it is with SEL-12, the proteins are related. Mutations in *spe-4* disrupt the fibrous body membrane organelle, an unusual organelle that is involved in spermatogenesis in the nematode (L'Hernault and Arduengo 1992). The function of this organelle is to package and deliver proteins to the spermatids during the unequal cytoplasmic partitioning that takes place during meiosis II. Unlike other organisms, the nematode spermatids do not contain ribosomes — they are discarded as the cells form, thus all of the proteins that are necessary for normal differentiation into functional sperm must be placed within the spermatid as it forms. Therefore, it is crucial, for normal development of spermatids that the orderly segregation of components takes place during meiosis II. *Spe-4* mutations disrupt the coordination of cytokinesis with meiotic nuclear divisions during spermatogenesis and result in the production of a spermatocyte-like cell that contains four haploid nuclei instead of four spermatids. Thus, SPE-4 appears to play a role in cytoplasmic partitioning of proteins.

Overall, the display of homology between PS1 and PS2 with the *C. elegans* proteins suggests that the presenilins may be involved in intracellular trafficking or localization of proteins. Mutations in APP lead to relative increases in the ratio of Aβ1–42:Aβ1–40 and this may be a result of altered intracellular trafficking and/or sorting of APP. This hypothesis gains further support from the observation that the levels of Aβ1–42 are increased in fibroblasts from patients with specific mutations in *PS1* or *PS2* (Scheuner *et al.* 1996).

3.5 **Apolipoprotein E**

Examination of a subset of late-onset FAD pedigrees has led to the observation that these families inherit a genetic risk factor located on chromosome 19 (Pericak-Vance *et al.* 1991). The defect involved in these particular pedigrees appears to be a susceptibility defect as opposed to a causative defect such as those present in the genes coding for APP and the pre-senilins. The inheritance of a susceptibility gene defect alone is not sufficient to cause the disease, and one or more secondary events, either environmental or genetic, must accompany the inheritance of the primary defect to cause the disease. Association studies have shown that the chromosome 19 susceptibility gene, which has been localized to band 19q13.2, is at the *APOE* gene locus (Pericak-Vance *et al.* 1991).

ApoE is encoded by a polymorphic gene that exists in three alleles: *APOE-ε2. APOE -ε3*, and *APOE -ε4* (reviewed in Mahley 1988). All three alleles encode a protein of 299 amino acids. The molecular basis of the *apoE* polymorphism is the substitution of amino acids at positions 112 and 158. Thus, whereas the apoE2 polypeptide has a cysteine at both of these positions, apoE3 has a cysteine at 112 and an argenine at 158, and apoE4 has arge-nine at both positions. These substitutions create a charge difference that allows the iso-forms to be separated by isoelectric focusing. The frequency of these alleles in the Caucasian population is 0.08 for ε2, 0.78 for ε3 and 0.14 for ε4, making ε3 the most common allele (Utermann *et al.* 1980). The expression of any two of the three alleles in a particular individual results in both homozygous (ε2/ε2, ε3/ε3, ε4/ε4) or heterozygous (ε2/ε3, ε2/ε4, ε3/ε4) phenotypes.

In 1991, Namba and colleagues reported that apoE antibodies were able to interact with both vesicular and plaque amyloid deposits and neurofibrillary tangles in the AD brain (Namba *et al.* 1991). This report was followed by the observations that apoE was able to interact with amyloid outside of the CNS as well (Wisniewski and Frangione 1992) and with synthetic Aβ (Strittmatter *et al.* 1993). These findings, in combination with the physical location of both the *APOC* and *APOE* genes within the region of chromosome 19 demonstrated to be linked to a subset of late-onset FAD, led investigators to ask whether a particular *APOE* allele segregated with the disease. Ultimately, genetic disequilibrium of the *APOE -ε4* allele with specific late-onset FAD pedigrees was demonstrated, indicating that a defect at or genetically near (within one million base pairs) the *APOE* gene locus was in disequilibrium with these forms of FAD (Corder *et al.* 1993). In this study, the likelihood of developing AD correlated with the *APOE -ε4* allele dosage — ε4 homozygote individuals displayed a greater risk of developing AD than ε4 heterozygote individuals, who in turn, displayed a greater risk than individuals with no ε4 allele. These results have been confirmed by a number of groups, and have been extended to sporadic AD by Rebeck and colleagues (Rebeck *et al.* 1993), who also found that *APOE -ε4/4* patients had more senile plaques than *APOE -ε3/3* patients. In contrast to the effects of *APOE -ε4*, the *APOE -ε2* allele has been suggested to have a protective effective on AD, as evidenced by a decreased frequency of this allele in late-onset cases (Corder *et al.* 1994). However, given the relative infrequency of this allele in the general population, and its association with cardiovascular disease in the homozygous state, the apparent protective effect could be a result of age censoring. Ongoing studies aimed at directly addressing this possibility should resolve this issue.

A series of studies have addressed the effect that the *APOE -ε4* allele has on the age of onset and progression of AD. A multicentre analysis by Blacker and colleagues (Blacker *et al.*

1997) indicates that the effect of the ε4 allele on the incidence of AD was strongest in individuals under 70 years of age. The results of a study by Gomez-Isla *et al.* (Gomez-Isla *et al.* 1996) indicate that the presence of an ε4 allele correlates with earlier onset of AD but has no effect on progression of dementia. A number of studies indicate that ε4 homozygotes with a mutation in *APP* have a lower age of onset than those with no ε4 alleles (St George-Hyslop *et al.* 1994; Schellenberg 1995). In contrast, *APOE* genotype does not appear to have any affect in the age-of-onset in families carrying *PS1* mutations (Van Broeckhoven 1995; Houlden *et al.* 1998).

Between 14 and 16% of normal aged individuals who do not have AD have at least one ε4 allele, and, even in chromosome 19-linked late-onset FAD families, there are occasional individuals who have only ε2 or ε3 alleles but are affected with AD. Thus although the presence of *APOE* -ε4 alone is neither necessary nor sufficient to cause the disease, it results in a marked increase in the probability of developing AD. In addition, surveys that have confirmed the over-representation of the *APOE* -ε4 allele in certain late-onset pedigrees and other AD populations also indicate that the association of an ε4 allele and AD may be sensitive to the choice of population that is examined (Kukull and Martin 1998). These observations indicate that the inheritance of an ε4 allele is best classified as a genetic risk factor, perhaps because the presence of the apoE4 protein isoforms itself causes an increase in the biological susceptibility to the disease, or because the *APOE* -ε4 allele is in disequilibrium with an as-of-yet unidentified polymorphism elsewhere in the *APOE* gene. Finally, although the presence of an ε4 allele results in a marked increase in the probability of developing AD it is unlikely that diagnostic testing assessing the presence of this allele alone would be of value as an effective screening tool. However, in combination with cognitive testing and other potential diagnostics, an *APOE* genotype can help to diagnose a case of probable AD more accurately.

The mechanism of action for the increased susceptibility of individuals with one or more *APOE* -ε4 alleles remains unclear. It may involve a biological effect of the protein produced by the allele, analogous to the manner by which the decrease in the avidity of the binding of apoE2 to the LDL-receptor results in an increase in plasma cholesterol levels in *APOE* -ε2 homozygotes. Strittmatter and colleagues have proposed that it is not the presence of apoE4, but the lack of the other apoE isoforms that result in the increased predisposition to AD (Strittmatter *et al.* 1994). They have hypothesized that apoE3 normally interacts with the microtubule associated protein tau, blocks its phosphorylation and subsequently blocks it from being incorporated into neurofibrillary tangles (NFT), and that apoE4 is unable to perform this function (Strittmatter *et al.* 1994). This hypothesis was based on the differing abilities of purified apoE3 and apoE4 to interact with purified tau *in vitro*, however these studies were neither carried out under physiological conditions, nor have affinity constants or saturation curves been performed to assess physiological relevance.

The apoE protein is found associated with lipid particles in the plasma and the cerebrospinal fluid (CSF) (Mahley 1988). It is a component of VLDL that is synthesized in the liver and transports triglycerides from the liver to peripheral tissues. It is also a component of the high-density lipoprotein (HDL) complex that is involved in the redistribution of cholesterol within cells. ApoE complexes bind to at least two receptors, the LDL receptor, which is the principal cholesterol-ester transporter in plasma (Mahley 1988), and the LRP (Kowal *et al.* 1989; Strickland *et al.* 1990). There are a number of additional receptors that are related to LDL receptor that may be involved in uptake of CSF lipoproteins into the cells of the CNS, via distinct subset of CNS cells or under specific conditions. These include the VLDL receptor, which is located on microglia, and megalin (gp330) which is present on epididymal cells. The scavenger receptors, which bind oxidized and acetylated forms of lipoproteins, may also act to take up apoE.

The amino acid substitutions that are a result of the *apoE* polymorphisms are located in the receptor- binding domain of the protein. Thus, apoE2 binds to the LDL receptor with significantly less avidity than apoE3 and apoE4, which interact with equal affinity (Mahley 1988). As a result, the plasma cholesterol and triglyceride levels of apoE2 homozygote individuals are elevated, and they display an increased susceptibility of hyperlipoproteinemia and cardiovascular diseases. ApoE4 is also associated with higher levels of plasma cholesterol, lower levels of plasma apoE, and an increase in heart disease.

In the CNS, apoE is produced by astrocytes and can be detected in CSF. ApoE that is produced by astrocytes in culture is found in association with lipids as small HDL (LaDu *et al.* 1998). ApoE is not produced by neurons, therefore any effect that it has on this cell type is presumed to be mediated by the uptake of the molecule in association with lipids by the LDL receptor or by LRP. The increased production of apoE in response to neuronal damage appears to allow for the redistribution of lipid breakdown products and cholesterol during neuronal regeneration. *In vitro*, apoE3 has been shown to be more effective than apoE4 in promoting neurite sprouting and extension in cultured dorsal root ganglion neurons (Nathan *et al.* 1994), primary hippocampal cells (Narita *et al.* 1997) and neuronal cell lines (Bellosta *et al.* 1995; Nathan *et al.* 1994; Fagan *et al.* 1996). In fact the addition of purified apoE4 to cultures of dorsal root ganglion decreased outgrowth (Nathan *et al.* 1994). Because of the role that apoE plays in lipid redistribution during development and regeneration, apoE may not be involved in the actual aetiology of AD, but instead, may affect the manner by which neurons are able to cope with a neurodegenerative physiological insult originating from other genetic or environmental factors.

3.6 Other genes and risk factors

Although most early-onset FAD can be attributed to mutations in *APP*, *PS1*, or *PS2*, these mutations do not appear to account for all known cases of this form of the disease. Ongoing studies to determine the exact prevalence of the mutations in the three known genes should provide clues regarding the possibility of inherited defects in other genes.

A series of genetic linkage analyses, which generally involved a complete genomic scan, indicate that there is a late-onset AD risk factor locus located on chromosome 12 (Pericak-Vance *et al.* 1998; Wu *et al.* 1998; Zubenko *et al.* 1998; Rogeava *et al.* 1999). Two attractive candidate genes, coding for LRP and α2M, are located on this chromosome. As described earlier, LRP appears to bind and internalize KPI-containing forms of APP as well as encode the neural receptor for apoE, while α2M is present in senile plaques and binds Aβ (Du *et al.* 1997).

Some recent studies have focused on polymorphisms in LRP and their potential association with AD. A series of conflicting studies assessing a tetranucleotide repeat located within the 5 prime end of the gene report that a specific allele of the repeat was more (Lendon *et al.* 1997), less (Wavrant-DeVriee *et al.* 1997), or equally (Clathworthy *et al.* 1997; Fallin *et al.* 1997) frequent in AD patients compared to controls. A second LRP polymorphism, which results in a silent mutation in exon 3 has also been reported to be associated with an increased risk for AD (Kang *et al.* 1997), although a series of conformational studies indicate that the association is not strong (Baum *et al.* 1998; Lambert *et al.* 1998b; Beffet *et al.* 1999).

The candidacy of α2M as a late onset risk factor has also been addressed in a number of studies. A family based study by Blacker *et al.* (1998) found an association between late-onset AD and the presence of a polymorphism in exon 2 of α2M that results in the deletion of a splice acceptor site in the gene. Three conformational follow up studies indicate that although family based association studies show a positive association between α2M and AD, case control studies do not (Dow *et al.* 1999; Rogeava *et al.* 1999; Rudrasingham *et al.* 1999). Liao *et al.* (1998) have demonstrated an association of increased amyloid burden with α2M. Taken together, these findings indicate that the association of α2M with AD may be conditional upon the existence of other shared genetic factors, suggesting that α2M is acting as a genetic modifier.

A series of polymorphisms in the *APOE* promoter have also been examined as potential modulators of the risk associated with *APOE* -ε4. The hypothesis driving these studies is that polymorphisms in the promoter may be genetically associated with the *APOE* -ε4 allele and may alter expression levels of apoE. There are three common polymorphisms in the *APOE* gene promoter regions (−491, −427, and −210) as well as one in the *APOE* intron-1 enhancer region (+113). Although several studies have demonstrated genetic associations between AD and these polymorphisms (Bullido *et al.* 1998; Lambert *et al.* 1998a), others have not supported the association between either the −219 or the +113 polymorphisms (Rebeck *et al.* 1999).

Finally, a study indicating that a specific allele of a common insertion polymorphism of the gene encoding the angiotensin converting enzyme (ACE) was associated with longevity (Schacter *et al.* 1994) was the impetus for looking for an association of the corresponding deletion polymorphism with an increased risk for AD (Kehoe *et al.* 1999). The study found a significant association of this allele with AD in two independent case-control samples. Conformational studies must be carried out to confirm this finding as well as those described for the LRP, α2M, and *APOE* polymorphism, and future efforts must investigate potential mechanisms for polymorphism-associated increases in the risk for AD.

References

Baum, L., Chen, L., Ng, H. K., *et al.* (1998). Low density lipoprotein receptor related protein gene exon 3 polymorphism association with Alzheimer's disease in Chinese. *Neuroscience Letters*, **247**, 33–6.

Baum, L., Dong, Z. Y., Choy, K. W., *et al.* (1998). Low density lipoprotein receptor related protein gene amplification and 766T polymorphism in astrocytomas. *Neuroscience Letters*, **256**, 5–8.

Baumeister, R., Leimer, U., Zweckbronner, I., *et al.* (1997). Human presenilin-1, but not familial Alzheimer's disease (FAD) mutants, facilitate *Caenorhabditis elegans* Notch signalling independently of proteolytic processing. *Gene Function*, **1**, 149–59.

Beffert, U., Arguin, C., and Poirier, J. (1999). The polymorphism in exon 3 of the low density lipoprotein receptor-related protein gene is weakly associated with Alzheimer's disease. *Neuroscience Letters*, **259**, 29–32.

Bellosta, S., Nathan, B. P., Orth, M., *et al.* (1995). Stable expression and secretion of apolipoproteins E3 and E4 in mouse neuroblastoma cells produces differential effects on neurite outgrowth. *Journal of Biological Chemistry*, **270**, 27063–71.

Benovic, S. A., McGowan, E. M., Rothwell, N. J., *et al.* (1997). Regional and cellular localization of presenilin-2 RNA in rat and human brain. *Experimental Neurology*, **145**, 555–64.

Berezovska, O., Xia, M. Q., Page, K., *et al.* (1997). Developmental regulation of presenilin mRNA expression parallels notch expression. *Journal of Neuropathology and Experimental Neurology*, **56**, 40–4.

Bird, T. D., Levy-Lahad, E., Poorkaj, P., *et al.* (1996). Wide range in age of onset form chromosome 1-related familial Alzheimer's disease. *Annals of Neurology*, **40**, 932–6.

Blacker, D. and Tanzi, R. E. (1998). The genetics of Alzheimer disease, current status and future prospects. *Archives of Neurology*, **55**, 294–6.

Blacker, D., Haines, J. L., Rodes, L., *et al.* (1997). APOE-4 and age of onset of Alzheimer's disease. The NIMH., Genetics Initiative. *Neurology*, **48**, 139–47.

Blacker, D., Wilcox, M. A., Laird, N. M., *et al.* (1998). Alpha-2 macroglobulin is genetically associated with Alzheimer disease. *Nature Genetics*, **19**, 357–60.

Blanchard, V., Cxeck, C., Bonci, B., *et al.* (1997). Immunohistochemical analysis of presenilin 2 expression in the mouse brain, distribution pattern and co-localization with presenilin 1 protein. *Brain Research*, **758**, 209–17.

Boissiere, F., Pradier, L., Delaere, P., *et al.* (1996). Regional and cellular presenilin 2 (STM2) gene expression in the human brain. *Neuroreport*, **7**, 2021–5.

Boulianne, G. L, Livne-Bar, I., Humphreys, J. M., *et al.* (1997). Cloning and characterization of the Drosophila presenilin homologue. *Neuroreport*, **8**, 1025–9.

Buee, L, Ding, W., Anderson, J. P., *et al.* (1993). Binding of vascular heparan sulfate proteoglycan to Alzheimer's amyloid precursor protein is mediated in part by the N-terminal region of A4 peptide. *Brain Research*, **627**, 199–204.

Bullido, M. J, Artiga, M.J, Recuero, M., *et al.* (1998). A polymorphism in the regulatory region of APOE associated with risk for Alzheimer's dementia. *Nature Genetics*, **18**, 69–71.

Bush, A. I., Pettingell, W. H. J. R., de Paradis, M., *et al.* (1994). The amyloid beta-protein precursor and its mammalian homologues. Evidence for a zinc-modulated heparin-binding superfamily. *Journal of Biological Chemistry*, **269**, 26618–21.

Buxbaum, J. D., Liu, K. N., Luo, Y., *et al.* (1998). Evidence that tumor necrosis factor alpha converting enzyme is involved in regulated alpha-secretase cleavage of the Alzheimer amyloid protein precursor. *Journal of Biological Chemistry*, **273**, 27765–7.

Caporaso, G. L., Gandy, S. E., Buxbaum, J. D., *et al.* (1992). Protein phosphorylation regulates secretion of Alzheimer beta/A4 amyloid precursor protein. *Proceedings of the National Acadamy of Sciences (USA)*, **89**, 3055–9.

Chartier-Harlin, M., Crawford, F., Hamandi, K., *et al.* (1991*a*). Screening for the β-amyloid precursor protein mutation (APP717, Val-Ile) in extended pedigrees with early onset Alzheimer's disease. *Neuroscience Letters*, **129**, 134–5.

Chartier-Harlin, M., Crawford, F., Houlden, H., *et al.* (1991*b*). Early-onset Alzheimer's disease caused by mutations at codon 717 of the β-amyloid precursor protein gene. *Nature*, **353**, 844–6.

Clark, R. F., Hutton, M., Fuldner, R. A. *et al.* (Alzheimer's Disease Collaboration Group) (1995). The structure of the presenilin 1 (S182) gene and identification of six novel mutations in early onset AD families. *Nature Genetics*, **11**, 219–22.

Clatworthy, A. E., Gomez-Isla, T., Rebeck, G. W., *et al.* (1997). Lack of association of a polymorphism in the low-density lipoprotein receptor-related protein gene with Alzheimer disease. *Archives of Neurology*, **54**, 1289–92.

Cook, D. G., Sung, J. C., Golde, T. E., *et al.* (1996). Expression and analysis of presenilin 1 in a human neuronal system, Localization in cell bodies and dendrites. *Proceedings of the National Academy of Sciences (USA)*, **93**, 9223–8.

Corder, E. H., Saunders, A. M., Strittmatter, W. J., *et al.* (1993). Gene dose of apolipoprotein E type 4 allele and the risk of Alzheimer's disease in late onset families. *Science*, **261**, 921–3.

Corder, E. H., Saunders, A. M., Risch, N. J., *et al.* (1994). Protective effect of apolipoprotein E type 2 allele for late onset Alzheimer disease. *Nature Genetics*, 7, 180–4.

Crook, R., Ellis, R., Shanks,M., Thal, L. J., Perez-Tur, J., Baker, M., *et al.* (1997). Early-onset Alzheimer's disease with a presenilin-1 mutation at the site corresponding to the Volga German presenilin-2 mutation. *Annals of Neurology*, 42, 124–8.

Daigle, I. and Li, C. (1993). apl-1, a *Caenorhabditis elegans* gene encoding a protein related to the human β-amyloid protein precursor. *Proceedings of the National Academy of Sciences (USA)*, 90, 12045–9.

Deng, G., Pike, C. J., and Cotman, C. W. (1996). Alzheimer-associated presenilin-2 confers increased sensitivity to apoptosis in PC12 cells. *FEBS Letters*, 397, 50–4.

Dewji, N. and Singer, S. J. (1997). Cell surface expression of the Alzheimer's disease-related presenilin proteins. *Proceedings of the National Academy of Sciences (USA)*, 94, 9926–31.

Doan, A., Thinakaran, G., Borchelt, D. R., *et al.* (1996). Protein topology of presenilin 1. *Neuron*, 17, 1023–30.

Dow, D. J., Lindsey, N., Cairns, N. J., *et al.* (1999). Alpha-2 macroglobulin polymorphism and Alzheimer disease risk in the UK. *Nature Genetics*, 22, 16–7.

Du, Y., Ni, B., Glinn, M, *et al.* (1997). Alpha2-Macroglobulin as a beta-amyloid peptide-binding plasma protein. *Journal of Neurochemistry*, 69, 299–305.

Du, Y., Bales, K. R., Dodel, R. C., *et al.* (1998). Alpha2-macroglobulin attenuates beta-amyloid peptide 1–40 fibril formation and associated neurotoxicity of cultured fetal rat cortical neurons. *Journal of Neurochemistry*, 70, 1182–8.

Duff, K., Eckman, C., Zehr, C., *et al.* Increased amyloid beta42(43) in brains of mice expressing mutant presenilin 1. *Nature*, 383, 710–13.

Esch, F. S., Keim, P. S., Beattie, E. C., *et al.* (1990). Cleavage of amyloid β peptide during constitutive processing of its precursor. *Science*, 248, 1122–4.

Fagan, A. M., Bu, G., Sun, Y., *et al.* (1996). Apolipoprotein E-containing high density lipoprotein promotes neuriteoutgrowth and is a ligand for the low density lipoprotein receptor-related protein. *Journal of Biological Chemistry*, 271, 30121–5.

Fallin, D., Kundtz, A., Town, T., *et al.* (1997). No association between the low density lipoprotein receptor-related protein (LRP) gene and late-onset Alzheimer's disease in a community-based sample. *Neuroscience Letters*, 233, 145–7.

Gandy, S. E. and Greengard, P. (1994). Processing of Aβ-amyloid precursor protein, Cell biology, regulation and role in Alzheimer's disease. *International Review of Neurobiology*, 36, 29–50.

Gandy, S. E., Buxbaum, J. D., Suzuki, T., *et al.* (1992). The nature and metabolism of potentially amyloidogenic carboxyl-terminalfragments of the Alzheimer beta/A4-amyloid precursor protein, some technical notes. *Neurobiology of Ageing*, 13, 601–3.

Gandy, S., Caporaso, G., Buxbaum, J., Frangione, B., and Greengard, P. *et al.* (1994). APP processing, Aβ amyloidogenesis, and the pathogenesis of Alzheimer's disease. *Neurobiology of Ageing*, 15, 253–6.

Goate, A. M. (1998). Monogenetic determinants of Alzheimer's disease, APP mutations. *Cellular and Molecular Life Sciences*, 54, 897–901.

Goate, A., Chartier-Harlin, M., Mullan, M., *et al.* (1991). Segregation of a missense mutation in the amyloid precursor protein gene with familial Alzheimer's disease. *Nature*, 349, 704–6.

Golde, T. E., Estus, S., Younkin, L. H., *et al.* (1992). Processing of the amyloid protein precursor to potentially amyloidogenic derivatives. *Science*, 255, 728–30.

Goldgaber, D., Lerman, M. I., McBride, O. W., *et al.* (1987). Characterization and chromosomal localization of a cDNA encoding brain amyloid of Alzheimer's disease. *Science*, 235, 877–80.

Gomez Isla, T., West, H. L, Rebeck, G. W., *et al.* (1996). Clinical and pathological correlates of apolipoprotein E epsilon 4 in Alzheimer's disease. *Annals of Neurology*, 39, 62–70.

Haass, C., Koo, E. H, Mellon, A., *et al.* (1992). Targeting of cell-surface beta-amyloid precursor protein to lysosomes: alternative processing into amyloid-bearing fragments. *Nature*, 357, 500–3.

Hardy J. (1997). Amyloid, the presenilins and Alzheimer's disease. *Trends in Neurosciences*, **20**, 154–9.

Hendriks, L., van Duijn, C. M., Cras, P., *et al.* (1992). Presenile dementia and cerebral haemorrhage caused by a mutation at codon 692 of the β-amyloid precursor protein gene. *Neurobiology of. Ageing*, **13** (suppl. 1), S67.

Hong, C. S. and Koo, E. H. (1997). Isolation and characterization of Drosophila presenilin homolog, *Neuroreport*, **8**, 665–8.

Houlden, H., Crook, R., Backhovens, H., *et al.* (1998). ApoE genotype is a risk factor in nonpresenilin early-onset Alzheimer's disease families. *American Journal of Medical Genetics*, **81**, 117–21.

Iwatsubo, T., Odaka, A., Suzuki, N., *et al.* (1994). Visualization of Aβ42(43)-positive and Aβ40-positive senile plaques with end-specific Aβ-monoclonal antibodies, evidence that an initially deposited Aβ species is Aβ1–42(43). *Neuron*, **13**, 45–53.

Jin, L. W., Ninomiya, H., Roch, J. M., *et al.* (1994). Peptides containing the RERMS sequence of amyloid β/A4 protein precursor bind cell surface and promite neurite extension. *Journal of Neuroscience*, **14**, 5461–70.

Kang, D. E., Saitoh, T., Chen, X., *et al.* (1997). Genetic association of the low-density lipoprotein receptor-related protein gene (LRP), an apolipoprotein E receptor, with late-onset Alzheimer's disease. *Neurology*, **49**, 56–61.

Kang, J., Lemaire, H., Unterbeck, A., *et al.* (1987). The precursor of Alzheimer's disease amyloid A4 protein resembles a cell-surface receptor. *Nature*, **325**, 733–6.

Kehoe, P. G., Russ, C., McIlory, S., *et al.* (1999). Variation in DCP1, encoding ACE., is associated with susceptibility to Alzheimer disease. *Nature Genetics*, **21**, 71–2.

Kibbey, M. C., Jucker, M., Weeks, B. S., *et al.* (1993). beta-Amyloid precursor protein binds to the neurite-promoting IKVAV site of laminin. *Proceedings of the National Academy of Sciences (USA)*, **90**, 10150–3.

Kim, T. W., *et al.* (1995). Neuronal apoliprotein E receptor, LRP, in the human central nervous system synaptic nerve terminal. *Society for Neuroscience Abstracts*, **21**.

Kim, T. -W., Pettingell, W. H., Hallmark, O. G., *et al.* (1997*a*). Endoproteolytic cleavage and proteasomal degradation of presenilin 2 in transfected cells. *Journal of Biological Chemistry*, **272**, 11006–10.

Kim, T. W, Pettingell, W. H., Jung, Y. K., *et al.* (1997*b*). Alternative cleavage of Alzheimer-associated presenilins during apoptosis by a caspase-3 family protease. *Science*, **277**, 373–6.

Knops, J., Lieberburg, I., and Sinha, S. (1992). Evidence for a nonsecretory, acidic degradation pathway for amyloidprecursor protein in 293 cells. Identification of a novel, 22-kDa,beta-peptide-containing intermediate. *Journal of Biological Chemistry*, **267**, 16022–4.

Kounnas, M., Moir, R. D., Rebeck, G. W. *et al.* (1995). LDL-receptor regulated protein, a multifunctionsl Apo-E receptor, binds secreted β-amuloid precursor protein and mediates its degradation. *Cell*, **82**, 331–340.

Kovacs, D. M. and Tanzi, R. E. (1998). Monogenic determinants of familial Alzheimer's disease, presenilin-1 mutations. *Cellular and Molecular Life Sciences*, **54**, 902–9.

Kovacs, D. M., Fausett, H. J., Page, K. J., *et al.* (1996). Alzheimer associated presenilins 1 and 2, Neuronal expression in brain and localization to intracellular membranes in mammalian cells. *Nature Medicine*, **2**, 224–9.

Kowal, R. C., Herz, J., Goldstein, J. L., *et al.* (1989). Low density lipoprotein receptor-related protein mediates uptake of cholesteryl esters derived from apoprotein E-enriched lipoproteins. *Proceedings of the National Academy of Sciences (USA)*, **86**, 5810–4.

Kukull, W. A. and Martin, G. M. (1998). APOE polymorphisms and late-onset Alzheimer disease, the importance of ethnicity. *Journal of the American Medical Association*, **279**, 788–9.

LaDu, M. J., Gilligan, S. M., Lukens, J. R., *et al.* (1998). Nascent astrocyte particles differ from lipoproteins in CSF. *Journal of Neurochemistry*, **70**, 2070–81.

Lah, J. J., Heilman,C. J., Nash, N. R., *et al.* (1997). Light and electron microscopic localization of presenilin-1 in primate brain. *Journal of Neuroscience*, 17, 1971–80.

Lambert, J. C., Berr, C., Pasquier, F., *et al.* (1998a). Pronounced impact of Th1/E47cs mutation compared with -491 AT mutation on neural APOE gene expression and risk of developing Alzheimer's disease. *Human Molecular Genetics*, 7, 1511–16.

Lambert, J. C., Wavrant-De Vrieze, F., Amouyel P., and Chartier-Harlin, M. C. (1998b). Association at LRP gene locus with sporadic late-onset Alzheimer's disease. *Lancet*, 351, 1787–8.

Lee, M. K., Slunt, H. H., Martin, L. J., *et al.* (1996). Expression of presenilin 1 and 2 (PS1 and PS2) in human and murine tissues. *Journal of Neuroscience*, 16, 7513–25.

Lehmann, S., Chiesa, R., and Harris, D. A. (1997). Evidence for a six-transmembrane domain structure of presenilin 1. *Journal of Biological Chemistry*, 272, 12047–51.

Lendon, C. L., Talbot, C. J., Craddock, N. J., *et al.* (1997). Genetic association studies between dementia of the Alzheimer's type and three receptors for apolipoprotein E in a Caucasian population. *Neuroscience Letters*, 222, 187–90.

Levitan, D. and Greenwald, I. (1995). Facilitation of lin-12-mediated signalling by sel-12, a *Caenorhabditis elegans* S182 Alzheimer's disease gene. *Nature*, 377, 351–4 .

Levitan, D., Doyle, T. G., Brousseau, D., *et al.* (1996). Assessment of normal and mutant human presenilin function in *Caenorhabditis elegans*. *Proceedings of the National Academy of Sciences (USA)*, 93, 14940–4.

Levy, E., Carman, M. D., Fernandez-Madrid, I. J., *et al.* (1990). Mutation of the Alzheimer's disease amyloid gene in hereditary cerebral haemorrhage, Dutch type. *Science*, 248, 1124–6.

Levy-Lahad, E., Wasco, W., Poorkaj, P., *et al.* (1995). Candidate gene for the chromosome 1 familial Alzheimer's disease locus. *Science*, 269, 973–7.

Levy-Lahad, E., Poorkaj, P., Wang, K., *et al.* (1996). Genomic structure and expression fo STM2, the chromosome 1 familial Alzheimer disease gene *Genomics*, 34, 196–204.

L'Hernault, S. W. and Arduengo, P. M. (1992). Mutation of a putative sperm membrane protein in *Caenorhabditis elegans* prevents sperm differentiation but not its associated meiotic divisions. *Journal of Cell Biology*, 119, 55–68.

Li, X. and Greenwald, I. (1996). Membrane topology of C. elegans SEL-12 protein. *Neuron*, 17, 1015–21.

Li, X. and Greenwald, I. (1997). HOP-1, a *Caenorhabditis elegans* presenilin, appears to be functionally redundant with SEL-12 presenilin and to facilitate LIN-12 and GLP-1 signaling. *Proceedings of the National Academy of Sciences (USA)*, 94, 12204–9.

Li, J., Ma, J., and Potter H (1995). Identification and expression analysis of a potential familial Alzheimer disease gene on chromosome 1 related to AD3. *Proceedings of the National Academy of Sciences (USA)*, 92, 12180–4.

Li, J., Xu, M., Zhou, H., Ma, J., and Potter, H. (1997). Alzheimer presenilins in the nuclear membrane, interphase kinetochores, and centrosomes suggest a role in chromosome segregation. *Cell*, 90, 917–27.

Liao, A., Nitsch, R. M., Greenberg, S. M., *et al.* (1998). Genetic association of an alpha2-macroglobulin (Val1000lle) polymorphism and Alzheimer's disease. *Human Molecular Genetics*, 7, 1953–6

Loetscher, H., Deuschle, U., Brockhaus, M. *et al.* (1997). Presenilins are processed by caspase-type proteases. *Journal of Biological Chemistry*, 272, 20655–9.

McMillan, P. J., Leverenz, J. B., Poorkaj, P., *et al.* (1996). Neuronal expression of STM2 mRNA in human brain is reduced in Alzheimer's disease. *Journal of Histochemistry and Cytochemistry*, 44, 1215–22.

Mahley, R. W. (1988). Apolipoprotein E, cholesterol transport protein with expanding role in cell biology. *Science*, 240, 622–30.

Mattson, M. P., Rydel, R. E., Lieberburg, I., *et al.* (1993). Altered calcium signalling and neuronal injury: stroke and Alzheimer's disease as examples. *Annals of the New York Academy of Science*, 679, 1–21.

Meyer, M. R., Tschanz, J. T., Norton, M. C., *et al.* (1998). APOE genotype predicts when-not whether - one is predisposed to develop Alzheimer disease. *Nature Genetics*, 19, 321–2.

Mills, J. and Reiner, P. B. (1999). Regulation of amyloid precursor protein cleavage. *Journal of Neurochemistry*, 72, 443–60.

Mullan, M., Crawford, F., Axelman, K., *et al.* (1992). A pathogenic mutation for probable Alzheimer's disease in the N-terminus of β-amyloid. *Nature Genetics*, 1, 345–7.

Murrell, J., Farlow, M., Ghetti, B., and Benson, M. D. (1991). A mutation in the amyloid precursor protein associated with hereditary Alzheimer disease. *Science*, 254, 97–9.

Namba, Y., Tomonaga, M., Kawasaki, H., *et al.* (1991). Apolipoprotein E immunoreactivity in cerebral amyloid deposits and neurofibrillary tangles in Alzheimer's disease and kuru plaque amyloid in Creutzfeldt-Jakob disease. *Brain Research*, 541, 163–6.

Narindrasorasak, S., Lowery, D. E., Altman, R. A., *et al.* (1992). Characterization of high affinity binding between laminin and Alzheimer's disease amyloid precursor proteins. *Laboratory Investigations*, 67, 643–52.

Narita, M., Bu G., Holtzman, D. M., and Schwartz, A. L. The low-density lipoprotein receptor-related protein, a multifunctional apolipoprotein E receptor, modulates hippocampal neurite development. *Journal of Neurochemistry*, 68, 587–95.

Narita, M., Holtzman, D. M., Schwartz, A. L., and Bu, G. (1997). Alpha2-macroglobulin complexes with and mediates the endocytosis of beta-amyloid peptide via cell surface low-density lipoprotein receptor-related protein. *Journal of Neurochemistry*, 69, 1904–11.

Nathan, B. P., Bellosta, S., Sanan, D. A., *et al.* (1994). Differential effects of apolipoproteins E3 and E4 on neuronal growth in vitro. *Science*, 264, 850–2.

Nordstedt ,C., Caporaso, G. L., Thyberg, J., *et al.* (1993). Identification of the Alzheimer beta/A4 amyloid precursor protein in clathrin-coated vesicles purified from PC12 cells. *Journal of Biological Chemistry*, 268, 608–12.

Oltersdorf, T., Fritz, L. C., Schenk, D. B., *et al.* (1989). The secreted form of the Alzheimer's amyloid precursor protein with the Kunitz domain is protease nexin-II. *Nature*, 341, 144–7.

Perez-Tur, J., Froelich, S., Prihar, G., *et al.* (1995). A mutation in Alzheimer's disease destroying a splice acceptor site in the presenilin-1 gene. *Neuroreport*, 7, 297–301.

Pericak-Vance, M. A., Bebout, J. L., Gaskell, P. C., Jr., *et al.* (1991). Linkage studies in familial Alzheimer disease, evidence for chromosome 19 linkage. *American Journal of Human Genetics*, 48, 1034–50.

Pericak-Vance, M. A., Bass, M. L., Yamaoka, L. H., Gaskell, P. C., Scott ,W. K., Terwedow, H. A., *et al.* (1998). Complete genomic screen in late-onset familial Alzheimer's disease. *Neurobiology of Ageing*, 19, S39–42.

Podlisny, M. B., Mammen, A. L., Schlossmacher, M. G., *et al.* (1990). Detection of soluble forms of the β-amyloid precursor protein in human plasma. *Biochemical Biophysical Research Communications*, 167, 1094–101.

Prihar, G., Fuldner, R. A., Perez-Tur, J., *et al.* (1996). Structure and alternative splicing of the Presenilin-2 gene. *Neuroroport*, 7, 1680–4.

Ramabhadran, T. V., Gandy, S. E., Ghiso, J., *et al.* (1993). Proteolytic processing of human amyloid beta protein precursor in insect cells. Major carboxyl-terminal fragment is identical to its human counterpart. *Journal of Biological Chemistry*, 268, 2009–12.

Ratovitski, T., Slunt, H. H., Thinakaran, G., *et al.* (1997). Endoproteolytic processing and stabilization of wild-type and mutant presenilin. *Journal of Biological Chemistry*, 272, 24536–41.

Rebeck, G. W. (1998). ApoE and its role in late onset Alzheimer's disease *In Molecular biology of Alzheimer s disease.* (Ed. C. Haass), pp. 295–308. Harwood Academic Publishers.

Rebeck, G. W., Reiter, J. S., Strickland, D. K., and Hyman, B. T. (1993). Apolipoprotein E in sporadic Alzheimer's disease, allelic variation and receptor interactions. *Neuron*, 11, 575–580.

Rebeck, G. W., Cheung, B. S., Growden, W. B., *et al.* (1999). Lack of independent associations of APOE promoter and intron 1 polymorphisms with Alzheimer's disease *Neuroscience Letters*, in press.

Robakis, N. K., Ramakrishna, N., Wolfe, G., and Wisniewski, H. M. (1987). Molecular cloning and characterization of a cDNA encoding the cerebrovascular and neuritic plaque amyloid peptides. *Proceedings of the National Academy of Sciences (USA)*, **84**, 4190–4.

Rogaev, E. I., Sherrington, R., Rogaeva, E. A., *et al.* (1995). Familial Alzheimer's disease in kindreds with missense mutations in a gene on chromosome 1 related to the Alzheimer's disease type 3 gene. *Nature*, **376**, 775–8.

Rogaev, E. I., Sherrington, R., Wu, C., *et al.* (1997). Analysis of the 5' sequence, genomic structure, and alternative splicing of the presenilin-1 Gene (PSEN1). Associated with early onset Alzheimer disease. *Genomics*, **40**, 415–24.

Rogaeva, E., Premkumar, S., Song, Y., *et al.* (1998). Evidence for an Alzheimer disease susceptibility locus on chromosome 12 and for further locus heterogeneity. *Journal of the American Medical Association*, **280**, 614–18.

Rogaeva, E. A., Premkumar, S., Grubber, J., *et al.* (1999). An alpha-2-macroglobulin insertion-deletion polymorphism in Alzheimer disease. *Nature Genetics*, **22**, 19–22.

Rosen, D. R., Martin-Morris, L., Luo, L., and White, K. (1989). A drosophila gene encoding a protein resembling the human β-amyloid protein precursor. *Proceedings of the National Academy of Sciences (USA)*, **86**, 2478–82.

Rudrasingham, V., Wavrant-DeVrieze F., Lambert, J. C., *et al.* (1999). Alpha-2 macroglobulin gene and Alzheimer disease. *Nature Genetics*, **22**, 17–9.

Schachter, F., Faure-Delanef, L., Guenot, F., *et al.* (1994). Genetic associations with human longevity at the APOE and ACE loci. *Nature Genetics*, **6** , 29–32.

Schellenberg, G. D. (1992). Genetic linkage for a novel familial Alzheimer's disease locus on chromosome 14. *Science*, **258**, 868–71.

Schellenberg, G. D. (1995). Progress in Alzheimer's disease genetics. *Current Opinions in Neurology*, **8**, 262–7.

Scheuner, D., Eckman, C., Jensen, M., *et al.* (1996). Aβ42(43) is increased in vivo by the PS1/2 and APP mutations linked to familial Alzheimer's disease. *Nature Medicine*, **2**, 865–70.

Selkoe, D. J. (1996). Amyloid β-protein and the genetics of Alzheimer's disease. *Journal of Biological Chemistry*, **271**, 18295–8.

Selkoe, D. J. (1998). The cell biology of beta-amyloid precursor protein and presenilin in Alzheimer's disease. *Trends in Cell Biology*, **8**, 447–53.

Seubert, P., Vigo-Pelfrey, C., Esch, F., *et al.* (1992). Isolation and quantification of soluble Alzheimer's beta-peptide from biological fluids. *Nature*, **359**, 325–7.

Sherrington, R., Rogaev, E. I., Liang, Y., *et al.* (1995). Cloning of a gene bearing missense mutations in early-onset familial Alzheimer's disease. *Nature*, **375**, 754–60.

Sisodia, S. S., Koo, E. H., Beyreuther, K., *et al.* (1990). Evidence that β-amyloid protein in Alzheimer's disease is not derived by normal processing. *Science*, **248**, 492–5.

Slunt, H.,H., Thinakaran, G., Von Koch, C., *et al.* (1994). Expression of a ubiquitous, cross-reactive homologue of the mouse β-amyloid precurspr protein (APP). *Journal of Biological Chemistry*, **269**, 2637–44.

Slunt, H. H., Thinakaran, G., Lee, M. K., and Sisodia, S. S. (1995). Nucleotide sequence of the chromosome 14-encoded S182 cDNA and revised secondary structure prediction. *International Journal of Experimental and Clinical Investigation*, **2**, 188–90.

Small, DH., Nurcombe, V., Reed, G., *et al.* (1994). A heparin-binding domain in the amyloid protein precursor of Alzheimer's disease is involved in the regulation of neurite outgrowth. *Journal of Neuroscience*, **14**, 2117–27.

Sprecher, C. A., Grant, F. J., Grimm, G., *et al.* (1993). Molecular cloning of the cDNA for a human amyloid precursor protein homolog, evidence for a multigene family. *Biochemistry*, 32, 4481–6.

St George-Hyslop, P., Crapper McLachlan, D., Tuda, T., *et al.* (1994). Alzheimer's disease and possible gene interaction. *Science*, 263, 537.

Steiner, H., Romig H., Grim, M. G., *et al.* (1999). The biological and pathological function of the presenilin-1 Delta exon 9 mutation is independent of its defect to undergo proteolytic processing. *Journal of Biological Chemistry*, 27, 7615–8.

Strickland, D. K, Ashcom, J. D., Williams, S., *et al.* (1990). Sequence identity between the alpha 2-macroglobulin receptor and low density lipoprotein receptor-related protein suggests that this molecule is a multifunctional receptor. *Journal of Biological Chemistry*, 265, 17401–4.

Strittmatter, W. J., Saunders, A. M., Schmechel, D., *et al.* (1993). Apolipoprotein E, high avidity binding to β-amyloid and increased frequency of type 4 allele in late-onset familial Alzheimer disease. *Proceedings of the National Academy of Sciences (USA)*, 90, 1977–81.

Strittmatter, W. J., Saunders, A. M., Goedert, M., *et al.* (1994). Isoform-specific interactions of apolipoprotein E with microtubule-associated protein tau, implications for Alzheimer disease. *Proceedings of the National Academy of Sciences (USA)*, 91, 11183–6.

Takano, T., Sahara, N., Yamanouchi, Y., and Mori, H. (1997). Assignment of Alzheimer's presenilin-2 (PS-2) gene to 1q42.1 by fluorescence *in situ* hybridization. *Neuroscience Letters*, 211, 205–7.

Tamaoka, A., Fraser, P. E., Ishii, K., *et al.* (1998). Amyloid-beta-protein isoforms in brain of subjects with PS1-linked, betaAPP-linked and sporadic Alzheimer disease. *Molecular Brain Research*, 56, 178–85.

Tanzi, R. E., Gusella, J. F., Watkins, P. C., *et al.* (1987). Amyloid β protein gene, cDNA., mRNA distribution and genetic linkage near the Alzheimer locus. *Science*, 235, 880–4.

Tanzi, R. E., Vaula, G., Romano, D., *et al.* (1992). Assessment of APP gene mutations in a large set of familial and sporadic AD patients. *Neurobiology of Ageing*, 13 (suppl. 1), S65.

Tanzi, R., Gaston, S., Bush, A., *et al.* (1994). Genetic heterogenity of gene defects responsible for familial Alzheimer disease. *Genetica*, 91, 255–63.

Thinakaran, G., Borchelt, D. R., Lee, M. K., *et al.* (1996). Endoproteolysis of presenilin 1 and accumulation of processed derivatives *in vivo*. *Neuron*, 17, 181–90.

Thinakaran, G., Harris, C. L., Ratovitski, T., *et al.* (1997). Evidence that levels of presenilins (PS1 and PS2) are coordinately regulated by competition for limiting cellular factors. *Journal of Biological Chemistry*, 272, 28415–22.

Tomika, T., Maruyama, K., Saido, T. C., *et al.* (1997). The presenilin 2 mutation (N141I) linked to familial Alzheimer disease (Volga German families) increases the secretion of amyloid beta protein ending at the 42nd (or 43rd) residue. *Proceedings of the National Academy of Sciences (USA)*, 94, 2025–30.

Tsuang, D., Kukull, W., Sheppard, L., *et al.* (1996). Impact of sample selection on APOE epsilon 4 allele frequency, a comparison of two Alzheimer's disease samples. *Journal of the American Geriatric Society*, 44, 704–7.

Tsujimura A., Yasojima K, and Hashimoto-Gotoh T. (1997). Cloning of Xenopus presenilin-alpha and -beta cDNAs and their differential expression in oogenesis and embryogenesis. *Biochemical Biophysical Research Communications*, 231, 392–6.

Utermann, G., Langenbeck, U., Beisiegel, U., and Weber, W. (1980). Genetics of the apolipoprotein E system in man. *American. Journal of Human Genetics*, 32, 339–47.

Van Broeckhoven, C. (1995). Presenilins and Alzheimer disease. *Nature Genetics*, 11, 230–2.

Van Nostrand, W. E., McKay, L. D., Baker, J. B., and Cunningham, D. D. (1988). Functional and structural similarities between protease nexin I and C1 inhibitor. *Journal of Biological Chemistry*, 263, 3979–83.

Van Nostrand, W. E., Wagner, S. L., Shankle, W. R., *et al.* (1992). Decreased levels of soluble amyloid beta-protein precursor in cerebrospinal fluid of live Alzheimer disease patients. *Proceedings of the National Academy of Sciences (USA)*, **89**, 2551–5.

Vito, P., Wolozin, B., Ganjei, J. K., *et al.* (1996a). Requirement of the familial Alzheimer's disease gene PS2 for apoptosis. Opposing effect of ALG-3. *Journal of Biological Chemistry*, **271**, 31025–8.

Vito., P., Lancana, E., and D'Adamio, L. (1996b). *Science*, **271**, 521–5.

Walter, J., Capell, A., Grunberg, J., *et al.* (1996). The Alzheimer's disease-associated presenilins are differentially phosphorylated proteins located predominantly within the endoplasmic reticulum. *Molecular Medicine*, **2**, 673–91.

Wasco, W., Bupp, K., Magendantz, M., *et al.* (1992). Identification of a mouse brain cDNA that encodes a protein related to the Alzheimer disease-associated β precursor protein. *Proceedings of the National Academy of Sciences (USA)*, **89**, 10758–62.

Wasco, W., Gurubhagavatula, S., Paradis, M. d., *et al.* (1993). Isolation and characterization of the human APLP2 gene encoding a homologue of the Alzheimer's associated amyloid β protein precursor. *Nature Genetics*, **5**, 95–100.

Wavrant-DeVrieze, F., Perez-Tur, J., Lambert, J. C., *et al.* (1997). Association between the low density lipoprotein receptor-related protein (LRP) and Alzheimer's disease. *Neuroscience Letters*, **227**, 68–70.

Weidemann, A., König, G., Bunke, D., *et al.* (1989). Identification, biogenesis and localization of precursors of Alzheimer's disease A4 amyloid protein. *Cell*, **57**, 115–26.

Wisniewski, T. and Frangione, B. (1992). Apolipoprotein E, a pathological chaperone protein in patients with cerebral and systemic amyloid. *Neuroscience Letters*, **135**, 235–8.

Wolozin, B., Iwasaki, K., Vito, P., *et al.* (1996). Participation of presenilin 2 in apoptosis, enhanced basal activity conferred by an Alzheimer mutation. *Science*, **274**, 1710–3.

Wu, W. S., Holmans, P., Wavrant-DeVrieze, F., *et al.* (1998). Genetic studies on chromosome 12 in late-onset Alzheimer disease. *Journal of the American Medical Association*, **280**, 619–22.

Zubenko, G. S., Hughes, H. B., Stiffler, J. S., *et al.* (1998). A genome survey for novel Alzheimer disease risk loci, results at 10-cM resolution. *Genomics*, **50**, 121–8.

Chapter 4

The biology and molecular neuropathology of β-amyloid protein

D. R. Howlett, D. Allsop, and E. H. Karran

4.1 Introduction

The basic doctrine of the so-called 'amyloid hypothesis' is that the deposition of the beta-amyloid (Aβ) peptide in the brain parenchyma is fundamental to the neuronal loss and associated dementia characteristic of Alzheimer's disease (AD). This hypothesis draws on support from a number of perspectives: (i) the brains of all AD patients exhibit many amyloid-containing senile plaques surrounded by degenerating nerve endings; the number of senile plaques far outweighs that found in normal aged brain; (ii) the senile plaque count in specific brain areas correlates with the degree and type of mental impairment (Cummings *et al.* 1995); (iii) genetic factors which either cause or increase the risk of AD (mutations in the amyloid precursor protein (APP), apolipoprotein E4 (apoE4) status, presenilin-1 (PS1), presenilin-2 (PS2)) are all known to either increase Aβ deposition and/or Aβ production; (iv) Down syndrome sufferers (with three copies of chromosome 21 and hence of the gene coding for APP) show brain Aβ deposits as early as age 12, long before they develop other pathology (such as neurofibrillary tangles (NFT)) and usually go on to develop Alzheimer-like dementia (Iwatsubo *et al.* 1995); (v) in apoE4 patients, there is an excessive build up of Aβ before symptoms of AD develop(Polvikoski *et al.* 1995); (vi) transgenic mice expressing mutant human APP genes develop diffuse and later fibrillar Aβ deposits together with neuronal and microglial damage and behavioural abnormalities (Games *et al.* 1995; Hsiao *et al.* 1996); (vii) aggregated or fibrillar Aβ is toxic to cultured neurones and neuronal-like cell lines: inhibiting the aggregation prevents the toxicity. Hence, there is compelling evidence to portray the deposition of Aβ as the seminal causative event in AD. This chapter explores recent advances in our understanding of the biology of Aβ from production to deposition or clearance.

4.2 Processing of amyloid precursor protein

The processing of APP (Fig 4.1) to the 40 or 42 amino acid Aβ1–40 or Aβ1–42 involves the cleavage, at the N- and C- termini of Aβ, by β- and γ secretases, respectively. Cleavage of APP within the Aβ fragment by α-secretase precludes the formation of Aβ and leads to the release of secreted forms of APP (sAPPα). (see Appendix I for sequence and mutations of APP). Nevertheless, Aβ is a normal product of neuronal cells and is found in the CSF and

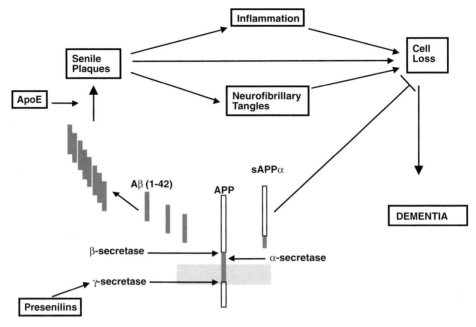

Fig. 4.1 Processing of the amyloid precursor protein and the amyloid cascade.

plasma. In AD, however, it fibrillizes to form insoluble deposits within the parenchyma and vasculature of specific vulnerable brain regions. The presence of degenerating neurones associated with the Aβ deposits has led to the belief that the neurodegeneration is a consequence of either the deposition itself or processes associated with the deposition. As commented earlier, the fact that familial forms of the disease are associated with mutations within or around the Aβ fragment, which affect processing or fibrillization, has further causally substantiated the link between Aβ and AD. In addition to promoting Aβ production, such mutations also lead to decreases in the neuroprotective sAPPα fragment (Mattson *et al.* 1993). Whilst in cell lines and primary cultures Aβ is directly neurotoxic, the disease is also associated with the appearance of activated complement components, microglia and paired helical filaments (PHF). The role that these factors play in the pathology is not clear although the injection of fibrillar Aβ into the cerebral cortex of aged rhesus monkey brains results in neuronal loss, microglial proliferation and tau hyperphosphorylation (Geula *et al.* 1998).

4.2.1 Secretases and inhibitors

The identity of the α, β-, and γ-secretases is still unknown, but it is becoming increasingly likely that α-secretase is a member of the ADAMs (a disintegrin and metalloprotease-like) family of membrane-associated zinc metalloproteinases that are similar to (but distinct from) the matrix metalloproteinases (Parvathy *et al.* 1998*a*; *b*). The ADAMs family are responsible for the 'shedding' of a diverse range of different membrane-bound proteins, such as angiotensin converting enzyme (ACE), tumour necrosis factor-α (TNFα), L-selectin, transforming growth factor-α, (TGFα) and the interleukin-6 (IL-6) receptor.

The suggestion that α-secretase is the matrix metalloproteinase gelatinase A (Miyazaki *et al.* 1993) has not been substantiated (Walsh *et al.* 1994; Lepage *et al.* 1995).

There are numerous reports in the academic and patent literature claiming identification of β-secretase and/or γ-secretase, but the evidence in support of any of these candidates is still inconclusive. The metallopeptidase 'thimet' and the aspartyl proteinase cathepsin D, which were once considered as candidates for β-secretase, can now be discounted (Saftig *et al.* 1996; Chevallier *et al.* 1997).

Recently, there has been considerable interest in similarities between the proteolytic cleavage of APP and cleavage of the sterol regulatory element binding protein (SREBP) (Manni *et al.* 1998; Ross *et al.* 1998; Tomita *et al.* 1998). SREBP has an N-terminal, cytosolic domain of 480 amino acids, a hydrophobic domain containing two membrane-spanning sequences, and a C-terminal cytosolic domain. This protein is cleaved sequentially by two proteinases, with the first cleavage (site 1) occurring in the region between the two transmembrane sequences (β-secretase-like) and the second cleavage (site 2) occurring within the transmembrane domain closest to the N-terminus (γ-secretase-like). The latter cleavage releases an N-terminal transcription factor that turns on genes associated with cholesterol biosynthesis and uptake. The cleavage at site 1 is facilitated by SREBP cleavage activation protein (SCAP), which is a multiple membrane-spanning protein, with a structure reminiscent of the presenilins (Nohturfft *et al.* 1998). Cleavage at site 2 is dependent on prior cleavage at site 1, which mirrors the dependence of γ-secretase on the prior action of α- or β-secretase. Given this striking similarity, the enzyme involved in cleavage of SREBP at site 2 (or one very similar to it) is an obvious candidate for γ-secretase. This enzyme is referred to as S2P (Rawson *et al.* 1997) and is a metalloproteinase possessing four or five transmembrane domains. It has been reported that production of Aβ1–40 and Aβ1–42 is the same in CHO variant M19 cells that lack S2P as in wild-type cells, suggesting that S2P cannot be γ-secretase (Ross *et al.* 1998; Tomita *et al.* 1998). In contrast, Aβ production may be inhibited in M19 cells, as demonstrated by ^{35}S[Met] metabolic labelling followed by immunoprecipitation of Aβ (Manni *et al.* 1998). However, transient transfection of S2P back into the M19 cells failed to restore the ability of the cells to produce Aβ. Further work is required in order to resolve the differences in these studies.

So far there are no studies on whole cells using metalloproteinase inhibitors that would support a role for S2P in Aβ formation. In fact, such studies have shown that metalloproteinase inhibitors are ineffective at reducing Aβ, whereas peptide aldehyde inhibitors of serine/cysteine proteinases and boronic acid inhibitors of serine proteinases have been found to block Aβ production, apparently through inhibition of the γ-secretase pathway (Higaki *et al.* 1995; Citron *et al.* 1996; Klafki *et al.* 1996; Allsop *et al.* 1998; Christie *et al.* 1999). We have shown that the activity of these compounds as inhibitors of Aβ secretion correlates with their potency as inhibitors of the chymotrypsin-like activity of the proteasome, suggesting that the proteasome may be involved directly or indirectly in the γ-secretase cleavage (Allsop *et al.* 1998; Christie *et al.* 1999).

In the case of γ-secretase, there is the additional complication that there could be separate enzymes responsible for generation of Aβ1–40 and Aβ1–42 (Citron *et al.* 1996; Klafki *et al.* 1996). APP is synthesized in the rough endoplasmic reticulum (ER), and follows the conventional secretory pathway through the Golgi where it is tyrosyl sulphated and sialylated (Weidemann *et al.* 1989), and then to secretory vesicles and the cell surface. Studies on the subcellular compartments where the α-, β-, and γ-secretase cleavages take place are complicated by the fact that the sites of processing could be different in neuronal and non-neuronal cells, and also the fact that many published data were obtained using APP-transfected cells where the overexpressed APP could be forced into a non-physiological compartment. Current evidence suggests that in differentiated neuronal cells the formation of Aβ1–40 occurs in the trans-Golgi network, whereas Aβ1–42 is synthesized within the ER and closely-associated nuclear envelope (Hartmann *et al.* 1997). This finding that Aβ1–40 and Aβ1–42 appear to be formed in different subcellular compartments has strengthened the possibility that they might be derived by different γ-secretases, as have reports that peptide aldehyde inhibitors affect the production of Aβ1–40 and not Aβ1–42 (Citron *et al.* 1996; Klafki *et al.* 1996). However, a likely explanation for the latter phenomenon is that in addition to their effects on Aβ production, inhibitors of this type also selectively block the C-terminal degradation of Aβ1–42, but not Aβ1–40, in culture medium (Hamazaki 1998). Thus, the different subcellular localizations of Aβ1–40 and Aβ1–42 in neuronal cells might be due to the same γ-secretase acting at different peptide bonds in the membrane-spanning domain of APP due to slight differences in the thicknesses of the ER and Golgi intracellular membranes (Weidemann *et al.* 1989).

4.2.2 Amyloid precursor protein structure/functions

The potential functions of full-length or sAPP have now been expanded to include membrane receptor, protease inhibitor, cell adhesion molecule, neurite outgrowth regulator, promoter of cell survival, neuroprotective molecule, stimulator of synaptogenesis, and modulator of synaptic plasticity (see Mattson 1997*a* for comprehensive review).

Kang *et al.* (1987) pointed out similarities between full-length APP and cell-surface receptors. One line of support for this has stemmed from the claim that the cytoplasmic domain of APP catalyses GTP exchange with G_0, suggesting that APP might function as a G_0-coupled receptor (Nishimoto *et al.* 1993). This has been followed by the observation that antibody stimulation of APP results in the activation of mitogen-activated protein kinases (MAP kinases), suggesting that APP might indeed have a signalling function (Murayama *et al.* 1996). The same workers have also claimed that the APP mutants V642 to I, G, or F (V717 using APP770 notation; V717I is also known as the London mutation) are constitutively active, and give signalling outputs by a G_0-independent mechanism (Okamoto *et al.* 1996). These various findings remain to be confirmed by others. The other line of support stems from the finding of more than one laboratory that the cytoplasmic domain of APP interacts with certain phosphotyrosine binding proteins (Fe65, X11 and homologues) (Fiore *et al.* 1995; Borg *et al.* 1996; Mcloughlin and Miller 1996; Zambrano *et al.* 1997; Duilio *et al.* 1998). These proteins bind to the sequence Asn-Pro-X-Tyr (present in the APP cytoplasmic domain) only when the Tyr residue is phosphorylated, and are consistent with a role for APP in signal transduction mechanisms. However, APP is not a conventional seven-transmembrane G_0-protein-coupled receptor, and signal transduction through the phosphotyrosine binding motif on APP may be related to its role in cell adhesion (see below).

The secreted form of APP containing the KPI insert was found some time ago to be identical to protease nexin II, a growth regulatory molecule produced by fibroblasts (Van Nostrand *et al.* 1989). Protease nexin II is an inhibitor of serine proteinases, including factor XIa of the blood clotting cascade (Smith *et al.* 1990). APP has also been found to inhibit the matrix metalloproteinase gelatinase A (Miyazaki *et al.* 1993) possibly through a small homologous motif between residues 407–417 of APP-695 and Cys³-Cys¹³ of TIMP (tissue inhibitor of matrix metalloproteinases) (Allsop *et al.* 1994). However, since the original report of Miyazaki *et al.* (1993) there have been no further publications on the ability of APP to inhibit matrix metalloproteinases.

Evidence that APP might function as an adhesion molecule promoting cell–cell or cell–extracellular matrix interactions continues to grow (Mattson 1997*a*; Coulson *et al.* 1997). APP has two or more heparin binding regions (Clarris *et al.* 1997), a collagen binding site (Beher *et al.* 1996), and an integrin binding motif (RHDS) at residues 5–8 of the Aβ sequence (Ghiso *et al.* 1992) and has been shown to bind to collagen type I, laminin and heparan sulphate proteoglycans (Coulson *et al.* 1997).

A growth promoting effect of soluble APP has been shown for fibroblasts and cultured neurons, and this activity has been claimed to reside in the amino acid sequence 'RERMS' at residues 328–332 of APP_{695} (Ninomiya *et al.* 1993; Jin *et al.* 1994). Synthetic 'RERMS' peptide and a 17-mer peptide containing this sequence were reported to retain the neu-rotrophic properties of soluble APP. In addition, the bioactivity of these peptides was reversed by the antagonist peptide 'RMSQ' which overlaps the active 'RERMS' pentapeptide at the C-terminal end. Specific and saturable binding for soluble APP and the 17-mer has been detected on a rat neuronal cell line (B103) after heparinase treatment (Kd = 20 nM) (Ninomiya *et al.* 1994). Thus the beneficial trophic effects of soluble APP would appear to be mediated via an unknown membrane receptor.

Soluble APP has also been reported to be neuroprotective (Mattson 1997*a*), which might explain its rapid upregulation in response to heat-shock, ischaemia, and neuronal injury. Soluble APP can protect against Aβ- or glutamate-mediated neuronal damage (Mattson *et al.* 1993; Goodman and Mattson 1994), and the 17-mer peptide mentioned above has been claimed to retain these properties. Soluble APP or the 17-mer peptide have also been reported to protect against neurological damage *in vivo* (Smith-Swintosky *et al.* 1994; Masliah *et al.* 1997). However, not all of the neurotrophic and neuroprotective activities of soluble APP can be attributed to the 'RERMS' pentapeptide region (Ohsawa *et al.* 1997). Soluble APP released by cleavage at the α-secretase site (sAPPα) seems to be ~100-fold more potent than sAPPβ in protecting hippocampal neurons against excitotoxicity or Aβ-mediated toxicity (Furukawa *et al.* 1996). This may be due to the 'VHHQK' heparin binding domain (residues 12–16 of Aβ) which is present on sAPPα but not sAPPβ. Most recently, secreted forms of APP have been reported to have memory enhancing effects (Meziane *et al.* 1998).

4.3 **Presenilins and amyloid precursor protein**

The discovery that mutations to a gene located on chromosome 14 (14q24.3), and since named presenilin 1 (*PS1*) were responsible for most early-onset familial AD (FAD) cases opened up a whole new area of research into the molecular mechanisms that subserve the pathology of AD. Shortly after the discovery of *PS1* (Sherrington *et al.* 1995), searching of gene sequence data-bases led to the identification of a homologous gene (named presenilin 2; *PS2*), mutations to which also resulted in FAD in the so-called Volga German kindred (Levy-Lahad *et al.* 1995). *PS2* was mapped to chromosome 1 (1q41.2). Currently, missense mutations to 35 codons; a mutation to a splice acceptor site leading to the in-frame deletion of exon 9/10 (Cruts and Van Broeckhoven 1998), an unidentified intronic mutation also leading to the deletion of exon 9/10 (Crook *et al.* 1998), and a deletion mutation from the splice donor site of intron 4 leading to truncated PS1 mRNA transcripts (Tysoe *et al.* 1998) have been described for PS1. Three missense mutations have been described for *PS2* (Cruts and Van Broeckhoven 1998).

PS1 is a 467 amino acid protein with 10 hydrophobic domains. PS2 has 448 amino acids and is 67% identical to PS1, with most of the sequence dissimilarity being in the hydrophilic domains of the proteins. Although a number of topological models have been proposed for PS1, the consensus view, based on experiments performed with PS1 and the *C. elegans* homologue *sel 12*, would favour an 8 transmembrane model in which the N-terminus, a large hydrophilic loop domain between transmembrane domains 6 and 7 and the C-terminus all face the cytosol (Doan *et al.* 1996; Li and Greenwald 1996; 1998). Given that the hydrophobic regions of PS1 and PS2 are highly conserved, it is very likely that PS2 adopts the same topology across the membrane as does PS1.

An important aspect of the biochemistry of the presenilins is their endoproteolytic processing to produce, in the case of PS1, 28 kDa N-terminal and 18 kDa C-terminal cleavage products from the 46 kDa holoprotein, and in the case of PS2, 35 kDa N-terminal and 20 kDa C-terminal cleavage products from the 55 kDa holoprotein (Mercken *et al.* 1996; Thinakaran *et al.* 1996; Ward *et al.* 1996; Kim *et al.* 1997*a*; Shirotani *et al.* 1997). From a number of studies, it is clear that the cleavage of the presenilin proteins is a highly regulated event with the levels of cleaved products being tightly controlled (Thinakaran *et al.* 1997). Most studies have shown that the presenilins reside predominantly within the ER and Golgi (Kovacs *et al.* 1996; Walter *et al.* 1996), and recent data suggest that while the holoprotein is restricted to the ER, cleavage allows the trafficking of the N-and C-terminal products to the Golgi (Zhang *et al.* 1998*a*).

To date, the functionality of the presenilin proteins remains obscure. It has been demonstrated in *C elegans* that sel 12 facilitates cell fate decisions via *Notch* signalling (Levitan and Greenwald, 1995), and further that presenilin can functionally substitute for *sel 12* (Levitan *et al.* 1996). The relationship between presenilin and *Notch* signalling has been supported by the very similar phenotypes induced by PS1, *Notch 1* and *Dll1* knockout mice (Delta-like ligand 1 (*Dll1*) is a *Notch* ligand) (Conlon *et al.* 1995; Shen *et al.* 1997; Wong *et al.* 1997; Hrabe *et al.* 1997). However, it remains to be determined whether the functional interaction between *Notch* and *sel 12* in development in *C. elegans* is important and relevant to higher order species and to the pathogenesis of AD. Indeed, one striking difference is that whereas presenilin proteins harbouring FAD mutations are not able to substitute functionally for *sel 12* in *C. elegans* (with the exception of the PS1 exon 9 deletion mutant, PS1Δ9), they are able to rescue the developmental abnormalities in PS1 null mice (Davis *et al.* 1998; Qian *et al.* 1998).

Other workers have demonstrated a role for presenilins in apoptosis. Over-expression of PS2 in PC-12 cells augments programmed cell death in response to apoptotic stimuli (Deng *et al.* 1996) and expression of a PS2 FAD mutant increases the basal level of apoptosis (Wolozin *et al.* 1996). A pro-apoptotic role for PS1 has also been proposed: over-expression of a PS1 FAD mutant increases the susceptibility of PC-12 cells to trophic factor withdrawal (Guo *et al.* 1997). In addition, several studies have demonstrated that the presenilins can also be substrates for caspases, the proteinases activated as part of the apoptotic response (Kim *et al.* 1997*b*; Loetscher *et al.* 1997; Vito *et al.* 1997; Grunberg *et al.* 11998) . Although these studies are intriguing, it is difficult to determine to what extent their results reflect the *in vivo* effects mediated by presenilin mutants in FAD patients. If augmentation of apoptosis was a primary pathological mechanism mediated by presenilin mutations, one might expect to reveal such effects in mice expressing mutant presenilin transgenes — and to date, this remains to be demonstrated.

Several proteins that interact with the presenilins have been identified, including filamin (Zhang et al. 1998b) tau and glycogen synthase kinase-3β (Takashima et al. 1998); and Δ- and β-catenin (Zhou et al. 1997; Yu et al. 1998). The interaction with the catenins is especially interesting, as these proteins form part of the wnt/frizzled signalling pathway together with glycogen synthase kinase-3β which has been implicated in tau phosphorylation (Lovestone et al. 1996). Recently, data has been published demonstrating that PS1 FAD mutants destabilized the interaction with β-catenin compared with PS1 wild type, and further that β-catenin is subject to increased degradation in cells expressing PS1 FAD mutants (Zhang et al. 1998c). It has also been demonstrated that loss of signalling through the β-catenin pathway is associated with increased susceptibility to the pro-apoptotic effects of fibrillized Aβ.

The most striking effect mediated by the presenilin FAD mutants concerns their effects on Aβ secretion. Seminal data has been published demonstrating that fibroblasts obtained from PS1 and PS2 FAD patients produce increased amounts of the longer, 42 amino acid, form of Aβ (Aβ1–42) relative to the 40 amino acid form (Aβ1–40) (Scheuner et al. 1996). Indeed, an absolute or relative increase in Aβ1–42 production is shared by all the known FAD mutations in the presenilins and APP. This observation is striking as it is well documented that Aβ1–42 is highly fibrillogenic compared with the more abundantly produced Aβ1–40 (Jarrett et al. 1993b). This work has since been replicated by a number of other groups, in a range of experimental paradigms. Thus, cells transfected with PS1 or PS2 FAD mutants (Borchelt et al. 1996; Citron et al. 1997; Mehta et al. 1998), and mice expressing human transgenes for PS1 or PS2 FAD mutants (Borchelt et al. 1996; Duff et al. 1996; Oyama et al. 1998) all show increased Aβ1–42 production or deposition. The relevance of this finding to the disease pathogenesis has been confirmed by studies in Down syndrome (Iwatsubo et al. 1995), AD (Iwatsubo et al. 1994) and FAD patients (Lemere et al. 1996), which have all shown the preferential and early deposition of Aβ1–42 in the brain parenchyma.

Of all the mechanisms and biochemical interactions currently proposed for the presenilins, the augmentation of Aβ1–42 production will probably remain an important aspect of their role in the aetiopathology of AD. What is unclear is how this effect is mediated at the molecular biochemical level, although some key observations have begun to address this question. Both PS2 (Weidemann et al. 1997) and PS1 (Xia et al. 1997) are able to associate physically with APP. As the interaction was with immature APP, this probably occurs within the ER. The site of interaction is important, as production of Aβ1–42 may be predominantly within the ER, and particularly prevalent in cells with a neuronal phenotype (Cook et al. 1997; Hartmann et al. 1997). The inference from these data is that presenilins in some way mediate the production of Aβ1–42 within the ER. This hypothesis has been strengthened by data from neuronal cultures derived from PS1 knockout mice, where γ-secretase activity was markedly suppressed, although there was no differential effect on the production of Aβ1–40 versus Aβ1–42 (DeStrooper et al. 1998).

Collectively, these data argue that presenilins play an important role in mediating the γ-secretase cleavage of APP. Whether this is a direct or indirect effect remains to be elucidated. Thus, it could be that presenilins act to control the transit of APP through the ER. However, recent data suggest that PS1 FAD mutants do not affect the ER-to-Golgi transport of the LDL receptor, or the secretion of α- or β-secretase-cleaved APP (Tan et al. 1998). Alternatively, presenilin, APP and γ-secretase may form a macromolecular complex that mediates the cleavage of APP, and all of the presenilin mutations are able to change subtly the conformation of the protein in the membrane and thereby alter the apposition of APP to γ-secretase — in turn altering the position of the cleavage. An extension of this hypothesis would be that the APP FAD mutants at the C-terminus of the Aβ sequence in APP would likewise alter the conformation of a PS-APP-γ-secretase complex with a similar outcome.

4.4 Aβ and neurodegeneration

There is an emerging consensus that the aggregation state of the Aβ peptide is a key factor in determining the toxicity of Aβ. Indeed, data have confirmed that fibrillized Aβ is neurotoxic, whereas freshly-prepared soluble peptide exhibits little toxicity (Simmons *et al.* 1994; Howlett *et al.* 1995). However, how fibrillized Aβ mediates cell death still remains to be elucidated, partly because data have been collected in a wide range of model systems (i.e. primary cultures vs. cell lines) and different endpoints have been used to assess the degree of neurotoxicity. Although the role of Aβ deposition in initiating cell death in AD has been pre-eminent in recent years, nothing is known with a high degree of confidence concerning the mechanism through which neuronal cells die. Attention has focused on apoptotic cell death with cell lines and primary cultures exposed to Aβ peptides and postmortem tissue from AD patients showing neurones displaying signs of apoptosis (Su *et al.* 1994; Mattson *et al.* 1998). However, the current transgenic animal models of AD do not show significant signs of apoptotic neuron death.

A common theme that has emerged from a range of studies is the importance of Aβ-induced oxidative stress as a toxic mechanism. Aβ has been implicated in reactive oxygen species (ROS) generation directly (Hensley *et al.* 1994) but there is also considerable evidence that Aβ in proto- or fibrillar form disturbs the membrane environment of metabolic pathway enzymes giving rise to increased leakage from their redox chains leading to ROS toxicity (Goodman and Mattson. 1994; Behl and Holsboer 1998). Since oxidative stress in cells can lead to apoptosis there are possibilities for synergies between this and anti-apoptotic theories. Early data on Aβ toxicity *in vitro* showed a protective effect of vitamin E (Behl *et al.* 1992) and clinical data suggests a protective effect of vitamin E. Oestrogens are another group of molecules whose antioxidant properties have been studied in the context of Aβ toxicity (Xu *et al.* 1998). This data may relate to epidemiological findings suggesting that hormone replacement therapy delays the onset of AD (Tang *et al.* 1996). The role of oxidative stress in the mechanism of Aβ toxicity has been reviewed extensively elsewhere (Mattson 1997*b*).

The brain has a high rate of oxygen consumption and relatively low levels of protective, anti-oxidant enzymes which makes it especially vulnerable to free radical damage (Behl 1997). In both cell lines and primary cortical neuronal cultures, exposure to Aβ results in an increase in intracellular H_2O_2 that correlates with toxicity (Behl *et al.* 1994). H_2O_2 can, via the Fenton reaction, lead to the production of the highly reactive hydroxyl radical. Aβ-resistant clonal PC12 cells have been shown to be highly resistant to the direct toxic effects of exogenous H_2O_2 (Mazziotti and Perlmutter 1998) and this protective effect has subsequently been shown to be mediated by an increase in the constitutive levels of nuclear factor-κβ (NF-κβ). NF-κβ is a redox-sensitive transcription factor. DNA-binding motifs for NF-κB are present in the promoter or enhancer regions of a wide range of genes that are up-regulated during an inflammatory response (Baeuerle and Baichwal 1997). This protective role of NF-κB has been further supported by data showing that Aβ reduces the levels of constitutive NF-κB activity in rat primary neurons and that this correlates with Aβ-mediated toxicity. This effect was in turn mediated by an increase in the endogenous NF-κβ inhibitor, IκB (Bales *et al.* 1998). However, this study also demonstrated opposite effects of Aβ on microglia, where Aβ caused an increase in NF-κB activation. Aβ-mediated activation of NF-κB has also been demonstrated in primary neurons, and has been shown in neurons and astroglia vicinal to amyloid plaques in AD brains (Kaltschmidt *et al.* 1997). Thus, given the different responses of microglia and neurons, it is not yet clear whether the activation of NF-κB acts in a neuroprotective, or a neurotoxic fashion, in AD.

While events downstream of Aβ exposure to cells are beginning to be unravelled, there is still considerable uncertainty with regard to the very early events in Aβ-mediated neurotoxicity. For example: what are the biochemical systems that result in oxidative stress; does Aβ interact with a receptor, or is there a non-specific association with the cell membrane? It has been suggested that a receptor for advanced glycation end products (RAGE) is involved in binding Aβ and inducing oxidative stress (Yan *et al.* 1996). However, although the binding of Aβ to RAGE results in the generation of ROS from microglia, it has not been conclusively demonstrated that this mechanism is directly involved in neuronal cell death.

The amphiphilic nature of Aβ allows it to associate and intercalate with membranes (McLaurin and Chakrabartty 1996) which may allow 'uncoupling' of enzymatic systems leading to leakage of ROS. An intriguing report (Yan *et al.* 1997) has highlighted the effects of cell exposure to Aβ on the endoplasmic reticulum Aβ-binding protein (ERAB), a novel protein with homology to a hydroxysteroid dehydrogenase. In this study, Aβ treatment of cells was shown to cause a translocation of ERAB from the ER to the plasma membrane and the toxic effects of Aβ could be ameliorated using anti-ERAB antibodies introduced into the cells using liposomes. However, precisely how ERAB mediated Aβ toxicity has not been elucidated. Further details of RAGE and ERAB are given in Chapter 9 by Shi Du Yan.

The effects of Aβ on cells and the mechanism of neurotoxicity is still an area of active research and debate. One striking aspect of this work has been the relative lack of neuronal death evident in mice over-expressing human APP FAD mutations, that nevertheless have abundant evidence of amyloid plaques (Hsiao *et al.* 1996; Irizarry *et al.* 1997). This conundrum has been partly explained by recent data showing that primate brains are inherently more sensitive than rodent brains to the toxic effects of fibrillized Aβ, and that primate brains in turn show increased susceptibility with increasing age (Geula *et al.* 1998). Alternatively, most transgenic mouse models have increased levels of sAPPα which could be acting to protect against Aβ-mediated damage.

4.5 Aβ fibrillization

4.5.1 Monomers, oligomers, fibrils, and neurotoxicity

The progressive deposition of Aβ in AD is generally considered to be fundamental to the development of neurodegenerative pathology. The description of cell toxicity associated with Aβ appeared to explain the neuronal cell loss found in AD (Yankner *et al.* 1989, 1990). In particular, the neurotoxic effects in cell culture systems were found to be dependent on the fibrillar state of the peptide (Pike *et al.* 1991; May *et al.* 1992) and on the degree and rate of fibril formation (Howlett *et al.* 1995). *In vitro* studies have demonstrated that the carboxy-terminus of the Aβ peptide is a critical determinant for the kinetics of fibrillization. Aβ1–42 fibrillizes several orders of magnitude faster than the Aβ1–40 isoform (Jarrett *et al.* 1993*b*) and as all of the FAD genes have in common the ability to induce the production of Aβ1–42 relative to Aβ1–40, it seems likely that Aβ fibrillization is an important aspect of the pathology of AD. However, the precise nature of the toxic species of Aβ peptide is unclear with both small oligomers (Oda *et al.* 1995; Roher *et al.* 1996; Stine *et al.* 1996; Lambert *et al.* 1998) and protofibrils (Harper *et al.* 1997; Walsh *et al.* 1997) being implicated. A serious problem in assessing the relevance of many such studies is the difference in fibrillization rate and toxic product which occur between synthetic batches of peptide (May *et al.* 1992; Howlett *et al.* 1995). The inherent aggregatory properties of Aβ, superimposed on a chemically difficult synthetic target exhibiting an ability to be synthesizedwith differing degrees of seed content and conformational substructure lead to effectively different pre-aggregatory Aβ molecules being studied between laboratories. The picture is further complicated by variations in the conditions under which the Aβ is fibrillized, as variations in buffer composition and pH are known to influence the process. For instance, although Aβ aggregates at pH 5.8, in that it exhibits Congo red binding characteristic of beta-sheet formation, the peptide does not form fibrils (Wood *et al.* 1996c). Furthermore, Aβ1–40 aggregated at pH 5.8 is not toxic in cell culture and aggregation at pH 3.0 gives a product which is neither toxic nor Congo red positive but which is positively immunoreactive in an aggregate-specific immunoassay (Fig 4.2). Hence, the identification of Aβ, as in senile plaque, classically stained with the dye Congo red, does not necessarily confer pathological properties on the peptide and the need to confer physiologic activity on any preparation is critical. Overall, however, the end result of the variability in Aβ preparations and aggregation protocols is that the Aβ aggregation/toxicity literature is not reproducible.

Nevertheless, a greater understanding of the Aβ fibrillization process has been achieved leading to a questioning of the physiological and pathological relevance of the fibrillar

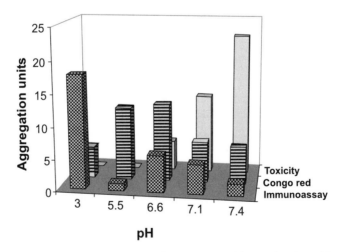

Fig. 4.2 pH profile of aggregation products of Aβ1–40. Peptide was incubated for 18 h over the pH range 3–7.4. Products were assessed by Congo red binding assay (Wood *et al.* 1996) or fibrillization-dependent immunoassay and cell toxicity assay (Howlett *et al.* 1997).

Aβ1–40 peptide and has led to suggestions that smaller peptide oligomers may be the toxic derivatives (Roher et al. 1996; Lambert et al. 1998; Podlisny et al. 1998) although, equally, there are proponents of the toxic fibril theory (Seilheimer et al. 1997; Malinchik et al. 1998). Analysis of AD and normal brains has demonstrated the presence of both water-soluble, non-filamentous Aβ1–40 and Aβ1–42 forms from less than 10 kDa to greater than 100 kDa (Kuo et al. 1996) and stable dimeric and trimeric species (Roher et al. 1996). Although in the latter case, the peptides were separated in the presence of 80% formic acid and 5 M guanidine, the oligomers were reported to be stable and to have pathogenic effects in cell culture systems. The formation of small oligomers of Aβ has also been demonstrated in cell culture (Podlisny et al. 1995; 1998) although the relevance of these forms to cell toxicity have yet to be established. Non-fibrillar toxic oligomers have also been derived from synthetic Aβ, initially as slowly sedimenting soluble forms in the presence of the secreted glycoprotein clusterin (also known as apolipoprotein J) (Oda et al. 1995) and more recently as neurotoxic 20–40 kDa forms (Lambert et al. 1998).

Data on the actual fibrillogenesis process are drawn almost entirely from work with synthetic peptides and are consistent with Aβ monomers combining to form nuclei which themselves combine to form an early fibrillar intermediate or protofibril (Walsh et al. 1997) with eventual fibril formation occurring via end-to-end association of fibrils or by monomer/dimer addition (Naiki and Nakakuki 1996). It is also possible that deposited Aβ forms a template upon which Aβ monomers continue to build by first-order kinetics, thus allowing the process to proceed at physiological concentrations (Maggio and Mantyh 1996). The slow formation of nuclei is considered to be the rate limiting step in the process. However, this step can be by-passed or greatly accelerated by the presence of amyloid seed (Jarrett and Lansbury 1993), where the seed can be fibrils of Aβ (Jarrett et al. 1993a) or of the non-amyloid component (NAC — a 35-amino acid peptide from plaques, found to be a fragment of α-synuclein) peptide of senile plaque core (Han et al. 1995). Thus, the removal of seeds from Aβ preparations drastically reduces their propensity to fibrillize, whereas the addition of seeds to supersaturated solutions of Aβ monomer induces rapid fibrillization (Wood et al. 1996b). Hence, control or lack of control of nucleation-dependent oligomer formation may be the determinant of disease development in AD. A slow nucleation phase is characteristic of nucleation-dependent protein polymerization (Jarrett and Lansbury 1993) where the reaction only proceeds once a 'critical concentration' is exceeded. The critical concentration is about 10 μM for Aβ1–40 (Jarrett et al. 1993a) and 2 μM for Aβ1–42 (Soreghan et al. 1994). This raises the issue of the concentration which Aβ may achieve in the AD brain and whether any cellular compartment ever attains micromolar Aβ concentrations. Studies of APP processing suggest that Aβ1–42, in particular, may be produced within discrete cellular compartments (Hartmann et al. 1997; Wild Bode et al. 1997), where pH is low. However, although Aβ rapidly aggregates at low pH, it does not form fibrils (Wood et al. 1996c) and, as commented above, is neither Congo red positive or neurotoxic. Estimations of Aβ concentrations in plasma or CSF suggest that nucleation of peptide is unlikely to occur (Van Gool et al. 1994; Jensen et al. 1995) and the secretion of Aβ even by cells over-expressing APP is only of the order of 1 pmole per million cells (Howlett, unpublished). In vivo, however, the nucleation process may be facilitated by association of Aβ with chaperones such as apoE (Hyman et al. 1995) which would effectively lower the critical concentration.

4.5.2 Factors regulating fibrillization

The enzyme acetylcholinesterase (AChE) has been found to be colocalized with Aβ in both diffuse and mature plaques in AD brain tissue (Carson *et al.* 1991; Moran *et al.* 1993). The presence of the enzyme in diffuse plaque suggests that it is present at an early stage in amyloid deposition and hence may be involved in the process itself. In line with this suggestion is the demonstration that *in vitro*, AChE accelerates Aβ aggregation and appears to decrease the critical concentration some threefold (Inestrosa *et al.* 1996). Aβ peptides have also been shown to interact with the plasma membrane lipid bilayer matrix (Arispe *et al.* 1993) and in the presence of ganglioside-containing membranes (Choosmith *et al.* 1997), membrane phospholipid metabolites (Klunk *et al.* 1997) and phosphatidylinositol (McLaurin *et al.* 1998) fibril formation is enhanced. Metal ion presence also regulates aggregation. Cu^{2+}, Fe^{2+} and Zn^{2+} all increase the rate of aggregate formation of Aβ1–40 in a pH-dependent manner, which may be linked to inflammatory responses (Atwood *et al.* 1998). Other materials which bind to and increase the rate of aggregation of Aβ include apoE, proteoglycans and glucose. Although such agents may lower the critical concentration for Aβ fibrillization, the lack of other materials which naturally destabilize fibril formation may influence deposition. As examples, melatonin, laminin, transthyretin, and hemin all inhibit fibrillization (Schwarzman *et al.* 1994; Bronfman *et al.* 1996; Howlett *et al.* 1997; Pappolla *et al.* 1998) and laminin inhibits apoE4-dependent fibrillization (Monji *et al.* 1998). Clusterin has been shown to interfere with the aggregation process although it is not clear whether *in vivo* this would promote or attenuate the production of neurotoxic peptide species (Lambert *et al.* 1998).

Aβ deposition in AD may be a delicate balance, probably involving enhanced production of Aβ, decreased clearance, and the presence or absence of factors regulating the fibrillization process. There are many approaches which can be taken to limit Aβ deposition in AD. To date, however, drug intervention has almost totally been confined to inhibiting the proteases that regulate APP processing to Aβ (see Section 4.2.1) and to inhibitors of Aβ self-aggregation.

4.5.3 Drug inhibitors of Aβ fibrillization

Binding of a compound to Aβ, particularly to the hydrophobic core region which is believed to be fundamental to the peptides ability to aggregate, is an obvious means of preventing fibrillization, although to be clinically suitable, the binding stoichiometry between inhibitor and Aβ would probably have to be less than 1:1. Until the fibrillization process is fully understood however, the discovery of inhibitors is likely to be achieved more by serendipity than design.

Nevertheless, a number of series of compounds have now been described which effectively inhibit Aβ fibrillization, albeit usually at micromolar concentrations. We have recently described a series of benzofurans which bind to Aβ and inhibit the formation of cell toxic Aβ aggregates (Howlett *et al.* 1998; Swatton *et al.* 1998) (Fig. 4.3). Other inhibitors, such as β-cyclodextrin, rifamycins, sulphonates, nicotine, quaternary ammonium salts, and the anthracycline 4′-deoxy-4′-iododoxorubicin (IDOX), have been reviewed elsewhere (Bandiera *et al.* 1997). There have been no reports of the effects of any of these compounds on Aβ deposition *in vivo* although peripheral amyloid formation has been attenuated by sulphonates (Kisilevsky *et al.* 1995) and IDOX (Tagliavini *et al.* 1997). Short peptide

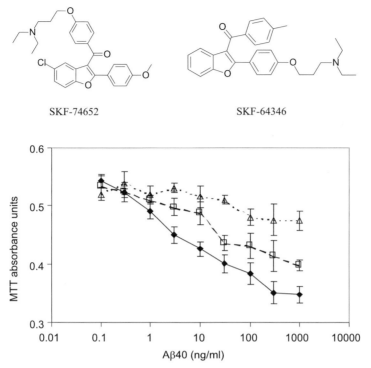

Fig. 4.3 Effects of SKF-74652 and SKF-64346 on Aβ1–40 fibrillization-dependent toxicity in IMR32 cells. Aβ1–40 (11.6 μmole/litre) was fibrillized in the presence of 100μmole/litre SKF-74652 □, 100 μmole/litre SKF-64346 △ or drug vehicle (♦) before challenging of cells with the incubate over the range 0.1–1000 ng/ml Aβ1–40. Cell viability was assessed by MTT assay. Data are means and SEM of three experiments. p<0.05 for all SKF-74652 or SKF-64346 data points over the Aβ1–40 range 3–1000 ng/ml compared to Aβ1–40 alone.

fragments, primarily based on the central hydrophobic region of Aβ, have been proposed as being capable of preventing beta-sheet formation (Soto *et al.* 1996; Tjernberg *et al.* 1997) and peptides of this type may inhibit fibrillogenesis in a rat brain model of amyloidosis where both Aβ1–42 and peptide inhibitor were injected directly into rat brain amygdala (Soto *et al.* 1998). Although transgenic mouse models of AD with Aβ deposits have now been described (Games *et al.* 1995; Hsiao *et al.* 1996), there are no published reports describing the effects of fibrillization inhibitor administration in these models.

4.6 **Aβ clearance and degradation**

Several peptidases have been shown to degrade Aβ *in vitro*, including a non-matrix metalloprotease secreted by neuronal and non-neuronal cell lines, particularly microglia (Qiu *et al.* 1997), cathepsin D (McDermott and Gibson 1996), and insulin degrading enzyme (EC 3.4.22.11) from human brain (McDermott and Gibson 1997). In aggregated form, however, Aβ appears to be resistant to proteolysis (Norstedt *et al.* 1994; Paresce *et al.* 1997; Qiu *et al.*

1997); suggesting that once the critical concentration of Aβ is attained to facilitate aggregation, protease-dependent clearance becomes ineffective and peptide is able to accumulate and forms neurotoxic species.

α2-macroglobulin (α2M) is an acute phase protein normally found in plasma and tissues, including brain, which is able to form complexes with a wide variety of secreted endoproteases. A number of lines of evidence link α2M to AD: (a) α2M is associated with senile plaques (Van Gool *et al.* 1993); (b) α2M binds to Aβ and prevents the formation of toxic peptide species (Du *et al.* 1998; Hughes *et al.* 1998) and (c) mutations in the α2M gene increase the risk of developing AD (Blacker *et al.* 1998). In this latter report, Tanzi and colleagues suggest that α2M-protease complexes may either directly degrade Aβ or after binding Aβ are internalized by lipoprotein-receptor associated protein (LRP — acting as a scavenger receptor) and be targeted for lysosomal degradation. Apolipoprotein E may also fit into this model by competing at the LRP receptor for uptake into cells or by interfering in the α2M-mediated degradation of Aβ in some other way (Zhang *et al.* 1996).

Apolipoprotein E genotype is a major risk factor for the development of AD. The presence of the E4 allele is strongly associated with both early and late-onset AD although the precise mechanism by which this is mediated is not known. As well as possibly interfering with Aβ/α2M internalization, apoE has also been shown to affect fibril formation (Evans *et al.* 1995; Wood *et al.* 1996a; Naiki *et al.* 1997) and, by binding with high affinity to Aβ (Golabek *et al.* 1996) may restrict the blood–brain-barrier clearance of the peptide (Zlokovic *et al.* 1993). Apolipoprotein J has also been shown to bind to Aβ (Matsubara *et al.* 1996) and to facilitate internalization and lysosomal degradation of the peptide via the LRP-2 receptor (Hammad *et al.* 1997).

4.7 Aβ-mediated inflammation

The brain does not sustain typical inflammatory responses characterized by pain, swelling, and infiltration of inflammatory cells. Nevertheless, several findings have suggested that the inflammatory response may play an important part in the neurodegenerative process of AD. Thus, rheumatoid arthritis patients (often treated with anti-inflammatory agents) have been shown to be less likely to have AD (McGeer *et al.* 1990); an inverse relationship between the use of anti-inflammatory treatments and AD has been demonstrated in a co-twin study (Breitner *et al.* 1994); and indomethacin treatment delayed cognitive decline in AD patients in a 6 month, double-blind placebo-controlled study (Rogers *et al.* 1993). The connection between NF-kβ activation and Aβ may provide the link between one of the key features of the pathology of AD and the inflammatory process.

Activation of microglia around the amyloid plaque is a common feature of AD pathology, leading to the release of cytokines such as interleukin-1 (IL-1) and IL-6 (Griffin *et al.* 1989; Bauer *et al.* 1991), that in turn can up-regulate the activity of the cycloxygenase-2 (COX-2) enzyme which is responsible for the production of inflammatory prostaglandins. COX-2 is produced by both glial cells and neurons and this may provide an explanation for the apparent beneficial effects of non-steroidal anti-inflammatory drugs in AD.

Of considerable interest currently is the role of the complement system in mediating neuronal cell death. All of the components of the complement system, including the membrane attack complex (MAC) have been found to co-localize with Aβ in amyloid plaques (McGeer *et al.* 1989). Several reports have shown that fibrillized Aβ is able to bind C1q, which initiates the classical complement cascade (Rogers *et al.* 1992; Jiang *et al.* 1994). Recent data have shown that Aβ-activated complement produces a functional MAC that can insert into the membranes of NT2 cells (Bradt *et al.* 1998). Neurons express the complement inhibitor CD59 which inhibits the formation of the MAC, but if this is removed by phospholipase C treatment, Aβ-mediated cell death is markedly enhanced (Shen *et al.* 1998). Thus, in AD, Aβ may cause neurotoxicity via complement activation with the extent of neuronal cell death being a function of the amount of MAC compared with the expression levels of CD59.

4.8 **Relation between Aβ and tau**

The relative importance of senile plaques and neurofibrillary tangles in the pathogenesis of AD has been debated ever since Alzheimer himself first discovered them. As noted above, biochemical analysis of the effects of the APP, PS1, and PS2 mutations responsible for early-onset FAD has provided powerful evidence that the formation and aggregation of Aβ (particularly Aβ1–42) in the brain are crucial events in the pathogenesis of AD. However, mutations in the tau gene have now been discovered, not in families with inherited forms of AD, but in families with so-called fronto-temporal dementia and Parkinsonism linked to chromosome 17 (or FTDP-17) (Hutton *et al.* 1998; Poorkaj *et al.* 1998; Spillantini *et al.* 1998). For further information on tau see Chapter 5 by Claude Wischik and Appendix 5. This finding has renewed interest in tau and neurodegeneration. Hutton *et al.* (1998) have identified three missense mutations in the tau gene, namely Gly272Val (within exon 9), Pro301Leu (exon 10), and Arg406Trp (exon 13), and Poorkaj *et al.* (1998) have identified an additional Val339Met mutation (exon 12). Since the alternative splicing of exon 10 generates the 3-repeat and 4-repeat isoforms of tau (referring to the number of microtubule binding domains) the Pro301Leu mutation can affect 4-repeat tau only, whereas the other mutations can affect all of the tau isoforms. Families with FTDP-17 have also been identified with mutations in the 5′ splice site of exon 10 (Hutton *et al.* 1998), and these mutations have been shown to result in an increase in the proportion of tau mRNA encoding the 4-repeat isoforms. The discovery of these mutations indicates that disruption of tau structure/function can lead to neurodegeneration, which is not surprising given the important role of tau in maintaining the integrity of the neuronal cytoskeleton. However, the neuropathological picture resulting from these tau mutations is distinct from that seen in AD, and so the mechanism of neuronal loss in FTDP-17 and AD may be different. Thus tau mutations can result in the formation of tau-derived inclusions and neurodegenerative disease, but they do not give rise to typical AD, unlike the APP, PS1, and PS2 mutations. Of particular note is the absence of significant numbers of senile plaques with associated Aβ deposits in most cases of FTDP-17.

The presence of neurofibrillary tangles or tau-derived inclusions in a wide range of neurodegenerative conditions (e.g. post-encephalitic Parkinsonism, progressive supranuclear palsy, amyotrophic lateral sclerosis) suggests that formation of this type of lesion is a relatively non-specific response of the brain to a variety of neurotoxic insults. In typical AD, the amyloid cascade hypothesis would predict that neurofibrillary tangles are formed as a consequence of significant deposits of Aβ in the brain, whereas in FTDP-17 mutations in the tau gene can lead directly to formation of pathological tau inclusions. A number of studies have shown that exposure of cells, including human primary neuronal cultures, to fibrilized forms of Aβ can lead to tau phosphorylation (Busciglio *et al.* 1995; Takashima *et al.*

1996), and more recently (Geula *et al.* 1998). The latter group has reported that microinjection of fibrillar Aβ into aged rhesus monkey cerebral cortex can lead to tau phosphorylation *in vivo*. These observations support the idea of a direct link between Aβ deposition and NFT formation in AD. However, in considering AD, it might not be the amyloid fibrils themselves that initiate the cascade of events leading to tangle formation, neurodegeneration, and dementia. The real culprit in AD may be a form of intermediate Aβ aggregate (e.g. amyloid protofibrils) en route to fibril formation.

4.9 Aβ **and the cerebral vasculature**

Although Aβ deposits in senile plaque are considered a hallmark of AD, the majority of sufferers also demonstrate vascular amyloid deposition which results in cerebral amyloid angiopathy (Premkumar *et al.* 1996). The apoE e4 allele, whilst posing a risk factor for AD, also presents a risk for stroke patients with dementia (Slooter *et al.* 1997). Deposition of Aβ in the walls of the cerebral vasculature results in smooth muscle cell degeneration and in an increased production of APP and Aβ by the cells themselves (Pierce *et al.* 1998). The deposition, however, is of nonfibrillar, monomeric, and oligomeric Aβ (Frackowiak *et al.* 1995). Hence, the smooth muscle cells may actively contribute to the degenerative process. However, in contrast to neuronal-type, cells from the cerebrovasculature appear to be sensitive to non-fibrillar Aβ. Thus, soluble nonfibrillar Aβ1–42 and the E22Q (also known as APP693 HCHWA-D locus) mutated Aβ1–40 (but not Aβ1–40 itself) have been shown to cause degeneration of cultured human cerebrovascular smooth muscle cells (Davis-Salinas *et al.* 1995). These authors report that re-aggregation of the Aβ1–42 abolishes the degenerative effects of this peptide on the cells suggesting different cytotoxic mechanisms for the differing cell types, although internalization of Aβ by cerebrovascular smooth muscle cells may be mediated by complexation with apolipoprotein E and uptake by the LRP receptor (Urmoneit *et al.* 1997), in a manner similar to that suggested for neuronal cells. Smooth muscle cells, however, may play a role in facilitating the assembly of the soluble Aβ into a pathogenic species on their cell surface (Van Nostrand *et al.* 1998).

Freshly solubilized Aβ has also been shown to have contractile effects on blood vessels, demonstrating both direct vasoconstriction and enhancement of contraction to phenylephrine (Thomas *et al.* 1996) and endothelin (Crawford *et al.* 1998). In contrast to endothelial cells, where Aβ1–42 is more cytotoxic than Aβ1–40, in terms of vasoactivity, Aβ1–40 is considerably more potent than the longer form of the peptide and the highly neurotoxic Aβ 25–35 is inactive (Suo *et al.* 1997). These data may point to different mechanisms for Aβ actions, not just between neurones and vascular cells but even from endothelium to its juxtaposed vascular smooth muscle cell. However, the generally deleterious effects of Aβ in the vasculature suggest that the pathology of AD could be due, to some extent, to a break down of vascular physiology.

4.10 **Conclusion**

There is no doubt that there are criticisms of the amyloid hypothesis, many of which have been discussed elsewhere (Neve and Robakis 1998). Difficulties in reaching a consensus on issues such as the identity of the toxic form of Aβ have no doubt confused and complicated the literature, which deal with the neurotoxic properties of this ill-defined species. The original belief that toxic Aβ had to be congophilic, fibrillar, and extracellular has been refuted by recent findings cited in the above chapter. Furthermore, a corresponding disbelief, by amyloid proponents, in the involvement of tau in the aetiology of AD has now been overcome in a re-evaluation of the hypothesis (Hardy *et al.* 1998). For a large proportion of workers in the field, however, amyloid remains the target and, for the pharmaceutical industry, the prevention of deposition, directly or indirectly, is a therapeutic goal.

Editor's note added in proof

Please see Appendix VI for new discoveries on α-, β- and γ- secretases.

References

Allsop, D., Clements, A., Kennedy, H., *et al.* (1994). Mechanism of cerebral amyloidosis in Alzheimer's disease. In *Amyloid protein precursor in development, aging and Alzheimer's disease,* (ed. C. L. Masters, K. Beyereuther, M. Trillet, and Y. Christen), pp. 47–59. Springer-Verlag, Berlin.

Allsop, D., Howlett, D. R., Christie, G., and Karran, E. (1998). Fibrillogenesis of beta-amyloid. *Biochemical Society Transactions*, **26**, 459–63.

Arispe, N., Rojas, E., and Pollard, H. B. (1993). Alzheimer disease amyloid beta protein forms calcium channels in bilayer membranes: blockade by tromethamine and aluminum. *Proceedings of the National Academy of Sciences (USA)*, **90**, 567–71.

Atwood, C. S., Moir, R. D., Huang, X. D., *et al.* (1998). Dramatic aggregation of Alzheimer a-beta by cu(ii) is induced by conditions representing physiological acidosis. *Journal of Biological Chemistry*, **273**, 12817–26.

Baeuerle, P. A. and Baichwal, V. R. (1997). NF-kB as a frequent target for immunosuppressive and anti-inflammatory molecules. *Advances in Immunology*, **65**, 111–37.

Bales, K. R., Du, Y. S., Dodel, R. C., *et al.* (1998). The NF-kappa-b/rel family of proteins mediates A-beta-induced neurotoxicity and glial activation. *Molecular Brain Research*, **57**, 63–72.

Bandiera, T., Lansen, J., Post, C., and Varasi, M. (1997). Inhibitors of A-beta peptide aggregation as potential anti- alzheimer agents. *Current Medicinal Chemistry*, **4**, 159–70.

Bauer, J., Strauss, S., Schreiter-Gasser, U., *et al.* (1991). Interleukin-6 and alpha-2-macroglobulin indicate an acute-phase state in Alzheimer's disease cortices. *FEBS Letters*, **285**, 111–4.

Beher, D., Hesse, L., Masters, C. L., and Multhaup, G. (1996). Regulation of amyloid protein precursor (APP) binding to collagen and mapping of the binding sites on APP and collagen type I. *Journal of Biological Chemistry*, **271**, 1613–20.

Behl, C. (1997). Amyloid beta-protein toxicity and oxidative stress in Alzheimer's disease. *Cell Tissue Research*, **290**, 471–80.

Behl, C. and Holsboer, F. (1998). Oxidative stress during the pathogenesis of alzheimers-disease and antioxidant neuroprotection. *Fortschritte der Neurologie Psychiatrie*, **66**, 113–21.

Behl, C., Davis, J., Cole, G. M., and Schubert, D. (1992). Vitamin E protects nerve cells from amyloid beta protein toxicity. *Biochemical and Biophysical Research. Communications*, **186**, 944–50.

Behl, C., Davis, J. B., Lesley, R., and Schubert, D. (1994). Hydrogen peroxide mediates amyloid beta protein toxicity. *Cell*, **77**, 817–27.

Blacker, D., Wilcox, M. A., Laird, N. M., *et al.* (1998). Alpha-2-macroglobulin is genetically associated with Alzheimer-disease. *Nature Genetics*, **19**, 357–60.

Borchelt, D. R., Thinakaran, G., Eckman, C. B., *et al.* (1996). Familial Alzheimer's-disease-linked pre-senilin-1 variants elevate a-beta-1–42/1–40 ratio *in-vitro* and *in-vivo*. *Neuron*, **17**, 1005–13.

Borg, J. P., Ooi, J., Levy, E., and Margolis, B. (1996). The phosphotyrosine interaction domains of x11 and fe65 bind to distinct sites on the YENPTY motif of amyloid precursor protein. *Molecular And Cellular Biology*, **16**, 6229–41.

Bradt, B. M., Kolb, W. P., and Cooper, N. R. (1998). Complement-dependent proinflammatory properties of the Alzheimer's disease beta-peptide. *Journal of Experimental Medicine*, **188**, 431–8.

Breitner, J. C., Gau, B. A., Welsh, K. A., *et al.* (1994). Inverse association of anti-inflammatory treatments and Alzheimer's disease: initial results of a co-twin control study. *Neurology*, **44**, 227–32.

Bronfman, F. C., Garrido, J., Alvarez, A., *et al.* (1996). Laminin inhibits amyloid-beta-peptide fibrillation. *Neuroscience Letters*, **218**, 201–3.

Busciglio, J., Lorenzo, A., Yeh, J., and Yankner, B. A. (1995). Beta-amyloid fibrils induce tau phosphorylation and loss of microtubule binding. *Neuron*, **14**, 879–88.

Carson, K. A., Geula, C., and Mesulam, M. M. (1991). Electron microscopic localization of cholinesterase activity in Alzheimer brain tissue. *Brain Research*, **540**, 204–8.

Chevallier, N., Jiracek, J., Vincent, B., *et al.* (1997). Examination of the role of endopeptidase 3. 4. 24. 15 in A beta secretion by human transfected cells. . *British Journal of Pharmacology*, **121**, 556–62.

Choosmith, L. P., Garzonrodriguez, W., Glabe, C. G., and Surewicz, W. K. (1997). Acceleration of amyloid fibril formation by specific binding of a-beta-(1–40) peptide to ganglioside-containing membrane-vesicles. *Journal of Biological Chemistry*, **272**, 22987–90.

Christie, G., Markwell, R. E., Gray, C. W., *et al.* (1999). Alzheimer's disease: correlation of the suppression of Aβ peptide secretion from cultured cells with inhibition of the chymotrypsin-like activity of the proteasome. *Journal of Neurochemistry*, **73**, 195–204.

Citron, M., Diehl, T. S., Gordon, G., *et al.* (1996). Evidence that the 42- and 40-amino acid forms of amyloid beta protein are generated from the beta-amyloid precursor protein by different protease activities. *Proceedings of the National Academy of Sciences (USA)*, **93**, 13170–5.

Citron, M., Westaway, D., Xia, W., *et al.* (1997). Mutant presenilins of Alzheimer's disease increase production of 42-residue amyloid beta-protein in both transfected cells and transgenic mice. *Nature Medicine*, **3**, 67–72.

Clarris, H. J., Cappai, R., Heffernan, D., *et al.* (1997). Identification of heparin-binding domains in the amyloid precursor protein of alzheimers-disease by deletion mutagenesis and peptide-mapping. *Journal of Neurochemistry*, **68**, 1164–72.

Conlon, R. A., Reaume, A. G., and Rossant, J. (1995). Notch1 is required for the coordinate segmentation of somites. *Development*, **121**, 1533–45.

Cook, D. G., Forman, M. S., Sung, J. C., *et al.* (1997). Alzheimer's A beta(1–42) is generated in the ER/intermediate compartment of NT2N cells. . *Nature Medicine*, **3**, 1021–3.

Coulson, E. J., Barrett, G. L., Storey, E., *et al.* (1997). Down-regulation of the amyloid protein precursor of Alzheimer's disease by antisense oligonucleotides reduces neuronal adhesion to specific substrata. *Brain Research*, **770**, 72–80.

Crawford, F., Suo, Z. M., Fang, C. H., and Mullan, M. (1998). Characteristics of the *in-vitro* vasoactivity of beta-amyloid peptides. *Experimental Neurology*, **150**, 159–68.

Crook, R., Verkkoniemi, A., Perez Tur, J., *et al.* (1998). A variant of Alzheimer's disease with spastic paraparesis and unusual plaques due to deletion of exon 9 of presenilin 1. *Nature Medicine*, **4**, 452–5.

Cruts, M. and Van Broeckhoven, C. (1998). Presenilin mutations in Alzheimer's disease. *Human Mutation*, **11**, 183–90.

Cummings, B. J. and Cotman, C. W. (1995). Image analysis of beta-amyloid load in Alzheimer's disease and relation to dementia severity. *Lancet*, **346**, 1524–8.

Davis, J. A., Naruse, S., Chen, H., *et al.* (1998). An Alzheimers-disease-linked ps1 variant rescues the developmental abnormalities of ps1-deficient embryos. *Neuron*, **20**, 603–9.

Davis-Salinas, J., Saporito-Irwin, S. M., Cotman, C. W., and Van Nostrand, W. E. (1995). Amyloid beta-protein induces its own production in cultured degenerating cerebrovascular smooth muscle cells. *Journal of Neurochemistry*, **65**, 931–4.

Deng, G., Pike, C. J., and Cotman, C. W. (1996). Alzheimer-associated presenilin-2 confers increased sensitivity to apoptosis in PC12 cells. *FEBS Letters*, **397**, 50–4.

DeStrooper, B., Saftig, P., Craessaerts, K., *et al.* (1998). Deficiency of presenilin-1 inhibits the normal cleavage of amyloid precursor protein. *Nature*, **391**, 387–90.

Doan, A., Thinakaran, G., Borchelt, D. R., *et al.* (1996). Protein topology of presenilin 1. *Neuron*, **17**, 1023–30.

Du, Y., Bales, K. R., Dodel, R. C., Li *et al.* (1998). Alpha2-macroglobulin attenuates beta-amyloid peptide 1–40 fibril formation and associated neurotoxicity of cultured fetal rat cortical neurons. *Journal of Neurochemistry.*, **70**, 1182–8.

Duff, K., Eckman, C., Zehr, C., *et al.* (1996). Increased amyloid-beta 42(43) in brains of mice expressing mutant presenilin 1. *Nature*, **383**, 710–3.

Duilio, A., Faraonio, R., Minopoli, G., *et al.* (1998). Fe65l2 — a new member of the fe65 protein family interacting with the intracellular domain of the alzheimers beta-amyloid precursor protein. *Biochemical Journal*, **330**, 513–9.

Evans, K. C., Berger, E. P., Cho, C. G., *et al.* (1995). Apolipoprotein E is a kinetic but not a thermodynamic inhibitor of amyloid formation: implications for the pathogenesis and treatment of Alzheimer disease. *Proceedings of the National Academy of Sciences (USA)*, **92**, 763–7.

Fiore, F., Zambrano, N., Minopoli, G., *et al.* (1995). The regions of the Fe65 protein homologous to the phosphotyrosine interaction phosphotyrosine binding domain of shc bind the intracellular domain of the alzheimers amyloid precursor protein. *Journal of Biological Chemistry*, **270**, 30853–6.

Frackowiak, J., Mazur-Kolecka, B., Wisniewski, H. M., *et al.* (1995). Secretion and accumulation of Alzheimer's beta-protein by cultured vascular smooth muscle cells from old and young dogs. *Brain Research*, **676**, 225–30.

Furukawa, K., Sopher, B. L., Rydel, R. E., *et al.* (1996). Increased activity-regulating and neuroprotective efficacy of alpha-secretase-derived secreted amyloid precursor protein conferred by a c-terminal heparin-binding domain. *Journal of Neurochemistry*, **67**, 1882–96.

Games, D., Adams, D., Alessandrini, R., *et al.* (1995). Alzheimer-type neuropathology in transgenic mice overexpressing V717F beta-amyloid precursor protein. *Nature*, **373**, 523–7.

Geula, C., Wu, C. K., Saroff, D., *et al.* (1998). Aging renders the brain vulnerable to amyloid beta-protein neurotoxicity. *Nature Medicine*, **4**, 827–31.

Ghiso, J., Rostagno, A., Gardella, J. E., *et al.* (1992). A 109-amino-acid C-terminal fragment of Alzheimer's-disease amyloid precursor protein contains a sequence, -RHDS-, that promotes cell adhesion. *Biochemical Journal*, **288**, 1053–9.

Golabek, A. A., Soto, C., Vogel, T., and Wisniewski, T. (1996). The interaction between apolipoprotein E and Alzheimer's amyloid beta- peptide is dependent on beta-peptide conformation. *Journal of Biological Chemistry*, **271**, 10602–6.

Goodman, Y. and Mattson, M. P. (1994). Secreted forms of β-amyloid precursor protein protect hippocampal neurons against amyloid β-peptide-induced oxidative injury. *Experimental Neurology*, **128**, 1–12.

Griffin, W. S., Stanley, L. C., Ling, C., *et al.* (1989). Brain interleukin 1 and S-100 immunoreactivity are elevated in Down syndrome and Alzheimer disease. *Proceedings of the National Academy of Sciences (USA)*, **86**, 7611–5.

Grunberg, J., Walter, J., Loetscher, H., *et al.* (1998). Alzheimers-disease associated presenilin-1 holoprotein and its 18–20 kDa C-terminal fragment are death substrates for proteases of the caspase family. *Biochemistry*, **37**, 2263–70.

Guo, Q., Sopher, B. L., Furukawa, K., *et al.* (1997). Alzheimers presenilin mutation sensitizes neural cells to apoptosis induced by trophic factor withdrawal and amyloid beta- peptide — involvement of calcium and oxyradicals. *Journal of Neuroscience*, **17**, 4212–22.

Hamazaki, H. (1998). Carboxy-terminal truncation of long-tailed amyloid beta-peptide is inhibited by serine protease inhibitor and peptide aldehyde. *FEBS Letters*, **424**, 136–8.

Hammad, S. M., Ranganathan, S., Loukinova, E., *et al.* (1997). Interaction of apolipoprotein J-amyloid beta-peptide complex with low density lipoprotein receptor-related protein-2/megalin. A mechanism to prevent pathological accumulation of amyloid beta- peptide. *Journal of Biological Chemistry*, **272**, 18644–9.

Han, H., Weinreb, P. H., and Lansbury, P. T., Jr. (1995). The core Alzheimer's peptide NAC forms amyloid fibrils which seed and are seeded by beta-amyloid: is NAC a common trigger or target in neurodegenerative disease? *Chemistry and Biology*, **2**, 163–9.

Hardy, J., Duff, K., Hardy, K. G., *et al.* (1998) Genetic dissection of Alzheimer's disease and related dementias: amyloid and its relationship to tau. *Nature Neuroscience*, **1**, 355–8.

Harper, J. D., Lieber, C. M., and Lansbury, P. T. (1997). Atomic-force microscopic imaging of seeded fibril formation and fibril branching by the Alzheimers-disease amyloid-beta protein. *Chemistry and Biology*, **4**, 951–9.

Hartmann, T., Bieger, S. C., Bruhl, B., *et al.* (1997). Distinct sites of intracellular production for Alzheimer's disease A beta40/42 amyloid peptides. *Nature Medicine*, **3**, 1016–20.

Hensley, K., Carney, J. M., Mattson, M. P., *et al.* (1994). A model for beta-amyloid aggregation and neurotoxicity based on free radical generation by the peptide: relevance to Alzheimer disease. *Proceedings of the National Academy of Sciences (USA)*, **91**, 3270–4.

Higaki, J., Quon, D., Zhong, Z. Y., and Cordell, B. (1995). Inhibition of beta-amyloid formation identifies proteolytic precursors and subcellular site of catabolism. *Neuron*, **14**, 651–9.

Howlett, D. R., Jennings, K. H., Lee, D. C., *et al.* (1995). Aggregation state and neurotoxic properties of alzheimer beta- amyloid peptide. *Neurodegeneration*, **4**, 23–32.

Howlett, D., Cutler, P., Heales, S., and Camilleri, P. (1997). Hemin and related porphyrins inhibit beta-amyloid aggregation. *FEBS Letters*, **417**, 249–51.

Howlett, D. R., Markwell, R. E., and Wood, S. J. (1998). Identification of a novel class of inhibitor of beta-amyloid peptide aggregation. *British Journal of Pharmacology*, **123**, 25.

Hrabe, d. A., McIntyre, J., and Gossler, A. (1997). Maintenance of somite borders in mice requires the Delta homologue DII1. *Nature*, **386**, 717–21.

Hsiao, K., Chapman, P., Nilsen, S., *et al.* (1996). Correlative memory deficits, Abeta elevation, and amyloid plaques in transgenic mice. *Science*, **274**, 99–102.

Hughes, S. R., Khorkova, O., Goyal, S., *et al.* (1998). Alpha(2)-macroglobulin associates with beta-amyloid peptide and prevents fibril formation. *Proceedings of the National Academy of Sciences (USA)*, **95**, 3275–80.

Hutton, M., Lendon, C. L., Rizzu, P., *et al.* (1998). Association of missense and 5'-splice-site mutations in tau with the inherited dementia FTDP-17. *Nature*, **393**, 702–5.

Hyman, B. T., West, H. L., Rebeck, G. W., *et al.* (1995). Quantitative-analysis of senile plaques in alzheimer-disease — observation of log-normal size distribution and molecular epidemiology of differences associated with apolipoprotein-E genotype and trisomy-21 (down-syndrome). *Proceedings of The National Academy of Sciences (USA)*, **92**, 3586–90.

Inestrosa, N. C., Alvarez, A., Perez, C. A., *et al.* (1996). Acetylcholinesterase accelerates assembly of amyloid-beta- peptides into alzheimers fibrils — possible role of the peripheral site of the enzyme. *Neuron*, **16**, 881–91.

Irizarry, M. C., Soriano, F., Mcnamara, M., *et al.* (1997). Abeta deposition is associated with neuropil changes, but not with overt neuronal loss in the human amyloid precursor protein V717F (PDAPP) transgenic mouse. *Journal of Neuroscience*, **17**, 7053–9.

Iwatsubo, T., Mann, D. M., Odaka, A., *et al.* (1995). Amyloid beta protein (A beta) deposition: A beta 42(43) precedes A beta 40 in Down syndrome. *Annals of Neurology*, **37**, 294–9.

Jarrett, J. T. and Lansbury, P. T., Jr. (1993). Seeding 'one-dimensional crystallization' of amyloid: a pathogenic mechanism in Alzheimer's disease and scrapie? *Cell*, **73**, 1055–8.

Jarrett, J. T., Berger, E. P., and Lansbury, P. T., Jr. (1993a). The C-terminus of the beta protein is critical in amyloidogenesis. *Annals of the New York Academy of. Science*, **695**, 144–8.

Jarrett, J. T., Berger, E. P., and Lansbury, P. T., Jr. (1993b). The carboxy terminus of the beta amyloid protein is critical for the seeding of amyloid formation: implications for the pathogenesis of Alzheimer's disease. *Biochemistry*, **32**, 4693–7.

Jensen, M., Song, X. H., Suzuki, N., *et al.* (1995). The delta-NL Alzheimer mutation (swedish) increases plasma amyloid-beta protein-concentration. *Journal of Neurochemistry*, **65**, S136.

Jiang, H., Burdick, D., Glabe, C. G., *et al.* (1994). β-Amyloid activates complement by binding to a specific region of the collagen-like domain of the C1q A chain. *Journal of Immunology*, **152**, 5050–9.

Jin, L. W., Ninomiya, H., Roch, J. M., *et al.* (1994). Peptides containing the RERMS sequence of amyloid beta/A4 protein precursor bind cell surface and promote neurite extension. *Journal of Neuroscience*, **4**, 5461–70.

Kaltschmidt, B., Uherek, M., Volk, B., *et al.* (1997). Transcription factor nf-kappa-b is activated in primary neurons by amyloid-beta peptides and in neurons surrounding early plaques from patients with Alzheimer-disease. *Proceedings of the National Academy of Sciences (USA)*, **94**, 2642–7.

Kang, J., Lemaire, H. G., Unterbeck, A., *et al.* (1987). The precursor of Alzheimer's disease amyloid A4 protein resembles a cell-surface receptor. *Nature*, **325**, 733–6.

Kim, T. W., Pettingell, W. H., Hallmark, O. G., *et al.* (1997a). Endoproteolytic cleavage and proteasomal degradation of presenilin 2 in transfected cells. *Journal of Biological Chemistry*, **272**, 11006–10.

Kim, T. W., Pettingell, W. H., Jung, Y. K., *et al.* (1997b). Alternative cleavage of Alzheimer-associated presenilins during apoptosis by a caspase-3 family protease. *Science*, **277**, 373–6.

Kisilevsky, R., Lemieux, L. J., Fraser, P. E., *et al.* (1995). Arresting amyloidosis *in vivo* using small-molecule anionic sulphonates or sulphates: implications for Alzheimer's disease. *Nature Medicine*, **1**, 143–8.

Klafki, H., Abramowski, D., Swoboda, R., *et al.* (1996). The carboxyl termini of beta-amyloid peptides 1–40 and 1–42 are generated by distinct gamma-secretase activities. *Journal of Biological Chemistry*, **271**, 28655–9.

Klunk, W. E., Xu, C. J., McClure, R. J., *et al.* (1997). Aggregation of beta-amyloid peptide is promoted by membrane phospholipid metabolites elevated in Alzheimer's disease brain. *Journal of Neurochemistry*, **69**, 266–72.

Kovacs, D. M., Fausett, H. J., Page, K. J., *et al.* (1996). Alzheimer-associated presenilins 1 and 2: neuronal expression in brain and localization to intracellular membranes in mammalian cells. *Nature Medicine*, **2**, 224–9.

Kuo, Y. M., Emmerling, M. R., Vigo Pelfrey, C., *et al.* (1996). Water-soluble Abeta (N-40, N-42) oligomers in normal and Alzheimer disease brains. *Journal of Biological Chemistry*, **271**, 4077–81.

Lambert, M. P., Barlow, A. K., Chromy, B. A., *et al.* (1998). Diffusible, nonfibrillar ligands derived from A-beta(1–42) are potent central-nervous-system neurotoxins. *Proceedings of the National Academy of Sciences (USA)*, **95**, 6448–53.

Lemere, C. A., Lopera, F., Kosik, K. S., *et al.* (1996). The E280A presenilin-1 Alzheimer mutation produces increased A- beta-42 deposition and severe cerebellar pathology. *Nature Medicine*, **2**, 1146–50.

Lepage, R. N., Fosang, A. J., Fuller, S. J., *et al.* (1995). Gelatinase A possesses A beta-secretase-like activity in cleaving the amyloid protein precursor of Alzheimer's disease. *FEBS Letters.*, **377**, 267–70.

Levitan, D. and Greenwald, I. (1995). Facilitation of lin-12-mediated signalling by sel-12, a Caenorhabditis elegans S182 Alzheimer's disease gene. *Nature*, **377**, 351–4.

Levitan, D., Doyle, T. G., Brousseau, D., *et al.* (1996). Assessment of normal and mutant human presenilin function in Caenorhabditis elegans. *Proceedings of the National Academy of Sciences (USA)*, **93**, 14940–4.

Levy-Lahad, E., Wasco, W., Poorkaj, P., *et al.* (1995). Candidate gene for the chromosome 1 familial Alzheimer's disease locus. *Science*, **269**, 973–7.

Li, X. and Greenwald, I. (1996). Membrane topology of the C. elegans SEL-12 presenilin. *Neuron*, **17**, 1015–21.

Li, X. and Greenwald, I. (1998). Additional evidence for an eight-transmembrane-domain topology for Caenorhabditis elegans and human presenilins. *Proceedings of the National Academy of Sciences (USA)*, **95**, 7109–14.

Loetscher, H., Deuschle, U., Brockhaus, M., *et al.* (1997). Presenilins are processed by caspase-type proteases. *Journal of Biological Chemistry*, **272**, 20655–9.

Lovestone, S., Hartley, C. L., Pearce, J., and Anderton, B. H. (1996). Phosphorylation of tau by glycogen synthase kinase-3 beta in intact mammalian cells: the effects on the organization and stability of microtubules. *Neuroscience*, **73**, 1145–57.

McDermott, J. R. and Gibson, A. M. (1996). Degradation of alzheimers beta-amyloid protein by human cathepsin-D. *Neuroreport*, **7**, 2163–6.

McDermott, J. R. and Gibson, A. M. (1997). Degradation of alzheimers beta-amyloid protein by human and rat brain peptidases — involvement of insulin-degrading enzyme. *Neurochemical Research*, **22**, 49–56.

McGeer, P. L., Akiyama, H., Itagaki, S., and McGeer, E. G. (1989). Activation of the classical complement pathway in brain tissue of Alzheimer patients. *Neuroscience Letters*, **107**, 341–6.

McGeer, P. L., McGeer, E., Rogers, J., and Sibley, J. (1990). Anti-inflammatory drugs and Alzheimer disease. *Lancet*, **335**, 1037.

McLaurin, J. and Chakrabartty, A. (1996). Membrane disruption by Alzheimer beta-amyloid peptides mediated through specific binding to either phospholipids or gangliosides. Implications for neurotoxicity. *Journal of Biological Chemistry*, **271**, 26482–9.

McLaurin, J., Franklin, T., Chakrabartty, A., and Fraser, P. E. (1998). Phosphatidylinositol and inositol involvement in alzheimer amyloid-beta fibril growth and arrest. *Journal of Molecular Biology*, **278**, 183–94.

Mcloughlin, D. M. and Miller, C. C. (1996). The intracellular cytoplasmic domain of the Alzheimer's disease amyloid precursor protein interacts with phosphotyrosine-binding domain proteins in the yeast two-hybrid system. *FEBS Letters*, **397**, 197–200.

Maggio, J. E. and Mantyh, P. W. (1996). Brain amyloid — a physicochemical perspective. *Brain Pathology*, **6**, 147–62.

Malinchik, S. B., Inouye, H., Szumowski, K. E., and Kirschner, D. A. (1998). Structural analysis of Alzheimer's beta(1–40) amyloid: protofilament assembly of tubular fibrils. *Biophysical Journal*, **74**, 537–45.

Manni, M. E., Cescato, R., and Paganetti, P. A. (1998). Lack of beta-amyloid production in m19 cells deficient in site-2 processing of the sterol regulatory element-binding proteins. *FEBS Letters*, **427**, 367–70.

Masliah, E., Westland, C. E., Rockenstein, E. M., *et al.* (1997). Amyloid precursor proteins protect neurons of transgenic mice against acute and chronic excitotoxic injuries *in vivo*. *Neuroscience*, **78**, 135–46.

Matsubara, E., Soto, C., Governale, S., *et al.* (1996). Apolipoprotein J and Alzheimer's amyloid beta solubility. *Biochemical Journal*, **316**, 671–9.

Mattson, M. P. (1997a). Cellular actions of beta-amyloid precursor protein and its soluble and fibrillogenic derivatives. *Physiological Reviews*, **77**, 1081–132.

Mattson, M. P. (1997b). Central role of oxyradicals in the mechanism of amyloid beta-peptide cytotoxicity. *Alzheimer's Disease Review*, **2**, 1–14.

Mattson, M. P., Cheng, B., Culwell, A. R., *et al.* (1993). Evidence for excitoprotective and intraneuronal calcium- regulating roles for secreted forms of the beta-amyloid precursor protein. *Neuron*, **10**, 243–54.

Mattson, M. P., Partin, J., and Begley, J. G. (1998). Amyloid beta-peptide induces apoptosis-related events in synapses and dendrites. *Brain Research*, **807**, 167–76.

May, P. C., Gitter, B. D., Waters, D. C., *et al.* (1992). β-Amyloid peptide in vitro toxicity: lot-to-lot variability. *Neurobiology of Aging*, **13**, 605–7.

Mazziotti, M. and Perlmutter, D. H. (1998). Resistance to the apoptotic effect of aggregated amyloid-beta peptide in several different cell-types including neuronal- derived and hepatoma-derived cell-lines. *Biochemical Journal*, **332**, 517–24.

Mehta, N. D., Refolo, L. M., Eckman, C., *et al.* (1998). Increased Abeta42(43) from cell lines expressing presenilin 1 mutations. *Annals of Neurology*, **43**, 256–8.

Mercken, M., Takahashi, H., Honda, T., *et al.* (1996). Characterization of human presenilin 1 using N-terminal specific monoclonal antibodies: Evidence that Alzheimer mutations affect proteolytic processing. *FEBS Letters*, **389**, 297–303.

Meziane, H., Dodart, J. C., Mathis, C., *et al.* (1998). Memory enhancing effects of secreted forms of the beta-amyloid precursor protein innormal and amnestic mice. *Proceedings of the National Academy of Sciences (USA)*, **95**, 12683–8.

Miyazaki, K., Hasegawa, M., Funahashi, K., and Umeda, M. (1993). A metalloproteinase inhibitor domain in Alzheimer amyloid protein precursor. *Nature*, **362**, 839–41.

Monji, A., Tashiro, K., Yoshida, I., *et al.* (1998). Laminin inhibits a beta-42 fibril formation *in-vitro*. *Brain Research*, **788**, 187–90.

Moran, M. A., Mufson, E. J., and Gomez-Ramos, P. (1993). Colocalization of cholinesterases with beta amyloid protein in aged and Alzheimer's brains. *Acta Neuropathologie (Berlin)*, **85**, 362–9.

Murayama, Y., Takeda, S., Yonezawa, K., *et al.* (1996). Cell surface receptor function of amyloid precursor protein that activates Ser/Thr kinases. *Gerontology*, **42**, 2–11.

Naiki, H. and Nakakuki, K. (1996). First-order kinetic model of Alzheimer's beta-amyloid fibril extension in vitro. *Laboratory Investigation*, **74**, 374–83.

Naiki, H., Gejyo, F., and Nakakuki, K. (1997). Concentration-dependent inhibitory effects of apolipoprotein E on Alzheimer's beta-amyloid fibril formation *in vitro*. *Biochemistry*, **36**, 6243–50.

Neve, R. L. and Robakis, N. K. (1998). Alzheimers-disease — a re-examination of the amyloid hypothesis. *Trends in Neurosciences*, **21**, 15–9.

Ninomiya, H., Roch, J. M., Sundsmo, M. P., *et al.* (1993). Amino acid sequence RERMS represents the active domain of amyloid beta/A4 protein precursor that promotes fibroblast growth. *Journal of Cell Biology*, **121**, 879–86.

Ninomiya, H., Roch, J. M., Jin, L. W., and Saitoh, T. (1994). Secreted form of amyloid beta/A4 protein precursor (APP) binds to two distinct APP binding sites on rat B103 neuron-like cells through two different domains, but only one site is onvolved in neurotrophic activity. *Journal of Neurochemistry*, **63**, 495–500.

Nishimoto, I., Okamoto, T., Matsuura, Y., *et al.* (1993). Alzheimer amyloid protein precursor complexes with brain GTP- binding protein G(o). *Nature*, **362**, 75–9.

Nohturfft, A., Brown, M. S., and Goldstein, J. L. (1998). Topology of SREBP cleavage-activating protein, a polytopic membrane protein with a sterol-sensing domain. *Journal of Biological Chemistry*, **273**, 17243–50.

Norstedt, C., Lannfelt, L., and Winblad, B. (1994). Alzheimer's disease: a molecular perspective. *Journal of Internal Medicine*, **235**, 195–8.

Oda, T., Wals, P., Osterburg, H. H., *et al.* (1995). Clusterin (apoJ) alters the aggregation of amyloid beta-peptide (A beta 1–42) and forms slowly sedimenting A beta complexes that cause oxidative stress. *Experimental Neurology*, **136**, 22–31.

Ohsawa, I., Takamura, C., and Kohsaka, S. (1997). The amino-terminal region of amyloid precursor protein is responsible for neurite outgrowth in rat neocortical explant culture. *Biochemical Biophysical Research Communications*, **236**, 59–65.

Okamoto, T., Takeda, S., Giambarella, U., *et al.* (1996). Intrinsic signaling function of app as a novel target of 3 v642 mutations linked to familial Alzheimer's-disease. *European Molecular Biology Organisation Journal*, **15**, 3769–77.

Oyama, F., Sawamura, N., Kobayashi, K., *et al.* (1998). Mutant presenilin-2 transgenic mouse — effect on an age-dependent increase of amyloid beta-protein-42 in the brain. *Journal of Neurochemistry*, **71**, 313–22.

Pappolla, M., Bozner, P., Soto, C., *et al.* (1998). Inhibition of Alzheimer beta-fibrillogenesis by melatonin. *Journal of Biological Chemistry*, **273**, 7185–8.

Paresce, D. M., Chung, H., and Maxfield, F. R. (1997). Slow degradation of aggregates of the Alzheimer's disease amyloid beta-protein by microglial cells. *Journal of Biological Chemistry*, **272**, 29390–7.

Parvathy, S., Hussain, I., Karran, E. H., *et al.* (1998a). Alzheimers amyloid precursor protein alpha-secretase is inhibited by hydroxamic acid-based zinc metalloprotease inhibitors — similarities to the angiotensin-converting enzyme secretase. *Biochemistry*, **37**, 1680–5.

Parvathy, S., Karran, E. H., Turner, A. J., and Hooper, N. M. (1998b). The secretases that cleave angiotensin-converting enzyme and the amyloid precursor protein are distinct from tumor-necrosis-factor- alpha convertase. *FEBS Letters*, **431**, 63–5.

Pierce, J. S., Smith, D. H., Trojanowski, J. Q., and Mcintosh, T. K. (1998). Enduring cognitive, neurobehavioral and histopathological changes persist for up to one-year following severe experimental brain injury in rats. *Neuroscience*, **87**, 359–69.

Pike, C. J., Walencewicz, A. J., Glabe, C. G., and Cotman, C. W. (1991). *In vitro* aging of beta-amyloid protein causes peptide aggregation and neurotoxicity. *Brain Research*, **563**, 311–4.

Podlisny, M. B., Ostaszewski, B. L., Squazzo, S. L., *et al.* (1995). Aggregation of secreted amyloid beta-protein into sodium dodecyl sulfate-stable oligomers in cell-culture. *Journal of Biological Chemistry*, **270**, 9564–70.

Podlisny, M. B., Walsh, D. M., Amarante, P., *et al.* (1998). Oligomerization of endogenous and synthetic amyloid beta-protein at nanomolar levels in cell-culture and stabilization of monomer by congo red. *Biochemistry*, **37**, 3602–11.

Polvikoski, T., Sulkava, R., Haltia, M., *et al.* (1995). Apolipoprotein-E, dementia, and cortical deposition of beta-amyloid protein. *New England Journal of Medicine*, **333**, 1242–7.

Poorkaj, P., Bird, T. D., Wijsman, E., *et al.* (1998). Tau is a candidate gene for chromosome 17 frontotemporal dementia. *Annals of Neurology*, **43**, 815–25.

Premkumar, D. R., Cohen, D. L., Hedera, P., *et al.* (1996). Apolipoprotein E-epsilon4 alleles in cerebral amyloid angiopathy and cerebrovascular pathology associated with Alzheimer's disease. *American Journal of Pathology*, **148**, 2083–95.

Qian, S., Jiang, P., Guan, X. M., *et al.* (1998). Mutant human presenilin 1 protects presenilin 1 null mouse against embryonic lethality and elevates Abeta1–42/43 expression. *Neuron*, **20**, 611–7.

Qiu, W. Q., Ye, Z., Kholodenko, D., *et al.* (1997). Degradation of amyloid beta-protein by a metalloprotease secreted by microglia and other neural and nonneural cells. *Journal of Biological Chemistry*, **272**, 6641–6.

Rawson, R. B., Zelenski, N. G., Nijhawan, D., *et al.* (1997). Complementation cloning of S2P, a gene encoding a putative metalloprotease required for intramembrane cleavage of SREBPs. *Molecular Cell*, 1, 47–57.

Rogers, J., Cooper, N. R., Webster, S., *et al.* (1992). Complement activation by beta-amyloid in Alzheimer disease. *Proceedings of the National Academy of Sciences (USA)*, 89, 10016–20.

Rogers, J., Kirby, L. C., Hempelman, S. R., *et al.* (1993). Clinical trial of indomethacin in Alzheimer's disease. *Neurology*, 43, 1609–11.

Roher, A. E., Chaney, M. O., Kuo, Y. M., *et al.* (1996). Morphology and toxicity of Aβ-(1–42) dimer derived from neuritic and vascular amyloid deposits of Alzheimerís disease. *Journal of Biological Chemistry*, 271, 20631–5.

Ross, S. L., Martin, F., Simonet, L., *et al.* (1998). Amyloid precursor protein processing in sterol regulatory element-binding protein site-2 protease-deficient chinese-hamster ovary cells. *Journal of Biological Chemistry*, 273, 15309–12.

Saftig, P., Peters, C., von Figura, K., *et al.* (1996). Amyloidogenic processing of human amyloid precursor protein in hippocampal neurons devoid of cathepsin D. *Journal of Biological Chemistry*, 271, 27241–4.

Scheuner, D., Eckman, C., Jensen, M., *et al.* (1996). Secreted amyloid beta-protein similar to that in the senile plaques of alzheimers-disease is increased in-vivo by the presenilin-1 and presenilin-2 and APP mutations linked to familial alzheimers-disease. *Nature Medicine*, 2, 864–70.

Schwarzman, A. L., Gregori, L., Vitek, M. P., *et al.* (1994). Transthyretin sequesters amyloid β protein and prevents amyloid formation. *Proceedings of the National Academy of Sciences (USA)*, 91, 8368–72.

Seilheimer, B., Bohrmann, B., Bondolfi, L., *et al.* (1997). The toxicity of the alzheimers beta-amyloid peptide correlates with a distinct fiber morphology. *Journal of Structural Biology*, 119, 59–71.

Shen, J., Bronson, R. T., Chen, D. F., *et al.* (1997). Skeletal and CNS defects in Presenilin-1-deficient mice. *Cell*, 89, 629–39.

Shen, Y., Sullivan, T., Lee, C. M., *et al.* (1998). Induced expression of neuronal membrane attack complex and cell-death by Alzheimers beta-amyloid peptide. *Brain Research*, 796, 187–97.

Sherrington, R., Rogaev, E. I., Liang, Y., *et al.* (1995). Cloning of a gene bearing missense mutations in early-onset familial Alzheimer's disease. *Nature*, 375, 754–60.

Shirotani, K., Takahashi, K., Ozawa, K., *et al.* (1997). Determination of a cleavage site of presenilin 2 protein in stably transfected SH-SY5Y human neuroblastoma cell lines. *Biochemical and Biophysical Research Communications*, 240, 728–31.

Simmons, L. K., May, P. C., Tomaselli, K. J., *et al.* (1994). Secondary structure of amyloid beta-peptide correlates with neurotoxic activity *in vitro*. *Molecular Pharmacology*, 45, 373–9.

Slooter, A. J., Tang, M. X., van Duijn, C. M., *et al.* (1997). Apolipoprotein E epsilon4 and the risk of dementia with stroke. A population-based investigation. *Journal of the American Medical Association*, 227, 818–21.

Smith-Swintosky, V. L., Pettigrew, C., Craddock, S. D., *et al.* (1994). Secreted forms of beta-amyloid precursor protein protect against ischaemic brain injury. *Journal of Neurochemistry*, 63, 781–4.

Smith, R. P., Higuchi, D. A., and Broze, G. J. J. (1990). Platelet coagulation factor Xia-inhibitor, a form of Alzheimer amyloid precursor protein. *Science*, 248, 1126–8.

Soreghan, B., Kosmoski, J., and Glabe, C. (1994). Surfactant properties of Alzheimer's A beta peptides and the mechanism of amyloid aggregation. *Journal of Biological Chemistry*, 269, 28551–4.

Soto, C., Kindy, M. S., Baumann, M., and Frangione, B. (1996). Inhibition of Alzheimers amyloidosis by peptides that prevent beta-sheet conformation. *Biochemical and Biophysical Research Communications*, 226, 672–80.

Soto, C., Sigurdsson, E. M., Morelli, L., *et al.* (1998). Beta-sheet breaker peptides inhibit fibrillogenesis in a rat- brain model of amyloidosis — implications for Alzheimer's therapy. *Nature Medicine*, **4**, 822–6.

Spillantini, M. G., Murrell, J. R., Goedert, M., *et al.* (1998). Mutation in the tau gene in familial multiple system tauopathy with presenile dementia. *Proceedings of the National Academy of Sciences (USA)*, **95**, 7737–41.

Stine, W. B., Snyder, S. W., Ladror, U. S., *et al.* (1996). The nanometer-scale structure of amyloid-beta visualized by atomic-force microscopy. *Journal of Protein Chemistry*, **15**, 193–203.

Su, J. H., Anderson, A. J., Cummings, B. J., and Cotman, C. W. (1994). Immunohistochemical evidence for apoptosis in Alzheimer's disease. *Neuroreport*, **5**, 2529–33.

Suo, Z., Fang, C., Crawford, F., and Mullan, M. (1997). Superoxide free radical and intracellular calcium mediate A beta(1–42) induced endothelial toxicity. *Brain Research*, **762**, 144–52.

Swatton, J. E., Howlett, D. R., and Spitzfaden, C. (1998). The use of a scintillation proximity assay to determine the interactions between beta-amyloid aggregation inhibitors and beta- amyloid peptide. *British Journal of Pharmacology*, **123**, P181

Tagliavini, F., Mcarthur, R. A., Canciani, B., *et al.* (1997). Effectiveness of anthracycline against experimental prion disease in Syrian hamsters. *Science*, **276**, 1119–22.

Takashima, A., Noguchi, K., Michel, G., *et al.* (1996). Exposure of rat hippocampal neurons to amyloid beta peptide (25- 35) induces the inactivation of phosphatidyl inositol-3 kinase and the activation of tau protein kinase I/glycogen synthase kinase-3 beta. *Neuroscience Letters*, **203**, 33–6.

Takashima, A., Murayama, M., Murayama, O., *et al.* (1998). Presenilin 1 associates with glycogen synthase kinase-3beta and its substrate tau. *Proceedings of the National Academy of Sciences (USA)*, **95**, 9637–41.

Tan, Y. Z., Hong, J., Doan, T., *et al.* (1998). Presenilin-1 mutations associated with familial alzheimers-disease do not disrupt protein-transport from the endoplasmic- reticulum to the golgi-apparatus. *Biochimica et Biophysica Acta-Molecular Basis of Disease*, **1407**, 69–78.

Tang, M. X., Maestre, G., Tsai, W. Y., *et al.* (1996). Relative risk of Alzheimer disease and age-at-onset distributions, based on APOE genotypes among elderly African Americans, Caucasians, and Hispanics in New York City. *American Journal of Human Genetics*, **58**, 574–84.

Thinakaran, G., Borchelt, D. R., Lee, M. K., *et al.* (1996). Endoproteolysis of presenilin 1 and accumulation of processed derivatives *in vivo*. *Neuron*, **17**, 181–90.

Thinakaran, G., Harris, C. L., Ratovitski, T., *et al.* (1997). Evidence that levels of presenilins (PS1 and PS2) are coordinately regulated by competition for limiting cellular factors. *Journal of Biological Chemistry*, **272**, 28415–22.

Thomas, T., Thomas, G., Mclendon, C., *et al.* (1996). Beta-amyloid-mediated vasoactivity and vascular endothelial damage. *Nature*, **380**, 168–71.

Tjernberg, L. O., Lilliehook, C., Callaway, D. J., *et al.* (1997). Controlling amyloid beta-peptide fibril formation with protease- stable ligands. *Journal of Biological Chemistry*, **272**, 12601–5.

Tomita, T., Chang, T. Y., Kodama, T., and Iwatsubo, T. (1998). Beta-app gamma-secretase and srebp site-2 protease are 2 different enzymes. *Neuroreport*, **9**, 911–3.

Tysoe, C., Whittaker, J., Xuereb, J., *et al.* (1998). A presenilin-1 truncating mutation is present in two cases with autopsy-confirmed early-onset Alzheimer disease. *American Journal of Human Genetics*, **62**, 70–6.

Urmoneit, B., Prikulis, I., Wihl, G., *et al.* (1997). Cerebrovascular smooth muscle cells internalize Alzheimer amyloid beta protein via a lipoprotein pathway: implications for cerebral amyloid angiopathy. *Laboratory Investigation*, **77**, 157–66.

Van Gool, D., De Strooper, B., Van Leuven, F., *et al.* (1993). α2-Macroglobulin expression in neuritic-type plaques in patients with Alzheimer's disease. *Neurobiology of Aging*, **14**, 233–7.

Van Gool, W. A., Schenk, D. B., and Bolhuis, P. A. (1994). Concentrations of amyloid-beta protein in cerebrospinal fluid increase with age in patients free from neurodegenerative disease. *Neuroscience Letters*, **172**, 122–4.

Van Nostrand, W. E., Wagner, S. L., Suzuki, M., *et al.* (1989). Protease nexin-II, a potent antichymotrypsin, shows identity to amyloid beta-protein precursor. *Nature*, **341**, 546–9.

Van Nostrand, W. E., Melchor, J. P., and Ruffini, L. (1998). Pathological amyloid beta-protein cell-surface fibril assembly on cultured human cerebrovascular smooth-muscle cells. *Journal of Neurochemistry*, **70**, 216–23.

Vito, P., Ghayur, T., and D'Adamio, L. (1997). Generation of anti-apoptotic presenilin-2 polypeptides by alternative transcription, proteolysis, and caspase-3 cleavage. *Journal of Biological Chemistry*, **272**, 28315–20.

Walsh, D. M., Williams, C. H., Kennedy, H. E., *et al.* (1994). Gelatinase A not alpha-secretase? *Nature*, **367**, 27–8.

Walsh, D. M., Lomakin, A., Benedek, G. B., *et al.* (1997). Amyloid beta-protein fibrillogenesis — detection of a protofibrillar intermediate. *Journal of Biological Chemistry*, **272**, 22364–72.

Walter, J., Capell, A., Grunberg, J., *et al.* (1996). The Alzheimer's disease-associated presenilins are differentially phosphorylated proteins located predominantly within the ER. *Molecular Medicine*, **2**, 673–91.

Ward, R. V., Davis, J. B., Gray, C. W., *et al.* (1996). Presenilin-1 is processed into two major cleavage products in neuronal cell lines. *Neurodegeneration*, **5**, 293–8.

Weidemann, A., Konig, G., Bunke, D., *et al.* (1989). Identification, biogenesis, and localization of precursors of Alzheimer's disease A4 amyloid protein. *Cell*, **57**, 115–26.

Weidemann A., Paliga K., Durrwang U., *et al.* (1997). Formation of stable complexes between two Alzheimer's disease gene products: presenilin-2 and beta-amyloid precursor protein. *Nature Medicine*, **3**, 328–32.

Wild Bode, C., Yamazaki, T., Capell, A., *et al.* (1997). Intracellular generation and accumulation of amyloid beta- peptide terminating at amino acid 42. *Journal of Biological Chemistry*, **272**, 16085–8.

Wolozin, B., Iwasaki, K., Vito, P., *et al.* (1996). Participation of presenilin 2 in apoptosis: enhanced basal activity conferred by an Alzheimer mutation. *Science*, **274**, 1710–3.

Wong, P. C., Zheng, H., Chen, H., *et al.* (1997). Presenilin 1 is required for Notch1 and DII1 expression in the paraxial mesoderm. *Nature*, **387**, 288–92.

Wood, S. J., Chan, W., and Wetzel, R. (1996a). An apoE-A-beta inhibition complex in A-beta fibril extension. *Chemistry And Biology*, **3**, 949–56.

Wood, S. J., Chan, W., and Wetzel, R. (1996b). Seeding of A-beta fibril formation is inhibited by all 3 isotypes of apolipoprotein-E. *Biochemistry*, **35**, 12623–8.

Wood, S. J., Maleeff, B., Hart, T., and Wetzel, R. (1996c). Physical, morphological and functional differences between ph 5. 8 and 7. 4 aggregates of the Alzheimer's amyloid peptide AP. *Journal of Molecular Biology*, **256**, 870–7.

Xia, W., Zhang, J., Perez, R., *et al.* (1997). Interaction between amyloid precursor protein and presenilins in mammalian cells: implications for the pathogenesis of Alzheimer disease. *Proceedings of the National Academy of Sciences (USA)*, **94**, 8208–13.

Xu, H., Gouras, G. K., Greenfield, J. P., *et al.* (1998). Estrogen reduces neuronal generation of Alzheimer beta-amyloid peptides. *Nature Medicine*, **4**, 447–51.

Yan, S. D., Chen, X., Fu, J., *et al.* (1996). RAGE and amyloid-beta peptide neurotoxicity in Alzheimer's disease. *Nature*, **382**, 685–91.

Yan, S. D., Fu, J., Soto, C., *et al.* (1997). An intracellular protein that binds amyloid-beta peptide and mediates neurotoxicity in alzheimers-disease. *Nature*, **389**, 689–95.

Yankner, B. A., Dawes, L. R., Fisher, S., *et al.* (1989). Neurotoxicity of a fragment of the amyloid precursor associated with Alzheimer's disease. *Science*, **245**, 417–20.

Yankner, B. A., Duffy, L. K., and Kirschner, D. A. (1990). Neurotrophic and neurotoxic effects of amyloid beta protein: reversal by tachykinin neuropeptides. *Science*, **250**, 279–82.

Yu, G., Chen, F. S., Levesque, G., *et al.* (1998). The presenilin-1 protein is a component of a high-molecular- weight intracellular complex that contains beta-catenin. *Journal of Biological Chemistry*, **273**, 16470–5.

Zambrano, N., Buxbaum, J. D., Minopoli, G., *et al.* (1997). Interaction of the phosphotyrosine interaction/phosphotyrosine binding-related domains of Fe65 with wild-type and mutant alzheimers beta-amyloid precursor proteins. *Journal of Biological Chemistry*, **272**, 6399–405.

Zhang, J., Kang, D. E., Xia, W., *et al.* (1998a). Subcellular distribution and turnover of presenilins in transfected cells. *Journal of Biological Chemistry*, **273**, 12436–42.

Zhang, W. J., Han, S. W., Mckeel, D. W., *et al.* (1998b). Interaction of presenilins with the filamin family of actin- binding proteins. *Journal of Neuroscience*, **18**, 914–22.

Zhang, Z., Hartmann, H., Do, V. M., *et al.* (1998c). Destabilization of β-catenin by mutations in presenilin-1 potentiates neuronal apoptosis. *Nature*, **395**, 698–702.

Zhang, Z. Y., Drzewiecki, G. J., May, P. C., *et al.* (1996). Inhibition of alpha(2)-macroglobulin/proteinase-mediated degradation of amyloid-beta peptide by apolipoprotein-E and alpha(1)-antichymotrypsin — evidence that the alpha(2)- macroglobulin/proteinase complex mediates degradation of the A- beta peptide. *Amyloid-International Journal of Experimental and Clinical Investigation*, **3**, 156–61.

Zhou, J., Liyanage, U., Medina, M., *et al.* (1997). Presenilin 1 interaction in the brain with a novel member of the Armadillo family. *Neuroreport*, **8**, 2085–90.

Zlokovic, B. V., Ghiso, J., Mackic, J. B., *et al.* (1993). Blood-brain barrier transport of circulating Alzheimer's amyloid beta. *Biochemical. and Biophysical Research. Communications*, **197**, 1034–40.

Chapter 5

The molecular basis of tau protein pathology in Alzheimer's disease and related neurodegenerative dementias

Claude M. Wischik, Franz Theuring, and
Charles R. Harrington

5.1 Introduction

Alzheimer discovered flame-shaped fibrillary structures (neurofibrillary tangles: NFT) in about a quarter of the large cortico-cortical association neurons (pyramidal cells) in a 51-year-old woman who presented with a paranoid syndrome and progressed rapidly to severe cognitive deterioration and death over a period of $4\frac{1}{2}$ years (Alzheimer 1907). These lesions were revealed by a silver staining technique that was developed by Bielschowsky, variations of which remain in use by neuropathologists today. Essentially the same pathology can be revealed immunohistochemically by antibodies directed against the microtubule-associated protein tau. Figure 5.1 shows such a preparation using the monoclonal antibody 6.423 (mAb 423) which recognizes a C-terminally truncated form of tau protein. The tau protein pathology encompasses NFT, neuritic plaques, and dystrophic neurites.

Tau protein pathology is therefore a prominent and defining histological feature of the Alzheimer's disease (AD) phenotype, regardless of fundamental aetiology. The recent discovery that a range of primary mutations in the *TAU* gene cause dementing syndromes with histological features overlapping with AD simply reinforces the strong correlations between tau pathology and dementia which have been known for many years. A revised view of molecular pathogenesis must increasingly acknowledge that altered processing of the amyloid β-protein precursor (APP) represents one, but not necessarily the only or even the most important cause, of a characteristic abnormality in the processing of tau protein which leads to the dementia of AD (Fig. 5.2).

In this chapter, we review the structural and biochemical basis of the tau pathology in AD and discuss the recently discovered mutations in tau that cause frontotemporal dementias and related disorders (Sections 5.2–5.7). Although mutations in the *TAU* gene have not been reported for AD, mutations in APP and the presenilin proteins are still the pathogenic cause of a small proportion of the total number of AD cases. It is necessary, therefore, to determine how such mutations and other non-genetic factors impinge on the genesis of tau

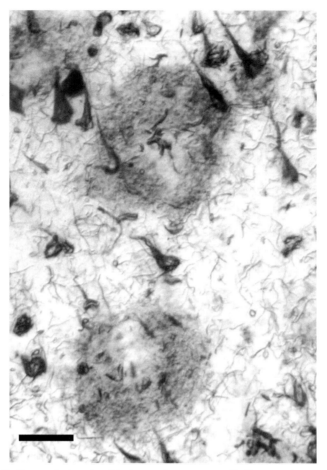

Fig. 5.1 Neurofibrillary pathology in Alzheimer's disease. Neurofibrillary tangles, dystrophic neurites throughout the neuropil and neuritic plaques, are all sites at which PHFs accumulate. Here they are shown by immunohistochemistry, using mAb 423 that recognises PHF-tau protein that has been truncated by endogenous proteases at position Glu-391. Scale bar, 50 μm

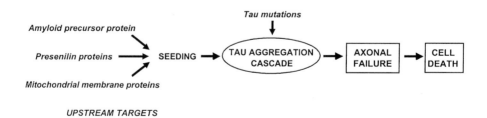

Fig. 5.2 Tau aggregation as a central process in neurodegeneration. Tau aggregation is a proximal process prior to failure of axonal transport and consequent neuronal death. The tau aggregation cascade can be triggered either by a seeding/nucleation event arising from upstream changes or from primary mutations in the tau gene.

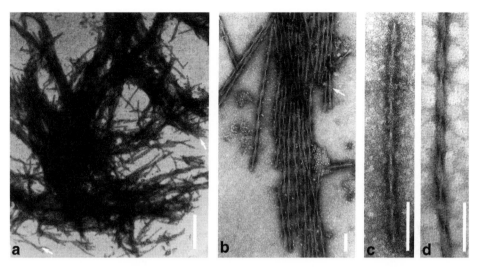

Fig. 5.3 Neurofibrillary tangles and PHFs. A single neurofibrillary tangle (a) and its constituent PHFs (b-d) visualized by electronmicroscopy. PHFs isolated without an exogenous protease digestion step retain a fuzzy outer coat (c) that is removed by proteases (d). Scale bars: 1 µm (a); 100 nm (b–d).

pathology in order to prevent symptoms of dementia. In Sections 5.9–5.14, we discuss the modifications that occur in tau protein and the importance of tau–tau interactions and truncation in the development of neurofibrillary pathology. Molecules have been discovered which disrupt this process and these serve as potential therapeutic agents for AD. The detection of biological markers in CSF has yet to provide a diagnostic tool for AD. Recent advances, however, in the measurement of tau and other proteins in CSF are summarized in Section 5.15.

5.2 The neurofibrillary tangles of Alzheimer's disease

Electron microscopical studies of NFT showed that their main structural constituent was an abnormal fibre, which differed in appearance from the normal fibrous constituents of the neuronal cytoplasm (Fig. 5.3). Kidd (1963) observed that there were more of these abnormal fibres inside dystrophic neurites scattered throughout the neuropil than there were in tangles. This morphological impression has been confirmed biochemically in severe cases using techniques which permit the direct measurement of paired helical filament (PHF) content in the brain (Harrington *et al.* 1991; Mukaetova-Ladinska *et al.* 1993; Holzer *et al.* 1994;). Thus, the unifying feature of neurofibrillary pathology is the presence of the same pathological 'neurofibres' or PHFs in tangles, in neuritic plaques, in dystrophic neurites throughout the neuropil, and in neuritic plaques (Braak *et al.* 1986, 1988).

Early attempts to determine the ultrastructure of the PHF using electron microscopy of embedded sections stained with heavy metals were limited by the quality of resolution attainable (Wischik *et al.* 1995c). Better resolution was achieved by negative staining of PHFs, which had been isolated from the brain (Crowther *et al.* 1985; Wischik *et al.* 1985) (Fig. 5.3). A single isolated tangle consists of a dense whirl of PHFs (Fig. 5.3a). When viewed

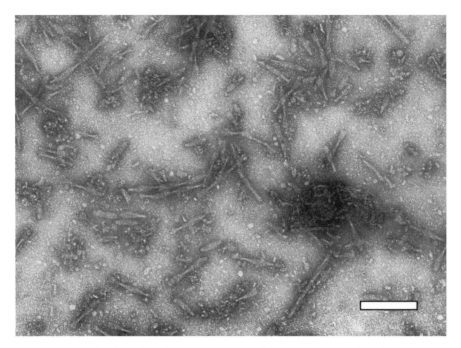

Fig. 5.4 Proteolytically stable PHF fragments. Fragmentation, as a result of sonication, occurs transversely and there is no indication of extended molecules underlying the axial striation pattern. Scale bar: 200 nm.

at higher magnification, the PHF has a clear helical morphology with a characteristic modulation in the transverse diameter with a periodicity of ~80 nm (Fig. 5.3b). This axial periodicity is variable, ranging from 60 nm at one extreme to almost complete flattening and loss of modulation at the other. The transverse diameter varies from 7 nm at the narrowest part to 19 nm at the widest. PHFs fragment at random intervals, with no evidence of a favoured longitudinal unit. Short fragments can be found in all PHF preparations, although their apparent contribution to the preparation can be enhanced by initial selection of low-speed supernatant fractions (Rubenstein *et al.* 1986; Lee *et al.* 1991; Goedert *et al.* 1992*b*; Greenberg *et al.* 1990). Conversely, bulk PHF preparations can be converted into short fragments by sonication (Fig. 5.4).

The presence of these short fragments has led to speculations about different classes of PHFs in extracts from AD brain tissues, some 'soluble' and some 'resistant'. Although some PHFs appear to be more resistant to chemical degradation, fragmented PHFs isolated on the basis of low sedimentation velocity and insolubility in 1% sarkosyl are no less proteolytically stable than PHFs isolated from fractions which initially sediment with higher velocity (Wischik *et al.* 1995*a*).

PHFs consist of two structurally distinct parts. There is an external fuzzy region (Fig. 5.3c) which can be removed by proteases, leaving behind a proteolytically stable core which has smoother outlines, but retains the characteristic structural features of the PHF (Fig. 5.3d). The mean mass of the core PHF is relatively homogenenous, at ~65 kDa/nm. The mass of PHFs with an intact fuzzy coat is variable, with the majority having a mass of ~77 kDa/nm, and minor species (approximately 10%) having a mass as high as 104 kDa/nm.

For the majority of PHFs isolated from the brain, the core therefore accounts for ~85% of the mass of the filament, with a variable addition of fuzzy coat material which contributes, maximally, ~ 40 kDa/nm (Wischik *et al.* 1997).

The characteristic transverse and axial fragmentation patterns, and morphology of untwisted PHFs, indicate that the PHF is a double helical stack of transversely oriented subunits each of limited axial extent, giving the overall shape of a ribbon twisted into a left-handed helix. There are regularly repeating 3/4 longitudinal striations, suggesting the presence of two C-shaped subunits, each containing three domains. Image reconstruction of macromolecular assemblies confirmed the presence of three domains within the C-shaped transverse features with a large central cleft. From data on the longitudinal fragmentation patterns, it is likely that when the two halves of a PHF separate, the cleavage occurs in the region of contact between the C-shaped features (Fig. 5.5) rather than this cleft repre-

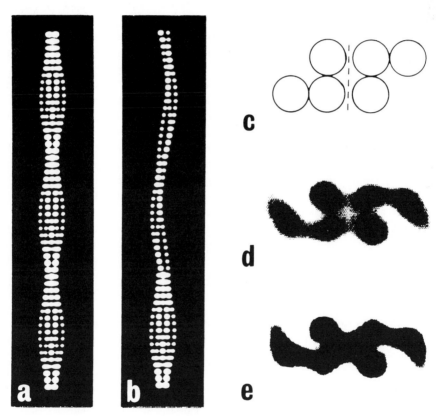

Fig. 5.5 Subunit composition of the PHF. The PHF is a left-handed helical ribbon consisting of two symmetrical C-shaped subunits each containing 3 domains (c–e). In the course of the helical rotation, superimposition produces an impression of 3 or 4 longitudinal elements as shown in (a). 'Straight filaments' are structural variants in which the same C-shaped subunits are joined base-to-base, along the longer side of the 'C', rather than back-to-back as in the standard PHF. This gives lower aspect ratio, with the transverse breadth of the filament more comparable to its depth.

senting a subunit boundary. The so-called 'straight filament' variant of the PHF, has a lower aspect and a lower transverse diameter of 15 nm (that is, the transverse breadth of the filament is more comparable to its depth than in the standard PHF) (Crowther 1991).

5.3 'PHF-tau' and tau content of PHFs

5.3.1 Biochemical and ultrastructural analyses

Immunohistochemical studies demonstrated that NFT contain neurofilament proteins, vimentin, actin, ubiquitin, MAP2, tau, and β-amyloid (see review Wischik 1989). Isolated PHFs could be immunodecorated with antibodies against MAP2, neurofilament, ubiquitin, and tau. Antibodies raised against PHF preparations included those with reactivity against tau, MAP2, and β-amyloid. Biochemical studies of isolated PHFs showed that many of the immunological ambiguities arising from histological studies of tangles could be resolved by removing a fuzzy coat that surrounds the PHF-core (Wischik *et al.* 1988a). The PHF-core lacks immunoreactivity for many of the proteins which had been claimed as tangle/PHF constituents on immunohistochemical grounds, including the N-terminal half of the tau molecule (Wischik *et al.* 1988a). A protocol was developed for preparing a highly enriched PHF-core preparation. Acid treatment was found to release an essentially pure preparation of a 12-kDa protein. This protein was labelled by mAb 423, as were PHFs isolated in the presence or absence of exogenous proteases (Novak *et al.* 1993). Sequence analysis of this protein showed that it was derived from the tandem repeat region of the microtubule-associated protein tau. This established that tau protein represents at least one constituent of the core structure of the PHF (Wischik *et al.* 1988a).

Human tau protein in the CNS exists in 6 isoforms, ranging from 352–441 amino acids in length, that are derived by alternative mRNA splicing from a single gene located on chromosome 17q21-q22 (Fig. 5.6). Each isoform contains either 3- or 4- tandem repeats of 31- or 32- amino acids located in the C-terminal half of the molecule. The repeats are rich in basic amino acids and capable of binding to an acidic domain of tubulin (Fig. 5.7). The extra repeat in the 4-repeat isoform is inserted within the first repeat in a way that preserves the periodic pattern. Similar microtubule-binding repeats are found in the carboxy-terminal domain of high molecular weight microtubule associated proteins, MAP2 and MAP-U (Goedert *et al.* 1988,1989a, b). The 12-kDa tau peptides, derived from the PHF core, originate from the tandem repeat region of both 3- and 4-repeat isoforms (Jakes *et al.* 1991; Fig. 5.8).

Although PHFs isolated without protease digestion can be immunolabelled by tau antibodies directed against epitopes located in the N-terminal half of the molecule, this immunoreactivity is lost after proteolytic removal of the fuzzy coat (Wischik *et al.* 1988a, b). Further biochemical and immunochemical studies of PHF-core preparations have failed to reveal any amino acid sequence or immunoreactivity derived from the N-terminal half of the molecule (Caputo *et al.* 1992b). The N-terminus is rich in acidic amino acid residues and interacts with the plasma membrane (Brandt *et al.* 1995). Furthermore, the N-terminal half of the tau molecule can be removed proteolytically from the fuzzy coat without affecting the structural integrity of the PHF or the characteristic ultrastructural features of the core (Wischik *et al.* 1988b). Thus, the only tau fragments isolated from the proteolytically stable core of the PHF originate from the tandem repeat region. The N-terminal half of the

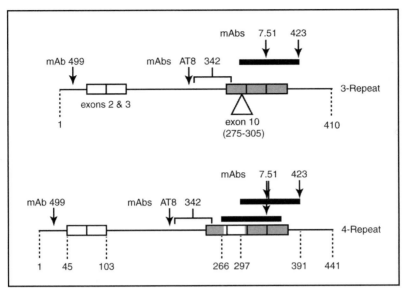

Fig. 5.6 Tau protein isoforms. Six isoforms arise due to alternative splicing of three exons (2, 3, and 10). Inclusion of exon 10 within the tandem repeat region gives rise to 4-repeat isoforms. Exons 2 and 3 encode for adjacent segments within the N-terminus. Two of the six isoforms are shown, each containing both the N-terminal inserts; the other four isoforms lack one or both of these. The 10-kDa fragment isolated from the proteolytically stable core of the PHF was found to correspond to fragments of tau derived from the tandem repeat regions of both 3- and 4-repeat isoforms (black bars). The approximate locations of the epitopes of several monoclonal antibodies are also shown. mAb 499 recognizes a human-specific epitope between Gly-14 and Gln-26 near the N-terminus of the molecule. mAb AT8 recognizes a phosphorylation-dependent epitope at Ser-199/202. mAb 342 recognizes a segment between Ser-208 and Pro-251. mAb 7.51 recognizes an epitope in the last repeat which undergoes acid-reversible occlusion when tau is in the assembled configuration in the PHF. mAb 423 recognizes a characteristic C-terminal truncation at Glu-391 in the core PHF-tau fragment.

tau molecule is located entirely in the fuzzy outer coat of the PHF, and makes no structural contribution to the repeating C-shaped structural subunits of the PHF core.

It is possible to deduce the relative contributions of tau protein to the core and the fuzzy coat of the PHF by relating these biochemical and immunochemical observations to the scanning transmission electron microscope (STEM) measurements of PHF mass referred to above. The mean molecular mass of the protease-resistant core of the PHF is 65.2 ± 0.7 kDa/nm (Wischik *et al.* 1988*b*). The only tau species identified after extensive biochemical (Jakes *et al.* 1991; Wischik *et al.* 1988*a*) and immunochemical (Caputo *et al.* 1992*b*) analyses of such PHF-core preparations are tau fragments. These have a predicted mass of ~10 kDa, with a variable contribution of fragments from the extreme C-terminus of the tau molecule. If the PHF-core mass is to be accounted for entirely by tau, there must be 6 or 7

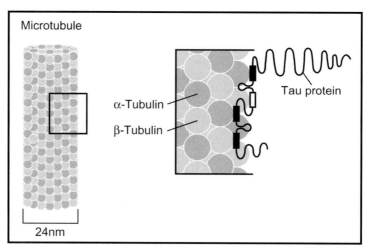

Fig. 5.7 Tau protein and microtubules. Microtubules consist of α- and β-tubulin subunits. Tau binds to tubulin through the binding domains in the 3- or 4-tandem repeats and helps in the assembly and stabilization of the neuronal, microtubular cytoskeleton.

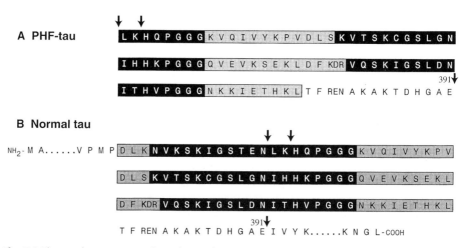

Fig. 5.8 The tandem repeat region of tau. The segments shown in black are the tubulin-binding segments, and those shown in grey are flexible linker segments. The vertical arrows show the N- and C-terminal boundaries of the tau fragments from the 3-repeat isoform found within the proteolytically stable core of the PHF. There is an alternative phasing of the repeat region in core PHF-tau (A) which is shifted by half a repeat (15 residues) relative to that shown in normal tau (B). The core PHF-tau fragment extends by the equivalent of half a repeat, to Glu-391. The net effect of the phase shift is the apparent replacement of the linker segments (grey) by the tubulin-binding segments (black).

tandem-repeat fragments per nm to account for the observed mass. The N-terminal domain of tau, found only in the fuzzy outer coat of the PHF and removed during Pronase digestion, has a predicted mass in excess of 24 kDa. If each of the core tau fragments were to extend to the N-terminus in the intact PHF, this would add a further 6×24 kDa/nm (144 kDa/nm), and the predicted mass of the intact PHF would therefore exceed 209 (65 + 144) kDa/nm. As discussed above, the maximum measured mass of the fuzzy coat is ~ 45 kDa/nm, equivalent to the N-terminal domains from, at most, two tau molecules per nm. However, most PHFs isolated without exogenous proteases have much lower fuzzy coat mass, equivalent to one N-terminal tau domain every 2 nm. The mass data for intact PHFs imply that, if tau were the sole constituent of the PHF, most of the tau molecules that contribute to its structure must have undergone N-terminal truncation. Fewer than 1 or 2 tau molecules in 7 that contribute to the PHF extend to the N-terminus. If tau is the sole constituent of the PHF, most of this must be in a truncated form (Fig. 5.9c).

5.3.2 **Immunochemical analyses**

Amongst evidence to support the presence of truncated tau within most PHFs in the brain is a recent study which compared three different measures of tau protein in the PHF preparation isolated from an initial low-speed supernatant on the basis of insolubility in 1% sarkosyl (Wischik *et al.* 1995*a*). PHFs in this preparation, variously referred to as 'soluble PHFs', 'dispersed PHFs' or 'A68-PHFs', are composed of full-length hyperphosphorylated tau protein (Greenberg and Davies 1990; Lee *et al.* 1991; Goedert *et al.* 1992*b*). Although tau proteins are a minor constituent of the SDS-soluble species present in this material, these can be visualized selectively by immunoblot using antibodies which recognize phosphorylated forms of tau protein as a characteristic triplet of bands of gel mobility 60, 64, and 68 kDa, the so-called 'A68-proteins'. However, determining the proportion of PHF-bound tau protein in this preparation, which contains a hyperphosphorylated N-terminal domain, requires not only the measurement of phosphorylated tau, but also a method which would permit total PHF-tau to be measured irrespective of its state of phosphorylation. No relevant quantitative statement, therefore, can be made from measurement of phosphorylated tau content alone.

Total tau protein, bound in a PHF-like configuration, can be measured by an antibody (mAb 7.51) which detects a generic tau epitope located in the tandem repeat region. The epitope is located within the sequence 350–368 (Fig. 5.6). This antibody can detect PHF-bound tau only after the epitope has been revealed by acid treatment of the preparation (Harrington *et al.* 1990, 1991). Normal soluble tau, on the other hand, is detected by this antibody without acid treatment. Measurements of PHF-bound tau protein using either acid-dependent mAb 7.51 immunoreactivity, or mAb 423 reactivity, are highly correlated with each other.

SDS-soluble phosphorylated tau protein in the sarkosyl-insoluble preparation was first measured by densitometry of immunoblots developed with a phosphorylation-dependent anti-tau antibody (mAb AT8), a method frequently claimed to measure PHF-content in AD brain tissues. This was compared both with measurement of mAb AT8 immunoreactivity by competitive immunoassay in the sarkosyl preparation, and with protease-resistant PHF-content measured by mAb 423 immunoreactivity in the if-II preparation (Harrington *et al.* 1994*b*; Wischik *et al.* 1995*a*). The immunoblot data from the sarkosyl preparation was

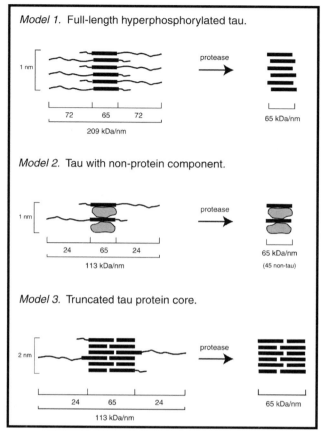

Fig. 5.9 The composition of PHFs. Three models can be proposed to explain the composition of PHFs and these are represented schematically. In model 1, PHFs are composed of intact, full-length tau molecules. In model 2, an unidentified, non-protein component would account for a substantial proportion of the PHF mass. Finally, in model 3, a PHF built up with truncated tau in the core, contains occasional molecules with full-length N-termini. Following extensive proteolysis, the resistant structure remaining has an observed mass of 65 kDa/nm. Based upon ultrastructural, biochemical, and immunochemical analyses described in the text, the third model remains the only one that is consistent with the data. The only tau species isolated from the proteolytically stable core of the PHF correspond to the phase-shifted core PHF-tau fragments from the tandem repeat region. If tau protein is the sole or major constituent of the PHF-core, the observed mass of ~ 65 kDa/nm must be accounted for by ~ 6 core PHF-tau fragments per nm. If each of these were to be N-terminally intact in PHFs which retain the fuzzy coat, the mass of the fuzzy coat would have to exceed 6 × 24 kDa/nm, as the N-terminal half of the tau molecule has a predicted mass of ~ 24 kDa. However, even for the highest mass PHFs isolated without exogenous proteases, the mass of the fuzzy coat is no more than 45 kDa/nm, and for the majority of PHFs is 15–30 kDa/nm. Therefore, only 1 in 7 of the tau molecules that make up the PHFs and which retain N-terminal tau immunoreactivity extends to the N-terminus.

found to correlate neither with the mAb AT8 immunoreactivity, as determined by immunoassay assay using the same sarkosyl preparation, nor with PHF-content determined by mAb 423 immunoreactivity. However, the immunoassay measure of mAb AT8 immunoreactivity was significantly correlated with PHF content. Therefore, the SDS-solubility of phosphorylated tau species released from the sarkosyl preparation is not quantitative, and cannot be used to determine the tau composition of PHFs in the sarkosyl preparation (Wischik *et al.* 1995*a*).

It is possible, however, to determine how much of the total tau protein in either the sarkosyl or the if-II PHF preparations is phosphorylated by comparing acid-dependent mAb 7.51 and mAb AT8 immunoreactivity in a large number of preparations (Wischik *et al.* 1995*a*). Both parameters increase in parallel with the tangle count in the corresponding brain tissues. In the if-II preparation, phosphorylated tau accounts for less than 5% of total PHF-bound tau at any stage of pathology, including those stages that immediately precede the appearance of NFT. Similar studies undertaken in the sarkosyl preparation again show that both parameters increase in parallel with tangle count, but in this preparation, the phosphorylated tau protein accounts for some 14% of total PHF-bound tau (Lai *et al.* 1995; Wischik *et al.* 1995*a*).

As the sarkosyl preparation contains no N-terminally intact tau protein which is not hyperphosphorylated, the estimate of 14% also provides a measure of total N-terminally intact tau in this preparation. This estimate agrees very closely with model 3 depicted in Fig. 5.9, based on an independent body of evidence relating to biochemical analysis and mass measurements of PHFs. If tau protein is the main constituent of the PHF (and even this has not been proven), then only 1 in 7 of the tau molecules which are incorporated into PHFs is either N-terminally intact or hyperphosphorylated, that is 'PHF-tau'. The remaining tau molecules that make up the core structure of the PHF must be truncated, even in PHFs, which retain N-terminally intact tau in the fuzzy outer coat. Nevertheless, immunochemical measures of 'PHF-tau' are highly correlated with the brain content of PHFs (Lai *et al.* 1995). Although the literature continues to refer to PHFs as being composed entirely of 'PHF-tau' (that is full-length phosphorylated tau, or A68-tau), this is not the case.

5.4 Normal functions of tau protein

The critical functions of neurons as information processing and transfer units depend on characteristic morphological adaptations, typified at the extreme by spinal motor neurones, where the axon can be 1000-fold longer than the diameter of the cell body (Brandt 1998). The cell biology of the cytoskeleton remains a fast-moving research area and only a few points can be highlighted here. The intracellular determinants of morphology are the three filament structures that constitute the neuronal cytoskeleton: microfilaments (made from actin), microtubules (produced from tubulin α/β-dimers), and intermediate filaments (neurofilaments in neurones, composed of 3 proteins). Although these were earlier conceived as discrete structural entities, their interconnections are increasingly being recognized (Klymkowsky 1999). The most obvious example is the 'collapse' of intermediate filament organization following the depolymerization of microtubules, in a process which itself is dependent on microfilaments. The formation of circuitry in the developing nervous system is a process in which neurons initially undergo an exploratory phase, this depends on an actively motile growth cone, followed by consolidation, involving the formation of more stable axons and dendrites. The former depends on the assembly and disassembly of actin filaments in conjunction with actin-based motor proteins (Brandt 1998). Consolidation depends on the assembly of microtubules, regulated by microtubule-associated proteins (MAPs) that stabilize tubulin dimers in the polymerized configuration. Dynamic interactions between the actin and microtubule filament systems also underlie cytoskeletal reorganization occurring within dendritic spines during neurotransmitter receptor activation, contributing the changes in spine shape that participate in memory consolidation (van Rossum *et al.* 1999).

In addition to morphogenesis, microtubules play a critical role in cell division and intracellular trafficking, functions which both depend on establishing polarity at the molecular level, and in which deeper similarities can be discerned (Baas 1999). Microtubules in axons are uniformly oriented with the plus ends facing the axon terminal (that is those ends at which preferential addition of tubulin subunits occurs), whereas the microtubules in dendrites are present in both orientations. In either orientation, microtubules serve as tracks for transport of organelles (synaptic vesicles, endocytotic vesicles, mitochondria, lysosomes, peroxisomes, and phagosomes) via microtubule-dependent motor proteins, such as the plus-end directed motor kinesin and the minus-end directed motor dynein. Kinesin and MAPs are also involved in the alignment of neurofilaments. Overexpression of tau and MAP2 has been shown to suppress organelle movement (Sato-Harada *et al.* 1996), particularly by interfering with the attachment and detachment of organelles to the microtubule tracks. In the presence of excess tau bound to microtubules, there is inhibition of kinesin binding and facilitation of dynein detachment (Trinczek *et al.* 1999), with the effect that mitochondria accumulate near the microtubule-organizing centre, the endoplasmic reticulum (ER) retracts to the periphery and the exocytosis of vesicles is retarded (Ebneth *et al.* 1998). Thus tau has a dual role. At physiological concentrations it stabilizes microtubules as tracks for intracellular transport, but in excess it interferes with transport down the axon. These findings may have relevance for understanding the movement abnormalities seen in mice overexpressing human tau protein (Ishihara *et al.* 1999).

Microtubule stability is regulated by the binding of several types of MAPs, proteins possessing the ability to stimulate tubulin polymerization *in vitro*. MAPs are classified into two groups: neural MAPs and non-neural MAPs. The three important neural MAPs are MAP1A, MAP2, tau, and MAP5 (MAP1B). The main non-neural MAP is MAP4. Tau and MAP2 are characteriztically distributed *in situ*, with tau localized to the axon, and MAP2 in the somatodendritic compartment. A form of MAP2 is present in somatic and germ cells of the rat testis, where its predominant localization is nuclear (Loveland *et al.* 1999). MAP2, MAP5, and tau are expressed early during neuronal differentiation, where axon development coincides with a transition from a MAP2-actin filament interaction to a predominant MAP2-microtubule interaction, with preferential binding of tau to the distal axon (Kwei *et al.* 1998).

The view that tau is essential for determining axonal identity, stability, and function was based on several lines of evidence. First, the close temporal correlation between the expression of tau, microtubule assembly and axon extension (Drubin *et al.* 1985); and second, results from anti-sense experiments which showed that tau is essential for the establishment of axonal polarity (Caceres *et al.* 1990, 1991, 1992). This view has had to be revised following the surprising observation that mice lacking the *tau* gene are entirely viable and show only minor axonal abnormalities (Harada *et al.* 1994). *In vitro*, the principal effect of tau is to stabilize microtubules by reducing the frequency of rapid shrinkage ('catastrophe') and promoting the transition back to the growing phase ('rescue') (Bre *et al.* 1990; Pryer *et al.* 1992; Itoh *et al.* 1998). Within living cells, overexpression of MAP2 and tau leads to increased microtubule rigidity, and a paradoxical increase in the stability of microtubules while preserving their dynamic properties (capacity for catastrophe and rescue) (Kaech *et al.* 1996). Cells microinjected with anti-tau antibodies prior to the extension of axons showed no detectable effects on the dynamics of axonal microtubules (Tint *et al.* 1998). In developing neurones, tau functions in the terminal axon and growth cone appear to pre-dominate.

5.5 **Tau protein and dementia in Alzheimer's disease**

The density of NFT is closely linked to intellectual status before death (Wilcock and Esiri 1982; Duyckaerts *et al.* 1987; Delaère *et al.* 1989, 1990, 1991; McKee *et al.* 1991; Arriagada *et al.* 1992*b*; Nagy *et al.* 1995; Giannakopoulos *et al.* 1997). The link is stronger than that found with the density of Aβ deposits, although the latter correlation can be improved by measuring the 'amyloid load' or the area occupied by Aβ deposits in the neocortex (Cummings *et al.* 1995). Deposition of diffuse amyloid can be extensive in intellectually normal elderly cases (Giannakopoulos *et al.* 1997); however, there are no reports of preservation of normal cognitive functioning in the presence of numerous neocortical tangles. 'Plaque only' arose during efforts to define neuropathological criteria for AD in terms of age-related Aβ plaque counts. This concept is now explained better in terms of either abundant Lewy bodies (Hansen *et al.* 1993) or extensive tau pathology occurring in the absence of NFT (Mukaetova-Ladinska *et al.* 1992). Neuritic plaque densities tend to correlate better both with the biochemical measure of PHF-burden (see below), and also with cognitive dysfunction. Other studies confirm that Aβ load does not predict neuronal loss (Gómez-Isla *et al.* 1997), synapse loss (Terry *et al.* 1991), or dementia (Gómez-Isla *et al.* 1997). Furthermore, there is considerable overlap in the levels of Aβ deposition found in AD and non-demented patients (Harrington *et al.* 1994*a*) that is not the case for the accumulation of PHFs (Mukaetova-Ladinska *et al.* 1993). The PHF content in AD tissue is 19-fold greater than that found in control tissue, and the difference is even greater in brain regions such as temporal cortex (Fig. 5.10a). The accumulation of PHFs is accompanied by a corresponding loss of normal soluble tau, in excess of that found in normal ageing (Mukaetova-Ladinska *et al.* 1996). In contrast, the levels of Aβ in nearly half of the cases of AD are found to overlap the levels found in controls, regardless of *APOE* genotype (Fig. 5.10b). These findings argue against the hypothesis that Aβ deposition induces a direct toxic effect on neurons in the human brain.

The relationship between dementia and neurofibrillary degeneration is being refined further, and will provide an explanatory basis for those complexities of clinical presentation that are obscured by relatively crude global measures of dementia. For example, in a recent study of apraxia, tangle densities in the anterior cingulate cortex were found to predict ideomotor and dressing apraxia, whereas tangle densities in the posterior neocortex (superior parietal, occipital and posterior cingulate) were correlated with constructional apraxia (Giannakopoulos *et al.* 1998).

The evaluation of tau pathology in the brain has been helped by the introduction of the stageing method proposed by Braak (Braak and Braak 1991) (Fig. 5.11). The first two stages

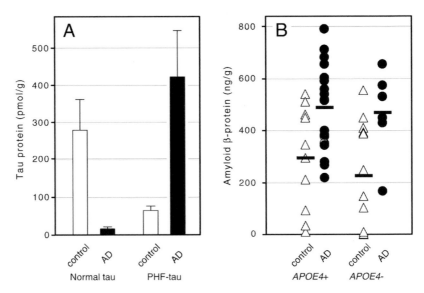

Fig. 5.10 Distribution of tau protein and amyloid β-protein in brain tissue. (A) Tau protein accumulates in AD in hippocampus and neocortical areas with concomitant loss of normal soluble tau when compared with non-demented controls (Mukaetova-Ladinska *et al.* 1993). *APOE* genotype does not affect the distribution of tau (Harrington *et al.* 1994). (B) Although insoluble Aβ protein accumulates in AD tissue, there is considerable overlap of individual cases with controls, regardless of whether *APOE* genotype is taken into account (Harrington *et al.* 1994)

are characterized by the presence of tau pathology in layer II of the transentorhinal cortex, occasional pathology in CA1 of hippocampus, and none in neocortical regions. Stages 3 and 4 (limbic stages) are characterized by more severe pathology in transentorhinal and entorhinal cortices, CA1, amygdala, and early pathology in temporal association neocortex. In the isocortical stages (5 and 6), there is extensive pathology in all neocortical association areas and also in the primary sensory areas such as striate cortex.

The stageing method in practice requires the use of only two brain sections (one at the level of the entorhinal cortex and the second from the striate area). The validity of the stageing system, which represents a qualitative judgement, depends on an underlying quantitative principle that progression of pathology can be described systematically in two dimensions: number of regions affected and density of pathology in affected regions. There are three possible correlations which empirically test the validity of the concept: stage *vs.* global tangle count, stage *vs.* number of regions affected, and global tangle count *vs.* number of regions affected. All three correlations are highly significant statistically (Gertz *et al.* 1998). Furthermore, 90% of a prospectively studied series of cases conformed to the expected neuroanatomical hierarchy of vulnerability to pathology, provided two order violations or less were tolerated. That is, the regional hierarchy is a reasonable, but not absolute, approximation to the qualitative anatomical progression of pathology that is linked in a stereotyped manner with global pathological load in the brain.

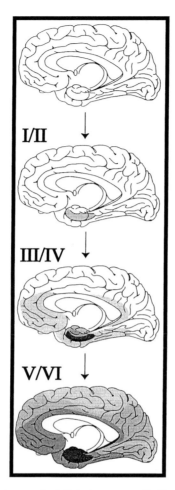

Fig. 5.11 Neuroanatomical development of Alzheimer neurofibrillary pathology. The staging method, introduced by Braak and Braak (1991), is based upon the spread of neurofibrillary pathology from the transentorhinal cortex and hippocampus (stages I/II) to the temporal association cortex and amygdala (stages III/IV) and, finally, most neocortical association areas (stages V/VI).

The existence of this stereotyped hierarchy presents difficulties in formulating a simplistic anatomical theory of the pathophysiology of 'clinical dementia'. Paradoxically, this is due to the validity of the hierarchical model itself, because it carries with it the implication that advanced pathology in medial temporal lobe structures is necessarily associated with the early appearance of pathology in neocortex. The question then arises as to whether the transition to overt clinical dementia is to be explained by cortical pathology *per se*, or by the fact that this is simply a statistical marker of severe neurodegeneration in medial temporal lobe structures. The role for the disconnection of the medial temporal lobe from neocortical association areas via neuronal destruction as the direct anatomical substrate for memory impairment and dementia has been emphasized by some (Van Hoesen *et al.* 1990). Thus,

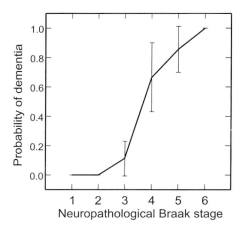

Fig. 5.12 Dementia according to Braak stage. Frequency of clinical dementia by DSMIV criteria in the 12 months prior to death is plotted against neuropathological stage post-mortem according to the criteria of Braak and Braak (1991). If cases with any evidence whatsoever of vascular pathology are excluded, there is a robust relationship between the transition from stage 3 to stage 4 and the appearance of clinical dementia, with fewer than 15% of cases wrongly classified.

AD patients with very mild cognitive impairment were found to have more than 50% neuronal loss in layer II of the entorhinal cortex (Arriagada *et al.* 1992*a*).

Pathology in the medial temporal lobe structures is widespread in the cognitively normal ageing population (see below) and there is a progressive increase in the probability of clinical dementia with advancing Braak stage (Fig. 5.12). However, this remains a probability rather than a diagnostic statement. Although the transition from stage 3 to stage 4 is associated in a statistically significant manner with the appearance of clinical dementia, there is considerable overlap (Gertz *et al.* 1996). In a recent study of 59 cognitively normal people of mean age 84, 15 (25%) were found to be at stage 4 or beyond, and 6 (10%) of these were at stages 5 or 6 (Davis *et al.* 1999*a*). In another study, tangles were found to present in hippocampus and entorhinal cortex in more than 94% of an elderly cohort of mean age 86 (Haroutunian *et al.* 1999). Furthermore, the tangle density in entorhinal cortex of more than half of the subjects who were normal on the Clinical Dementia Rating Scale was rated as moderate or severe. This represents the most recent restatement of a well established clinico-pathological finding (Wilcock and Esiri 1982; Crystal *et al.* 1988; Price *et al.* 1991; Bouras *et al.* 1993; Giannakopoulos *et al.* 1995; Khachaturian 1995; Gómez-Isla *et al.* 1996), and indicates that tangles appear to be reasonably well tolerated in medial temporal lobe structures without clinical evidence of impairment.

The total number of brain regions with at least one tangle, or the 'diffusion index', was found to be more highly correlated ($r = 0.93$) with the Blessed Test Score than measures of the total 'tangle burden' (Duyckaerts *et al.* 1997). However, this parameter may represent a surrogate for both Braak stage and global burden of neurofibrillary pathology. The strong correlation with the diffusion index suggests that even a few tangles in a given cortical region is associated with a significant functional deficit and that the appearance of a tangle is a late event in a more generalized disturbance of functional activity (Salehi *et al.* 1995).

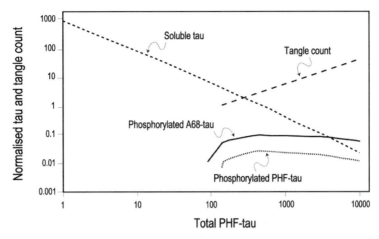

Fig. 5.13 Redistribution of tau species in AD. The relative changes in various tau pools, as a proportion of total PHF-tau, are shown during disease progression. The data show that the redistribution of soluble tau into PHFs precedes the first appearance of phosphorylated tau species, and also precedes the appearance of neurofibrillary tangles (Lai *et al.* 1995). Tangles appear at the point when the PHF-tau and soluble tau pools are approximately equivalent; presumably the point at which cytoskeletal transport can no longer be maintained.

The molecular basis of this can be understood better from studies relating the number of NFT to direct biochemical measurements of PHF accumulation and loss of normal soluble tau protein (Lai *et al.* 1995). The point at which NFT first begin to appear in histological preparations can be defined in terms of the point at which there is, in the corresponding tissue, an approximate equivalence between the total PHF-bound tau pool and the residual free tau pool (Fig. 5.13). The appearance of a single NFT implies that extensive transfer of the normal soluble tau pool into PHFs has already occurred, but is not necessarily visible histologically. This probably indicates a critical threshold for failure of normal cytoskeletal transport. The cytoplasmic volume of the neuronal processes of pyramidal cells exceeds the volume of the cell body by at least 10-fold, and perhaps by as much as 40-fold (Blinkov *et al.* 1968). The point at which PHFs begin to accumulate visibly in the cell soma is one at which either transport into processes has failed, or at which the capacity of neuronal processes to absorb PHFs has been exceeded. Either way, the appearance of a single tangle in a given brain tissue is already a late event in terms of redistribution of the normal tau protein pool into PHFs, and indicates an advanced state of failure of systems essential for cortico-cortical connectivity.

In regard to the question of the relationship between tangles, dementia, and neuronal loss, there is a direct correlation between neurofibrillary pathology and loss of neurons in CA1 of hippocampus (Bondareff *et al.* 1993), in the hippocampus (Bobinski *et al.* 1997), and superior temporal sulcus (Gómez-Isla *et al.* 1997). However, the extent of neuronal loss exceeds NFT count by a factor of 7-fold (Gómez-Isla *et al.* 1997), leading the authors to conclude that most neuronal loss in advanced AD occurs through non-Aβ and non-tangle mechanisms. Attempts to model the relationships between tangle count and neuronal loss in CA1 has lead other workers to conclude that tangle formation is not obligatory for cell death (Morsch *et al.* 1999).

Even if the tangle itself were an epiphenomenon, it would not follow that the aggregation of tau protein is irrelevant to cell death or dysfunction. The tangle count in a given tissue provides only an indirect measure of the balance between PHF assembly and loss of normal tau occurring in brain tissue. The relationships between PHF assembly, tangle count, and tau loss are non-linear. At the stage of relatively modest neurofibrillary pathology, as measured by tangle count, there is already very extensive loss of soluble tau. For example, soluble tau levels have already decreased by half when tangle formation has reached only 3% of maximum. It is not known how much loss of normal tau can be tolerated in the ageing brain before neuronal function is terminally compromised. Furthermore, the toxicity of early tau aggregates (proto-filaments, in amyloid terminology, see below) has yet to be addressed.

Tau pathology is strongly linked with loss of synapses. Loss of synapses may provide a better correlate of cognitive deficit than NFT; when comparing tangles and Aβ plaques, Terry and colleagues (1991) found that only tau pathology was associated with synapse loss. Others have confirmed these findings (DeKosky *et al.* 1990; Price *et al.* 1991; White *et al.* 1995). More recently, the extent of synapse loss has been found to be as great in 'Lewy body variant' cases as in AD, but in the former synapse loss is not linked to tau pathology (Brown *et al.* 1998). This may imply that in dementia with Lewy bodies, synapse and neuronal loss are mediated by different mechanisms (Harrington *et al.* 1994*a*).

The relationship between tau pathology and cholinergic dysfunction has been subject to more extensive analysis. Loss of cholinergic activity is more severe in temporal cortex than in primary sensory areas such as visual cortex, a similar pattern to that of the tau pathology (Davies 1979; Rossor *et al.* 1980; Rossor *et al.* 1982; Wilcock *et al.* 1982; Henke and Lang 1983; Reinikainen *et al.* 1988). Cholinergic loss was correlated with 'senile plaques' and/or tangles in some reports (Perry *et al.* 1978, 1981; Wilcock *et al.* 1982; Mountjoy *et al.* 1984; Zubenko *et al.* 1989) but not others (Wilcock *et al.* 1982; Brashear *et al.* 1988; Zubenko *et al.* 1989; DeKosky *et al.* 1992; Ransmayr *et al.* 1992). Some of these discrepancies can be resolved by direct biochemical measurement of PHF accumulation. There is a strong correlation, both in terms of quantity and regional pattern of loss, between choline acetyltransferase activity and level of insoluble phosphorylated tau in neocortical areas, hippocampus and nucleus basalis of Meynert (nbM) (Arendt *et al.* 1999). Although these findings strongly link the cholinergic deficit with tau pathology, the causative mechanism remains unclear. Tau pathology in nbM is highly correlated with neocortical tau pathology, but precedes the latter. Therefore, loss of cholinergic activity most probably provides neurotransmitter evidence of tau-mediated functional disconnection of the nbM from neocortex; that is neocortical cholinergic loss is the consequence of tau pathology in the nbM. Alternatively, aberrant tau-reactive neurites in neocortex are predominantly cholinergic fibres. However, this seems less likely, as PHF content in neocortex is highly correlated with neuritic pathology in neocortex.

5.6 Tau protein in fronto-temporal and other neurodegenerative dementias

5.6.1 Clinicopathological spectrum

Pick originally described a syndrome characterized by progressive aphasia and personality changes over 100 years ago (Pick 1892). The use of the term Pick's disease defines a strict clinico-pathological entity with characteristic argyophyllic inclusions in ballooned neurons

(Pick bodies), originally described by Alzheimer (Alzheimer 1911). Their presence distinguishes a small subset of a broad range of clinical presentations of dementing disorders, that are characterized by varying combinations of behavioral disturbance, cognitive decline, personality change, and progressive language deficit. Unlike AD, episodic memory and visuospatial functions are notably spared until relatively late in the disease (Gustafson 1987; The Lund and Manchester Groups 1994; Miller *et al.* 1997). Indeed 'the relative preservation of spatial orientation and praxis in FTD [is] the single feature that may be most important in distinguishing FTD from AD and vascular dementia' (Wilhelmsen 1997). This broad clinical presentation tends to be covered by the term 'fronto-temporal dementia (FTD)'. The relationship between FTD and Pick's disease as a pure neuropathological entity is unclear, but the latter is increasingly thought to represent a particular histological variant of non-Alzheimer fronto-temporal lobar atrophy (Armstrong *et al.* 1998).

The broad diagnostic distinction with respect to AD would be supported in a given case by the presence of fronto-temporal atrophy demonstrated by computerized tomography (CT) or magnetic resonance imageing (MRI) scan, frontal hypoperfusion on a single photon emission computed tomography (SPECT) scan, and absence of NFT and senile plaques in the neocortex at post-mortem. The histopathology is non-specific, with microvacuolation, gliosis, and neuronal loss (Mann *et al.* 1993*a*, *b*). Atrophy measured during life by MRI scan shows that tissue loss in the entorhinal cortex can be as severe as in AD, but hippocampal atrophy may be less prominent (Frisoni *et al.* 1999).

The only population-based study to date found the prevalence of FTD to vary from 1.2 per million at age 30–40 to 28 per million at age 60–70 (Stevens *et al.* 1998). This should be compared with a prevalence of AD of at least 50 000 per million over the age of 65 (Hofman *et al.* 1991). Although FTD occurs sporadically in ~60% of cases, there is increased familial clustering versus elderly controls (15%), to a level comparable with AD (~30%) (Khachaturian 1995; Baker *et al.* 1997; Heutink *et al.* 1997). The age of onset in first-degree relatives occurs 11 years earlier than dementia in relatives of controls (Stevens *et al.* 1998).

In 1996, a consensus conference agreed the common features of a group of 13 kindreds linked to chromosome 17q21-q22, and characterized in some kindreds by the combination of FTD and parkinsonism (Foster *et al.* 1997). Although clinically and pathologically heterogeneous, common pathological features included variable neuronal loss and gliosis in frontal and temporal cortices and variable involvement of limbic and subcortical structures. This grouping has come to be termed frontotemporal dementia and parkinsonism linked to chromosome 17 or FTDP-17 (Wilhelmsen *et al.* 1994; Petersen *et al.* 1995; Wijker *et al.* 1996; Yamaoka *et al.* 1996; Baker *et al.* 1997; Foster *et al.* 1997; Heutink *et al.* 1997; Murrell *et al.* 1997; Lendon *et al.* 1998; Poorkaj *et al.* 1998; Froelich *et al.* 1999). Several of these cases have been linked to mutations in the *TAU* gene, located on chromosome 17q21-q22 (Clark *et al.* 1998; Dumanchin *et al.* 1998; Hutton *et al.* 1998; Poorkaj *et al.* 1998; Spillantini *et al.* 1998*b*; Bugiani *et al.* 1999; Iijima *et al.* 1999; Rizzu *et al.* 1999). Mutations in the *TAU* gene have been identified in 18% of familial FTD cases, and in 40% of cases with FTD who have a positive family history of dementia of any type (Rizzu *et al.* 1999). Although the frequency of tau mutations in hereditary FTD is relatively high, no mutations in the *TAU* gene have yet been identified in 60% of hereditary FTD cases. There appears to be at least one dementia kindred linked to chromosome-17 in which no mutation in the tau locus has been found and in which there is no immunohistochemical evidence of tau pathology (Rizzu *et al.* 1999).

The clinical spectrum of neurodegenerative syndromes linked to mutations at the *TAU* locus is not restricted to the FTD phenotype. The first two families genetically mapped to 17q21-q22 were called disinhibition-dementia-parkinsonism-amyotrophy complex (DDPAC) and pallido-ponto-nigral degeneration (PPND). The DDPAC presentation is dominated by personality changes, progressing to motor extrapyramidal/parkinsonian features and amyotrophic pyramidal features (atrophic weakness, spasticity, and hyperreflexia). In the PPND phenotype, patients present in their fifth decade with parkinsonism and personality changes, progressing to dementia, ocular dysfunction (supranuclear gaze paresis), dystonia, pyramidal signs, mutism, aphagia, and cachexia.

Progressive supranuclear palsy (PSP), the most common degenerative form of parkinsonism after Parkinson's disease with a prevalence of 14 per million, has also been linked to allelic variation at or near the *TAU* locus (Conrad *et al.* 1998). PSP is characterized by supranuclear down-gaze paresis, akinesia, dystonia, dysarthria, dysphagia, and postural instability, with later progression to dementia. There are numerous NFT in subcortical and brain stem nuclei (including the superior colliculus), in both neurons and glia, with relatively minor involvement of the neocortex. The number of TG repeats between exons 9 and 10 of the *TAU* gene defines five alleles (A0, 11 repeats; A1, 12 repeats; A2, 13 repeats; A3, 14 repeats; A4, 15 repeats). Although 95% of Caucasian PSP subjects are homozygous for the A0 allele (Conrad *et al.* 1997; Higgins *et al.* 1998; Oliva *et al.* 1998), this allele was not over-represented in Japanese PSP patients (Conrad *et al.* 1998). The A0 allele is itself part of a more extensive haplotype (H1), covering ~100 kb of DNA. Nine different polymorphisms, in complete disequilibrium, appear to exist as two different haplotypes and H1 is over-represented in PSP cases (Baker *et al.* 1999). A change in the *TAU* promoter region, that could potentially alter tau expression, further extends the *TAU* haplotype (Ezquerra *et al.* 1999). A common extended haplotype was also found to co-segregate with a PSP phenotype in a small group of unrelated individuals carrying the disease but not in age-matched controls (Higgins *et al.* 1999*a*). The latter haplotype is characterized by a homozygous polymorphism in the 5' splice site UTR of exon 1, two mis-sense mutations in exon 4A (D285N, A289V) and a nonsense mutation in the 5' splice site of exon 8. Such genetic variants may predispose individuals to develop the neurofibrillary pathology of PSP. A significant increase in the A0 allele has since been reported in Parkinson's disease, suggesting an involvement of the *TAU* gene in some cases of PD (Pastor *et al.* 2000). This finding must be replicated to establish whether an association with either dementia or tau deposition exists.

Although a single family with an atypical clinicopathologic form of dominantly inherited PSP has been found with a mis-sense mutation in tau (R406W) (Hutton *et al.* 1998), neither this mutation nor any other exonic mutation in tau is a general feature of PSP (Baker *et al.* 1999; Bonifati *et al.* 1999; Higgins *et al.* 1999*b*). There is no evidence that altered splicing of exon 10 acts as a determinant of 4-repeat tau deposition in NFTs in PSP. An alternative hypothesis is that tau deposition reflects a selective vulnerability of neurons that express only exon 10-positive tau isoforms (Sergeant *et al.* 1999).

Many non-pathogenic polymorphisms have been identified in the *TAU* gene found in both AD and controls (Baker *et al.* 1999; Bonifati *et al.* 1999; Higgins *et al.* 1999*a*). Several of these are located in introns or result in amino acid substitutions in codons not contained in human CNS tau (exons 4A and 6). Others cause substitutions in coding exons 7, 9, and 14 (Fig. 5.14). Studies are needed to determine if and how these polymorphisms might influence AD-related pathology and to understand the expression of tau in disease states

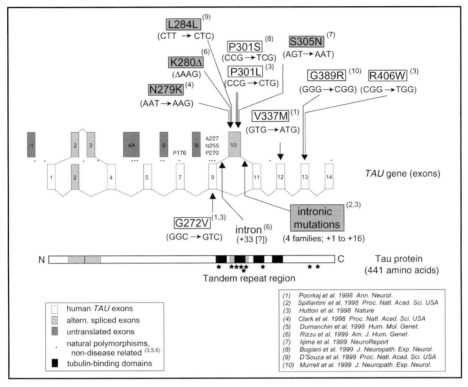

Fig. 5.14 Tau mutations in neurodegenerative diseases. The relative positions of mutations in the *TAU* gene are shown in this schematic figure. Mutations in exons 9 to 13 and in the introns adjoining exon 10 co-segregate with disease in FTD and other related tauopathies. The exon mutations (*) are clustered around the tandem repeat region, with six of these being unique to the 4-repeat tau isoforms. The mutations N279K, L284L, S305N and K280Δ are mutations in exons that affect the splicing of exon 10. The coding sequence is unaltered by the L284L mutation or the intronic mutations.

and in normal ageing. Transcription activity of the *TAU* gene decreases with age (Tohgi *et al.* 1999) and this may account for the decrease in normal tau protein levels that occurs with ageing (Mukaetova-Ladinska *et al.* 1996). A common tau haplotype may interact with *APOE4* to increase the risk of AD in a subgroup of the AD population (that is an early-onset, clinic-based population) (Lilius *et al.* 1999; Bullido *et al.* 2000). However, no such association was found in a sample where the age of onset was high and the *APOE4* frequency was low (Crawford *et al.* 1999; Roks *et al.* 1999).

The relationships between clinical phenotype, neuropathology, and patterns of expression of tau protein are not clear. There has been an attempt to group conditions according to amounts of the 3- or 4-repeat tau isoforms found in crude brain extracts containing insoluble tau (Table 5.1). These patterns do not appear to have any predictive power with respect to clinical phenotype, neuropathology, or filament morphology. Thus AD, which is primarily a dementing condition with relatively minor motor features, as well as post-

Table 5.1 Neurodegenerative syndromes associated with tau protein *

Disorder	Tau mutation	Insoluble tau extract		References
		4 repeat	3 repeat	
Alzheimer's disease	Sporadic	+	++	(Jakes et al. 1991)
Pick's disease	Sporadic	–	++	(Buée-Scherrer et al. 1996; Delacourzte et al. 1996)
	G272V			(Rizzu et al. 1999; Spillantini et al. 1998a)
	G389R	++	++	(Murrell et al. 1999)
DDPAC	Exon 10 splice + 3	++	±	(Clark et al. 1998)
FTDP-17	P301L	++	±	(Baker et al. 1997; Dumanchin et al. 1998;Heutink et al. 1997; Poorkaj et al. 1998; Rizzu et al. 1999; Spillantini et al. 1998a)
	N279K	++	±	(Hasegawa et al. 1999)
	S305N	++	±	(Hasegawa et al. 1999)
	V337M	+	++	(Lanska et al. 1994; Poorkaj et al. 1998; Spillantini et al. 1996; Spillantini et al. 1998a; Sumi et al. 1992)
	G272V			(Baker et al. 1997; Heutink et al. 1997; Poorkaj et al. 1998; Rizzu et al. 1999; Spillantini et al. 1998a)
	K280Δ			(Rizzu et al. 1999)
	Exon 9 splice + 33			(Rizzu et al. 1999)
	Exon 10 splice + 13			(Poorkaj et al. 1998)
	Exon 10 splice + 14			(Petersen et al. 1995; Poorkaj et al. 1998; Sima et al. 1996; Wilhelmsen et al. 1994)
	Exon 10 splice + 16			(Lendon et al. 1998; Poorkaj et al. 1998; Yamaoka et al. 1996)
	Exon 10 splice + 3			(Hutton et al. 1998)
PPND	P301L	++	±	(Clark et al. 1998)
	N279K	++	±	(Clark et al. 1998)

Table 5.1 Neurodegenerative syndromes associated with tau protein*   (continued)

Disorder	Tau mutation	Insoluble tau extract		References
		4 repeat	**3 repeat**	
Progressive supranuclear palsy	Sporadic	++		(Sergeant et al. 1999)
	A0 allele			(Conrad et al. 1997)
Parkinson's disease	Sporadic			
	A0 allele			(Pastor et al. 2000)
Multiple system tauopathy with presenile dementia	Exon 10 splice + 3	++	±	(Spillantini et al. 1998b)
	R406W	++	±	(Sergeant et al. 1999)
Corticobasal degeneration	Sporadic	++	−	(Sergeant et al. 1999)
Frontotemporal dementia & CBD	P301S	++	+	(Bugiani et al. 1999)
Guam-ALS	Sporadic	+	++	(Buée-Scherrer et al. 1995)
Postencephalitic parkinsonism	Sporadic	+	++	(Buée-Scherrer et al. 1997)

* Other tauopathies not listed include: Down syndrome, non-Guam ALS with tangles; Niemann-Pick Type C disease; subacute sclerosing panencephalitis; dementia pugilistica; myotonic dystrophy; Gerstmann-Sträussler-Scheinker syndrome with tangles; prion protein amyloid angiopathy; presenile dementia with tangles and calcification; Hallervorden-Spatz; argyrophilic grain disease; and tangle-only dementia. For individual references, see Tolnay et al. 1999.

encephalitic parkinsonism, and the Guam-ALS syndrome, syndromes in which motor abnormalities feature prominently, are all characterized by filamentous inclusions containing both 3- and 4-repeat tau isoforms. Conversely, subcortical dementing syndromes, such as PSP and cortico-basal degeneration (CBD), share with the FTDP-17 syndromes an excess of the 4-repeat tau isoform but have filaments of differing morphology accumulating in neurons and oligodendroglia. Pick's disease, the most classical FTD syndrome, appears to be characterized by the presence of the 3-repeat isoform in extracts of insoluble tau and neuronal tau deposits.

The significance of the tau isoform expression patterns is unknown. The proportions of tau protein visualized after SDS-gel electrophoresis of sarkosyl-insoluble extracts are not quantitative with respect to the tau protein composition of the filaments. In the case of AD, the PHFs have been characterized quantitatively (Wischik *et al.* 1995*a*). The phosphorylated tau extracted by these methods represents less than 5% of the total tau incorporated into the filaments (Lai *et al.* 1995). Thus depending on the relative stability of the filaments, that accumulate in the conditions listed, the tau protein, which constitutes the core structure of the filaments in the various disorders, may have a different composition from that so far reported.

5.6.2 Chromosome 3-linked frontotemporal dementia

A Danish family with frontotemporal dementia shares a similar clinical phenotype to that described for some FTDP-17 families. Dementia in this family is linked to a gene that lies in the pericentromeric region of chromosome 3 (Brown *et al.* 1995). The mean age of onset is 57 years. Limited post-mortem data indicates that dementia is associated with neuronal loss and gliosis, but accumulation of tau, Aβ, or prion proteins is not observed. Attempts to identify the locus on chromosome 3 are still in progress.

5.6.3 Mutations in the *tau* gene

Mutations in the *TAU* gene in FTDP-17 not only strengthen the relevance of tau pathology in neurodegenerative processes, but also provide an experimental framework on which to test the mechanism by which tau protein may be involved in neurodegeneration processes. The locations of the mutations identified to date are shown on Fig. 5.14. The most common of these mutations occur in a predicted stem loop structure in the 5′-splice site of exon 10. 5′-splice site mutations destabilize the intron 10 stem-loop structure, giving rise to an increased splicing in of exon 10, which increases production of the 4-repeat isoforms (Hutton *et al.* 1998; Spillantini *et al.* 1998*b*; Grover *et al.* 1999; Varani *et al.* 1999). At the ultrastructural level, the tau filaments in these patients consist mainly of twisted-ribbon filaments, rather than the PHFs typical of AD (Spillantini *et al.* 1998*b*).

Mutations that affect the coding sequence have been found in exons 9, 10, 12, and 13 of the *TAU* gene. These mutations are all clustered round the tandem repeat microtubule-binding region of the tau protein with the exception of R406W in the C-terminal segment (Fig. 5.14). The mis-sense mutations in exon 10 will only affect those tau isoforms with 4 repeats, but will not affect the 3-repeat forms. All tau isoforms will be affected by the mutations G272V, V337N, and R406W. Intronic mutations and mutations such as S305N, close to the exon-intron boundary, have destabilizing effects on the stem loop in the pre mRNA at the exon10 5'-intron boundary. Recombinant tau proteins carrying mis-sense mutations or the deletion mutation (K280Δ) have a decreased ability to promote microtubule assembly, which is more marked for 3- repeat than for 4- repeat isoforms (Bugiani *et al.* 1999; Hasegawa *et al.* 1998; Rizzu *et al.* 1999). A decrease in binding of tau to microtubules could destabilize them over time and disrupt axonal transport. The tau mutations could also result in a toxic gain of function because decreased binding of mutant tau leads to increases in free, cytosolic tau, and an increased propensity to form insoluble aggregates (Hong *et al.* 1998). Of the mutations tested, the P301L and K280Δ mutations in exon 10 have the greatest effect on microtubule assembly. The P301L mutant has the greatest potential for fibril formation, and spherical structures are obtained by incubation of the mutant protein in the absence of heparin (Nacharaju *et al.* 1999). However, the mutations N279K and S305N do not show a decreased ability to promote microtubule assembly. The latter mutations increase the splicing-in of exon 10: the N279K mutation creates an exon-spliced enhancer sequence, whereas the S305N mutation destabilizes the predicted stem loop (Clark *et al.* 1998; Hong *et al.* 1998; Delisle *et al.* 1999; Hasegawa *et al.* 1999; Iijima *et al.* 1999). The net effect of the intronic mutations increases the splicing-in of exon 10 thus increasing the ratio of 4- to 3-repeat tau expressed (Hutton *et al.* 1998; Spillantini *et al.* 1998*b*; Goedert 1999). Several splicing regulators affect the ratio of tau isoforms by inhibiting exon 10 inclusion, and both the flanking exons are involved in its regulation (Gao *et al.* 2000). *TAU* is one of only two genes known to cause disease if their alternative splicing is disturbed, even while they produce wild-type proteins. The other is Wilms tumour gene, in which incorrect isoform ratios result in Frasier syndrome (Barbaux *et al.* 1999).

Although the analyses have not been performed exhaustively, there is no data to suggest that mutations in the *TAU* gene are responsible for AD. No genetic association between polymorphisms in the *TAU* gene in AD in either clinic or population based samples was observed (Crawford *et al.* 1999; Roks *et al.* 1999) and the frequency of tau mutations in a community-based dementia series was less than the detection limit of 0.2% (Houlden *et al.* 1999*a*). A possible interaction between *APOE4* and *TAU* haplotypes (Bullido *et al.* 2000; Lilius *et al.* 1999), requires further study. In contrast to AD, tau mutations were present in 13.6% of cases from a pathologically confirmed FTDP-17 series and 43% of patients with FTD, with a positive family history of FTD, had mutations in the *TAU* gene (Rizzu *et al.* 1999). The ratio of 3- to 4-repeat tau isoforms in AD was identical to that found in control patients (Chambers *et al.* 1999). In contrast, the latter group noticed that the 4-repeat tau isoform was increased in those patients with PSP. Stochastic epigenic changes may occur for AD, that lead to the accumulation of abnormal aggregates of tau analagous to the postulated disease mechanism for sporadic prion disorders (Wischik *et al.* 1997).

The heterogeneity of FTDP-17 is exemplified by a family, in which the P301L mutation segregates with frontotemporal dementia. There is considerable neuropathological overlap between different disorders, and although significant pathological similarity was observed between two cases from the same family, the pattern of degenerative change in tau-positive inclusions was not identical. This suggests that other genetic or epigenetic factors modify the regional topology of neurodegeneration in this condition. A different mis-sense mutation of the same amino acid residue (P301S) has been found to lead to two distinct clinical phenotypes in a single family. One individual presented with FTD, whereas his son had CBD (Bugiani *et al.* 1999). Both individuals developed a rapidly progressive disease in their third decade. Pathologically, the father presented with an extensive filamentous pathology associated with hyperphosphorylated tau protein. This mutation provides an additional potential phosphorylation site within the tubulin-binding domain. Although it does not have as much of an effect on microtubule assembly as does P301L, patients with the P301S mutation have a greater amount of tau pathology than with P301L (Bugiani *et al.* 1999).

The varied ways in which mutations in tau affect the processing and function of this protein is probably responsible for the phenotypic heterogeneity observed in FTPD-17 (Bird *et al.* 1999; D'Souza *et al.* 1999; Goedert 1999). The characteristic hallmark of all these tauopathies is the presence of aggregated insoluble tau. Other factors are involved in the phenotypic variability are unknown. In contrast to the situation in AD, *APOE* genotype does not appear to be a factor influencing age of onset in FTDP-17 (Bird *et al.* 1999; Houlden *et al.* 1999*b*). The same mutation in different ethnic backgrounds may result in similar, if not identical, phenotypes. The N279K mutation occurs in both Caucasian and Japanese patients causing pallido-ponto-nigral degeneration (PPND) (Clark *et al.* 1998) and pallido-nigro-luysian degeneration (PNLD) (Yasuda *et al.* 1999).

The effect of mutations on the microtubule network *in vivo* has been examined using cells transfected with mutated tau proteins by several groups of workers. Although subtle changes in tau distribution have been observed in cells, no evidence of filament formation has been reported (Plate 1). The V337M mutation primarily affected the microtubules causing loss of cellular organization and function due to microtubule disruption rather than as the result of abnormal phosphorylation of tau (Arawaka *et al.* 1999). The microtubules in non-neuronal CHO cells transfected with G272V and P301L transfectants showed greater instability than wild-type tau, V337M, or R406W transfectants (Matsumara *et al.* 1999). Surprisingly, R406W showed negligible levels of phosphorylation at Thr231 and Ser396 in transfected cells. This is in sharp contrast to the observation that tau aggregates in R406W-affected brains are heavily phosphorylated at both of these two sites. This suggests that hyperphosphorylation at these sites cannot occur in the mutant tau bound to microtubules and that the hyperphosphorylated species of tau may be generated only after disruption of microtubules. Tau with the mutations V337M, R406W, and P301L all bind to microtubules (Dayanandan *et al.* 1999). However, microtubule extension was decreased in non-neuronal (CHO) and human neuroblastoma (M17 and SY-SH5Y) cells transfected with 3-repeat isoforms of these mutant proteins as compared with the 4-repeat isoforms. Microtubule extension was decreased also in cells carrying tau with the P301L and V337M mutations (Hasegawa *et al.* 1998). Subtle changes in the ratio between 4- and 3-repeat tau isoforms may be sufficient to cause neurodegeneration over a prolonged period. Using the baculovirus expression system, the microtubule organization was disrupted in the presence of tau with the V337M mutation. In this system, greater distances between the microtubules and fewer microtubules per process were observed with the mutant isoform (Frappier *et al.* 1999).

The regional distribution, ultrastructural and biochemical characteristics of the tau deposits in FTDP-17 differentiate them from those present in AD, CBD, PSP, and Pick's disease. In many families no β-amyloid deposits are present, indicating that FTDP-17 is a disorder distinct from AD. It also implies that the tau aggregation in the brain is not dependent upon prior deposition of β-amyloid. Conversely, intraneuronal tauopathy does not necessarily lead to the deposition of β-amyloid. If the tau and amyloid pathologies are to be linked in AD, then some other factor must account for their association in the brain in AD.

5.7 **Animal models of tau pathology**

Animal models of AD aid the understanding of the relationship between the biochemical and pathological changes in the brain and impairment of memory and behaviour. They enable the pathogenesis of the disease process to be followed *in vivo*, and provide a model in which therapeutic strategies can be tested. However, existing models fail to display the combination of tangles, plaques, and cognitive impairment characteristic of AD. Aged dogs and non-human primates develop β-amyloidosis, but tau pathology is not a feature in these animals (Walker 1997). Similarly, transgenic mice modelling amyloidosis have been created, but these fail to exhibit abnormal deposition of tau (Price *et al.* 1998).

The tangles that accumulate in the brains of rodents treated with aluminium differ in their ultrastructure from those found in AD (see Section 5.8.8). Accumulation of NFT and phosphorylated tau has been observed in the brains of elderly sheep and goats (Braak *et al.* 1994; Nelson *et al.* 1994,1995), an Asiatic brown bear, and an aged wolverine (Cork *et al.* 1988; Roertgen *et al.* 1996). Filamentous cytoskeletal changes associated with abnormally phosphorylated tau have recently been observed in aged baboons (Schultz *et al.* 2000). In addition to aberrant localization of tau in the somatodendritic compartment of neurons, glial tau pathology was observed in these animals. Furthermore, tau-positive straight filaments were observed in both neurons and glia using immunoelectron microscopy. This pattern of tauopathy is reminiscent of that observed in some of the patients with FTDP or argyrophilic grain disease.

Hyperphosphorylated tau accumulates in the somatodendritic compartment of neurons in rat brains following chronic intraventricular infusion of okadaic acid, an inhibitor of protein phospatase 2A (Arendt *et al.* 1995). Furthermore, the okadaic acid treatment also led to the formation of extracellular deposits of Aβ and memory impairment. Two other studies have implicated Aβ in the accumulation of tau in animal models. Microinjections of fibrillar Aβ in the cortex of aged rhesus monkeys resulted in focal accumulations of intra-cellular phosphorylated tau (Geula *et al.* 1998). This was dependent upon both age and species; the same result was not observed for rats or young rhesus monkeys. Second, focal deposits of tau have been observed in mice that were transgenic for APP carrying AD-associated mutations (Sturchler-Pierrat *et al.* 1997).

Chloroquine-induced myopathy provides a different model in which cognitive changes cannot be considered. Nevertheless, tau protein acumulates in rimmed vacuoles and as PHF-like fibrils in inclusion body myositis (Askanas *et al.* 1994) and in autophagic vacuoles in chloroquine-induced myopathy (Murakami *et al.* 1998). Tau is normally degraded in lysosomes and, by blocking the lysosomal degradation pathway, chloroquine might lead to the accumulation of increased levels of tau in the cytoplasm. Similar changes can be observed in rat hippocampal slices, where meganeurites are generated following treatment with lysosomal protease inhibitors (Bi *et al.* 1999). The precise relevance of these studies to the pathogenesis of AD remains to be established, but the accumulation of tau in these paradigms can be used. A suitable model for AD, however, is still needed. As the implication of other genetic determinants of AD become apparent (for example *APOE* genotype; see Section 5.8), these factors will need to be considered in any relevant animal models.

5.7.1 Transgenic animals

Advances in molecular genetics during the past decade using transgenic technology have begun to provide approaches for the establishment of animal models that mirror different aspects of several of the most important neurodegenerative diseases (Theuring *et al.* 1997). Their analysis will lead to a better understanding of disease pathogenesis and will be invaluable for the identification of new diagnostic and therapeutic agents, even for complex disorders such as AD. The ability to integrate genes into the germline of mice, either by DNA microinjection or homologous recombination in embryonic stem cells, and the successful expression of the inserted genes within an organism provides new opportunities and insights for neurodegenerative research. Therefore, transgenic technology constitutes an increasingly important tool for studying the regulation and function of given genes. Moreover, the different experimental strategies employing either gain-of-function or loss-of-function approaches, combined with the current pace of genomic research, will allow the generation of specific animal models, reproducing in full the pathology and symptoms of even complex disorders such as AD. Although the generation of animals transgenic for various forms of amyloid precursor protein (APP) and the presenilins has been given considerable attention (Price *et al.* 1998), none of the mice exhibit tau pathology.

To test the hypothesis that the tau protein is essential for neuronal cell morphogenesis, especially axonal elongation and maintenance, gene targeting in ES cells by homologous recombination was used to generate mice lacking the *TAU* gene (Harada *et al.* 1994). The brains of tau-deficient mice appeared normal immunohistochemically and axonal elongation was not affected in cultured neurons. However, microtubule stability was decreased and its organization altered in some small-calibre axons. An increase in MAP1A, which might compensate for a functional loss of tau in large-calibre axons, was found. Thus, tau seems to be crucial in the stabilization and organization of axonal microtubules in certain axons. Subsequent studies have shown that tau-deficient mice exhibit signs similar to certain symptoms characteristic of frontotemporal dementia patients, such as personality changes (disinhibition/aggression) and deterioration of memory and executive function. The mice showed muscle weakness and impaired balance control, hyperactivity in a new environment, and impairment in the contextual fear conditioning (Ikegami *et al.* 2000). Spatial learning tasks in the mice were unaffected, as is the memory function in FTDP-17 patients.

Transgenic mice expressing the largest human tau isoform, containing four repeats under the control of the murine *Thy1*-promoter, displayed phosphorylated tau immunoreactivity (mAb AT8) within the axons and the somatodendritic compartment of a few neurons, but no neurofibrillary lesions nor phenotypic abnormalities were reported (Götz *et al.* 1995). This suggested that additional factors are necessary for PHF generation. In mice harbouring a transgene encoding the human shortest (fetal-type) tau isoform, containing three repeats under the control of the 3-hydroxy-methyl-glutaryl CoA reductase promoter, marked changes in tau compartmentalization and phosphorylation were observed (Brion *et al.* 1999). In this case, the tau in neurons did not react with mAb AT8. Neither NFT nor phenotypic alterations were reported in the animals transgenic for 3-repeat tau when examined up to the age of 19 months. The failure of tau filament formation in the transgenic mouse brains may be due to the low level of human transgene expression. Transgenic human tau accounted for less than 15% of total mouse tau proteins.

The most advanced tau-driven pathology was observed in transgenic mice expressing the smallest human tau isoform containing three repeats under the control of the murine prion protein promoter (Ishihara *et al.* 1999). A 5–15-fold higher level of human fetal tau than endogenous mouse tau was expressed. These mice developed a progressive age-dependent accumulation of intraneuronal filamentous inclusions, associated with axon degeneration, gliosis, motor weakness, and tau protein abnormalities. Interestingly, highest tau transgene expression, for example in a homozygous state, caused lethality of the embryos *in utero*. However, these filamentous inclusions did not exhibit the ultrastructural features of PHFs in classic AD. In fact the distribution of tauopathy in these mice most closely resembles that found in ALS/PDC and PSP.

These data corroborate findings observed in transgenic mice expressing the four repeat human tau fragment only, or in combination with the full length human tau isoform, under the control of the NSE promoter (Thunecke *et al.* 2000). Several independent expressing transgenic lines were generated. The transgenic protein was reactive with several phosphorylation-dependent antibodies, implying again that the murine kinases are able to phosphorylate the human tau at several sites hyperphosphorylated in AD. The transgenic mice displayed a characteristic phenotype consisting of 'hind limb clenching'(Fig. 5.15). The most severe cases developed an abnormal gait. Transgenic mice expressing the four repeat fragment only also developed this phenotype. Hence the presence of this tau fragment, reportedly also found in the PHF-core of AD, causes some subtle alterations in the axons of motoneurons resembling an amyotrophic lateral sclerosis-like phenotype, leading to impairment of function. Furthermore, it provides evidence that both the three repeat and the four repeat fragment of human tau can induce tauopathies in transgenic mice. In both studies neurodegenerative alterations were obtained that partially recapitulate key features of these diseases. Overexpression of the four-repeat isoform in mice, under control of the *Thy-1* promoter, has been achieved recently (Spittaels *et al.* 1999). The resultant mice exhibited axonal degeneration in brain and spinal cord, and sensorimotor impairments and muscle atrophy accompanied the axonopathy.

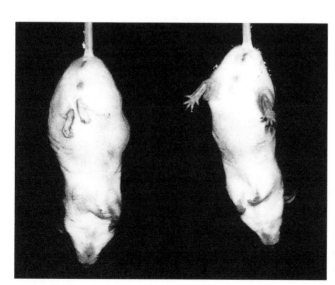

Fig. 5.15 Tau transgenic mice. Mice transgenic for the human truncated tau fragment (297–391) and full-length, four-repeat human tau develop a phenotype in which 'hind limb clenching' is observed (left). This is not apparent in control mice (right).

Merely increasing the concentration of tau was sufficient to injure neurons in the absence of NFTs. The effects were seen in mice expressing two- to three-fold more tau than wild-type mice, which only express the 4-repeat tau isoform (Kampers *et al.* 1999). Expression of tau isoforms and the mutant proteins at different levels should enable investigators to determine those factors that lead to neuronal degeneration and tangle formation and those that influence the selective vulnerability associated with the different tauopathy disorders.

The recent advances in genome sciences and the development of transgenic technologies have provided a unique opportunity to study how genes associated with neurodegenerative diseases alter normal brain function. One problem is the relevance of the animal phenotype to the disease state. This issue will remain a challenge for the interpretation of transgenic studies and must be considered carefully when extrapolating to human disease states. Nonetheless transgenic studies have already provided, and will continue to provide valuable information regarding the significance of certain candidate molecules in AD.

5.7.2 Niemann-Pick, type C disease

Niemann-Pick type C disease (NPC) is an autosomal recessive, cholesterol storage disease with defects in the intracellular trafficking of exogenous cholesterol derived from low density lipoproteins. In NPC cases with a chronic progressive course, NFTs that contain abnormally phosphorylated tau proteins have been identified (Auer *et al.* 1995; Love *et al.* 1995; Suzuki *et al.* 1995). Abnormally phosphorylated tau proteins extracted from tangle-rich NPC brains are indistinguishable from those extracted from AD brains (Auer *et al.* 1995). More importantly these findings suggest that, in NPC brains, the aggregation of tau proteins to form PHFs can occur without the presence of Aβ-rich senile plaques. These results confirm similar findings in dementias associated with primary tau mutations summarized above. Using positional cloning methods, a gene (*NPC1*) with insertion, deletion, and mis-sense mutations has been identified in NPC patients (Carstea *et al.* 1997). The gene encodes an integral membrane protein of 1278 amino acids. In parallel, an integrated human-mouse positional candidate approach was used to identify the gene responsible for the phenotypes observed in a mouse model of NPC disease (Loftus *et al.* 1997). The predicted murine NPC1 protein has sequence homology to the cholesterol-sensing regions of 3-hydroxy-3-methylglutaryl coenzyme A reductase and SREBP cleavage-activating protein (SCAP), and to the NPC1 orthologues identified in human, the nematode *Caenorhabditis elegans*, and the yeast *Saccharomyces cerevisiae*. Sequence analysis confirmed the putative mutation in the murine *NPC1* gene and demonstrated that the NPC phenotype observed in BALB/c $^{npc\ nih}$ mice resulted from a frame shift mutation of the *NPC1* gene. Both findings establish the role for the *NPC1* gene mutations in inducing NPC disease in humans. In the NPC mice, progressive emaciation and development of neurological symptoms such as tremor, ataxia, and hind limb weakness are principal signs. Pathological studies of brains of NPC mice revealed neuronal storage, axonal spheroids, which may precede NFT common in human NPC brains, hypomyelination, and myelin degradation (Suzuki *et al.* 1995). In summary the mouse model may provide an important resource for studying the role of NPC1 in cholesterol homeostasis and neurodegeneration.

5.8 Genetic heterogeneity in Alzheimer's disease

Although the tau mutations can cause degenerative dementia with tauopathy, no mutations in the *TAU* gene have been found to be causative of AD. Mutations in other proteins, however, do cause disease in a small proportion of all AD cases and it is important to determine how

Table 5.2 Factors involved in the heterogeneity of Alzheimer's disease

Gene	Chromosomal location	Gene defect	Number of mutations (kindreds)	Age of onset	Proportion of familial AD (%) *
AD1	21q22.1	APP mutations	8† (20)	Early	5
AD3	14q.24.3	PS1 mutations	>60 (>100)	Early	50
AD4	1q42.1	PS2 mutations	4 (10)	Early	1
AD2	19q13.2	APOE polymorphism	ε4 allele (risk factor)	Early/Late	
Others	?	?	?	?	40–80
Non-genetic	–	–	–	?	

* Familial AD represents approximately 10–20% of total AD, the remainder of cases being sporadic and, generally, of late onset. Only *APOE* has been associated with the sporadic form of AD.

Down syndrome (trisomy 21) is also associated with Alzheimer-type pathology in the third decade.

† Another mutation causes HCHWA-D

tau pathology in AD is related to these mutations. Recent advances in our understanding of the cell biology of various proteins provide much useful information. We shall also consider dementia with Lewy bodies, a condition in which there are areas of overlap with AD, and some other dementia syndromes in which genetic details are beginning to emerge.

From epidemiological studies, the established risk factors, which predispose individuals to an increased risk of acquiring AD, include: increased age, family history, head trauma, and Down syndrome. Mutations in three genes have been identified which cause AD: *APP*, and the presenilin genes, *PS1* and *PS2*. The biology of APP is covered in detail elsewhere (Selkoe 1999), and various aspects of the presenilin proteins have been reviewed (Mattson and Guo 1997; Cruts and Van Broeckhoven 1998; Selkoe 1998; Annaert and De Strooper 1999; Haass and De Strooper 1999; Wolfe *et al.* 1999a). Whereas APP is a glycoprotein with a single transmembrane domain, the two presenilin genes encode for homologous proteins that are predicted to have multiple transmembrane domains, a feature characteristic of many membrane receptor proteins. In all three instances, dominant mis-sense mutations co-segregate with AD (Table 5.2). This demonstrates the genetic heterogeneity of AD, and these forms could be classified as distinct conditions within a disorder syndrome. Molecular sub-classification of AD (Hardy *et al.* 1991), seems unnecessary, since there is no evidence for subtypes with distinct clinical and neuropathological profiles. Subtle differences in age of onset and duration of disease have been observed and these may be sufficient to account for the genetic heterogeneity seen in familial AD. However, a genetic cause in possibly as many as half of the early, familial AD cases has yet to be found (Tanzi *et al.* 1996). Although various mutations are associated with some differences in clinical presentation, the pathological changes at autopsy are relatively constant. Familial mutations in *APP*, *PS1*, and *PS2*, when combined, account for only a small percentage of the incidence of AD. The *APOE* polymorphism can account for as much as 60% of the susceptibility to AD and is the first gene identified in which 'normal' alleles predispose to dementia. Unlike mutations in the familial forms of AD, inheritance of an ε4 allele does not reliably predict whether or when a carrier will develop AD.

Independent genetic defects that lead to a similar clinical and neuropathological profile may share some part of a common neurodegenerative pathway. Thus, although the successful search for genes that cause AD provides important starting blocks for investigation, the common pathway(s) can provide critical points at which therapeutic strategies might be targeted. The genetic and biochemical approaches, therefore, provide complementary approaches to our understanding of a disease process and neither should be viewed in isolation.

5.8.1 Amyloid β-protein precursor

Mutations in the *APP* gene, near to or within the Aβ domain, are linked with AD in a few families throughout the world and in different ethnic populations (Table 5.2). The AD mutations are either within or flanking the Aβ domain of APP that gives rise to the deposits of Aβ in plaques throughout the cortex and, to a lesser extent, in the cerebellum (Selkoe 1999). APP exists in at least 5 isoforms, but its physiological role in the brain is not understood. In the numbering of the largest APP isoform (770 residues), the 42-residue Aβ domain corresponds to residues 672–713 encoded for by exons 16 and 17. Nine mutations in APP are associated with disease, eight with AD and one with hereditary cerebral haemorrhage with amyloidosis — Dutch type (HCHWA-D). In one family, a Swedish mutation results in the replacement of 2 amino acids (K670N and M671L). Other point mutations causing AD are: A692G, V715M, I716L, V717I, V717G, V717F and L723P (Hardy 1997; Ancolio *et al.* 1999; Kwok *et al.* 2000). HCHWA-D, which exhibits severe congophilic angiopathy in the absence of plaques and tangles, is caused by the mutation E693Q.

Although APP mutations are causative for AD in rare families, the mechanism by which such mutations cause disease is not clear. Some mutations result in over-production of longer Aβ1–42 forms that aggregate more readily than Aβ1–40. The ratio between Aβ peptides terminating at 40 and those with 42 or 43 residues is important, and may have an effect on the acceleration of plaque formation (Jarrett *et al.* 1993). The predominant form of Aβ in diffuse and neuritic plaques tend to be those that terminate after 42 residues (Iwatsubo *et al.* 1995) in contrast to the vascular deposits of Aβ that tend to be 40 residues in length (Suzuki *et al.* 1994). Aβ1–42 is also more resistant to proteolysis; diffuse Aβ deposits can be removed from rat brain by a neutral protease, similar to neprilysin, that is sensitive to specific inhibition by thiorphin (Iwata *et al.* 2000). Evidence that extracellular Aβ deposits can be cleared is supported by the finding that deposits of amyloid in transgenic APP mice are removed by immunization with Aβ1–42 (Schenk *et al.* 1999).

Degradation-resistant Aβ is found within neurons (Selkoe 1999) and these may be more important in AD than the extracellular deposits. Cells can respond abnormally to aggregated proteins or, alternatively, resistant Aβ could act as a focus for seeding the aggregation of other cellular proteins such as tau protein (see Section 5.13). Evidence that Aβ is toxic to neurons *in vivo* is unconvincing, and very elderly patients with abundant Aβ deposition can be found to be clinically normal (Delaère *et al.* 1993). Furthermore, the distribution of Aβ deposition does not follow the same pattern as that of neurofibrillary degeneration, which is more closely correlated with cognitive decline (Wilcock and Esiri 1982; Arriagada *et al.* 1992b). Models of amyloidosis in mice (Games *et al.* 1995) do not induce neurofibrillary tau pathology.

Three pathways for processing APP have been identified so far. There are two secretory pathways: one in which the Aβ domain is cleaved within the middle (α-secretase) and the second, a potentially amyloidogenic pathway which leaves the Aβ peptide intact (β-secretase). APP can also be internalized and degraded via the endosoma/lysosomal pathway (γ-secretase) to yield C-terminal fragments of APP that also contain an intact Aβ domain. The β-secretase (Hussain *et al.* 1999; Vassar *et al.* 1999) and γ-secretase (Wolfe *et al.* 1999*b*) cleaves APP to create Aβ peptides. β-secretase, which is also referred to as BACE (β-site APP cleaving enzyme) is an aspartic protease located in the ER and Golgi. APP processing is modulated by presenilin 1, which acts either as the γ-secretase itself or by increasing γ-secretase activity. γ-Secretase cleavage generates Aβ of different lengths — Aβ1–42 in pre-Golgi compartments and Aβ1–40 in later compartments and in the endocytic pathway. Aβ itself, when aggregated, posseses proteolytic activity and thus may be responsible for inactivation of other proteins (Elbaum *et al.* 2000).

The accumulation of misfolded proteins in the lumen of the ER results in an 'unfolded-protein response' in which increased production of chaperones alleviates the increased demand on the existing protein folding machinery. In neuroblastoma cells, mutations in PS1 downregulate the ER to nucleus signalling pathway that adjusts the levels of chaperones (Katayama *et al.* 1999). Altered chaperone levels may also influence the aggregation of other proteins. Further research could provide clues to a link between tau processing, and either APP or the presenilin proteins.

5.8.2 **Presenilin proteins**

The human presenilin proteins, PS1 and PS2, were identified in 1995 (Levy-Lahad *et al.* 1995; Rogaev *et al.* 1995; Sherrington *et al.* 1995). The *PS1* gene was identified by classical positional cloning techniques, while *PS2* was isolated on the basis of its homology to *PS1* (Table 5.2). More than 60 mutations in these two proteins have been identified to be causative of AD, most being in PS1. Patients with the earliest age of onset tend to be those with mutations in PS1. Onset in certain cases occurs by the age of 30 years. These include mis-sense and deletion mutants and truncated variants. The biology and function of the presenilin proteins at present, is relatively poorly understood, but is reviewed in greater detail elsewhere (Mattson and Guo 1997; Cruts and Van Broeckhoven 1998; Selkoe 1998; Annaert and De Strooper 1999; Haass and De Strooper 1999; Wolfe *et al.* 1999*a*). Both proteins are membrane spanning, with at least 6 transmembrane domains and a large hydrophilic loop. The two proteins show extensive homology with each other and both undergo proteolytic processing, with a cleavage site situated within the large hydrophilic loop. The full-length *PS1* and *PS2* genes encode predicted proteins of 467 and 448 amino acids, respectively. They are both cleaved into N- and C-terminal fragments of approximately 35 and 20 kDa. They are normally localized in the nuclear envelope, the ER and the Golgi, with PS2 appearing to be more predominant in the Golgi component than PS1.

Clues about their function in mammalian cells are derived from the observation that both presenilin proteins share significant amino acid homology with two *C.elegans* proteins: *sel-12* and *spe-4*. *Sel-12* interacts with *lin-12*, a member of the Notch family of receptors for intracellular signals that specify cell fate in the nematode (Levitan *et al.* 1995). *Sel-12* may play a role in receptor trafficking, localization, or recycling of *lin-12*. *Spe-4*, on the other hand, is involved in the cytoplasmic partitioning of proteins. Thus the presenilin proteins may play a role in the intracellular trafficking or localization/recycling of proteins in the brain. Just as mutations in APP lead to increases in the ratio of Aβ1–42:Aβ1–40, mutations in PS1 increase the levels of Aβ(1–42) in transfected cell lines (Citron *et al.*

1996), transgenic mice (Borchelt *et al.* 1996; Duff *et al.* 1996), and brain tissue from AD patients carrying PS mutations (Lemere *et al.* 1996). Recent studies suggest that γ-secretases involved in APP processing are aspartyl proteases that catalyse new intramembranous proteolysis. This proteolysis requires the presenilins, and two conserved aspartate residues in a transmembrane domain of PS1 appear to be essential for γ-secretase (Wolfe *et al.* 1999*a*). Presenilins also mediate the intramembraneous cleavage of the Notch receptor, an event critical for Notch signalling in embryonic development. This links both presenilin proteins to APP processing and to proteins involved in intracellular signal transduction.

PS1 mutations facilitate apoptotic neuronal death *in vitro* (Chui *et al.* 1999). A presenilin homologue in the mouse has been found, the apoptosis-linked gene 3 (*Alg-3*) (Vito *et al.* 1996). The *Alg-3* gene product is involved in apoptosis, functioning as an inhibitor of T-cell receptor-induced cell death by blocking death signal transduction. Mutations in *Alg-3* decrease blocking capacity and lead to an accelerated T-cell receptor-induced cell death. By analogy, PS mutations might account for some of the neurodegenerative process that occurs in the AD brain. There is also evidence that presenilin proteins may be involved in mitosis and that the mutations in the presenilin genes may predispose to chromosome mis-segregation (Geller *et al.* 1999).

Is there any evidence that presenilins interact with tau protein? PS1 is associated with both amyloid plaques and NFTs in AD. Both N- and C-terminal fragments of PS1 are found in NFT-bearing neurons and dystrophic neurites around plaques (Busciglio *et al.* 1997; Chui *et al.* 1998), but there is no co-localization of presenilins with PHF-tau positive neuropil threads or Aβ fibrils. No co-localization of presenilin and tau has been observed by immunohistochemical methods in one study (Hendriks *et al.* 1998) although an association between PHF-tau and the C-terminal fragments of PS1 was observed by others (Tomidokoro *et al.* 1999). In the latter study, however, the investigators only examined a dispersed, 'A68' PHF preparation from AD brain in which they observed smearing with C-terminal PS1-immunoreactive fragments. Further studies are necessary to establish a direct association between tau and PS1.

Two seemingly contradictory reports have examined the effect of presenilin mutations on the phosphorylation of tau protein. There was no evidence of increased tau phosphorylation in human and mouse neuroblastoma cell lines expressing PS1 proteins carrying either the I143T or G348A mutations PS1 (Julliams *et al.* 1999). In a separate study, however, PS1 was associated with glycogen synthase kinase-3β (GSK-3β) and bound to tau protein (Takashima *et al.* 1998). Deletion studies showed that tau and GSK-3β bound to the same domain of PS1 (residues 250–298) and that tau binds through its microtubule-binding domain. Mutations increased the ability of PS1 to bind GSK-3β and also increased its kinase activity toward tau. An association of this kinase with mutant PS1 may lead to increased phosphorylation of tau (Takashima *et al.* 1998). Although these interactions were all observed in transiently transfected COS-7 cells, which overexpress the individual proteins, the levels of PS1, tau protein, and GSK-3β are all increased in the brain suggesting that they could be linked *in vivo*.

5.8.3 Apolipoprotein E and other genetic susceptibility factors

An association between the apolipoprotein E ε4 allele and AD was first demonstrated at Duke University (Strittmatter *et al.* 1993). Although there may be some minor ethnic variations, the pattern of *APOE* genotype distribution for patients with AD in populations of diverse ethnic backgrounds indicates that it is the ε4 allele that is directly responsible for its association with AD. The ε4 allele frequency in AD and control populations is approximately 0.38 and 0.13, respectively (Harrington *et al.* 1994*a*), and an earlier age of onset is often associated with possession of an ε4 allele (Farrer *et al.* 1997). In the very old (> 85 years), however, the *APOE* gene does not influence cognitive decline or dementia (Farrer *et al.* 1997; Juva *et al.* 2000). A decreased risk of AD in those with the ε2 allele suggests that it is due to the *APOE* gene rather than a closely associated gene that is in linkage disequilibrium. In addition to AD, *APOE4* is associated with increased risk for dementia with Lewy bodies, a condition associated with minimal PHF accumulation (Harrington *et al.* 1994*a*). This has been supported by evidence from other studies which, taken together, indicate that *APOE* genotype does not influence tau pathology directly. Neither does it affect synapse loss (Corey-Bloom *et al.* 2000). Although many studies have now confirmed the *APOE* association in AD, testing populations for *APOE* genotype cannot be used to predict development of AD; presence of the ε4 allele is neither necessary nor sufficient to cause disease. Furthermore, distribution of the ε4 allele varies considerably between different populations (Uterman 1994).

ApoE is a plasma protein involved in cholesterol transport. In the CNS, it is secreted by astrocytes as a constituent of high-density lipoprotein complexes but is also found in neurons (Mahley *et al.* 1999). Three major alleles exist: ε2, ε3 and ε4, with ε3 being the most common. The ε4 allele is over-represented in AD patients with late-onset symptoms and *APOE* genotype represents an important biological marker for the disease, accounting for 45–60% of the genetic component of AD (Nalbantoglu *et al.* 1994). A recent study suggests that *APOE* represents less than 10% of the total variance in age at onset of familial AD and that it is but one of several important genes (Daw *et al.* 2000). At least four additional loci were identified that have an effect equal to or greater than that of *APOE*.

Possible biological explanations for the association of *APOE* genotype with AD have included isoform-specific neurotoxic and/or neuroprotective effects of apoE and the binding of apoE to Aβ or tau proteins in an isoform-dependent fashion (Strittmatter *et al.* 1994). Recent studies with transgenic mice indicate that apoE promotes the deposition and fibrillization of Aβ and that this is greatest in mice expressing the apoE4 isoform (Bales *et al.* 1999). This may result from decreased clearance of Aβ. Alternatively, apoE can influence neurite outgrowth: whereas apoE3 stimulates outgrowth in cell culture, apoE4 has the converse effect (Nathan *et al.* 1994). However, these explanations remain hypotheses whose relevance *in vivo* has yet to be established. The disease specificity of the association is uncertain and it is not known how apoE interacts with other gene products. Furthermore, other potential confounding factors such as cerebrovascular disease may impinge on the development of AD and its association with *APOE4* genotype (Harrington and Roth 1997). Linkage of AD with a locus on chromosome 12 (Pericak-Vance *et al.* 1997) remains to be defined.

Associations between AD and genetic polymorphisms other than *APOE* have been investigated extensively in recent years. These include α_1-antichymotrypsin (*ACT*) (Kamboh M.I. 1995), very low density lipoprotein receptor (Okuizumi *et al.* 1995), non-amyloid component precursor (Xia *et al.* 1996), butyrylcholinesterase (Lehmann *et al.* 1997), α_2-macroglobulin (Blacker *et al.* 1998), HLA-A (Payami *et al.* 1997); HLA-DR (Curran *et al.* 1997; Neill *et al.* 1999), bleomycin hydrolase (Montoya *et al.* 1998), the angiotensin converting enzyme, dipeptidyl carboxypeptidase I (*DCPI*) (Kehoe *et al.* 1999), oestrogen receptor α gene (*ERα*) (Brandi *et al.* 1999; Isoe *et al.* 1998), serotonin transporter (Li *et al.* 1997*a*), and endothelial nitric oxide synthase (*NOS3*) (Dahiyat *et al.* 1999) as well as polymorphisms in non-coding and regulatory regions of the *APOE* and *PS1* genes (Cruts and Van Broeckhoven 1998). A polymorphism in endothelial nitric oxide synthase (*NOS2A*) is associated with dementia with Lewy bodies, but not AD (Xu *et al.* 2000). The polymorphism in *ERα* at intron 1 was found to alter transcriptional activity of this gene (Maruyama *et al.* 2000). The latter group, however, were unable to confirm the previously reported associations between *ERα* gene polymorphisms and AD.

In some studies, polymorphisms have been found to modify the risk attributable to apoE. Polymorphisms in either *ACT* or *ERα* genes both increase the risk of AD, and is greatest in individuals possessing the *APOE-ε4* allele (Brandi *et al.* 1999; Kamboh M.I. 1995). In other studies, gender has been found to interact with genetic factors, for example *APOE* and *DCP1* (Crawford *et al.* 2000; Farrer *et al.* 1997). The presence of herpes simplex type 1 virus (HSV1) in the brains of many elderly people was reported to be a risk factor for AD in carriers of the *APOE-ε4* allele. On the basis of this result, and the finding that *APOE-ε4* is a risk factor for herpes labialis, a combination of viral and genetic factors has been considered to be detrimental in the CNS (Dobson *et al.* 1999).

None of these association studies has been established in subsequent investigations and so the role of the various factors listed above remains equivocal. Whether they play a role in a subset of AD patients cannot be excluded. Associations with certain polymorphisms may be the result of linkage disequilibrium such that it may be a nearby gene that is involved in AD. Genetic interactions may lead to stratification of sample populations into groups with different disease-associated risks and this may account for some of the controversial findings observed in genetic association studies.

5.8.4 Dementia with Lewy bodies

Lewy body pathology is pathognomic for a spectrum of disorders, the most familiar of which is Parkinson's disease (PD). PD is the prototypic Lewy body disease, characterized by extrapyramidal symptoms and the presence of Lewy bodies in the brainstem. Widespread Lewy bodies in the cerebral cortex of patients with dementia was first noted with significant frequency by Kosaka (Kosaka *et al.* 1984). Since then, this condition has emerged as the second most common form of degenerative dementia in the elderly after AD, accounting for 15–20% of demented patients. Immunohistochemical visualization of ubiquitin-positive Lewy bodies played an important part in revealing the extent of the prevalence of this condition. 'Dementia with Lewy bodies' (DLB) is the recently recommended term for a syndrome that has been ascribed numerous names during the last two decades, including cortical or diffuse Lewy body disease, senile dementia of Lewy body type and Lewy body variant of AD (Perry *et al.* 1996). Pathologically, it is defined by the formation of both brain stem and cortical Lewy bodies in the presence of sparse or absent neurofibrillary pathology. Although there is some overlap between DLB and both AD and PD, a fairly coherent picture of the clinical features of DLB is starting to emerge (McKeith *et al.* 1996; Perry *et al.* 1996; McKeith *et al.* 1999).

DLB is a progressive dementia, commonly accompanied by psychiatric symptoms and occasionally with mild extrapyramidal symptoms. The prevalence increases with advancing age. Most patients are characterized by a syndrome in which there is a fluctuating confusional state, behavioural disturbance, visual or auditory hallucinations, and progressive dementia (McKeith *et al.* 1996; Perry *et al.* 1996). Motor symptoms, characteristic of idiopathic PD, tend to be rare as a presenting feature in DLB. The fluctuating confusional states can lead to a misdiagnosis of vascular dementia. Patients often suffer transient episodes of loss of consciousness, and severe or fatal neuroleptic sensitivity is common. Cognitive decline and mortality tend to be accelerated in DLB when compared with AD. Revised clinical diagnostic criteria (McKeith et al. 1996), based on earlier sets of criteria from Nottingham and Newcastle, are being evaluated. Although the specificity of diagnosis remains high (>85%), improvements will be necessary to improve the sensitivity of the current criteria (McKeith et al. 1999). These criteria have even been employed recently to speculate that Cervantes' character of Don Quixote was based upon a real patient with DLB (Ruiz et al. 1999).

Changes at neuropathological, neurochemical, genetic, and molecular levels have all been observed in DLB. The extent to which each of these is involved in the pathogenesis of DLB still needs to be ascertained. Likewise, the seminal events which distinguish DLB from AD and PD remain to be elucidated.

The Lewy body is an intraneuronal, eosinophilic inclusion body, 5–25 μm in diameter. DLB is characterized by the presence of a moderate number of neocortical Lewy bodies and sparse or absent neurofibrillary lesions (Dickson et al. 1989; Perry et al. 1990). Although lacking the tau pathology characteristic of AD, DLB shares with AD the increased risk that is associated with possession of the apolipoprotein E ε4 allele (Harrington et al. 1994a). Lewy bodies in limbic and neocortical regions are smaller than those found in the brain stem and rarely have the electron dense cores of the latter. The Lewy body is composed of amorphous material and filaments, 10–20 nm in diameter. α-Synuclein, that has been identified recently as a major component of these filaments (Spillantini et al. 1997). Truncated fragments of α-synuclein have been found in isolated Lewy bodies (Baba et al. 1998). In addition, neurofilament subunits and ubiquitin and other related, cell-stress response proteins are present (Perry et al. 1996).

The quantity of amyloid β-protein deposits is similar to that found in AD, however, the relative proportion of plaques containing Aβ terminating at residues 40 or 42 distinguish DLB from that in AD. Although Aβ42 plaque numbers are similar in both conditions, the Aβ40 plaques are more frequent in AD than DLB (Lippa et al. 1999). In addition, Lewy-related neurites are found in the CA2/CA3 region of the hippocampus in DLB, that are absent in AD (Dickson et al. 1991), and these neurites also contain both α-synuclein and ubiquitin.

Neurochemically, DLB shows features of both PD and AD (Perry et al. 1996). Dopamine levels in DLB are decreased in the caudate and patients are particularly susceptible to typical neuroleptic drugs (dopaminergic D2-receptor antagonists). The cholinergic deficit in DLB is generally more severe than that found in AD, except for the hippocampus, which is usually spared. A correlation between choline acetyltransferase depletion and the prevalence of cortical Lewy bodies in DLB has not been found. This would support the notion that Lewy bodies themselves are not responsible for the clinical phenotype.

DLB may share common disease determinants with both AD and PD. The APOE ε4 allele is a risk factor for both AD and DLB (Harrington et al. 1994a). Although the cytochrome P-450 gene CYP2D6 was reported to be associated with both DLB and PD (Saitoh et al. 1995), this finding has not been substantiated. An elevated frequency of the CYP2D6*4 allele in PD, but no such elevations are found in either DLB or AD (Atkinson et al. 1999).

Lewy bodies may represent pathological end-products that simply serve as a marker for PD and DLB. Almost certainly cortical Lewy bodies themselves do not account for the clinical symptoms of DLB, since the number of affected neurons is approximately one thousandth of the number affected by neurofibrillary pathology in AD. Nevertheless, the process that leads to the formation of Lewy bodies may be central to the pathogenesis of DLB and other 'synucleinopathy' disorders. α-Synuclein is a soluble, presynaptic protein that is pathologically redistributed within intracellular lesions characteristic of several neurodegenerative diseases (Goedert 1999). Insoluble aggregates of α-synuclein in Lewy bodies are found not only in DLB, but also in familial AD patients with mutations in presenilin or APP genes (Lippa *et al.* 1998) and in patients with multiple system atrophy. Mutations in α-synuclein have been reported in a few families with PD (Polymeropoulos *et al.* 1997) and such mutations accelerate α-synuclein aggregation *in vitro* (Conway *et al.* 1998) to form filaments that are distinct from those formed from normal α-synuclein (Giasson *et al.* 1999). Mutations have not been found in sporadic PD or in DLB thus far and, in PD, they exhibit incomplete penetrance. Observations of additional axonal pathology and inclusions in DLB suggest that β- and γ-synucleins, in addition to α-synuclein, may be implicated in synaptic dysfunction (Galvin *et al.* 1999). The identification of a protein, synphilin-1, which interacts with α-synuclein and which produces cytoplasmic eosinophilic inclusions when the two proteins are introduced into mammalian cells provides a model to study the pathogenesis of α-synuclein aggregation (Engelender *et al.* 1999). The possibility that α-synuclein is not necessary for Lewy body formation but is still involved in the neurodegenerative process, is supported by the finding of α-synuclein-negative Lewy bodies in the cortex of a patient lacking the clinical signs of parkinsonism and/or dementia (van Duinen *et al.* 1999).

It will be important to determine whether or not the accumulation of filamentous inclusions is a key pathogenic event in DLB. If not, then is synaptic dysfunction a consequence of abnormal α-synuclein processing in these patients? These, and questions regarding the basis of selective neuronal vulnerability in DLB, require extensive clinical and biological research.

5.8.5 Chromosome 13 dementia

Familial British dementia (FBD) is an autosomal dominant disorder characterized by cerebral amyloid angiopathy, non-neuritic and perivascular plaques, and NFT. A unique 4-kDa protein subunit, termed ABri, has been isolated from amyloid fibrils (Vidal *et al.* 1999). The insoluble peptide is a fragment of a putative, single-spanning, transmembrane precursor encoded by a novel gene, *BRI*, located on chromosome 13q14. A single base substitution at the stop codon of this gene generates a longer open reading frame from which release of the 34 C-terminal amino acids generates the ABri amyloid sub-unit. The mutant ABri precursor is subject to enhanced proteolysis between Arg-243 and Glu-244 (Kim *et al.* 1999). Unlike Aβ fibrils, synthetic ABri fibrils comprise irregular fibrils containing branch points (Kim *et al.* 1999). The amyloid is co-localized immunohistochemically with plaques throughout the brain and no immunoreactivity is observed in brain sections of sporadic AD patients and other disorders. FBD bears similarities to AD and, in particular, to the PS1-Δexon9 variant. Both disorders have peptides of approximately 4-kDa; and the cytoskeletal pathology of FBD is indistinguishable from that observed in other neurodegenerative diseases, including sporadic and familial forms of AD and the vascular form of prion protein-congophilic amyloid angiopathy (Ghetti *et al.* 1996). Understanding of the pathogenisis of this rare disease may shed light on the cause of dementia in AD and other neurological disorders.

5.8.6 Familial encephalopathy with neuroserpin inclusion bodies

The genetic basis for a newly identified neurodegenerative disorder associated with dementia has recently been reported (Davis *et al.* 1999*c*). Affected subjects present with deficits in attention, concentration and oral fluency. Early learning and memory impairments do occur, but to a lesser extent than in early AD. This disorder has an autosomal-dominant pattern of inheritance and is characterized by the presence of new Collins bodies distributed throughout the cortex and in many sub-cortical nuclei. Mis-sense mutations (S49P and S52R) in the neuroserpin gene, located on chromosome 3q26, lead to the intracellular accumulation of a 57-kDa protein in the brain. This protein is a member of the serine protease inhibitor family and the disease has been accorded the name of familial encephalopathy with neuroserpin inclusion bodies (FENIB). The relationship between neuroserpin deposition and onset of clinical symptoms is not understood. In this disorder, tauopathy is not a feature. Instead, a point mutation leads to neuroserpin self association and aggregation into inclusions, with subsequent neuronal dysfunction. Other cases of familial dementia diagnosed as AD may have these neuroserpin aggregates. A better understanding of FENIB may shed light on the pathogenesis of neurodegenerative diseases in which protein aggregation is a key feature.

5.8.7 Mitochondrial DNA mutations

Evidence for oxidant stress in AD is less compelling than in Parkinson's disease. AD brains show evidence of iron dysregulation (that could promote free radical generation), changes in antioxidant levels, and oxidative damage (for example lipid peroxidation) (Beal 1995). The possibility that mitochondrial DNA mutations may be associated with a subset of AD (Hutchin *et al.* 1995) suggest that the bioenergetic capacity of neurons might be affected in these patients (Wallace 1994). Since many of the mitochondrial disorders occur sporadically, the common and sporadic, late-onset AD might be due, in part, to mitochondrial dysfunction and further genetic studies seem warranted.

5.8.8 Extrinsic factors in Alzheimer's disease pathogenesis

Genetic factors, so far identified, cannot account for all cases of AD, leaving the possibility that non-genetic, environmental factors could be involved in AD pathogenesis. Just as the late-onset nature of AD has hindered genetic analysis, so have the epidemiological studies designed to identify environmental factors been complicated.

5.8.8.1 Aluminium

Epidemiological evidence for a role of aluminium as a risk factor in AD remains inconclusive (Doll 1993). Aluminium has been reported to be found in both plaques (Candy *et al.* 1986) and tangles (Perl *et al.* 1980) in the brain and it can alter the metabolism of both tau protein (Yamamoto *et al.* 1990; Guy *et al.* 1991; Mesco *et al.* 1991; Kawahara *et al.* 1992; Abdel-Ghany *et al.* 1993; Scott *et al.* 1993) and Aβ (Exley *et al.* 1993; Mantyh *et al.* 1993; Kawahara *et al.* 1994). Aluminium interacts with PHF-tau through phosphorylated residues and, in so doing, masks the recognition of tau by phosphorylation-dependent antibodies (Murayama *et al.* 1999). Furthermore, aluminium-induced aggregation of phosphorylated tau *in vitro* could be inhibited by desferrioxamine (Murayama *et al.* 1999), an agent tested in clinical trials for the treatment of AD (Crapper-McLachlan *et al.* 1991).

The neurofibrillary degeneration observed in rabbits injected with aluminium is morphologically distinct from NFT-mediated degeneration found in AD (Klatzo *et al.* 1965; Terry and Peña 1965). PHF preparations injected with $AlCl_3$ into rat brains show that aluminium increases the resistance of PHF-tau to *in vivo* proteolysis (Shin *et al.* 1994), suggesting that aluminium might serve as a cofactor in the formation of neurofibrillary lesions. Likewise, evidence that aluminium might effect Alzheimer-like tau pathology in the human brain has been reported (Harrington *et al.* 1994c). AD-like changes to tau protein were observed in the absence of overt neurofibrillary pathology in the brains of patients with renal failure subjected to chronic aluminium exposure. These changes include: depletion of normal tau; the appearance of hyperphosphorylated tau, and a soluble form of truncated tau; and, in certain cases, the presence of PHFs in frontal cortex. These changes may represent early events similar to those involved in the formation of PHFs in AD, but it is unclear why overt neurofibrillary pathology is not found in those patients where excessive accumulation of aluminium occurs in the brain.

5.8.8.2 Head trauma

Dementia pugilistica in ex-boxers is associated with both the presence of large numbers of NFT (Corsellis *et al.* 1973) and the existence of both diffuse and neuritic Aβ plaques (Roberts *et al.* 1990). Aβ deposition may commence rapidly following head trauma (Roberts *et al.* 1991). A genetic susceptibility is associated with some of these individuals in that those possessing an *APOE* type ε4 allele are more susceptible to Aβ accumulation than those without (Nicoll *et al.* 1995).

5.8.8.3 Inflammatory response

Proteins and cells associated with the immune system are present in the brain and found in association with senile plaques (Eikelenboom *et al.* 1994; McGeer *et al.* 1995). These include activated microglia (the resident cerebral macrophages), components of the complement pathway, and inflammatory cytokines, especially interleukin-1 (Royston *et al.* 1992). In addition, the non-steroidal anti-inflammatory drug indomethacin has some protective effect in AD particularly in those patients lacking any *APOE* ε4 allele (Breitner *et al.* 1995). It is unknown how the inflammatory response is elicited and how it participates in the development of AD.

5.8.8.4 Other extrinsic factors

Other factors have been implicated in the pathogenesis of AD. The risk from these factors has not been established and space limits their discussion here. They include: trace metals such as iron, zinc, cobalt, mercury; neuroleptic treatment; infectious agents such as viruses (see above) and spirochaetes; pesticides; electromagnetic fields; organic solvents; and hypertension. Similarly, protective factors such as smoking, oestrogen replacement, and exposure to nonsteroidal anti-inflammatory drugs and H2-blocking drugs have been proposed. Evidence supporting an acquired environmental form of AD comes from monozygous twin studies. Twin pairs show clear discordance for AD (Breitner and Welsh 1995; Kumar *et al.* 1995), yet the critical factor responsible for this observation has not been found. An environmentally-based aetiology for the production of NFTs in Guam-ALS is suggested by two findings: decreased frequency of the disease and an altered pattern of neuropathology that has occured over a 30-year period since its discovery (Perl *et al.* 1999).

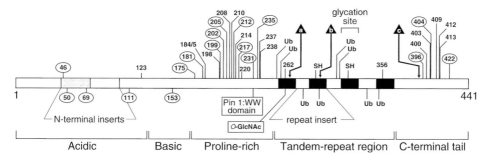

Fig. 5.16. The domains and post-translational modifications of tau protein. The largest tau isoform in the human brain is 441 amino acid residues in length, including two N-terminal inserts and a tandem repeat insert. Residue numbers above and below the sequence correspond to phosphorylation sites. The residues above are those which have been identified in PHF-tau by mass spectrometry or by the use of site-specific, phosphorylation-dependent antibodies (Morishima-Kawashima et al. 1995; Hanger et al. 1998). Most phosphorylation sites flank the tandem-repeat region and are outwith the PHF-core tau fragment (297–391). The latter truncated fragment coresponds to the region, indicated by the arrows, between Leu-266 (a), or Ile-297 (b), through to Glu-391 (c). The positions of putative phosphorylation sites that have not been identified in vivo are indicated below. There are 13 Ser-/Thr-Pro sites (encircled) that are phosphorylated by proline-directed protein kinases (with 4 further sites not identified in vivo). Ser-356 can be phosphorylated in vitro by the same enzyme (p110^{mark}) that phosphorylates Ser-262, but phosphorylation of the former has not been identified in vivo. SH denotes the two Cys residues in the repeat region that can potentially form both intra- or inter-chain disulfide bonds. At least four lysine residues in PHF-tau serve as ubiquitin acceptors and these are all in the microtubule-binding region (u; indicated above the sequence) (Morishima-Kawashima et al. 1993). Evidence of four other possible ubiquitination sites (u; below the sequence) has yet to be confirmed. A prominent site of glycation in PHF-tau has been identified within residues 317–335, a sequence containing three Lys residues (Ledesma et al. 1995). Other sites that have been found to be glycated in vitro (Nacharaju et al. 1997) are not shown. In addition to the binding regions (solid colour), an inter-repeat region between the first and second repeats in adult (but not fetal) tau also promotes tubulin polymerization and the binding is primarily derived from three lysine residues in this region (Goode and Feinstein 1994). A major site for O-glycosylation within the repeat region is shown (Arnold et al. 1996), while 11 other putative sites are not indicated. The WW domain of the prolyl isomerase Pin 1 binds to phosphorylated Thr-231, placing the isomerase site of the enzyme in the vicinity of its Ser-/Thr- Pro substrates (Lu et al. 1999).

5.9 **Modifications of tau protein in disease**

Tau protein is subject to a number of post-translational modifications. These include ubiquitination, phosphorylation, N- and O- glycosylation, non-enzymatic glycation, oxidation, proteolytic truncation, and aggregation. Several of these modifications are probably relevant to the insoluble, protease-resistant state of PHFs found in AD. Whether they occur as early events in the formation of the filaments that constitute tangles or are a secondary phenomena is less easy to demonstrate. Sites at which PHF-tau is modified by glycation, phosphorylation and ubiquitination are depicted schematically in Fig. 5.16.

5.9.1 **Non-enzymatic glycation in Alzheimer's disease**

Protein glycation occurs in diabetes and is a frequent feature of ageing. In AD the neuropathological lesions in the brain are glycated. Whether or not such glycation is a primary or secondary event in AD is uncertain. Tangles, plaques, Hirano and Lewy bodies, granulovacuolar degeneration, and lipofuscin are all structures in the brain that are modified by advanced glycation end products (AGEs) (Smith *et al.* 1994*b*; Vitek *et al.* 1994; Yan *et al.* 1994; Kimura *et al.* 1998; Münch *et al.* 1998; Sasaki *et al.* 1998; Takeda *et al.* 1998). A full qualitative and quantitative description of the cross links found in these pathological lesions has yet to be determined as their chemistry becomes known (Harrington and Colaco 1997). Oxidative reactions accelerate the Maillard reaction and AGEs are glycoxidants themselves (Yan *et al.* 1994; 1995; Münch *et al.* 1997). Although the antioxidant enzyme haemoxygenase 1 is upregulated in AD (Smith *et al.* 1994*a*, 1995), free radical damage to proteins, DNA, lipids in membranes in AD will continue unless the oxidative stress is prevented. AGEs are formed by spontaneous chemical reactions between carbohydrates and proteins. The AGEs are glycoxidation products formed by sequential glycation and oxidation reactions. AGEs can affect protein structure and function, induce oxidative stress, and lead to inflammation and tissue damage. Lesions containing AGE-modified protein aggregates are long lived and arise by abnormal processing of their constituent proteins. Tau protein has abundant lysine residues suitable for glycation (Ledesma *et al.* 1994; Nacharaju *et al.* 1997) and sites in tau capable of being glycated *in vitro* have been determined (Nacharaju *et al.* 1999). Using the longest isoform of tau, 13 sites were glycated and six of these were Lys residues located within the repeat regions (residues 259, 280, 281, 347, 353, and 369). Lysine residues within region 317–335 are glycated in PHF-tau (Ledesma *et al.* 1995). *In vitro* assays suggest that glycation is not involved in tau filament assembly but that subsequent cross-linking, as a result of glycation, could hinder the successful clearance of tau aggregates (Ledesma *et al.* 1995, 1996, 1998). Immunohistochemical evidence indicates that carboxymethyllysine adducts predominate in the aggregated species of tau (Ko *et al.* 1999), giving further support for the role of glycation in stabilizing PHFs in tangles. Normal tau function is altered by post-translational glycation (González *et al.* 1998). Other proteins involved in AD are glycated. Polymerization of Aβ is accelerated by AGEs *in vitro* (Vitek *et al.* 1994), and cytotoxicity of Aβ could be mediated by their presence (Yan *et al.* 1994, 1995). ApoE4 binds AGE more readily than apoE3 (Li *et al.* 1997*b*), an observation that may account for the increased risk for AD afforded to people possessing an ε4 allele.

Unlike diabetes, AGE modifications in AD are restricted to the CNS, and peripheral changes in AGE levels have not been observed (Münch *et al.* 1997). The selected neuronal vulnerability characteristic of AD may be dependent on a number of local factors. The relevance of risk factors for diabetes and vascular pathology in relation to AD has been explored with no clear consensus emerging (Finch *et al.* 1997; Stewart *et al.* 1999). Associations between diabetes and AD have been difficult to establish. Problems in determining risk factors for late-onset dementias make it hard to ascribe defined roles for protein glycation in their pathogenesis. The increased incidence of AD in diabetic patients in a large prospective study suggests that diabetes may have made a significant contribution to the risk for dementia (Ott *et al.* 1998). AGE-inhibitors may ameliorate disease progression by various mechanisms. Whether the mildly beneficial clinical effects of tenilsetam are due to its AGE-inhibitory capacity is not known (Münch *et al.* 1994, 1997). Anti-inflammatory compounds being considered in AD therapy, such as aspirin and ibuprofen, also have AGE inhibitory activity.

AGEs accumulate in pyramidal neurons in layer CA3/4 (Li *et al.* 1995). In the normal brain they have a granular, perinuclear distribution in humans, compared with a nuclear type of staining in rodent (Weber *et al.* 1998). AGEs accumulate with advancing age in the endosomes or lysosomes (Li *et al.* 1995; Kimura *et al.* 1996). In AD, AGEs are found in astrocytes and in activated microglial cells (Takeda *et al.* 1998). They are also involved in modifying long-lived protein deposits in both ageing and in AD. No peripheral changes in AGE levels have been observed although the nature of tau, found in increased amounts in AD CSF, has yet to be characterized (see 5.15 section). AGEs have been found in NFT (Ledesma *et al.* 1994; Smith *et al.* 1994*b*; Vitek *et al.* 1994; Yan *et al.* 1994). It is the intracellular tangles that tend to be immunoreactive for antibodies against AGE-tau. Reactivity is also associated with tau-positive neurites in plaques. Various antibodies reactive with pyrroline, pentosidine, carboxymethylysine, and NFC1 have been observed in tau (Ledesma *et al.* 1994; Smith *et al.* 1994*b*; Sims *et al.* 1996). The non-fluorescent glycation crosslink, NFC-1, was found to a greater extent in tau glycated *in vitro* than glycated Aβ (Sims *et al.* 1996) (tau and Aβ had 1 crosslink per 50 molecules and 1 in 1000, respectively). Furthermore, PHFs containing NFC-1 at 4 nmol/mg protein contained barely detectable levels of pentosidine. The AGE epitopes appear to be embedded within the core of the PHF (Harrington and Colaco 1997). The co-localization with NFTs of haemoxygenase 1, SOD1, and carbonyl content indicates that oxidative changes occur within the vicinity of NFTs (Smith *et al.* 1995). Experiments *in vitro* have shown that glycation of PHFs forms larger aggregates and can stabilize phosphorylated tau (Ledesma *et al.* 1996, 1998). Glycated tau affects normal tau function (González *et al.* 1998) and, in turn, glycated tau can induce cellular oxidative stress leading to the release of both amyloid and interleukin 6 and the production and activation of NFκB (Yan *et al.* 1994, 1995). Glycation of tau protein, rather than being involved in the assembly of PHFs, seems to be involved in the cross-linking of filaments which, in turn, leads to the increased insolubility and protease resistance associated with advanced neurofibrillary pathology (Smith *et al.* 1995; Harrington and Colaco 1997; Münch *et al.* 1997). Since AGEs can contribute to changes in protein conformation, induced changes in the tau molecule might enhance aggregation of further tau (see below). There are several features which argue against a central role for glycation in Alzheimer pathology. For example, pentosidine and CML levels were similar in frontal cortex from both AD, Down syndrome, and control patients (Seidl *et al.* 1997) and neither amyloid nor apoE extracted from Alzheimer cerebral cortex reacted with anti-pyrraline or anti-pentosidine antibodies (Tabaton *et al.* 1997). Nevertheless, intervention with antioxidants, metal chelators, and AGE-inhibitors may yet prove useful in minimizing the pathological consequences of Aβ.

5.9.2 Enzymatic glycosylation of tau protein

O-linked *N*-acetyl glucosamination is a dynamic and abundant post-translational modification that can be reciprocal with Ser-/Thr- phosphorylation (Hayes *et al.* 1994). In an initial study bovine tau was modified by *O*-linked glycosylation at multiple sites, and this modification may play a role in modulating tau function (Arnold *et al.* 1996). More than 12 different sites were glycosylated to the extent of at least 4 mols *O*-GlcNAC per mol of tau. One of these attachment sites resides within the first microtubule-binding domain. The phosphorylation of Ser-/Thr- residues in PHF-tau would decrease the chance of finding *O*-GlcNAc in PHFs. Modification of PHF-tau, but not normal tau by *N*-linked glycosylation, has also been reported (Wang *et al.* 1996). In contrast to *O*-linked glycosylation, *N*-linked glycosylation usually occurs co-translationally and is a considerably less dynamic modification. Deglycosylation of PHFs converts them into straight filaments, a property that suggested N-linked glycosylation may contribute to the maintenance of the PHF structure (Wang *et al.* 1996). *N*-glycosylation affected the helicity of PHFs as well as stabilizing tau. Immunohistochemical lectin-binding studies suggest that both tangles and neuritic plaques are sites of glycan addition. Intracellular neurofibrillary pathology, but not extracellular tangles, was positive for the lectin *Galanthus nivalis* agglutinin (Takahashi *et al.* 1999*a*). Similar changes in tangle-free neurons suggests that glycosylation may be involved early in AD pathogenesis (Guevara *et al.* 1998).

5.9.3 **Ubiquitination of tau protein**

Ubiquitin is a conserved, 76 amino acid polypeptide which binds to target proteins and is involved in the removal of abnormal or damaged proteins which become degraded in proteasome complexes (review: Alves-Rodrigues *et al.* 1998). The presence of ubiquitin in PHFs has been detected (Mori *et al.* 1987; Perry *et al.* 1987) and ubiquitinated PHF-tau fragments isolated from PHFs have been characterized (Morishima-Kawashima *et al.* 1993). Lys-254, 257, 311, and 317 in PHF-tau serve as acceptors for ubiquitin (Fig. 5.16). The amino-terminal portions of tau are cleared to a greater extent in those PHFs that have been ubiquitinated (Morishima-Kawashima *et al.* 1993). Most ubiquitin exists in the monoubiquitinated form and this form may not be such a good signal for degradation by the 26S proteasome complex. The long-lived ghost tangles in the brain are relatively resistant to degradation and removal. The proteasome complex fails to get access to the ubiquitinated sites located inside tightly packaged PHFs. However, from early immunohistochemical studies, ubiquitination probabaly occurs as a late event in the formation of NFT (Bancher *et al.* 1991).

Ubiquitin labelling of NFTs differs between AD and other neurodegenerative disorders (Lowe 1998). Although labelling of AD PHFs is more intense than CBD filaments, their solubility properties are unaffected (Yang *et al.* 1998). The proteasome, a multicatalytic protease complex, appears to be involved in the metabolism of some, but not all, ubiquitinated proteins in a variety of neurodegenerative disorders (Ii *et al.* 1997). Although found at sites of most dystrophic neurites in AD, the proteasome is not found in NFTs. The lysosomal protease cathepsin B, however, is associated with both dystrophic neurites and NFTs.

5.9.4 **Phosphorylation of tau protein**

Different tau isotypes exist, in part, due to different phosphorylation states of the proteins (Butler *et al.* 1986). Cloning of the different isoforms of tau has shown that their expression is under developmental regulation. Thus tau from neonate is phosphorylated at more sites than tau from adult brain and tau phosphorylation in developing brain is more dynamic than in adult brain (Burack *et al.* 1996). Multiple phosphorylation sites have been identified in tau using a combination of protein chemistry techniques and a variety of phosphorylation-dependent antibodies (for example T3P, AT8, tau-1, PHF1, AT270, AT180, 12E8, and AP422). The phosphate-dependent anti-PHF antibody AT100 is the only antibody that recognizes a site in PHF-tau that is not detected in normal tau. More than 20 phosphorylation sites have been identified in PHF-tau (Morishima-Kawashima *et al.* 1995*b*; Hanger *et al.* 1998; Fig. 5.16). After death, phosphate residues are lost quickly from normal tau protein. Normal tau isolated from fresh brain biopsies contains many sites that are phosphorylated although the extent of phosphorylation is much less than that found in PHF-tau (Matsuo *et al.* 1994).

A combination of kinase and phosphatase activity contributes to the extent of phosphorylation of tau both in normal situations and in AD. Protein phosphatases PP2A and PP2B regulate the phosphorylation state of human CNS-tau in a site-specific manner (Goedert *et al.* 1992*a*, 1995). Inhibition of phosphatase with okadaic acid causes hyperphosphorylation of tau protein in brain (Harris *et al.* 1993) and cultured cells (Harris *et al.* 1993; Vincent *et al.* 1994). In an adult rat model, chronic intraventricular infusion of okadaic acid, sufficient to inhibit PP2A, caused tau to become localized in the somatodendritic compartment of nerve cells, where it became hyperphosphorylated (Arendt *et al.* 1995). Furthermore, the okadaic acid treatment also led to the formation of extracellular Aβ deposits and memory impairment (Arendt *et al.* 1995). Likewise, phosphorylated tau was found in neurons in the brains of transgenic mice expressing the largest human tau isoform (Götz *et al.* 1995).

Many kinases are able to phosphorylate tau *in vitro* at both specific residues and at sites with less specificity. Some of these kinases are co-localized within the neurons affected by neurofibrillary pathology. These include mitogen-activated protein kinases (MAPK), also known as extracellular signal-regulated kinases (ERKs), proline-directed protein kinase (PDPK), glycogen synthase kinase-3α and 3β (GSK-3) and cyclin-dependent kinases, cdk2 and cdk5. Calcium-calmodulin-dependent protein kinase and cyclic AMP-dependent protein kinase can both phosphorylate normal tau *in vitro*, but not at sites that are phosphorylated in PHF-tau (Johnson *et al.* 1996).

Evidence that increased phosphorylation of MAPs decrease their ability to promote microtubule assembly was first presented 20 years ago (Jameson *et al.* 1980) and this was confirmed for bovine tau (Lindwall *et al.* 1984). Whereas most phosphorylation sites are away from the tandem-repeat microtubule-binding regions (Fig. 5.16), Ser-262 and Ser-356, in KXGS motifs, can be phosphorylated by p110^{mark}. When these sites are phosphorylated, tau loses its ability to bind microtubules (Drewes *et al.* 1995; Trinczek *et al.* 1995). Phosphorylation of tau also decreases the self-association of tau protein (Guttmann *et al.* 1995) and decreases the rate at which it can be degraded by the protease, calpain (Litersky *et al.* 1992).

The co-expression of tau and GSK3 in COS-7 cells resulted in a decrease in the electrophoretic mobility of tau and increased reactivity with a panel of monoclonal antibodies against phosphorylated tau (Lovestone *et al.* 1994). In contrast, neither ERK1 nor ERK2 phosphorylated tau in similarly transfected COS-7 cells. Whether the overexpression of protein kinases in these cellular models reflects what happens *in vivo* remains uncertain however.

Tau isolated from soluble, dispersed PHFs is extensively phosphorylated compared to both normal tau at both Ser-/Thr- Pro and other sites (Morishima-Kawashima *et al.* 1995*a*; Hanger *et al.* 1998; Fig. 5.17). The extent of tau phosphorylation in AD brain is in the region of 5–9 nmol of phosphate per mole of tau, which has over 20 different sites capable of being phosphorylated at any one time. The hyperphosphorylation of PHF-tau at many of the sites that are phosphorylated in normal adult and foetal tau and the stability of these phosphorylation sites post-mortem implies that, in AD, an abnormal phosphorylation-dephosphorylation equilibrium exists. There is no clear evidence that this is a primary event and that the subsequent stages of phosphorylation and dephosphorylation are not the result of localized activity around insoluble and intractable PHFs. Pools of normal tau, which are phosphorylated at certain epitopes, have been detected (Lu *et al.* 1993; Alonso *et al.* 1994). This has been considered to decrease the association of tau with axonal microtubules and its subsequent accumulation in the somatodendritic compartment (Lovestone *et al.* 1997). Phosphorylated tau accumulates in axonal PHFs early in AD (Bondareff *et al.* 1994*b*). It is

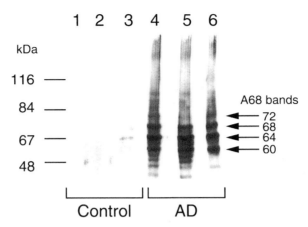

Fig. 5.17 Phosphorylated AD-tau. Sarkosyl-insoluble, 'dispersed' PHFs contain tau protein of abnormal gel mobility, that are not found in identical preparations from control brain tissues. 'A68 bands' run at positions corresponding to 60, 64, and 68 kDa and a minor band at 72 kDa. These revert to normal gel mobility after treatment of the preparation with alkaline phosphatase. Such species represent only 14% of the PHF-tau protein present in these preparations and, of the phosphorylated tau in this preparation, only 12% has the sedimentation properties of PHFs. Therefore, this phosphorylated tau represents a minor species, most of which is not in the form of PHFs.

important to establish whether phosphorylation or dephosphorylation of proteins is altered in AD and whether this arises through direct protein phosphorylation or via other signalling pathways within the cell. Alteration of signal transduction appears to be intimately involved in AD (Fowler 1998) and its effect could be mediated through many different pathways (Anderton *et al.* 2000). Whereas presenilin proteins are clearly implicated in the Notch signalling, a link through this pathway has not been documented for tau.

The antibody AT100 is unique and is dependent on the phosphorylation of two residues. This antibody requires the simultaneous phosphorylation of Thr-212 and Ser-214 (Zheng-Fischhöfer *et al.* 1998). A similar antibody, PHF27, requires the phosphorylation of the primary site Thr-231 and the subsite Ser-235 (Hoffmann *et al.* 1997). Both of these antibodies have reacted with PHF-tau but failed to recognize either foetal or biopsy-derived tau (Hoffmann *et al.* 1997; Zheng-Fischhöfer *et al.* 1998). Based on the distinct iso-electric points of tau fragments, it was determined that PHF-tau from older AD patients was less phosphorylated than PHF-tau from younger AD cases (Sergeant *et al.* 1997). The duration of disease may be an important factor when evaluating the characteristics of PHF-tau. Most of the phosphorylation sites that have been identified are concentrated in two regions N- and C- terminal to the tubulin-binding repeats (Fig. 5.16). Many kinases, particularly the proline-directed kinases, will phosphorylate recombinant tau *in vitro*. Brain extracts contain MAPKs as well as cyclin-dependent kinases and GSK-3. Both GSK-3 and MAPK incorporate phosphate, but it is only GSK-3 that has been shown to phosphorylate tau in intact cells. Several members of the stress-activated protein kinase family, phosphorylate tau *in vitro* (Goedert *et al.* 1997*a*; Reynolds *et al.* 1997). The cellular location and developmental regulation of such kinases *in vivo* is not known. Further kinases, yet to be identified, may play a role in tau phosphorylation. Tau phosphorylation by a number of kinases is stimulated in a substrate-dependent manner by sulphated glycosaminoglycans such as heparin and heparin sulphate (Mawal-Dewan *et al.* 1992; Brandt *et al.* 1994; Yang *et al.* 1994). Stress-activated protein kinase phosphorylates tau at many Ser-/Thr- Pro sites (Mertens *et al.* 1997).

PHF-tau is a poorer substrate *in vitro* for PP1, PP2A, and PP2B than foetal tau, although its ability to be dephosphorylated is increased after solubilization with guanidine (Wang *et al.* 1995; Yamamoto *et al.* 1995). The effects of individual kinases on the properties of recombinant tau *in vitro* have been studied, but have failed to provide evidence that phosphorylation at any one particular site or by any particular kinase, is critical for tau interaction with the microtubules. Phosphorylation at Ser-262 by p110^{mark} decreases the interaction of tau with microtubules (Biernat *et al.* 1993; Trinczek *et al.* 1995). The significance of this finding is less than convincing since tau in normal adult brain is phosphorylated at the same site (Seubert *et al.* 1995a; Lovestone *et al.* 1996). Expression of GSK-3β in mammalian cells co-expressing tau alters the properties of tau protein, with a decrease in microtubule bundling, a reduction in tau binding to microtubules and a loss in the stability of microtubules (Lovestone *et al.* 1996).

Tau transiently expressed in non-neuronal mammalian cell lines is not phosphorylated significantly at sites that are phosphorylated in PHF-tau. However, when GSK-3β is co-expressed with tau in these cells, numerous Ser-/Thr- Pro sites found in PHF-tau become phosphorylated (Lovestone *et al.* 1996; Irving *et al.* 1997). Co-expression of tau with GSK-3β also resulted in less stable microtubules than when the cells were transfected with tau alone. A decrease in microtubule bundling was also observed when tau transfected cells were co-transfected with GSK-3β (Wagner *et al.* 1996). Transgenic mice with the highest levels of GSK-3β activity show the greatest extent of tau phosphorylation (Brownlees *et al.* 1997). Lithium, a selective inhibitor of GSK-3β, inhibits GSK-3β activity in cultured neurons and decreases tau phosphorylation (Hong *et al.* 1997). Lithium treatment decreases both the amount of tau associated with microtubules and tau phosphorylation in cultured rat neurons (Muñoz-Montano *et al.* 1999).

Proline-directed phosphorylation of tau increases during mitosis and correlates with other markers of mitosis (Vincent *et al.* 1997). Degeneration could therefore be the response of a differentiated neuron to inappropriate mitotic signals forcing the neuron to undergo apoptotic death. Since proline-directed phosphorylation does not influence binding of tau to microtubules, other kinases may be more important in the phosphorylation of tau *in vivo*. Cdk5 is a candidate kinase that is deregulated in AD (Patrick *et al.* 1999). It is activated by the binding of a membrane-anchored partner protein, p35. p35 is cleaved to yield p25, which forms a cdk-p25 complex that is a highly active, long-lived form of the enzyme. This complex is capable of phosphorylating tau *in vivo* and is detected in degenerating neurons in AD (Patrick *et al.* 1999).

Although highly speculative, several threads of evidence suggest that the different pathologies of AD might be interlinked (Lovestone and Reynolds 1997). Protein kinase C (PKC) can activate APP metabolism leading to a decrease in Aβ production. Since PKC activates MAP kinases and leads to an inhibition of GSK-3, increasing PKC activity would decrease tau phosphorylation. This is supported by the observation that tau phosphorylation is decreased in response to indirect activation of PKC in PC12 cells transfected with tau

(Sadot *et al.* 1996) or in response to glutamate on primary cortical cultures (Davis *et al.* 1995). PKC could provide a link between tau phosphorylation and APP metabolism; a small decrease in PKC over an extended period would increase both the levels of Aβ and the phosphorylation of tau. The activity of specific signal transduction cascades in neurons is too complicated to determine at this stage. Tau interacts with the key enzyme in the phosphatidyl inositol signalling pathway, phospholipase C-γ (PLC-γ) (Hwang *et al.* 1996). In human neuroblastoma cells, tau selectively associated with PLC-γ, and PLC-γ that co-precipitated with tau is enzymatically active (Jenkins *et al.* 1998). Tau acts as a phosphatidyl inositol bisphosphate binding protein, which may make the latter a more favourable substrate for PLC-γ (Flanagan *et al.* 1997). These data indicate that tau may play a role in signal transduction. A link between the cholinergic signal transduction pathway in tau phosphorylation was indicated recently (Sadot *et al.* 1996). PC12 cells transfected with M1 muscarinic acetylcholine receptor, when stimulated with acetylcholine agonists were found to have decreased levels of tau phosphorylation at sites recognized by tau-1 and AT8 (that is a site in the vicinity of Ser-202).

Phosphorylation on Ser-/Thr-Pro motifs decreases the rate of isomerization of the Ser-/Thr-Pro bonds, and proteins with these motifs are substrates for the prolyl isomerase Pin 1. Recently, Pin 1 has been found to restore the microtubule-binding capacity of phosphorylated tau and Pin 1 is sequestered in NFTs in AD (Lu *et al.* 1999). Pin 1 also binds to several mitotic phosphoproteins that may be affected in AD. The capture of Pin 1 within tangles depletes the soluble pool of this enzyme in AD, a situation that mimics the triggering of mitotic arrest leading to apoptosis. Binding of Pin 1 to phosphorylated tau and subsequent isomerization of the peptide bonds may change the conformation of domains in tau protein. Pin 1 specifically binds to the phosphorylated Thr-231 site in tau (Fig. 5.16), via a WW domain that is separate from the domain involved with isomerase activity. Phosphorylation of Thr-231 is both necessary and sufficient for mediating the interaction between Pin 1 and tau. Thus Pin 1 might be needed to prevent abnormal activation of mitotic events in differentiated neurons. Inappropriate expression of mitotic proteins in AD brain (Vincent *et al.* 1997; Vincent *et al.* 1998) may contribute to hyperphosphorylation of tau and the neurodegenerative process in AD. Phosphorylated tau would also be capable of sequestering Pin 1, which itself can trigger apoptosis.

Thus phosphorylation of proteins, including both tau and mitotic proteins, occurs in AD. Whether this plays a central role in the pathogenesis of AD is less clear. The relevance of tau phosphorylation in the assembly of PHFs is discussed below (Sections 5.11 and 5.14).

5.9.5 Other post-translational modifications of tau protein.

Because of the insoluble nature of the PHF-tau aggregates in AD brain tissue, it is difficult to be certain whether modifications of tau are involved in PHF assembly or merely responsible for increasing their insoluble status. Aside from the modifications described above, transglutamination and racemization of amino acids can alter tau protein.

Transglutaminase-induced ε-(γ-glutamyl)lysine bonds covalently crosslink peptides into insoluble, high molecular weight aggregates, involving both inter- and intra- molecular bridges. Tau serves as a substrate for transglutaminase activity, leading to aggregation *in vitro* (Dudek *et al.* 1993). Enzyme activity is elevated in AD neocortex, as compared with tissue from control patients (Johnson *et al.* 1997*a*), and is present also in the hippocampal neurons affected in AD (Appelt *et al.* 1996). ε-(γ–Glutamyl)lysine crosslinks have also been identified in tau filaments purified from brains of patients with PSP (Lee *et al.* 1999). Such cross-linking may be involved in stabilizing insoluble neurofibrillary structures in neurons. Increased enzyme activity could arise as the result of disturbed neuronal calcium homeostasis, since transglutaminases are calcium-regulated zymogens (Johnson *et al.* 1997a).

Racemization of aspartic acid occurs in long-lived proteins, and the proportion of total Asp in PHF-tau in the D-Asp is 4.9% as compared with 2.8% in normal adult tau (Kenessey *et al.* 1995). The increased racemization is probably inversely associated with the rate of protein turnover that, in turn, reflects their insolubility. There has been no evidence to suggest that isomerization is implicated in formation of PHFs.

Normal tau is readily susceptible to proteolysis, insoluble PHF-tau is markedly resistant. Selective degradation of tau in neurons undergoing apoptosis has been observed in cerebellar granule cells (Canu *et al.* 1998). During this process, a 17-kDa N-terminal fragment (residues 45–229) accumulates in the perikarya of dying neurons. Whether this process occurs in AD is not known. Altered phosphorylation of tau during apoptosis in PC12 cells also results in the retention of tau, with reduced microtubule-binding capacity, in the nuclear/perinuclear region (Davis *et al.* 1999b). This is similar to the pattern observed for the accumulation of PHF-like tau material in PC12 cells subjected to heat shock (Bondareff *et al.* 1998) and would facilitate the possible interaction of abnormally located tau with proteins in mitochondria and other organelles (see Section 5.13).

5.9.6 Post-transcriptional modifications in Alzheimer's disease

In addition to the genetic factors implicated in AD (Section 5.8), post-transcriptionally modified proteins have been associated with sporadic AD and Down syndrome (van Leeuwen *et al.* 1998a; van Leeuwen *et al.* 1998b). Deletions in 'vulnerable' dinucleotide repeats in messenger RNA are found in the absence of changes in the genomic DNA sequence. This 'molecular misreading' results in the expression of '+1 proteins' in which the C-terminal sequence is altered and the protein becomes truncated. Both truncated APP[+1] and ubiquitin-B[+1] proteins are present in AD brain and found to be colocalized with the pathological lesions found in AD. Ubiquitin-B[+1] immunoreactivity is not unique to AD, but is associated with compact globose tangles in PSP (Fergusson *et al.* 2000). These arose due to dinucleotide deletions that occurred in, or adjacent to, a GAGAG motif. Nevertheless, deletions in other motifs (for example CUCU) were also detected in ubiquitin-B, suggesting that other deletions may occur. Although the GAGAG sequence is not found in tau, there are six GAGA motifs and a total of 40 different dinucleotide repeats within the tau coding sequence. Six of these have a further base continuing the repeat, that is CACAC (2), CGCGC (1) and GUGUG (3). Dinucleotide deletions at these sequence sites would result in proteins of 85 (8), 85 (11), 102 (32), 294 (4), 312 (7), and 329 (8) amino acids in length, where the number of residues in the altered, C-terminal +1 sequence is given in parentheses. None of the potential dinucleotide deletions result in proteins terminating with a C-terminal Glu that might make them reactive with mAb 423. It would be interesting to discover if tau[+1] proteins exist in AD and, in particular, those truncated within the repeated microtubule-binding domain that might be capable of interfering with the function of normal tau proteins. Post-mitotic neurons are less capable of compensating for transcript-modifying activity and are thus particularly sensitive to the accumulation of frameshift mutations. Thus, during aging, single neurons may accumulate abnormal proteins leading to cellular disturbances and degeneration.

5.10 **Staging the pathological assembly of truncated tau**

The antigenic features of the core PHF-tau fragment are C-terminal truncation at Glu-391 (detected by mAb 423), and acid-reversible occlusion of a generic tau epitope located in the tandem repeat region of tau (detected by mAb 7.51). Another useful histological property of the PHF is that it contains a high-affinity binding site for planar molecules such as thioflavin-S, or thiazin-red (Resch *et al.* 1991). The latter is commercially available as a more homogeneous chemical preparation, and is useful in confocal microscopy because its fluorescence can be visualized in the standard red channel (Mena *et al.* 1995). This makes it possible to compare dye labelling with immunohistochemical labelling. Double-labelling in high resolution confocal microscopy has shown that pathological tau and β-amyloid deposits contain binding sites for thiazin red only when they are in the fibrillar state of assembly (Mena *et al.* 1995). Amorphous β-amyloid deposits lack thiazin-red binding sites, and likewise, PHFs lose thiazin red binding sites during end-stage degradation in the extra-cellular space.

The earliest mAb 423 immunoreactivity seen in the brain takes the form of diffuse cytoplasmic staining in the somatodendritic compartment of pyramidal cells lacking PHFs (Mena *et al.* 1991; 1996) (Plate 2). When examined in greater detail in aged cases with and without a diagnosis of AD, these deposits were also found to be labelled with mAb 7.51, but only after formic acid treatment of the section (Mena *et al.* 1996). Ultrastructural investigation showed these deposits to be amorphous clumps either free in the cytoplasm, or associated with membranous organelles, including mitochondria. This amorphous ultrastucture is consistent with absent or weak labelling by thiazin red. Therefore, the earliest pathological deposits of core PHF-tau antigens in pyramidal cell cytoplasm are characterized by C-terminal truncation at Glu-391, acid-reversible occlusion of the mAb 7.51 epitope, indicating partial pathological assembly involving the tandem repeat region of tau, and absence of fibrillar structure.

More typical fibrillar deposits found in NFT continue to show acid-reversible occlusion of the mAb 7.51 epitope. However, as PHFs form within cells, the mAb 423 epitope also undergoes acid-reversible occlusion, whereas it is not occluded in the amorphous tau complexes described above. Typical PHF deposits are strongly labelled by thiazin red (Plate 2). After formic acid treatment, most neurofibrillary pathology (tangles), dystrophic neuropil threads, and neuritic plaques, show co-localization of labelling by thiazin red, mAb 423 and mAb 7.51 (Plate 2). This indicates that the same immunochemical features that characterize the early amorphous tau deposits, namely C-terminal truncation at Glu-391 and occlusion of the tandem repeat region, are preserved during the formation of PHFs (Mena *et al.* 1996).

The transition between these two states of tau aggregation can be seen within individual neurites with a distal to proximal polarity. In preparations not treated with formic acid, amorphous thiazin-red negative truncated tau can be seen in an unoccluded state at the more distal tip. Extending more proximally, the labelling changes into the type which is characteristic of PHFs, with acid-dependent occlusion of the truncated tau epitope, and presence of thiazin-red binding sites.

These findings demonstrate that the assembly of truncated tau complexes into PHFs is at least a two-stage process. At the first stage, structurally amorphous complexes of truncated tau which have self-associated in the tandem repeat region begin to accumulate in the cytoplasm, often in close association with membranous organelles, particularly abnormal mitochondria. There may be possible links with more general abnormalities in processing of membrane-bound proteins or mitochondria (see Section 5.9). As these truncated tau complexes are converted into PHFs, the C-terminal epitope recognized by mAb 423 is retained, but undergoes acid-reversible occlusion. In isolated preparations of PHFs it is not fibrillar assembly *per se*, but the presence of a coating of full-length tau molecules in the fuzzy coat of the intact PHF, which occludes the mAb 423 epitope. Thus in the course of assembly of truncated tau complexes into PHFs, the C-terminal epitope is occluded by the addition of full-length tau molecules in the fuzzy coat of the PHF (Novak *et al.* 1993; Mena *et al.* 1996).

The tau protein which forms the fuzzy coat remains N-terminally intact only while PHFs remain intracellular (Bondareff *et al.* 1994*a*; 1995). These intracellular NFT have been designated as Type 1 tangles (Bondareff *et al.* 1994*a*). Superficial fuzzy coat epitopes include those recognized by BR133 (residues 1–16), AT8 (phosphorylation sites at residues 199/202) and Alz 50 (a conformational epitope that includes residues 3–10). As pyramidal cells begin to degenerate, 'pre-ghost' tangles, or Type 2 tangles, can be distinguished by immunohistochemical and morphological criteria. Type 2 tangles, which have lost the pyramidal cell nucleus and plasma membrane, but are not yet swollen and dispersed, lose immunoreactivity associated with the extreme N-terminus of tau. As tangles degenerate further in the extracellular space, Type 3 tangles are produced. These are typically enlarged by invasion of astrocytic processes, and lose all immunoreactivity except for epitopes associated with the tandem repeat region and the extreme C-terminus of tau (Fig. 5.18). Degradation of tangles in the extracellular space continues to the point of loss of thiazin-red binding sites (Mena *et al.* 1995). However, these tangles remain immunoreactive with mAb 423.

In summary, the following stages in the pathological assembly and disassembly of truncated tau protein can be distinguished in AD brain tissues. (1) Amorphous deposits characterized by aggregation through the repeat domain, C-terminal truncation at Glu-391, lack of fibrillar structure, and in which the nature of association with hyperphosphorylated tau is unknown. (2) Fibrillar intracellular deposits characterized by aggregation through the repeat domain and occlusion of Glu-391 epitope by full-length tau molecules in the fuzzy coat, some of which are hyperphosphorylated. (3) Fibrillar extracellular deposits characterized by aggregation through the repeat domain, exposure of the Glu-391 epitope, and progressive loss of N-terminal half of tau molecule. (4) Loss of fibrillar structure in the extracellular space and preservation of Glu-391 epitope.

The Glu-391 epitope appears to be extremely stable to proteolytic degradation, persisting even after advanced stages associated with loss of fibrillar structure in the extracellular space. Its appearance at very early stages of tau aggregation in tangle-free neurons indicates the intracellular generation of a species that does not appear to be amenable to proteolytic degradation. This is discussed further below.

5.11 Tau protein aggregation

5.11.1 Tau aggregation as an amyloidosis

It has never been demonstrated crystallographically that PHFs have an underlying cross β-pleated structure. However, in view of the shared ability of PHFs to bind planar dyes, it seems likely that they share at least some of the generic ultrastructural features of amyloids. The approaches that have proved useful in the study of other amyloids have failed to produce comparable results when tau protein aggregation has been studied *in vitro*. Indeed the behaviour of tau protein in solution is remarkable for its lack of ordered secondary

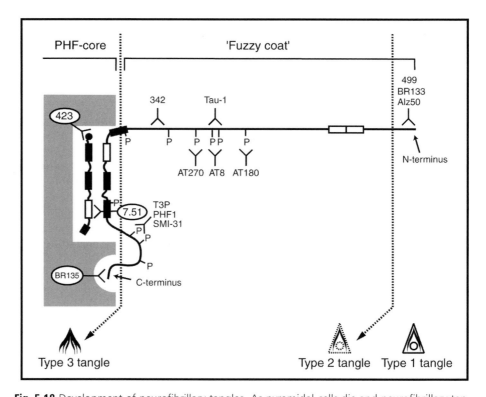

Fig. 5.18 Development of neurofibrillary tangles. As pyramidal cells die and neurofibrillary tangles become extracellular, the pattern of immunoreactivity reflects the removal of the N-terminus and C-terminal truncation of tau protein. This figure summarizes three identifiable stages in NFT development (Bondareff *et al.* 1994). Intracellular, Type 1 tangles contain N-terminally intact PHFs. C-Terminally truncated core PHF-tau fragment is still detected in these tangles after formic acid treatment, signifying its presence in an occluded configuration within the core of PHFs containing N-terminally intact tau in the fuzzy outer coat. Some intracellular PHFs contain N-terminally intact tau that is not phosphorylated, implying that phosphorylation is not an obligatory concomitant of PHF assembly (Bondareff *et al.* 1995). As pyramidal cells begin to degenerate, so-called 'pre-ghost' or Type 2 tangles lose immunoreactivity associated with the extreme N-terminus of tau. Such tangles are no longer associated with a plasma membrane or with a pyramidal cell nucleus, but have not as yet undergone invasion by astrocytes in the extracellular space. In Type 3 tangles, astrocytic invasion results in swelling of the extracellular tangle beyond the original outlines of the pyramidal cell body in which the tangle was assembled. Such tangles are immunoreactive only with antibodies which detect the repeat domain, and the extreme C-terminus of the tau molecule. The Glu-391 epitope detected by mAb 423 is not hidden in these tangles, and still can be demonstrated after PHFs lose their filamentous structure in the extracellular space. The preservation of the epitope in the course of severe end-stage degradation of PHFs in the extracellular space indicates the extreme proteolytic stability of this epitope.

structure, whether normal human tau, recombinant tau or hyperphosphorylated tau has been analysed (Lang *et al.* 1992*a,b*; Schweers *et al.* 1994). It is unlikely therefore that the aggregation of tau in PHFs is based on interactions between strands of β-sheets. Studies of the aggregation behaviour of individual microtubule-binding repeats have reached the same conclusion (Hoffmann *et al.* 1997). The only report of the expected β-pleated aggregation *in vitro* was obtained using fragments of tau restricted to the C-terminal tail, which are not the major component of the proteolytically stable core of the PHF (Yanagawa *et al.* 1998).

The aberrant aggregation of tau protein can best be understood within the broader context of neurodegenerative and other disorders characterized by aberrant protein aggregation. These have been termed 'conformational diseases' (Carrell *et al.* 1998), 'prionoses' (Wisniewski *et al.* 1998), or more simply, diseases characterized by protein misfolding. Thus the respective roles of β-amyloid versus tau protein converge on the more general problem of misfolding of two different proteins to form stable 'amyloids' in the generic sense. The aberrant protein deposits were originally identified pathologically by histochemical staining properties, hence the term 'amyloid' or 'starch-like'.

These deposits consist of highly ordered fibrils at the molecular level. The fibrils have a 'cross-β-pleated' structure: that is individual protein strands which make up the fibril are oriented transversely with respect to the fibril axis, and stabilized largely by hydrogen bonds oriented in the fibril axis. This bonding between the anti-parallel peptide β-sheets provides a binding site for flat molecules, such as Congo-red or thioflavin-S. A common feature of the 17 different human amyloid proteins deposited in disease conditions is the ultrastructure of the respective fibrils. Diffraction data derived from amyloid fibrils composed of different precursor proteins are virtually identical, suggesting that the structure of amyloid is common, despite the absence of homology in the primary structure (Kelly 1998).

The ability to form amyloid is a not a peculiarity of the relatively small group of proteins known to be implicated in human disease. By lowering the pH or otherwise partially denaturing/unfolding the protein, it is possible to generate conditions in which a large number of proteins can form amyloid fibrils (Dobson 1999). The critical factor appears to be the capacity under certain conditions to form an intermediate structure that is marginally stable relative to the correctly folded form of the protein. At sufficient concentration of the intermediate structure, however, aggregregation stabilizes the aberrant conformation, which now acts as a seed for further polymerization, recruiting more normal molecules into the aggregate (Wisniewski *et al.* 1998; Carrell and Gooptu 1998; Cohen *et al.* 1998; Kelly 1998; Lansbury 1999). This represents the 'conformational change' or 'induced conformational polymerization' hypothesis, as distinct from the 'nucleated condensation polymerization' hypothesis, in which there need not be any change in the conformation of the aggregating protein.

The mechanics of the induced conformational change have been modelled recently in an entirely artificial system (Takahashi *et al.* 1999*b*). Here a peptide forming a double α-helix in native conditions was susceptible to conversion into a β-fibril structure by addition of carbon chains of defined lengths to provide a site for initial hydrophobic interaction. The importance of the hydrophobic carbon-chain is to permit initial aggregation of unstable α-helix peptides, thereby favouring a transition to the β-sheet aggregate, a process that then becomes autocatalytic. This emphasizes the concentration-dependence of the transition. Whereas the normal folding of proteins is concentration independent, the formation of aberrant fibrils is highly concentration dependent (Lansbury 1999). This is thought to be due to the need to create conditions of co-operativity which permit partial ordering of the monomers prior to locking them into the stable cross-β configuration.

Once the β-fibril configuration has been achieved, the protein, or those parts forming the core of the fibril structure, becomes indestructible under physiological conditions, because of the large number of hydrogen bonds that must be disrupted in order to rescue the peptide chain from the aggregated state (Dobson 1999). The mechanics of transition to the proteolytically stable aggregate are perhaps best studied in the case of the prion protein. In this case, a normal transmembrane protein (PrP^C) is converted into a highly proteolytically stable shortened form (PrP^{Sc}) which, according to the 'prion hypothesis' has the capacity to propagate the Creutzfeldt-Jakob disease (CJD)-like neurodegenerative syndrome (Cohen and Prusiner 1998). PrP^C is composed of about 40% α-helix and little β-sheet, whereas PrP^{Sc} is composed of about 30% α-helix and 45% β-sheet (Prusiner *et al.* 1998). Evidence in favour of a templated conversion of PrP^C into PrP^{Sc} is provided by the recruitment of host PrP^C into the proteolytically stable aggregate after contact with the PrP^{Sc} form in cells (Horiuchi *et al.* 1999) and transgenic animals (Prusiner *et al.* 1998). The β-sheet structure is acquired rapidly by a dimeric species prior to polymerization (Post *et al.* 1998).

The possibility of a cause–effect relationship between the onset of fibril deposition and the onset of disease has been discussed by Kakizuka (1998), Koo *et al.* (1999), Lansbury (1999), and Tran *et al.* (1999). The main argument against has come from experiments attempting to model the neurodegeneration associated with the expression of proteins with an excessive number of glutamine repeats. The huntingtin protein is normally associated with between 6 and 34 glutamine repeats at the N-terminus. In individuals affected by Huntington's disease, the length of the repeat is increased to between 36 and 120 residues, with greater disease severity and generational anticipation associated with longer repeats. Ordway and colleagues (1997) showed that an otherwise innocuous protein linked to a 146-CAG repeat also produced a neurodegenerative phenotype. One possible explanation for this degenerative pathway is the formation of amyloid-like aggregates from proteins having an excessive number of repeats. The expanded glutamine repeats act as hydrogen-bonded polar zippers, forming β-fibrils held together by hydrogen bonds (Perutz *et al.* 1994). Inclusion formation, however, can be dissociated from cell death in at least one cellular model. Translocation of mutant huntingtin to the nucleus is considered to induce cell death via an apoptotic pathway, whereas formation of the aggregated protein merely reflects an epiphenomenon or perhaps a cellular mechanism to protect against cell death (Saudou *et al.* 1998). Given the abundant evidence that amyloid aggregates are almost always associated with disease states, Lansbury provides a way out of the paradox. He proposes that the protofibril (an intermediate in the assembly of the filament) is the toxic species, whereas the final assembled filament may represent a protective form of the aggregate in which the toxic protofilaments have been sequestered (Lansbury 1999). In this sense, the final filaments are indeed an epiphenomenon of the actual toxic species, namely the proto-aggregates.

5.11.2 Determinants of tau aggregation

Filament assembly in solution has been used widely as an experimental paradigm to study the aggregation properties of tau protein (Montejo de Garcini *et al.* 1986; Crowther *et al.*

1992, 1994; Wille *et al.* 1992; Garcia de Ancos *et al.* 1993; Ruben *et al.* 1993; Troncoso *et al.* 1993). However, such studies have yielded inconsistent results (Wille *et al.* 1992; Schweers *et al.* 1995; Wilson *et al.* 1995), probably because it has been difficult to induce tau aggregation experimentally. Full-length recombinant tau does not aggregate in physiological conditions (Yanagawa *et al.* 1998) even when the protein has been hyperphosphorylated *in vitro* (Crowther *et al.* 1994). Conversely, full-length tau and tau fragments restricted to the repeat domain can be made to assemble in non-physiological buffers and at high protein concentrations, irrespective of phosphorylation status (Wille *et al.* 1992). The conditions in which tau aggregation has been observed are highly artificial, including dialysis of urea-treated brain extracts, spraying of glycerol solutions of tau, and hanging drop crystallization conditions. Conversely, several non-tau proteins have also been shown to form PHF-like assemblies *in vitro*, including the C-terminal tail of APP (Caputo *et al.* 1992*a*) and α-1 antitrypsin (Lomas *et al.* 1992; Janciauskiene *et al.* 1995). As neither of these proteins is found in PHF-core preparations, the morphology of filaments produced *in vitro*, even when this closely resembles the PHF, is an insufficient criterion to establish disease relevance.

More recently, procedures have been developed whereby tau aggregation could be facilitated by co-incubation of tau protein with sulphated glycosaminoglycans (Goedert *et al.* 1996; Pérez *et al.* 1996). The N-terminal half of the protein inhibits aggregation, and this inhibition can be overcome by a range of polyanionic cofactors, including heparin, heparan sulphate, RNA, and polyglutamine (Goedert *et al.* 1993; Kampers *et al.* 1996; Hasegawa *et al.* 1997; Friedhoff *et al.* 1998*a*). Although tau assembly can be induced in more physiological buffers, using this manoeuvre, the concentrations of tau required are still very high. Typically, concentrations between 40 µM–100 µM are required, whereas direct measurements in the human brain indicate that tau protein concentrations are unlikely to exceed 1µM within pyramidal cells (Lai *et al.* 1995).

The initial nucleation step of all protein aggregation systems is rate-determining, whereas the elongation step is rapid, indeed autocatalytic. Mandelkow and co-workers have shown that tau aggregation can be seeded, greatly increasing the efficiency of the process in a concentration-dependent manner (Friedhoff *et al.* 1998*b*). This was achieved using crosslinked dimers or pre-formed tau aggregates extracted from the brain. Furthermore, in this system, N- and C-terminal truncation increases the rate of *in vitro* filament formation. Similarly, PHF-tau extracts from the brains of AD and CBD patients facilitate tau aggregation in the presence of high levels of Ca^{2+} and Mg^{2+} (Yang *et al.* 1999). With amyloids, aggregation clearly begins with dimer formation. There is no evidence that the dimer has an independent existence, as argued by Mandelkow in the case of the disulphide cross-linked form of truncated tau (Friedhoff *et al.* 1998*b*). In other studies, however, neither oxidation nor phosphorylation of truncated tau fragments enhance tau aggregation (Hoffmann *et al.* 1997).

In attempting to define further the mechanism of tau aggregation, two groups have shown that the third 18-residue tubulin-binding repeat (R3) is the shortest fragment capable of aggregating either following oxidation (Schweers *et al.* 1995) or in the presence of heparin (Goedert *et al.* 1996; Pérez *et al.* 1996). However, other studies have shown that oxidation-dependent homo-dimerization of R3 and R2 are equivalent, and that R2/R3 heterodimer formation may be more efficient (Hoffmann *et al.* 1997). Conversely, the aggregating activity of the other repeats is minimal, and the presence of an intact N-terminus, whether or not phosphorylated, is generally inhibitory to aggregation in a variety of settings (Friedhoff *et al.* 1998*b*; Yanagawa *et al.* 1998).

No further light on the molecular mechanism of aggregation has as yet been derived from the study of the pathogenic tau mutations. P301L (in R2), V337M (near R3), and R406W (C-terminal tail) all exhibit decreased microtubule binding and assembly properties (Hong *et al.* 1998). There is no clear unifying explanation for these effects. R1 and R2, and possibly the R1-R2 linker, have the strongest microtubule-binding activity (Chau *et al.* 1998), and cross-linking studies implicate R1 and the KK motif in the linker between R1-R2 as having particular importance (Chau *et al.* 1998). Likewise, full-length tau constructs having only R1-R2 in the microtubule-binding domain have the same tubulin-binding affinity as wild-type tau (Felgner *et al.* 1998). Structure prediction algorithms indicate that there would be reduced flexibility in the highly conserved PGGG motif (thought to act as a flexible hinge region during microtubule binding), but only for the G272V and P301L mutations. Full-length tau constructs bearing the mutations G272V, P301L, V337M, and R406W were all significantly more retarded in their elution profile in acetonitrile-HPLC, and all had greater α-helical character (Jicha *et al.* 1999), although these results were not confirmed by others (Goedert *et al.* 1999). These findings suggest that the mutations may make the repeat domain more rigid and less able to bind to microtubules.

According to these results, the role of the mutations in pathology would be mediated only by decreased microtubule binding, leading in some way to impaired microtubule function, and perhaps indirectly to tau aggregation. Arrasate and colleagues (1999) dealt with the self-aggregating propensity of the isolated repeats and showed that the P301L mutation in repeat 2 increases its tendency to aggregate, but that the G272V mutation in repeat 1 has no effect on the otherwise negligible aggregation of the first repeat in the presence of heparin or chondroitin sulphate.

The filaments generated *in vitro* are not PHFs, but rather artificial tau polymers. The ultrastructural differences between tau polymers and PHFs have been well documented by Ksiezak-Reding and co-workers (Ksiezak-Reding *et al.* 1998). The filaments produced *in vitro* differ from PHFs in morphology, mass per unit-length (44 kDa/nm *vs.* 104 kDa/nm), and mass density (50 kDa/nm *vs.* 40 kDa/nm). This implies that the precise packing of tau protein within the PHF is different from the aggregation of tau produced *in vitro*. A more important practical implication is that the use of the filament assembly protocols to discover inhibitory substances need not predict inhibitors of PHF-formation in AD.

5.11.3 Modelling tau aggregation

The tau–tau binding interactions that are critical for the stability of the PHF in AD have been reproduced. A relatively simple solid-phase assay is used to measure the properties of tau–tau binding through the repeat domain in physiological buffer conditions over a range of tau concentrations relevant to the neuronal cytoplasm (Wischik *et al.* 1996). A tau–tau binding interaction of very high affinity through the repeat domain can be demonstrated, with an affinity of ~20 nM, comparable to a strong antibody–antigen interaction. This binding confers proteolytic stability on the repeat domain, and reproduces the conditions required for the characteristic C-terminal truncation at Glu-391 found in the core of the PHF. Proteolytic digestion of the N-terminal domain of the molecule is accompanied by acquisition of immunoreactivity characteristic of the Glu-391 truncation (Fig. 5.19). The high affinity tau–tau binding interaction is therefore all that is required to induce the characteristic conformation of the repeat domain of tau found in the PHF-core.

Furthermore, this binding interaction is self-propagating. As shown in Fig. 5.19, the truncated tau aggregate generated after the first binding/digestion cycle retains the ability to

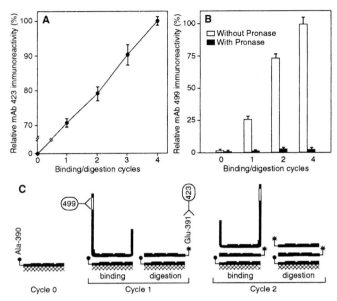

Fig. 5.19 Autocatalytic propagation of tau capture *in vitro*. A progressive increase in mAb 423 immunoreactivity is observed as full length tau is first captured by truncated tau before being exposed to proteolysis (A). After each digestion cycle, the mAb 499-immunoreactive N-terminus is removed (B). In this process, over 4 binding/digestion cycles, progressively more full-length tau is bound as truncated tau accumulates in the solid-phase.

bind full-length tau, and indeed with *higher* affinity than in the base-line condition. This progressive accumulation of the proteolytically stable species and the increasing binding capacity could be demonstrated over four binding/digestion cycles. In Prusiner's prion terminology, the repeat-domain binding interaction 'encrypts' a characteristic aberrant conformation which has the capacity to catalyse the further conversion of normal tau into the aggregated/truncated form.

Phosphorylation of tau is systematically inhibitory to tau–tau binding through the repeat domain, by factors in the range 24- to 50-fold for full-length tau species (Table 5.3). These inhibitory effects are in part reversible by adsorbtion of tau to a non-specific solid-phase substrate, implying that the effect is conformational. That is, phosphorylation stabilizes an aqueous-phase conformation of tau that restricts access to the repeat domain. These results

Table 5.3 Relative affinities for the tau–tau binding interaction through the repeat domain. After phosphorylation, this binding affinity is decreased by up to 50-fold when both binding partners are hyperphosphorylated.

	Unphosphorylated full-length tau	Phosphorylated full-length tau
Repeat domain	100%	8.9%
Unphosphorylated fetal tau	101%	4.2%
Phosphorylated fetal tau	3%	2.0%

are in agreement with the recent findings from Mandelkow and co-workers who demonstrated that phosphorylation protects tau against aggregation (Schneider *et al.* 1999). They contradict the earlier hypothesis that hyperphosphorylation is essential for tau aggregation through the repeat domain (Lee *et al.* 1991; Biernat *et al.* 1992, 1993; Goedert *et al.* 1992*b*, 1997*b*; Gustke *et al.* 1992; Lichtenberg-Kraag *et al.* 1992).

The mounting body of evidence that cannot be reconciled with the phosphorylation hypothesis is increasingly being recognized within the field. Few of the phosphorylation sites found in PHFs are abnormal (Baum *et al.* 1995). There is no evidence that phosphorylation potentiates tau polymerization *in vitro* (Wille *et al.* 1992; Crowther *et al.* 1994), and indeed tau polymers can be generated independently of phosphorylation. Hyperphosphorylation of tau protein in cells and in transgenic animals overexpressing tau has failed to produce PHFs (Baum *et al.* 1995; Götz *et al.* 1995). Insoluble forms of phosphorylated tau do not behave as PHF precursors at early stages of AD as predicted (Lai *et al.* 1995). Hyperphosphorylation of tau in intracellular tangles is variable (Bondareff *et al.* 1995) and is not even required heuristically as an explanation for the detachment of tau from microtubules. As the binding affinity at the tau–tau site is 20-fold higher than the tau–tubulin binding interaction, tau aggregation will be propagated at the expense of normal tubulin binding, once the relevant tau–tau site becomes available within the cell.

Phosphorylation can be seen as a mechanism not only for regulating tau–tubulin binding, but also for protecting tau protein from aberrant aggregation. Aberrant tau–tau binding, once initiated, locks the repeat domain in a proteolytically stable conformation which has the capacity to propagate further conversion of tau protein into the proteolytically stable form. As noted above for amyloids, tau–tau binding renders the repeat domain essentially indestructible in physiological conditions. Tau protein carrying the foetal complement of phosphorylation sites is a particularly poor aggregation substrate (Yang and Ksiezak-Reding 1999). In our assay, no binding was observed (Wischik *et al.* 1996). These findings directly contradict the hypothesis that reversion to a foetal state of phosphorylation is the key prerequisite for aggregation (Lee *et al.* 1991; Goedert *et al.* 1992*b*).

The mechanics of generation of the high-affinity tau–tau site within the cell can be understood from the intrinsic binding properties of tau. The binding behaviour of tau in solution is different from that observed when tau protein is adsorbed to a non-specific solid-phase and is most dramatically seen in the case of foetal tau. Whereas foetal tau protein in solution does not aggregate at all through the repeat domain, prior binding to a non-specific solid-phase permits high affinity tau–tau binding to occur. This might partly explain why polyanionic substrates help in artificial aggregation conditions. This is a non-specific phenomenon, and carries no implications as to the particular relevance of sulphated glycosaminoglycans, heparin, RNA, or polyglutamine in pathogenesis. Other substrates within the cell may mediate non-specific binding of tau in such a way as to expose the high affinity binding site in the repeat domain. Biochemical evidence to shed light on the identity of such substrates has yet to be forthcoming.

5.12 **Proteolytic stability and propagation of tau capture**

The core PHF-tau fragment contains a high-affinity tau capture site, with an affinity comparable to a strong antibody–antigen interaction. It now becomes possible to examine whether the binding interaction confers proteolytic stability on the bound segment of the molecule, but not those regions of the molecule outside the binding domain. The identity of the binding constants for full-length and truncated tau species indicate that the truncated core PHF-tau fragment contains the critical tau-binding domain.

This was achieved using proteolytic mapping with the aid of two further monoclonal antibodies that recognize epitopes depicted in Fig. 5.6. mAb 499 recognizes a human-specific segment between Gly-14 and Gln-26 near the N-terminus of full-length tau, whereas mAb 342 recognizes a segment between Ser-208 and Pro-251. These antibodies span the segment of the tau molecule N-terminal to the tandem repeat region. Full-length recombinant tau, which had bound to truncated tau in the solid phase, lost immunoreactivity associated with both of these antibodies in a protease concentration-dependent manner when digested with increasing concentrations of Pronase (Fig. 5.19). On the other hand, mAb 423 immunoreactivity was acquired in a protease concentration-dependent manner in the course of the same experiment (Wischik *et al.* 1996). As the truncated species on the solid phase terminates at Ala-390, it is not recognized by mAb 423, since Glu-391 is essential for this immunoreactivity. Furthermore, the Glu-391 epitope cannot be created by further digestion of the Ala-390 fragment. Likewise, full-length recombinant tau is not recognized by mAb 423, because it is not truncated at Glu-391. The appearance of mAb 423 immunoreactivity can only be explained by truncation of full-length tau in the bound configuration. Similar results were obtained when full-length tau was allowed to self-aggregate during binding to the solid phase. This indicates that the conformation required for C-terminal truncation at Glu-391 does not require a pre-existing truncated fragment, but is produced solely by the tau–tau binding interaction occurring in the solid phase. In general terms, the high affinity tau–tau binding interaction confers proteolytic stability on a short segment that excludes most of the tau molecule N-terminal to the repeat domain, and reproduces the characteristic truncation to Glu-391 at the C-terminus.

As the proteases used in these experiments come from a broad spectrum mixture ('Pronase', Calbiochem), it is unlikely that C-terminal truncation at Glu-391 is due to the proteolytic specificity of a particular endoprotease included in the mixture. The action of specific proteases, however, cannot be excluded. Two recently identified aggrecanase enzymes, which are expressed in brain tissue, cleave Glu-Ala bonds within the core protein of proteoglycans (Abbaszade *et al.* 1999; Tortorella *et al.* 2000) and deserve to be examined with tau as a substrate for generating Glu-391 truncation. The site of truncation, however, is most likely due to steric hindrance produced by the tau–tau binding interaction that limits access by non-specific exoproteases. Furthermore, the Glu-391 truncation in the PHF-core tau fragment is associated with a characteristic 15-residue shift in the tandem repeats (Fig. 5.8). The fact that the same truncation can be reproduced *in vitro* indicates that tau–tau binding through the tandem repeat region induces the conformational change responsible for the phase shift.

Although high affinity binding through the repeat domain could explain the production of the proteolytically stable core-PHF tau fragment, the binding studies indicate that the process is saturable. How do PHFs continue to accumulate in AD? In the phosphorylation hypothesis, filaments assemble directly from the aqueous phase. If this were so, then aqueous-phase aggregation must be extremely favourable with a negligible off-rate. Alternatively, the concentration of soluble tau would have to be maintained at a high level in the aqueous phase. As discussed above, neither of these conditions are met in the AD brain. That is, phosphorylation of tau, generally regarded as favouring aggregation, is in fact highly inhibitory in the aqueous phase. Second, the levels of soluble tau actually fall substantially below normal levels in the AD brain and, despite this, PHF assembly appears to continue relentlessly.

A possible factor which could make tau capture irreversible is some form of chemical post-translational modification and/or cross-linking. However, mass-spectroscopic analysis of preparations of the PHF-core tau fragment isolated from AD brain has failed to reveal any mass deviations from those predicted for the corresponding peptides (Poulter *et al.* 1993). In the tau species, which can be released by acid treatment from proteolytically stable PHFs, there is no evidence of chemical cross-linking or of any other post-translational modification other than the truncation described above.

The truncation itself may represent a post-translational modification, one which could both enhance further tau capture and reduce the off-rate for tau release from the bound complex. The truncated fragment generated after binding and digestion *in vitro* should retain the capacity to bind full-length tau presented in the aqueous phase, and should do so with a higher binding affinity. The progressive accumulation of tau and increased binding capacity has been demonstrated (Fig. 5.19c; Wischik *et al.* 1996).

There are two possible explanations for the propagation of incremental tau capture. The first is that the removal of regions of the tau molecule outside the binding domain has the effect of improving access to it, thereby increasing binding capacity for full-length tau. The second is the concentration-dependent increase in K_D and B_{max}. Increasing the concentration of tau protein in either the solid or the aqueous phases has the effect of producing concentration-dependent conformational changes at the binding interface which facilitate binding. The introduction of more truncated tau in the solid phase after the first binding/digestion cycle reproduces this phenomenon, increasing the effective K_D and B_{max} values. The results of these experiments demonstrate that tau capture can be propagated through proteolytic digestion cycles, that is in the presence of proteases, and also that the process has the intrinsic capacity for autocatalytic propagation of tau capture.

The findings of the *in vitro* binding experiments are in agreement with the apparent dynamics of tau protein redistribution into PHFs at early stages of AD. PHF-bound tau accumulation increases with the tangle count and is accompanied by a corresponding decrease in the level of soluble tau (Wischik *et al.* 1995a). As the tangle count measures disease progression over time in both cases, it is possible to examine directly the rate of transfer of soluble tau into the PHF-bound pool relative to tangle count by solving the relevant first order differential equations (Lai *et al.* 1995). The rate of transfer of soluble tau into the PHF-bound pool is exponential, with the highest rates observed at the earliest stages. It is assumed that the level of soluble tau depends on an equilibrium between newly synthesized tau entering the pool of soluble tau, and tau that is lost through PHF assembly. As the level of soluble tau falls below 580 pmol/g, progressively more new tau synthesis would be required to account for the level of soluble tau that is actually observed. Thus, there appears to be a negative feedback relationship, in which the loss of soluble tau via assembly of PHFs demands progressively higher levels of new tau synthesis. This analysis fits well with a model in which there is autocatalytic incorporation of soluble tau into PHFs which eventually exceeds the intrinsic capacity for new tau synthesis (Lai *et al.* 1995).

5.13 Mechanisms for initiation of tau aggregation in Alzheimer's disease

5.13.1 Links with APP via phosphorylation

APP undergoes cleavage and secretion by a number of cellular pathways (Selkoe 1999). Secretory processing of APP occurs either at the cell surface or intracellularly releasing the extracellular domain and cleaving within the Aβ domain. The so-called β-secretase pathway is thought to prevent Aβ deposition. Other processing pathways generate C-terminal APP fragments produced by complex endosomal/lysosomal processing or the secretion of Aβ via the β-secretory pathway (Selkoe 1999), perhaps through the action of presenilin proteins (Wolfe *et al.* 1999*a*).

The secretion of APP is regulated by protein phosphorylation (Buxbaum 1995). Thus increasing overall phosphorylation in the cell is associated with increased production of secreted APP and decreased production of Aβ and *vice versa*. Although initially it was assumed that the latter involved the phosphorylation of APP in the cytoplasmic domain by protein kinase C, it now appears that PKC regulates APP processing by the phosphorylation of some component of the processing pathway other than the APP. Various PKC/phospholipase C-linked first messengers have been shown to regulate APP processing. These include acetylcholine, interleukin-1, bradykinin, thrombin, and ATP. Whether these interactions are relevant *in vivo* is not yet known; cytoplasmic calcium levels and release of calcium from intracellular stores may also affect APP processing.

If APP molecules were to serve as aberrant tau-binding proteins in AD (see below) then their occurrence within the cell at an appropriate location would need to be altered from the normal situation. For example, direct phosphorylation of the C-terminal tail APP may affect its processing and/or cellular trafficking. In this respect Thr-743 of APP_{770} is phosphorylated by GSK-3β (Aplin *et al.* 1996), a kinase putatively involved in tau hyperphosphorylation.

Another link between Aβ and tau pathology has focused on the neurotoxicity of Aβ which induces tau phosphorylation (Busciglio *et al.* 1995) and which can be prevented by GSK-3β anti-sense oligonucleotides (Takashima *et al.* 1993). The *Drosophila* homologue of GSK-3β is also involved with an intracellular signalling pathway containing a gene product that is homologous to the two recently identified presenilins linked to familial AD.

It has been reported that the transmembrane region of APP just C-terminal to the Aβ domain is immunochemically associated with PHFs (Giaccone *et al.* 1996). A peptide, corresponding to this region, forms fibrils *in vitro* and dense fibrillary assemblies are generated in the presence of tau. Tau interacts with a conformation-dependent domain of APP encompassing residues 714–723. PHF-like structures were also assembled from the cytoplasmic APP peptide, consisting of residues 751–770 (Caputo *et al.* 1992*a*). Thus either of these peptides might conceivably act as 'seeds' for the nucleation of tau assembly into PHFs (Smith *et al.* 1995). In a disorder such as parkinsonism-dementia complex of Guam, where tangles occur in the absence of Aβ (Buée-Scherrer *et al.* 1995), alternative mechanisms would need to account for the aggregation of tau.

5.13.2 Pathological tau capture as an initiating mechanism

Normal tau protein has little in the way of physical structure: α-helical, β-sheet, and β-turns are absent (Schweers *et al.* 1994). PHF-tau does not show significant changes in structure

(Schweers *et al.* 1994). Although AD-like conformational epitopes, detected using mono-clonal antibodies with a specificity for PHF-tau (for example Alz50, MC1, and AT100 (Jicha *et al.* 1997; Zheng-Fischhöfer *et al.* 1998), still need to be established. Nevertheless, tau aggregation through the repeat domain confers proteolytic stability on a short segment of the molecule that corresponds closely to that isolated from the PHF-core. This fragment has the intrinsic capacity to propagate tau capture (Wischik *et al.* 1996), reproducing itself in the presence of proteases by a mechanism similar to that proposed for prion protein propagation (see Section 5.11). The proteolytically stable conformation depends on a high affinity tau–tau binding interaction which induces a characteristic phase-shift in the tubulin-binding repeats (discussed in Section 5.3.1). Although it has been proposed that 'aberrant' hyper-phosphorylation of tau appears to represent one, if not the, principal mechanism for its aggregation into PHF (Lovestone *et al.* 1992), the binding studies discussed earlier indicate that phosphorylation is inhibitory to tau aggregation through the repeat domain in all phase configurations. Furthermore, tau protein in an immature state of phosphorylation cannot form the proteolytically stable binding interaction through the repeat domain without prior non-specific binding to a solid-phase substrate (as discussed above). Macromolecules within the cell might provide the early pathological tau capture substrates required to initiate the propagation of high affinity tau capture through the repeat domain.

Extracellular matrix proteins may promote tau aggregation *in vitro* (Goedert *et al.* 1996; Pérez *et al.* 1996). However, facilitation of tau aggregation *in vitro* can be due to a general property of macromolecular substrates that bind tau non-specifically, including polyvinyl chloride. This property cannot therefore be used as a criterion for identification of relevant tau-binding substrates in AD brain. Since prior binding to such a substrate is required for C-terminal truncation at Glu-391, one possible way to identify endogenous macromole-cules involved in tau capture in AD would be on the basis of their co-elution with truncated tau in AD brain extracts and co-localization with endogenously truncated tau within pyra-midal cells.

We analysed non-tau proteins copurifying with proteolytically stable PHFs with the aim of identifying candidate macromolecular substrates relevant to tau capture in AD. ApoE and histone fragments were identified among proteins co-sedimenting with PHFs after Pronase digestion and dialysis. However, these were readily separated from PHFs by sonica-tion, and no tau sequences were found in fractions containing apoE. In contrast to proteins loosely associated with PHFs, the core PHF-tau fragment can be extracted by formic acid treatment (Wischik *et al.* 1988*a*). This procedure leaves an SDS-insoluble residue (more than 80% of protein present) which appears on immunoblots as a tau-immunoreactive smear (Novak *et al.* 1991). This material was found unsuitable for the further biochemical analysis necessary to identify candidate tau-binding macromolecules in AD brain. However, following a protocol developed for biochemical analysis of scrapie fibrils (Stahl *et al.* 1990), it was possible to discrete species, to isolate by preparative electrophoresis, that were suitable for sequence analysis.

The core PHF-tau fragment was found to co-elute with ubiquitin and two nuclear-encoded mitochondrial membrane proteins in the form of formic acid-, guanidine-, SDS-, and electrophoresis-resistant complexes. The mitochondrial outer membrane protein porin was identified with truncated tau in species migrating at 66 kDa and 34/32 kDa. Core protein 2 (CP2) of the mitochondrial cytochrome *bc₁* enzyme complex was identified with truncated tau in species migrating at 46/44 kDa and 26/24 kDa. The same associations with endogenously truncated tau could be demonstrated within pyramidal cells by double-labelling confocal microscopy (Plate 3). As indicated above, there is electron-microscopic evidence that truncated tau aggregates are associated with abnormal mitochondria in AD (Mena *et al.* 1996). Tau protein was not found in similar extracts from aged control brain that nevertheless contained the same proteolytically stable mitochondrial proteins identified by sequence analysis. Thus porin and CP2 accumulate in a proteolytically stable form in the ageing brain without tau binding, but form stable complexes with truncated tau in AD.

A third nuclear-encoded mitochondrial membrane protein, ATP-synthase subunit 9 (ATP9), co-eluted with four N-terminally distinct Aβ fragments in a species migrating at 5 kDa in the same preparation, but not with tau. Lipofuscin deposits and Aβ fibrils can be visualized by electronmicroscopy in these preparations (Wischik *et al.* 1988*b*). As ATP9 is known to accumulate in neuronal lipofuscin deposits in sheep (Palmer *et al.* 1989), co-elution of Aβ fragments with ATP9 is consistent with Aβ immunoreactivity reported in lipofuscin deposits in AD (Bancher *et al.* 1989; Wisniewski *et al.* 1990). No extracellular matrix proteins (Goedert *et al.* 1996; Pérez *et al.* 1996), bound or unbound to either tau or Aβ, were identified in these preparations.

MAPs including tau have been reported to interact with normal brain mitochondria through the repeat region (Rendon *et al.* 1990), but the specificity and nature of these inter-actions is unclear (Leterrier *et al.* 1990; Linden *et al.* 1996). Mitochondrial function is highly dependent on import of nuclear encoded structural proteins (Neupert 1997). Binding to endogenously truncated tau within pyramidal cells in AD raises the possibility that age-related defects in endosomal-lysosomal turnover of mitochondrial and other membrane-spanning proteins such as the presenilins and the Aβ precursor provide cytosolic substrates which initiate tau capture (Fig. 5.20). In such a scenario, quantitatively minor incremental changes associated with neuronal ageing could cross a threshhold required to initiate an exponential cascade mediated by autocatalytic propagation of tau capture, leading to the destruction of pyramidal cells in AD (Bondareff *et al.* 1993).

5.14 Tau-based therapeutic approaches to Alzheimer's disease

5.14.1 Phosphorylation-based approaches

The view that hyperphosphorylation of tau has a central role in PHF formation, and reviewed more extensively elsewhere (Wischik *et al.* 1995*b*, *c*; 1997), has led to several thera-peutic proposals for AD. Kinases thought to be particularly relevant include the 42-kDa MAP kinase, GSK-3α, GSK-3β, cdc2, cdk5, and one or more proline-directed kinases (Biernat *et al.* 1992; Drewes *et al.* 1992; Gustke *et al.* 1992; Hanger *et al.* 1992; Ishiguro *et al.* 1992; Ledesma *et al.* 1992; Lichtenberg-Kraag *et al.* 1992; Mandelkow *et al.* 1992; Vulliet *et al.* 1992; Wille *et al.* 1992). These kinases are capable of phosphorylating tau on at least some of the residues which are phosphorylated in PHF-tau. There has been interest in mod-elling the activation of some of these kinases by a further cascade of kinases (Howe *et al.* 1992; Lange-Carter *et al.* 1993; Nebreda *et al.* 1993; Zheng *et al.* 1993)

Four International Patent Applications have been filed in relation to hyperphosphoryla-tion as a process potentially amenable to therapeutic intervention in AD.

V. M. Ingram ('*Novel TAU/neurofilament protein kinases*', Publication Number WO 93/03177, Filing Date 09.08.91) reported the identification of two novel kinases, PK40 and PK36. These are not associated with the cytoskeleton, but are capable of phosphorylating neurofilament and tau proteins in a manner that is claimed to be relevant to AD by virtue of

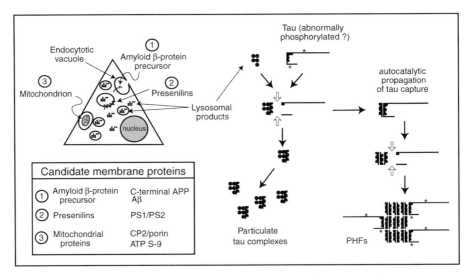

Fig. 5.20 Involvement of membrane proteins in the initiation of tau capture in AD. Diagrammatic representation of how abnormalities in the endosomal/lysosomal turnover of a number of different membrane proteins might converge to initiate and propagate tau capture, leading to overt neurofibrillary degeneration in Alzheimer's disease. The turnover of mitochondrial membrane proteins becomes increasingly defective in the course of neuronal ageing, leading to the accumulation of so-called aging pigments (lipofuscin), which are composed of incompletely degraded mitochondrial membrane proteins (ATP-synthase subunit 9, core protein 2 of the bc_1 enzyme complex and porin) accumulating in tertiary lysosomes. Mutations in the membrane proteins implicated in the genetic etiology of Alzheimer's disease (APP, presenilins) lead to an increased requirement for endosomal/lysosomal processing which in the ageing brain is increasingly unable to deal with the demands arising from turnover of mitochondria. At some point, these macromolecules provide the pathological substrates required to initiate tau capture. Once tau capture is initiated, the repeat domain exists in a stable conformation that is able to propagate the exponential capture of tau. Progressive redistribution of tau protein from the soluble pool to proteolytically stable aggregates could be prevented by blocking the high affinity tau–tau binding interaction through the repeat domain.

the appearance of immunoreactivity detected by SMI-31 and SMI-34 (Roder *et al.* 1991). Assays are proposed for the measurement of these kinase activities in a variety of cell lines, and it is further proposed that an inhibitor of these kinases will reduce the formation of PHFs in AD and normal aging.

E.-M. Mandelkow, E. Mandelkow, B. Lichtenberg-Kraag, J. Biernat, G. Drewes, and B. Steiner ('*Tools for the diagnosis and treatment of Alzheimer's disease*', Publication Number WO 93/11231, Filing Date 07.12.92) argued that as phosphorylation of tau protein lowers its affinity for microtubules this would lead to both microtubule disassembly and aggregation of tau protein into PHFs. The key proposal relates to the identification of critical phosphorylated epitopes and the characterization of the kinase which catalyse these phosphorylations, permitting the development of inhibitors of the relevant kinases. In the preferred embodiment, the critical epitopes include the serine residues at positions 262, 293, 324, and 409 which are phosphorylated by a 42 kDa-MAP (microtubule-associated protein or mitogen-activated) kinase. Further kinases which are proposed include GSK-3α or -3β or cdk2-cyclin A, capable of phosphorylating tau serine residues at positions 46, 199, 202, 235, 262, 396, 404, 422, and threonine residues at positions 50, 69, 111, 153, 175, 181, 205, 212, 217, and 231. However, phosphorylation at Ser-262 is regarded as critical, and diagnosis in AD brain biopsy or CSF specimens would depend on detection of this particular epitope (Biernat et al. 1993; Drewes et al. 1995). It is proposed that these kinases can be used for the conversion of tau protein, in vitro, into Alzheimer-like PHFs. Substances that inhibit these kinases should be capable of inhibiting the formation of PHFs. 'Moreover, they may be used for the development of drugs capable of dissolving PHFs or for converting Alzheimer tau protein into normal tau protein.'

B. H. Anderton and C. Miller ('Models of Alzheimer's disease', Publication Number WO 95/05466, Filing Date 01.08.94) propose that transgenic cell and animal models for Alzheimer's disease could be created by introducing DNA sequences encoding a protein kinase. This would enable the modulation of tau phosphorylation to be tested against potential therapeutic agents for AD. In the preferred embodiment they propose co-transfecting COS7 cells with tau and GSK-3α or GSK-3β, and monitoring the appearance of tau protein in cell extracts, using phosphorylation-dependent antibodies (Anderton et al. 1995). These include 8D8, RT97, 121.5, BF10 (Miller et al. 1986), AT8 (Biernat et al. 1992), SMI31, SMI34, SMI310 (Sternberger et al. 1983, 1985) and Alz-50 (Wolozin et al. 1986), which react with hyperphosphorylated tau from AD brain tissue. These results are complemented by in vitro phosphorylation of tau by isolated GSK-3β. The making of transgenic animal equivalents of these paradigms is also described (Brownlees et al. 1997; James et al. 1996).

P. Davies and I. J. Vincent ('Methods for treating and/or preventing Alzheimer's disease using phenothiazines and/or thioxanthenes', Publication Number WO 96/04915, Filing Date 07.08.95) used the phosphatase inhibitor okadaic acid to produce large amounts of hyperphosphorylated tau in neuroblastoma cell lines and hippocampal slices (Harris et al. 1993). These were detected using a range of phosphorylation-dependent tau antibodies. They demonstrated that the neuroleptics trifluoperazine and chlorpromazine reduced the amount of phosphorylated tau in such preparations and propose a wide range of standard antipsychotic compounds for the treatment or prevention of AD.

The main arguments which can be raised against these approaches centre on the weakness of the evidence that aberrant hyperphosphorylation of tau is the principal mechanism responsible for its aggregation into PHFs. In particular, few if any of the phosphorylation sites found in PHFs are abnormal (Matsuo et al. 1994). There is no evidence from any in vitro tau aggregation studies that phosphorylation potentiates tau polymerization (Crowther et al. 1992, 1994; Wille et al. 1992). Hyperphosphorylation of tau protein in either cells (Baum et al. 1995) or transgenic animals (Section 5.7) overexpressing tau has failed to produce PHFs. Insoluble forms of phosphorylated tau do not behave as PHF precursors at early stages of AD as predicted (Lai et al. 1995). Rather, phosphorylated PHF-tau was found to represent a relatively constant proportion (5%) of the PHF-tau pool at all stages of pathology, including the earliest (Wischik et al. 1995a). The phosphorylation that detaches tau from microtubules rather than priming it for PHF assembly, actually inhibits the process (Schneider *et al.* 1999). There is no data available to contradict the interpretation that hyperphosphorylation of tau protein occurs as a secondary phenomenon that occurs after pathological aggregation in AD.

Apart from these difficulties in theoretical rationale, the more practical difficulty of identifying and selectively inhibiting the putative pathogenic kinase has not been solved. Most of the kinases, referred to in these patent applications, have physiological functions. It would need to be demonstrated experimentally that these functions could be inhibited without detriment to other important cellular functions, such as cell-cycle control. Furthermore, hyperphosphorylation of tau protein *in vitro* inhibits both tau–tau and tau–tubulin binding interactions to a comparable extent (Wischik *et al.* 1996). There is as yet no evidence that inhibition of a relevant tau kinase could be achieved without impairment in the regulation of microtubule turnover. In any case, it can be shown from the binding studies *in vitro* that dephosphorylating tau would enhance tau aggregation. Indeed, the immature state of phosphorylation found in the neonatal brain, far from representing a risk factor for tau aggregation (Goedert *et al.* 1992*b*), is highly effective at blocking binding through the repeat domain entirely. A state of phosphorylation that protects against self-aggregation could be part of a physiologically important protective mechanism. This may occur not only in the immature brain, but also in response to injury, where tau protein accumulates in the somatodendritic compartment, as axonal transport and outgrowth is held in abeyance (Papasozomenos *et al.* 1991).

5.14.2 Direct inhibition of tau aggregation

The model of autocatalytic propagation of tau aggregation via high affinity binding and truncation implies that the pathological high affinity tau–tau binding interaction through the repeat domain is reponsible both for the propagation of tau capture, and for the creation of the proteolytically stable truncated intermediary which propagates tau capture. Furthermore, the model predicts that high affinity binding through the repeat domain is all that is necessary for the structural and proteolytic stability of the PHF-core. Therefore, a compound which blocked the high-affinity tau–tau binding interaction through the repeat domain would be expected to reverse the proteolytic stability of PHFs isolated from the brain.

Compounds that are able to disrupt the morphological ultrastructure of proteolytically stable PHFs have been isolated from advanced AD cases (Wischik *et al.* 1996). In the presence of increasing concentrations of methylene blue, PHFs are seen to coarsen, swell, untwist, fragment, and disappear (Fig. 5.21). This morphological disruption is associated with increased susceptibility to protease digestion. The tau–tau binding assay was used to identify compounds with higher inhibitory acitivity, which are active at 4:1 molar ratio with respect to tau. These compounds belong to the general class of diaminophenothiazines.

Methylene blue itself has been used in man in a variety of clinical indications. It was the first antiseptic dye to be used therapeutically, and has been used in the treatment of nephrolithiasis and methaemoglobininemia (Di Santo *et al.* 1972). It has been tried in the prophylaxis of manic depressive psychosis and severe depressive psychosis (Naylor 1986, 1987). Following systemic administration during life, methylene blue accumulates within cortical pyramidal cells (Muller 1992).

The mechanism of action of methylene blue on the tau–tau binding interaction is unknown, but it has two opposite actions on haemoglobin. At high concentations it

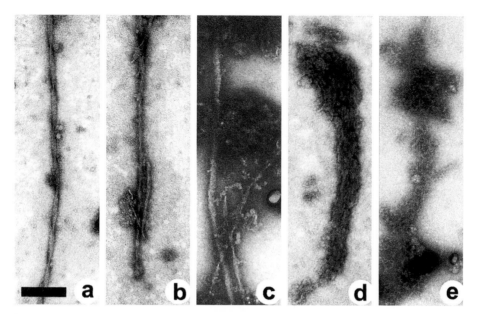

Fig. 5.21 Disruption of the structural integrity of PHFs. PHFs, isolated from AD brain tissues, are visualized after treatment with methylene blue (a: 0.01%; b: 0.1%; c–e: 1%). In the presence of increasing concentrations, PHFs are seen to coarsen (b & c), swell (c), fragment (d), and eventually disappear after longer incubation (e). Scale bar, 100 nm.

oxidizes the ferrous iron of reduced haemoglobin to the ferric form, and as a result methaemoglobin is produced. Conversely, *in vivo*, low concentrations of methylene blue, or its desmethyl derivatives thionine and tolonium chloride, are capable of hastening the conversion of methaemoglobin to haemoglobin. The reduction of methaemoglobin within the intact erythrocyte is accomplished by reductases which are pyridine-nucleotide dependent. Diaminophenothiazines act as electron acceptors in the transfer of electrons from reduced pyridine nucleotides to methaemoglobin. In this reaction, the compound is reduced by pyridine nucleotides to produce the leuko-form, which in turn reduces methaemoblobin to haemoglobin. These compounds do not affect methaemoglobin in persons with glucose-6-phosphate dehydrogenase deficiency, implying that prior reduction of the diaminophenothiazines is required. When the formation of reduced pyridine nucleotides is prevented, methylene blue acts purely as an oxidant (reviewed by Gilman *et al.* 1980).

Whatever the mechanism whereby the diaminophenothiazines inhibit the critical tau–tau binding interaction, the findings indicate that the development of a therapy based on this approach may be clinically feasible. A critical requirement is that an inhibitor of tau–tau binding should not interfere with normal binding of tau protein to tubulin. The diaminophenothiazines have this property (Fig. 5.22). Therefore, it is now technically feasible to optimize a treatment for AD based on prevention of the critical tau–tau binding interaction which underlies the formation of NFT.

The relevance of these findings to tau assembly is unknown. Several studies have shown that tau protein can form polymers *in vitro* (Montejo de Garcini *et al.* 1986; Crowther *et al.*

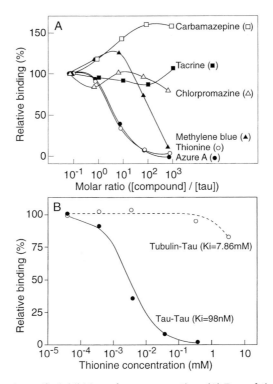

Fig. 5.22 Selective and specific inhibition of tau aggregation. (A) Two of the potent phenothiazine inhibitors (thionine and Azure A) inhibit tau-tau binding over the range 1:1 to 10:1 molar ratio with respect to tau. These are desmethyl derivatives of methylene blue that is itself inhibitory only at molar ratios greater than 30:1. The neuroleptic phenothiazine chlorpromazine and the anti-cholinesterase tacrine, are inactive. The anti-epileptic carbamazepine potentiated tau-tau binding. (B) Tau-tau binding is selectively inhibited by thionine, which does not affect tau-tubulin binding.

1992, 1994; Wille *et al.* 1992; Garcia de Ancos *et al.* 1993; Ruben *et al.* 1993; Troncoso *et al.* 1993). A feature common to assembly-competent fragments is the presence of the tandem repeat region. Tau fragments from PHFs encompassing this region form detergent-resistant dimers and trimers *in vitro* (Wischik *et al.* 1988*b*; Jakes *et al.* 1991; Novak *et al.* 1991). Aggregation involves anti-parallel dimerization (Wille *et al.* 1992) under non-reducing conditions (Schweers *et al.* 1995), whereas others have reported reducing conditions as necessary for filament assembly (Wilson and Binder 1995). In the latter case, straight filaments are formed in the presence of arachidonic acid, a fatty acid that has to bind to tau before filaments will assemble (King *et al.* 1999). After extended incubation of the straight filaments, however, extensive helical morphology becomes apparent (King *et al.* 1999). Straight filaments of various diameters have been formed following the incubation of tau with transglutaminase (Dudek and Johnson 1993). In the presence of glycosaminoglycans or RNA, 3-repeat tau isoforms form PHF-like polymers and 4-repeat tau form straight filaments (Goedert *et al.* 1996; Kampers *et al.* 1996; Pérez *et al.*1996). Studies of chemically cross-linked heparin-treated tau indicate that this treatment induces conformational change in tau protein (Paudel *et al.* 1999). Oxidization of PHF-core preparations has been shown to permit proteolytic cleavage by pepsin within the core tau fragment (Jakes *et al.* 1991), producing fragments similar in gel mobility to those obtained in the presence of methylene blue (Wischik *et al.* 1996). Furthermore, proteolytically stable PHFs have not been found to disassemble in the presence of DTT, although this blocks dimerization of repeat domain fragments (Wille *et al.* 1992).

Whatever the mechanism of action of methylene blue in inhibiting tau aggregation through the repeat domain, the concentrations required *in vitro* appear to exceed those which could be achieved in the brain. We determined the feasibility of using the tau–tau binding assay as a screening tool for identifying more potent inhibitors. Desmethyl derivatives of methylene blue, such as thionine, were 30-fold more potent, acting at concentrations close to equimolar with respect to tau, and with K_i values in the nM range. In contrast to the findings of Davies and Vincent, the side-groups added to the phenothiazine nucleus to achieve neuroleptic activity (for example chlorpromazine) abolished inhibitory activity in the tau–tau assay. Likewise, tacrine, a structurally related compound used as a symptomatic treatment for AD, had no activity in the assay. On the other hand, carbamazepine, an anti-epileptic considered to be safe in the elderly, was found to potentiate tau aggregation through the repeat domain. Thus the action of the diaminophenothiazines is chemically specific, and could in principle be optimized by further pharmaceutical chemistry.

A further concern in the potential therapeutic use of such compounds is selectivity with respect to tau–tubulin binding. A therapeutic strategy based on selective inhibition of putative pathogenic kinases would have the effect of enhancing both normal tau–tubulin binding and pathological tau–tau binding through the repeat domain. The tandem repeat region binds to microtubules via repeating 19-residue tubulin-binding segments which alternate with 12-residue linker segments. The 15-residue phase-shift in the organization of the repeats which characterizes the core PHF-tau fragment implies that tau–tau binding within PHFs is mediated by domains which differ from those involved in the normal interaction between tau and tubulin. This raises the possibility of distinguishing pharmaceutically between the two binding interactions. Inhibition of tau–tubulin binding was found to occur at concentrations of diaminophenothiazines 1000-fold higher than required to inhibit the tau–tau binding interaction (Fig. 5.22). This distinction is consistent with the findings indicating that the tau–tau binding required, for C-terminal truncation of the bound complex at Glu-391, is conformationally distinct from the physiological tau–tubulin binding.

5.15 Tau protein and other biological markers in cerebrospinal fluid

Autopsy studies indicate that clinical diagnosis of AD during life can be less than 80% accurate outside of established dementia research centres. A biological marker is needed both to aid diagnosis, especially in the detection of the early stages of AD, and in the development of disease-specific treatments. Many of the tests have been performed on patients with a clinical diagnosis of probable AD and where pathological confirmation has yet to be obtained. This lowers both the sensitivity and specificity of such tests and diagnosis of early AD is even less precise. Several investigators have examined cerebrospinal fluid (CSF) and serum samples in an effort to find appropriate biological markers for AD (Percy 1993). These would be of use both in confirming the probable diagnosis of AD during life and in providing further insight into the pathogenesis of the disease. Assays for both pathological hallmarks of AD, amyloid and tau protein, have been developed whereas the results from other tests have yet to be replicated.

5.15.1 Amyloid β-protein

Amyloid-related plaque constituents have been measured in CSF, but initial findings gave inconsistent evidence for any diagnostic potential in measuring Aβ in CSF. Although failing to detect changes in the levels of APP in CSF, Raby and colleagues (1998) found that $A\beta_{42}$ is elevated in the CSF after severe brain trauma, indicating that pathological amyloid can be released due to brain damage. The 1–42 peptide is the major species of Aβ in senile plaques in the brain. In contrast to the total levels of amyloid in CSF, which were unaltered, $A\beta_{42}$ concentrations in CSF are lower in AD patients than in control subjects (Andreasen et al. 1999a; Galasko et al. 1998; Kanai et al. 1998; Motter et al. 1995; Tamaoka et al. 1998). Decreased levels of $A\beta_{42}$ in CSF, however, are not specific for AD (Hulstaert et al. 1999). Measurement of their level in CSF in combination with other tests (see below) may still be productive. Four studies (Galasko et al. 1998; Hulstaert et al. 1999; Kanai et al. 1998; Shoji et al. 1998), have indicated improved sensitivity when combined analysis of $A\beta_{42}$ and tau levels in CSF are measured.

Aβ is found in a soluble form in plasma and tissues other than the brain (Seubert et al. 1995b). Both the major species, 1–40, and the more amyloidogenic form, of 42 residues, are increased two- to three-fold for patients carrying the Swedish APP mutation (Scheuner et al. 1996). Decreased levels of $A\beta_{42}$ in CSF are also correlated in a dose-dependent relationship with APOE4. Pirttilä and colleagues found soluble Aβ and apoE levels decreased during the progression of disease in patients carrying an ε4 allele but not in those without the ε4 allele (Pirttilä et al. 1998). In contrast, levels of APP were unchanged.

The decreased levels of $A\beta_{42}$ arise due to increased insolubility of the peptide, which forms deposits that accumulate in plaques in the brain. The decline in CSF-$A\beta_{42}$ need not necessarily be derived from progressive deposition of $A\beta_{42}$ within the brain parenchyma. CSF-$A\beta_{42}$ levels decline in those patients with diseases other than AD (Galasko et al. 1998; Kanai et al. 1998; Motter et al. 1995; Tamaoka et al. 1998; Andreasen et al. 1999a) and the decline is significantly correlated with temporal lobe glucose metabolism in both AD and non-AD patients (Okamura et al. 1999). CSF-$A\beta_{42}$ levels, but not $A\beta_{40}$, are decreased in Down syndrome patients (Tamaoka et al. 1999). CSF-$A\beta_{42}$ may reflect residual function of neurons, which constitutively produce and secrete Aβ protein into CSF (Okamura et al. 1999).

Elevated plasma $A\beta_{42}$ levels have been reported in an analysis with a small number of familial AD subjects (Scheuner et al. 1996) but not for sporadic AD (Mehta et al. 2000). Although $A\beta_{40}$ levels are elevated in sporadic AD and influenced by APOE genotype, their measurement is not helpful in diagnosis (Mehta et al. 2000). The levels of $A\beta_{42}$ may vary during progression of the disease and an increase in CSF $A\beta_{42}$ in the early stages of sporadic AD cases is followed by a decline as the disease progresses (Jensen et al. 1999). Further characterization of these changes is essential if therapeutic monitoring is to be undertaken.

5.15.2 **Tau protein**

Several groups have reported the presence of tau in CSF using different assays (Vandermeeren *et al.* 1993; Mori *et al.* 1995; Vigo-Pelfrey *et al.* 1995) and further trials with modified immunoassays have used a variety of anti-tau antibodies. The levels of tau in CSF range from 250 ng/g to in excess of 1000 ng/g protein in AD patients, which compares with levels of 50–70 ng/g in controls (Vanmechelen 1998). With tau being an intracellular protein, it is likely that CSF-tau levels are associated with neurodegeneration. CSF-tau levels correlate to the degree of temporal lobe atrophy and high levels of tau are observed in CSF from CJD patients (Otto *et al.* 1997). The latter also indicates the lack of disease specificity for such tests. Tau levels are elevated in both early onset (Arai *et al.* 1995; Vandermeeren *et al.* 1993) and in familial AD cases carrying APP or presenilin mutations (Jensen *et al.* 1999). Levels are relatively constant during the disease process (Blomberg *et al.* 1996; Isoe *et al.* 1996; Andreasen *et al.* 1999*b*; Sunderland *et al.* 1999), implying that tau protein appears in CSF early in the disease process. In a large community-based series of patients, CSF-tau showed high sensitivity and specificity to differentiate AD from normal ageing and depression (Andreasen *et al.* 1999*b*). CSF-tau is also increased for patients with vascular dementia (Arai *et al.* 1995; Blennow *et al.* 1995; Skoog *et al.* 1995; Tato *et al.* 1995; Andreasen *et al.* 1998), although many of these patients will have some degree of Alzheimer-type pathology. In a further study, however, no increase in CSF-tau was observed for patients with vascular dementia (Arai *et al.* 1998). Greater numbers of these vascular cases, with autopsy verification, need to be studied. Elevated CSF-tau has also been detected in FTD and in a group of CBD patients, whereas patients with PSP did not have elevated CSF-tau levels (Green *et al.* 1999; Urakami *et al.* 1999). In FTD, a concomitant increase in CSF S100β is observed (Green *et al.* 1997), which may reflect the marked astrocytosis observed in this condition. In contrast, however, a significant decrease in CSF-tau was observed in a group of 18 FTD patients (Molina *et al.* 1999). Further investigations are necessary to resolve these discrepancies.

CSF-tau levels correlated positively with the evolution of the disease and negatively with a MMSE state examination (Tato *et al.* 1995) and there was a decline in MMSE scores for patients possessing an *APOE* ε4 allele, which was associated with increased CSF-tau levels (Kanai *et al.* 1999). Others, however, have found no correlation between CSF-tau levels and degree of cognitive impairment or severity of dementia (Munroe *et al.* 1995; Nitsch *et al.* 1995; Riemenschneider *et al.* 1997; Sunderland *et al.* 1999) or with glucose metabolism, as measured by functional imaging (Okamura *et al.* 1999).

A combined assay of CSF-tau and Aβ in CSF provides a better discriminatory test for AD patients than the tests performed singly (Galasko *et al.* 1998; Kanai *et al.* 1998; Shoji *et al.* 1998; Hulstaert *et al.* 1999). In the biggest cross-centre study to date, Hulstaert and co-workers examined 250 CSF samples with ELISA tests for both $A\beta_{42}$ and tau protein (Hulstaert *et al.* 1999). At 85% sensitivity, specificity of the combined test was 86% in AD and 58% in non-AD dementias. Marker levels did not correlate with disease severity, as measured by MMSE. The combined measures of $A\beta_{42}$ and tau protein in CSF meet the requirements for clinical use in discriminating AD from normal ageing and specific neuro-logical disorders proposed by the working group for molecular and biochemical markers in AD (The Ronald and Nancy Reagen Research Institute of The Alzheimer's Association and The National Institute on Ageing Working Group 1998). In this study, half of the vascular dementia patients had assay levels comparable with AD, whereas the other half had values in the normal range (Hulstaert *et al.* 1999). An inverse correlation of CSF-tau with the progression of leukoaraiosis (Andreasen *et al.* 1998) suggests that patients with 'pure' vascular dementia have normal CSF-tau levels. Patients with mild cognitive impairment, who progressed to AD, also had high CSF-tau and/or low CSF-Aβ_{42} levels (Andreasen *et al.* 1999c), suggesting that these CSF-markers are abnormal before the onset of clinical symptoms. Further prospective studies will be needed to confirm whether these assays can provide a diagnostic test. Certain discrepancies between some of the studies depend on the use of different antibodies in different assay formats, while sample population and clinical diagnostic variation will also affect the outcome.

The high levels of CSF-tau observed in AD may be related to both neurodegeneration and to altered properties of the protein. Levels of phosphorylated tau correlate highly with the total tau measurements (Blennow *et al.* 1995). However, phosphorylation at sites recognized by the antibodies AT180 and AT270 indicate that CSF-tau is phosphorylated at both of these sites in both normal patients and in Alzheimer's patients (Blennow *et al.* 1995).

What then is the nature of the tau found in CSF? Most of the immunoassays have been performed by ELISA, in which the tau species being measured has not been characterized. These assays have used antibodies both to phospho-dependent and -independent epitopes. Two studies have demonstrated fragments of tau in CSF. A 32-kDa N-terminal fragment of tau, that was partially phosphorylated on Ser-199, Thr-231, and Ser-235, was found in CSF and a clear discrimination between levels of tau in AD patients and controls could be made when phosphorylated CSF-tau was measured rather than total CSF-tau (Ishiguro *et al.* 1999). Johnson failed to detect intact tau in any CSF samples examined, and reported that most of the tau fragments contained the N-terminus of the molecule (Johnson *et al.* 1997b). They found no difference in the electrophoretic properties of tau following alkaline phosphatase treatment suggesting that the tau was not phosphorylated. Detection of tau in serum samples (Mehta *et al.* 1999) from Down syndrome patients are harder to interpret. Big tau in the peripheral nervous system (Goedert *et al.* 1992c) may be a source of tau in the serum. In contrast to Down syndrome, elevated levels of this tau-like species was not detected in the serum from patients with AD (Mehta *et al.* 1999). Others, however, have found high molecular weight tau immunoreactivity in plasma from a small proportion of patients either with dementia or from healthy controls (Ingelson *et al.* 1999). Truncated tau proteins of 30–50 kDa have been observed in CSF-tau from head trauma patients (Zemlan *et al.* 1999). About 18 kDa of the protein has been cleaved and the remaining protein contains the repeated microtubule-binding domain with both its N- and C- termini cleaved (Zemlan *et al.* 1999).

The mechanism by which tau gets into CSF is uncertain, but may reflect neuronal destruction followed by subsequent release of tau into the brain. How it enters CSF, and in what form, remains uncertain due to the quantitative nature of the assays carried out. Further studies on the extent of tau truncation are still needed. The fact that several patients with AD do not have elevated CSF-tau levels suggests that other factors also play a role in determining the release of tau across the brain-CSF barrier.

5.15.3 Other markers related to pathology

Neuronal thread proteins (NTP) are a family of molecules expressed in the brain, which are immunologically related to pancreatic thread protein. Greater NTP immunoreactivity was found in brains from patients with AD compared with levels in the brains from control subjects (De La Monte and Wands1992). In advanced cases of AD, levels of NTP were increased in CSF and these levels correlated with the progression of dementia and neuronal degeneration (De La Monte *et al.* 1992). The NTP fragment in CSF is a 41-kDa protein, also referred to as AD 7C. Levels of NTP in excess of 3 ng/g identify 62% of patients with clinically diagnosed AD and 84% of neuropathologically verified cases (De La Monte *et al.* 1998). These studies have yet to be confirmed by independent studies.

We have screened a range of antibodies raised against PHF preparations to identify immunoreactive components in CSF specific for AD. The monoclonal antibody 11.57 recognized an 85-kDa protein that is both distinct from phosphorylated tau and synucleins, brain proteins that are known to cross-react with this antibody (Jakes *et al.* 1994). Levels of this antigen were decreased in those patients with dementia as compared with non-demented controls (Carretero *et al.* 1995). There was no difference in the level between patients with AD and those with non-Alzheimer-type dementias. In AD however, there was a significant relationship between disease progression and the amount of 85-kDa antigen. These results suggest that the level of 85-kDa antigen remains constant in those patients with non-Alzheimer-type dementia but that the level in AD continues to decrease as the disease progresses. If substantiated, these findings would suggest that monitoring the level of the 85-kDa band might be of use in clinical trials to assess the efficacy of drugs which have the potential to block the progression of neurodegeneration in AD. In combination with measurements of tau and Aβ, sensitivity and specificity for diagnostic assays may be improved by measuring a variety of markers related to AD pathology.

The use of elevated serum levels of an iron-binding protein in AD (Kennard *et al.* 1996), increased cAMP levels (correlated with CSF-tau) (Martínez *et al.* 1999), and the presence of glutamine synthetase (GS) in AD-CSF (Gunnersen *et al.* 1992) are further measures that await replication. In the latter study, GS was detected enzymatically. When measured immunochemically, the GS levels in CSF of patients with AD was increased five-fold but levels were also increased, to a lesser extent, in vascular dementia and amyotrophic lateral sclerosis (Tumani *et al.* 1999). GS enzymatic activity was not detected in either CSF or serum samples by these investigators (Tumani *et al.* 1999). Since GS in lumbar CSF is largely derived from the brain, its presence in CSF is likely to be related to astrogliosis in the CNS.

The presence of proteins that constitute pathological proteins in the brain in CSF is suggestive that neurodegeneration releases proteins into the CSF. This may also be the case for other related neurodegenerative disorders that remain to be examined. The levels of neither tau protein markers nor the native form of α-synuclein are altered in the CSF of patients with Parkinson's disease (PD) (Jakowec *et al.* 1998). An uncharacterized, 42-kDa protein in the CSF from both PD and control patients, however, was reported.

An ideal diagnostic test should reflect the pathophysiology of AD, be validated neuropathologically, and be able to detect AD early and differentiate it from other dementias. It should be reliable, non-invasive, and affordable (The Ronald and Nancy Reagen Research Institute of The Alzheimer's Association and The National Institute on Ageing Working Group 1998). None of the current biomarkers has achieved universal acceptance and none has yet met the consensus criteria decided by the working group in 1998. Amyloid, tau, and other tests can only be held as an adjunct to the psychometric and pathological diagnoses that are carried out at present. Markers may be more useful in future for tracking the course of the disease rather than being used for its diagnosis. At the moment, however, there is little benefit derived from testing these markers in a clinical situation.

5.16 **Concluding remarks**

There are rapid developments in recognizing the role of altered processing of tau protein in the molecular pathogenesis of AD. The discovery that tau mutations can cause a variety of dementing syndromes has confirmed the earlier clinico-pathological evidence showing that dementia in AD is closely linked with the tau pathology that is so prominent a histological feature of the AD phenotype. An understanding of how these mutations cause frontotemporal dementia should provide important information that can be applied to the mechanism whereby tau pathology arises in AD.

The real challenge at the theoretical level is to link the tau pathology with altered processing of the β-amyloid precursor protein and the presenilin proteins. At the clinical level, the most exciting possibility is that a therapy based on arresting the tau aggregation in AD has been shown to be theoretically feasible. The clinical success of a therapeutic strategy aimed at preventing PHF formation would finally establish the biological relevance of tau pathology in AD.

References

Abbaszade, I., Liu, R-Q., Yang, F., *et al.* (1999). Cloning and characterization of ADAMTS11, an aggrecanase from the ADAMTS family. *Journal of Biological Chemistry,* 274, 23443–50.

Abdel-Ghany, M., El-Sebae, A. K., and Shalloway, D. (1993). Aluminium-induced nonenzymatic phospho-incorporation into human tau and other proteins. *Journal of Biological Chemistry,* 268, 11976–81.

Alonso, A. D, Zaidi, T., Grundke-Iqbal, I., and Iqbal, K. (1994). Role of abnormally phosphorylated tau in the breakdown of microtubules in Alzheimer's disease. *Proceedings of the National Academy of Science (USA),* 91, 5562–6

Alves-Rodrigues, A., Gregori, L., and Figueiredo-Pereira, M. E. (1998). Ubiquitin, cellular inclusions and their role in neurodegeneration. *Trends in Neuroscience,* 21, 516–20

Alzheimer, A. (1907). Über eine eigenartige Erkrankung der Hirnrinde. *Allg. Z. Psychiat. Psych-Gerichtl. Med.* 64, 146–8

Alzheimer, A. (1911). Über eigenartige Krankheitsfälle des späteren Alters. *Z. Gesamte Neurol. Psychiatr.* 4, 356–85

Ancolio, K., Dumanchin, C., Barelli, H., *et al.* (1999). Unusual phenotypic alteration of beta amyloid precursor protein (βAPP). maturation by a new Val-715 → Met βAPP-770 mutation responsible for probable early-onset Alzheimer's disease. *Proceedings of the National Academy of Science (USA),* 96, 4119–24

Anderton, B. H., Brion, J. P., Couck, A. M, *et al.* (1995). Modulation of PHF-like tau phosphorylation in cultured neurons and transfected cells. *Neurobiology of Aging,* 16, 389–97

Anderton, B. H., Dayanandan, R., Killick, R., and Lovestone, S. (2000). Does dysregulation of the Notch and wingless/Wnt pathways underlie the pathogenesis of Alzheimer's disease? Molecular Medicine Today 6, 54–9

Andreasen, N., Hesse, C., Davidsson, P., *et al.* (1999a). Cerebrospinal fluid β-amyloid$_{(1-42)}$ in Alzheimer disease. Differences between early- and late-onset Alzheimer disease and stability during the course of disease. *Archives of Neurology,* 56, 673–80

Andreasen, N., Minthon, L., Clarberg, A., *et al.* (1999b). Sensitivity, specificity, and stability of CSF-tau in AD in a community-based patient sample. *Neurology,* 53, 1488–94

Andreasen, N., Minthon, L., Vanmechelen, E., *et al.* (1999c). Cerebrospinal fluid tau and Aβ42 as predictors of development of Alzheimer's disease in patients with mild cognitive impairment. *Neuroscience Letters,* 273, 5–8

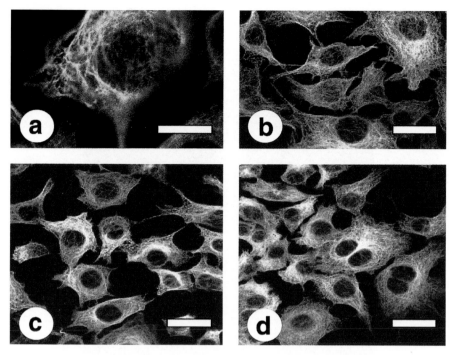

Plate 1 Expression of tau proteins in non-neuronal cells. 3T3 fibroblasts, which lack endogenous tau, express full-length tau when stably transfected with tau cDNA. Protein is seen co-localized with the microtubule network, using the anti-tau mAb 7.51 (Texas red-labelled) and anti-tubulin YL1/2 (green, FITC-labelled) (a). Cells which express tau carrying the pathogenic mutations G272V (b), S305N (c), and V337M (d) do not show any morphological differences from the wild-type protein at this level of resolution. Scale bar: 25 μm.

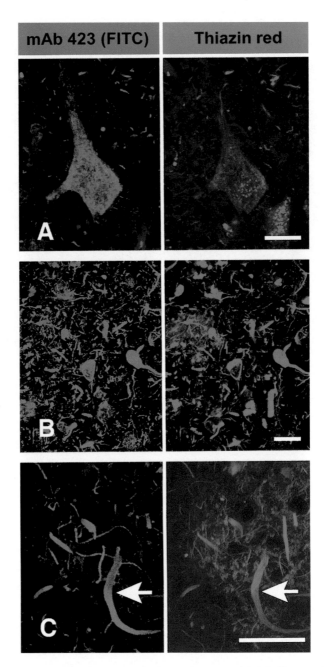

Plate 2 Truncated tau protein deposits in AD brain tissue. Double-labelling confocal microscopy using mAb 423 (left), labelled using goat anti-mouse:FITC, and thiazin red (right). (A) The earliest deposits of tau protein endogenously truncated at Glu-391, detected by mAb 423 immunoreactivity, take the form of amorphous cytoplasmic deposits appearing in cells prior to neurofibrillary tangles. These deposits are not filamentous when examined by electron

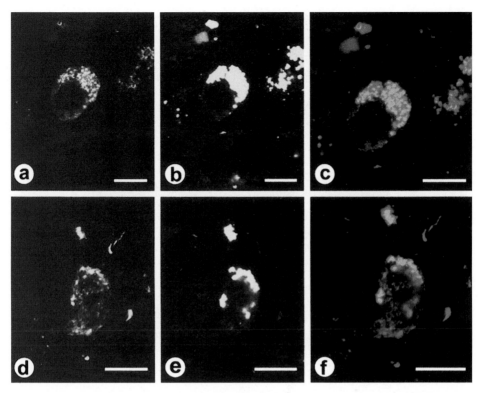

Plate 3 Co-localization of mitochondrial membrane proteins with truncated tau protein. Free-floating fixed frozen sections AD hippocampal brain tissue were double-labelled for tau protein endogenously truncated at Glu-391 (a; mAb 423) and an antiserum directed against core protein 2 of the mitochondrial bc_1 enzyme complex (b; anti-CP2). Tissues were also double-labelled with mAb 423 (d) and an antiserum directed against the outer mitochondrial membrane protein, porin (e; anti-porin). The composite images show colocalization of the two mitochondrial membrane proteins with endogenously truncated tau (c & f; yellow), as well as green amorphous deposits that were immunoreactive only with mAb 423.

Plate 2 (*contd*)

microscopy and lack binding sites for thiazin red. (B) As these amorphous deposits are transformed into filamentous PHFs, there is essentially complete co-localization of mAb 423 immunoreactivity and thiazin red labelling. This co-localization includes intracellular neurofibrillary tangles and dystrophic neuropil threads. (C) If formic acid treatment of the section is omitted, it is possible to visualize regions of transition from amorphous to filamentous stages of accumulation of C-terminally truncated tau within single neurites. The enlarged neurite in the centre of the field shows a complementary and partially overlapping distribution of double labelling, with the upper half, above the arrow, strongly labelled by thiazin red and the lower half, below the arrow, strongly labelled by mAb 423. The mAb 423 reactive portion is generally in the distal portion of the neurite, whereas that labelled with thiazin-red is generally nearer to the cell body. This suggests that the amorphous mAb 423-reactive aggregates are converted into the thiazin red-reactive filaments in the course of transport away from the cell body. Scale bar: 100 μm.

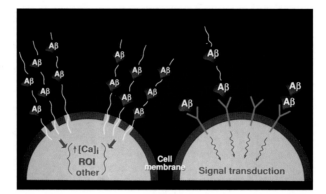

Plate 4 Schematic depiction of nonspecific (left) and specific (right) interactions of Aβ with cellular elements. Aβ monomer/oligomers/fibrils and cell binding proteins for Aβ (Y) are shown in relation to the cell membrane. Resulting increases in cytosolic free calcium [Ca]$_i$ and reactive oxygen intermediates (ROI) are also noted.

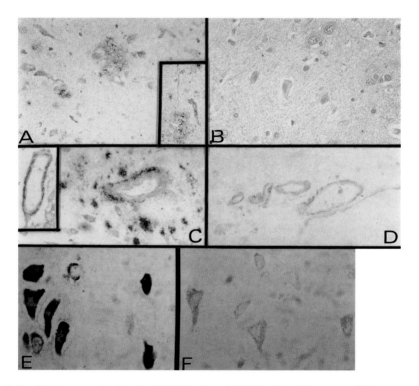

Plate 5 Double immunostaining for RAGE (red) and Aβ (black) in AD temporal lobe cortex (A) and vasculature (C) versus age-matched controls ((B), cortex; (D) vasculature). In panels A, E, and F, *in situ* hybridization with a human RAGE riboprobe is shown in affected AD temporal cortex (A and E) and age-matched control temporal cortex (F), (adapted from reference Yan *et al.* 1996).

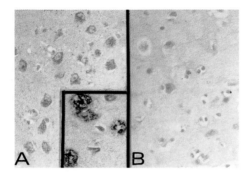

Plate 6 Immunostaining for M-CSF in affected temporal lobe of brain from a patient with AD (A) compared with staining of a comparable section from an age-matched, apparently normal control (B), (adapted from Yan *et al.* 1997*a*).

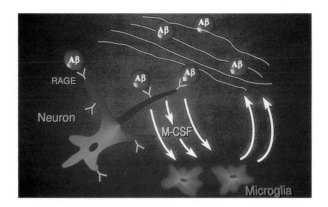

Plate 7 M-CSF and AD. Schematic depiction of Aβ-RAGE-dependent production of M-CSF by neurons, and its interaction with microglia.

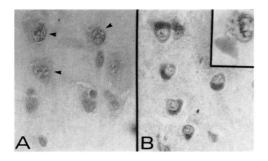

Plate 8 Immunostaining for ABAD in AD (A) versus age-matched control temporal lobe (B), (adapted from Yan *et al.* 1997*b*).

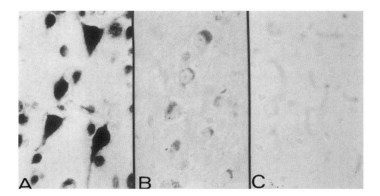

Plate 9 *In situ* hybridization for ABAD transcripts in affected temporal lobe from a patient with AD (A,C) and an age-matched apparently normal control (B). Panels A and B used ABAD antisense riboprobe and panel C used sense ABAD riboprobe (adapted from Yan *et al.* 1997).

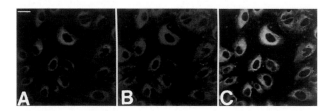

Plate 10 Dual confocal fluorescence microscopy of neuroblastoma cells for ABAD (red; A), protein disulfide isomerase (PDI; B) and both markers simultaneously (C). Marker bar is 25 µM (Adapted from Yan *et al.* 1997*b*).

Plate 11 Axial ^{99m}Tc-*d,l*-HMPAO SPECT images obtained at levels (i)53 and (ii)40 mm above the orbito-meatal plane in: (a) a 57-year-old healthy male. White and red colours represent high perfusion, whereas green and blue colours correspond to low perfusion. Note the symmetry of the perfusion pattern. (b) a 62-year-old female with AD. Note the typical bilateral temporo-parietal hypoperfusion, accompanied by slight bifrontal hypoperfusion, whereas primary motor and sensory cortex, basal ganglia and occipital cortex are relatively well preserved. (c) a 61-year-old female with frontotemporal dementia. Note the marked hypoperfusion of the frontotemporal cortex bilaterally, whereas the posterior parts of the cerebral cortex are relatively well preserved.

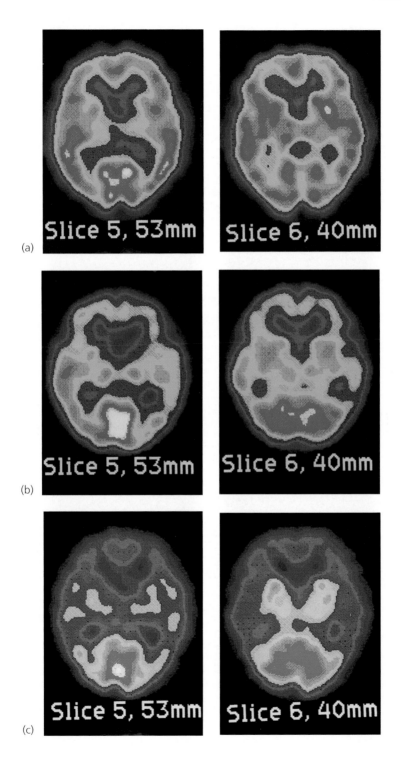

(a) Slice 5, 53mm   Slice 6, 40mm

(b) Slice 5, 53mm   Slice 6, 40mm

(c) Slice 5, 53mm   Slice 6, 40mm

Andreasen, N., Vanmechelen, E., Van de Voorde, A., *et al.* (1998). Cerebrospinal fluid tau protein as a biochemical marker for Alzheimer's disease: a community based follow up study. *Journal of Neurology, Neurosurgery and Psychiatry*, **64**, 298–305

Annaert, W., and De Strooper, B. (1999). Presenilins: molecular switches between proteolysis and signal transduction. *Trends in Neuroscience*, **22**, 439–43

Aplin, A. E., Gibb, G. M., Jacobsen, J. S., *et al.* (1996). In vitro phosphorylation of the cytoplasmic domain of the amyloid precursor protein by glycogen synthase kinase-3β. *Journal of Neurochemistry*, **67**, 699–707.

Appelt, D. M, Kopen, G. C, Boyne, L. J, and Balin, B. J. (1996). Localization of transglutaminase in hippocampal neurons: implications for Alzheimer's disease. *Journal of Histochemistry and Cytochemistry*, **44**, 1421–7

Arai, H., Satoh-Nakagawa, T., Higuchi, M., *et al.* (1998). No increase in cerebrospinal fluid tau protein levels in patients with vascular dementia. *Neuroscience Letters*, **256**, 174–6

Arai, H., Terajima, M., Miura, M., *et al.* (1995). Tau in cerebrospinal fluid: a potential diagnostic marker in Alzheimer's disease. *Annals of Neurology*, **38**, 649–52

Arawaka, S., Usami, M., Sahara, N., *et al.* (1999). The tau mutation (val337met) disrupts cytoskeletal networks of microtubules. *NeuroReport*, **10**, 993–7

Arendt, T., Holzer, M., Fruth, R., *et al.* (1995). Paired helical filament-like phosphorylation of tau, deposition of β/A4-amyloid and memory impairment in rat induced by chronic inhibition of phosphatase1 and 2A. *Neuroscience*, **69**, 691–8.

Arendt, T., Holzer, M., Gertz, H. J, and Bruckner, M. K. (1999). Cortical load of PHF-tau in Alzheimer's disease is correlated to cholinergic dysfunction. *Journal of Neural Transmission*, **106**, 513–23

Armstrong, R. A., Cairns, N. J., and Lantos, P. L. (1998). Clustering of Pick bodies in patients with Pick's disease. *Neuroscience Letters*, **242**, 81–4

Arnold, C. S., Johnson, G. V. W., Cole, R. N., *et al.* (1996). The microtubule-associated protein tau is extensively modified with O-linked N-acetylglucosamine. *Journal of Biological Chemistry*, **271**, 28741–4

Arrasate, M., Pérez, M., Armas-Portela, R., and Avila, J. (1999). Polymerization of tau peptides into fibrillar structures. The effect of FTDP-17 mutations. *FEBS Letters*, **446**, 199–202

Arriagada, P. V., Marzloff, K., and Hyman, B. T. (1992*a*). Distribution of Alzheimer-type pathologic changes in nondemented elderly individuals matches the pattern in Alzheimer's disease. *Neurology*, **42**, 1681–1688

Arriagada, P. W., Growdon, J. H., Hedley-White, E. T., and Hyman, B. T. (1992*b*). Neurofibrillary tangles but not senile plaques parallel duration and severity of Alzheimer's disease. *Neurology*, **42**, 631–9

Askanas, V., Engel, W. K., Bilak, M., *et al.* (1994). Twisted tubulofilaments of inclusion body myositis muscle resemble paired helical filaments of Alzheimer brain and contain hyperphosphorylated tau. *American Journal of Pathology*, **144**, 177–87

Atkinson, A., Singleton, A. B., Steward, A., *et al.* (1999). CYP2D6 is associated with Parkinson's disease but not with dementia with Lewy bodies or Alzheimer's disease. *Pharmacogenetics*, **9**, 31–5

Auer, I. A., Schmidt, M. L., Lee, V. M-Y., *et al.* (1995). Paired helical filament tau (PHF tau) in Neimann-Pick type C disease is similar to PHF tau in Alzheimer's disease. *Acta Neuropathologica*, **90**, 547–51

Baas, P. W. (1999). Microtubules and neuronal polarity: lessons from mitosis. *Neuron*, **22**, 23–31

Baba, M., Nakajo, S., Tu, P-H., *et al.* (1998). Aggregation of α-synuclein in Lewy bodies of sporadic Parkinson's disease and dementia with Lewy bodies. *American Journal of Pathology*, **152**, 879–84

Baker, M., Kwok, J. B. J., Kucera, S., *et al.* (1997). Localization of frontotemporal dementia with parkinsonism in an Australian kindred to chromosome 17q21–22. *Annals of Neurology*, **42**, 794–8

Baker, M., Litvan, I., Houlden, H., *et al.* (1999). Association of an extended haplotype in the *tau* gene with progressive supranuclear palsy. *Human Molecular Genetics*, 8, 711–15

Bales, K. R., Verina, T., Cummins, D. J., *et al.* (1999). Apolipoprotein E is essential for amyloid deposition in the APP^{V717F} transgenic mouse model of Alzheimer's disease. *Proceedings of the National Academy of Science (USA)*, **96**, 15233–8

Bancher, C., Grundke-Iqbal, I., Iqbal, K., *et al.* (1991). Abnormal phosphorylation of tau precedes ubiquitination in neurofibrillary pathology of Alzheimer's disease. *Brain Research*, **539**, 11–18

Bancher, C., Grundke-Iqbal, I., Iqbal, K., *et al.* (1989). Immunoreactivity of neuronal lipofuscin with monoclonal antibodies to the amyloid β-protein. *Neurobiology of Aging*, **10**, 125–32

Barbaux, S., Niaudet, P., Gubler, M-C., *et al.* (1999). Donor splice-site mutations in WT1 are responsible for Frasier syndrome. *Nature Genetics*, **17**, 467–70

Baum, L., Seger, R., Woodgett, J. R., *et al.* (1995). Overexpressed tau in cultured cells is phosphorylated without formation of PHF: implication of phosphoprotein phosphatase involvement. *Molecular Brain Research*, **34**, 1–17

Beal, M. F. (1995). Aging, energy, and oxidative stress in neurodegenerative diseases. *Annals of Neurology*, **38**, 257–66.

Bi, X., Zhou, J. and Lynch, G. (1999). Lysosomal protease inhibitors induce meganeurites and tangle-like structures in entorhinohippocampal regions vulnerable to Alzheimer's disease. *Experimental Neurology*, **158**, 312–27

Biernat, J., Mandelkow, E-M., Schröter, C., *et al.* (1992). The switch of tau protein to an Alzheimer-like state includes the phosphorylation of two serine-proline motifs upstream of the microtubule binding region. *EMBO Journal*, **11**, 1593–7

Biernat, J., Gustke, N., Drewes, G., *et al.* (1993). Phosphorylation of Ser262 strongly reduces binding of tau to microtubules: distinction between PHF-like immunoreactivity and microtubule binding. *Neuron*, **11**, 153–63

Bird, T. D., Nochlin, D., Poorkaj, P., *et al.* (1999). A clinical pathological comparison of three families with frontotemporal dementia and identical mutations in the tau gene (P301L). *Brain*, **122**, 741–56.

Blacker, D., Wilcox, M. A., Laird, N. M., *et al.* (1998). Alpha-2 macroglobulin is genetically associated with Alzheimer disease. *Nature Genetics*, **19**, 357–60

Blennow, K, Wallin, A, Ågren, M., *et al.* (1995). Tau protein in cerebrospinal fluid. A biochemical marker for axonal degeneration in Alzheimer disease. *Molecular and Chemical Neuropathology*, **26**, 231–46

Blinkov, S. M. and Glezer, I. I. (1968). *The human brain in figures and tables, a quantitative handbook.* Plenum Press, New York

Blomberg, M., Jensen, M., Basun, H., *et al.* (1996). Increasing cerebrospinal fluid tau levels in a subgroup of Alzheimer patients with apolipoprotein allele ε4 during 14 months follow-up. *Neuroscience Letters*, **214**, 163–6

Bobinski, M., Wegiel, J., Tarnawski, M., *et al.* (1997). Relationships between regional neuronal loss and neurofibrillary changes in the hippocampal formation and duration and severity of Alzheimer disease. *Journal of Neuropathology and Experimental Neurology*, **56**, 414–20

Bondareff, W., Mountjoy, C. Q., Wischik, C. M., *et al.* (1993). Evidence for subtypes of Alzheimer's disease and implications for etiology. *Archives of General Psychiatry*, **50**, 350–6

Bondareff, W., Harrington, C., Wischik, C. M., *et al.* (1994*a*). Immunohistochemical staging of neurofibrillary degeneration in Alzheimer's disease. *Journal of Neuropathology and Experimental Neurology*, **53**, 158–64

Bondareff, W., Harrington, C. R., McDaniel, S. W., Wischik, C. M., and Roth, M. (1994*b*). Presence of axonal paired helical filament tau in Alzheimer's disease: submicroscopic localization. *Journal of Neuroscience Research*, **38**, 664–9

Bondareff, W., Harrington, C. R., Wischik, C. M., *et al.* (1995). Absence of abnormal hyperphosphorylation of tau in intracellular tangles in Alzheimer's disease. *Journal of Neuropathology and Experimental Neurology*, **54**, 657–63

Bondareff., W, Matsuyama, S. S., and Dell'Albani, P. (1998). Production of paired helical filament, tau-like proteins by PC12 cells: a model of neurofibrillary degeneration. *Journal of Neuroscience Research*, **52**, 498–504

Bonifati, V., Joosse, M., Nicholl, D. J., *et al.* (1999). The tau gene in progressive supranuclear palsy: exclusion of mutations in coding exons and exon 10 splice sites, and identification of a new intronic variant of the disease-associated H1 haplotype in Italian cases. *Neuroscience Letters*, **274**, 61–5

Borchelt, D. R., Thinakaran, G., Eckman, C. B., *et al.* (1996). Familial Alzheimer's disease-linked presenilin 1 variants elevate $A\beta1$–$42/1$–40 ratio *in vitro* and *in vivo*. *Neuron*, **17**, 1005–13

Bouras, C., Hof, P. R., and Morrison, J. H. (1993). Neurofibrillary tangle densities in the hippocampal formation in a non-demented population define subgroups of patients with differential early pathologic changes. *Neuroscience Letters*, **153**, 131–5

Braak, H. and Braak, E. (1988). Neuropil threads occur in dendrites of tangle-bearing nerve cells. *Neuropathology and Applied Neurology*, **14**, 39–44

Braak, H. and Braak, E. (1991). Neuropathological stageing of Alzheimer-related changes. *Acta Neuropathologica*, **82**, 239–59

Braak, H., Braak, E., Grundke-Iqbal, I., and Iqbal, K. (1986). Occurrence of neuropil threads in the senile human brain and in Alzheimer's disease: a third location of paired helical filaments outside of neurofibrillary tangles and neuritic plaques. *Neuroscience Letters*, **65**, 351–355

Braak, H., Braak, E., and Strothjohann, M. (1994). Abnormally phosphorylated tau protein related to the formation of neurofibrillary tangles and neuropil threads in the cerebral cortex of sheep and goat. *Neuroscience Letters*, **171**, 1–4

Brandi, M. L., Gennari, L., Racchi, M., *et al.* (1999). Association of the oestrogen receptor α gene polymorphisms with sporadic Alzheimer's disease. *Biochemical and Biophysical Research Communications*, **265**, 335–8

Brandt, R. (1998). Cytoskeletal mechanism of axon outgrowth and pathfinding. *Cell and Tissue Research*, **292**, 181–9

Brandt, R., Lee, G., Teplow, D. B., *et al.* (1994). Differential effect of phosphorylation and substrate modulation on tau's ability to promote microtubule growth and nucleation. *Journal of Biological Chemistry*, **269**, 11776–82

Brandt, R., Léger, J., and Lee, G. (1995). Interaction of tau with the neuronal plasma membrane mediated by tau's amino-terminal projection domain. *Journal of Cell Biology*, **131**, 1327–40

Brashear, H. R., Godec, M. S., and Carlsen, J. (1988). The distribution of neuritic plaques and acetylcholinesterase staining in the amygdala in Alzheimer's disease. *Neurology*, **38**, 1694–9

Bre, M. H. and Karsenti, E. (1990). Effects of brain microtubule-associated proteins on microtubule dynamics and the nucleating activity of centrosomes. *Cell Motility and the Cytoskeleton*, **15**, 88–98

Breitner, J. C. S. and Welsh, K. A. (1995). Genes and recent developments in the epidemiology of Alzheimer's disease and related dementia. *Epidemiologic Reviews*, **17**, 39–47

Brion, J-P., Tremp, G., and Octave, J-N. (1999). Transgenic expression of the shortest human tau affects its compartmentalization and its phosphorylation as in the pretangle stage of Alzheimer's disease. *American Journal of Pathology*, **154**, 255–70

Brown, D. F., Risser, R. C., Bigio, E. H., *et al.* (1998). Neocortical synapse density and Braak stage in the Lewy body variant of Alzheimer disease: A comparison with classic Alzheimer disease and normal aging. *Journal of Neuropathology and Experimental Neurology*, **57**, 955–60

Brown, J., Ashworth, A., Gydesen, S., *et al.* (1995). Familial non-specific dementia maps to chromosome 3. *Human Molecular Genetics*, **4**, 1625–8

Brownlees, J., Irving, N. G., Brion, J-P., *et al.* (1997). Tau phosphorylation in transgenic mice expressing glycogen synthase-3β transgenes. *NeuroReport*, **8**, 3251–5

Buée-Scherrer, V., Buée, L., Hof, P. R., *et al.* (1995). Neurofibrillary degeneration in amyotrophic lateral sclerosis/parkinsonism-dementia complex of Guam. Immunochemical characterization of tau proteins. *American Journal of Pathology*, **146**, 924–32

Buée-Scherrer, V., Buée, L., Leveugle, B., *et al.* (1997). Pathological tau proteins in postencephalitic parkinsonism: comparison with Alzheimer's disease and other neurodegenerative disorders. *Annals of Neurology*, **42**, 356–9

Buée-Scherrer, V., Hof, P. R., Buée, L., *et al.* (1996). Hyperphosphorylated tau proteins differentiate corticobasal degeneration and Pick's disease. *Acta Neuropathologica*, **91**, 351–9

Bugiani, O., Murrell, J. R., Giaccone, G., *et al.* (1999). Frontotemporal dementia and corticobasal degeneration in a family with a P301S mutation in *Tau*. *Journal of Neuropathology and Experimental Neurology*, **58**, 667–77

Bullido, M., Aldudo, J., Frank, A., *et al.* (2000). A polymorphism in the tau gene associated with risk for Alzheimer's disease. *Neuroscience Letters*, **278**, 49–52

Burack, M. A. and Halpain, S. (1996). Site-specific regulation of Alzheimer-like tau phosphorylation in living neurons. *Neuroscience*, **72**, 167–84

Busciglio, J., Hartmann, H., Lorenzo, A., *et al.* (1997). Neuronal localization of presenilin-1 and association with amyloid plaques and neurofibrillary tangles in Alzheimer's disease. *Journal of Neuroscience*, **17**, 5101–7

Busciglio, J. and Yankner, B. A. (1995). Apoptosis and increased generation of reactive oxygen species in Down syndrome. *Nature*, **378**, 776–9

Butler, M. and Shelanski, M. L. (1986). Microheterogeneity of microtubule-associated tau protein is due to differences in phosphorylation. *Journal of Neurochemistry*, **47**, 1517–22

Buxbaum, J. D. (1995). Post-translational control of the amyloid β-protein precursor processing. In *Pathobiology of Alzheimer's disease* (ed. A. Goate and F. Ashall) pp. 99–114. Academic Press, London

Caceres, A. and Kosik, K. S. (1990). Inhibition of neurite polarity by tau antisense oligonucleotides in primary cerebellar neurons. *Nature*, **343**, 461–3

Caceres, A., Mautino, J., and Kosik, K. S. (1992). Suppression of MAP2 in cultured cerebellar macroneurons inhibits minor neurite formation. *Neuron*, **9**, 607–18

Caceres, A., Potrebic, S., and Kosik, K. S. (1991). The effect of tau antisense oligonucleotides on neuritic formation of cultured cerebellar macroneurons. *Journal of Neuroscience*, **11**, 1515–23

Candy, J. M., Klinowski, J., Perry, R. H., *et al.* (1986). Aluminosilicate and senile plaque formation in Alzheimer's disease. *Lancet*, **i**, 354–6

Canu, N., Dus, L., Barbato, C., *et al.* (1998). Tau cleavage and dephosphorylation in cerebellar granule neurons undergoing apoptosis. *Journal of Neuroscience*, **18**, 7061–74

Caputo, C. B., Sobel, I. R. E., Scott, C. W., *et al.* (1992*a*). Association of the carboxy-terminus of β-amyloid protein precursor with Alzheimer paired helical filaments. *Biochemical and Biophysical Research Communications*, **185**, 1034–40

Caputo, C. B., Wischik, C., Novak, M., *et al.* (1992*b*). Immunological characterization of the region of tau protein that is bound to Alzheimer paired helical filaments. *Neurobiology of Aging*, **13**, 267–74

Carrell, R. W. and Gooptu, B. (1998). Conformational changes and disease — serpins, prions and Alzheimer's. *Current Opinion in Structural Biology*, **8**, 799–809

Carretero, M. T., Harrington, C. R., and Wischik, C. M. (1995). Changes in a CSF antigen associated with dementia. *Dementia*, **6**, 281–5

Carstea, E. D., Morris, J. A., Coleman, K. G., *et al.* (1997). Niemann-Pick C1 disease gene: homology to mediators of cholesterol homeostasis. *Science*, **277**, 228–31

Chambers, C. B., Lee, J. M., Troncoso, J. C., *et al.* (1999). Overexpression of four-repeat tau mRNA isoforms in progressive supranuclear palsy but not in Alzheimer's disease. *Annals of Neurology*, **46**, 325–32

Chau, M-F., Radeke, M. J., de Inés, C., *et al.* (1998). The microtubule-associated protein tau cross-links to two distinct sites on each α and β tubulin monomer via separate domains. *Biochemistry*, **37**, 17692–703

Chui, D-H., Shirotani, K., Tanahashi, H., *et al.* (1998). Both N-terminal and C-terminal fragments of presenilin 1 colocalize with neurofibrillary tangles in neurons and dystrophic neurites of senile plaques in Alzheimer's disease. *Journal of Neuroscience Research*, **53**, 99–106

Chui, D-H., Tanahashi, H, Ozawa, K., *et al.* (1999). Transgenic mice with Alzheimer presenilin 1 mutations show accelerated neurodegeneration without amyloid plaque formation. *Nature Medicine*, **5**, 560–4

Citron, M., Diehl, T. S., Gordon, G., *et al.* (1996). Evidence that the 42- and 40-amino acid forms of amyloid β protein are generated from the β-amyloid precursor protein by different protease activities. *Proceedings of the National Academy of Science (USA)*, **93**, 13170–5

Clark, L. N., Poorkaj, P., Wszolek, Z., *et al.* (1998). Pathogenic implications of mutations in the tau gene in pallido-ponto-nigral degeneration and related neurodegenerative disorders linked to chromosome 17. *Proceedings of the National Academy of Science (USA)*, **95**, 13103–7

Cohen, F. E. and Prusiner, S. B. (1998). Pathologic conformations of prion proteins. *Annual Review of Biochemistry*, **67**, 793–819

Conrad, C., Andreadis, A., Trojanowski, J. Q., *et al.* (1997). Genetic evidence for the involvement of τ in progressive supranuclear palsy. *Annals of Neurology*, **41**, 277–81

Conrad, C., Amano, N., Andreadis, A., *et al.* (1998). Difference in a dinucleotide repeat polymorphism in the tau gene between caucasian and Japanese populations: implication for progressive supranuclear palsy. *Neuroscience Letters*, **250**, 135–7

Conway, K. A., Harper, J. D., and Lansbury, P. T. (1998). Accelerated *in vitro* fibril formation by a mutant α-synuclein linked to early-onset Parkinson disease. *Nature Medicine*, **4**, 1318–20

Corey-Bloom, J., Tiraboschi, P., Hansen, L. A., *et al.* (2000). E4 allele dosage does not predict cholinergic activity or synapse loss in Alzheimer's disease. *Neurology*, **54**, 403–6

Cork, L. C., Powers, R. E., Selkoe, D., *et al.* (1988). Neurofibrillary tangles and senile plaques in aged bears. *Journal of Neuropathology and Experimental Neurology*, **49**, 629–41

Corsellis, J. A. N., Bruton, C. J., and Freeman-Browne, D. (1973). The aftermath of boxing. *Psychological Medicine*, **3**, 270–303

Crapper-McLachlan, D. R., Dalton, A. J., Kruck, T. P. A., *et al.* (1991). Intramuscular desferroxamine in patients with Alzheimer's disease. *Lancet*, **337**, 1304–8

Crawford, F., Freeman, M., Town, T., *et al.* (1999). No genetic association between polymorphisms in the Tau gene and Alzheimer's disease in clinic or population based samples. *Neuroscience Letters*, **266**, 193–6

Crawford, F., Abdullah, L., Schinka, J., *et al.* (2000). Gender-specific association of the angiotensin converting enzyme gene with Alzheimer's disease. *Neuroscience Letters*, **280**, 215–19

Crowther, R. A. (1991). Straight and paired helical filaments in Alzheimer disease have a common structural unit. *Proceedings of the National Academy of Science (USA)*, **88**, 2288–92

Crowther, R. A. and Wischik, C. M. (1985). Image reconstruction of the Alzheimer paired helical filament. *EMBO Journal*, **4**, 3661–3665

Crowther, R. A., Olesen, O. F., *et al.* (1992). The microtubule binding repeats of tau protein assemble into filaments like those found in Alzheimer's disease. *FEBS Letters*, **309**, 199–202

Crowther, R. A., Olesen, O. F., Smith, M. J., *et al.* (1994). Assembly of Alzheimer-like filaments from full-length tau protein. *FEBS Letters*, **337**, 135–8

Cruts, M. and Van Broeckhoven, C. (1998). Presenilin mutations in Alzheimer's disease. *Human Mutation*, 11, 183–90

Crystal, H., Dickson, D., Fuld, P., *et al.* (1988). Clinico-pathologic studies in dementia: non-demented subjects with pathologically confirmed Alzheimer's disease. *Neurology*, 38, 1682–7

Cummings, B. J., and Cotman, C. W. (1995). Image analysis of β-amyloid load in Alzheimer's disease and relation to dementia severity. *Lancet*, 346, 1524–8

Curran, M., Middleton, D., Edwardson, J., *et al.* (1997). HLA-DR antigens associated with major genetic risk for late-onset Alzheimer's disease. *NeuroReport*, 8, 1467–9

Dahiyat, M., Cumming, A., Harrington, C., *et al.* (1999). Association between Alzheimer's disease and the *NOS3* gene. *Annals of Neurology*, 46, 664–7

Davies, P. (1979). Neurotransmitter-related enzymes in senile dementia of the Alzheimer type. *Brain Research*, 171, 319–27

Davis, D. G., Schmitt, F. A., Wekstein, D. R., and Markesbery, W. R. (1999a). Alzheimer neuropathologic alterations in aged cognitively normal subjects. *Journal of Neuropathology and Experimental Neurology*, 58, 376–88

Davis, D. R., Brion, J.-P., Couck, A. -M., Gallo, J. -M., *et al.* (1995). The phosphorylation state of microtubule-associated protein tau as affected by glutamate, colchicine and b-amyloid in primary rat cortical neuronal cultures. *Biochemical Journal*, 309, 941–9

Davis, P. K. and Johnson, G. V. W. (1999b). The microtubule binding of tau and high molecular weight tau in apoptotic PC12 cells is impaired because of altered phosphorylation. *Journal of Biological Chemistry*, 274, 35686–92

Davis, R. L., Shrimpton, A. E., Holohan, P. D., *et al.* (1999c). Familial dementia caused by polymerization of mutant neuroserpin. *Nature*, 401, 376–9

Daw, E. W., Payami, H., Nemens, E. J., *et al.* (2000). The number of trait loci in late-onset Alzheimer disease. *American Journal of Human Genetics*, 66, 196–204

Dayanandan, R., Van Slegtenhorst, M., Mack, T. G. A., *et al.* (1999). Mutations in tau reduce its microtubule binding properties in intact cells and affect its phosphorylation. *FEBS Letters*, 446, 228–32

De La Monte, S. M. and Wands, J. R. (1992). Neuronal thread protein overexpression in brains with Alzheimer's disease lesions. *Journal of the Neurological Sciences*, 113, 152–64

De La Monte, S. M., Volicer, L., Hauser, S. L., and Wands, J. R. (1992). Increased levels of neuropil thread protein in cerebrospinal fluid of patients with Alzheimer's disease. *Annals of Neurology*, 32, 733–42

De La Monte, S. M., Ghanbari, K., Frey, W. H., *et al.* (1998). Characterization of the AD7C-NTP cDNA expression in Alzheimer's disease and measurement of a 41-kD protein in cerebrospinal fluid. *Journal of Clinical Investigation*, 100, 3093–104

DeKosky, S. T. and Scheff, S. W. (1990). Synapse loss in frontal cortex biopsies in Alzheimer's disease: correlation with cognitive severity. *Annals of Neurology*, 27, 457–64

DeKosky, S. T., Harbaugh, R. E., Schmitt, F. A., *et al.* (1992). Cortical biopsy in Alzheimer's disease: diagnostic accuracy and neurochemical, neuropathological, and cognitive correlations. *Annals of Neurology*, 32, 625–32

Delacourte, A., Robitaille, Y., Sergeant, N., *et al.* (1996). Specific pathological tau protein variants characterize Pick's disease. *Journal of Neuropathology and Experimental Neurology*, 55, 159–68

Delaère, P., Duyckaerts, C., Brion, J. P., *et al.* (1989). Tau, paired helical filaments and amyloid in the neocortex: a morphometric study of 15 cases with graded intellectual status in ageing and senile dementia of the Alzheimer type. *Acta Neuropathologica*, 77, 645–53

Delaère, P., Duyckaerts, C., Masters, C., *et al.* (1990). Large amounts of neocortical βA4 deposits without neuritic plaques nor tangles in a psychometrically assessed, non-demented person. *Neuroscience Letters*, 116, 87–93

Delaère, P., Duyckaerts, C., He, Y., Piette, F., and Hauw, J. J. (1991). Subtypes and differential laminar distributions of βA4 deposits in Alzheimer's disease: relationship with the intellectual status of 26 cases. *Acta Neuropathologica*, **81**, 328–35

Delaère, P., He, Y., Fayet, G., *et al.* (1993). βA4 deposits are constant in the brain of the oldest old, an immunocytochemical study of 20 French centenarians. *Neurobiology of Aging*, **14**, 191–4

Delisle, M. B., Murrell, J. R., Richardson, R., *et al.* (1999). A mutation at codon 279 (N279K). in exon 10 of the *Tau* gene causes a tauopathy with dementia and supranuclear palsy. *Acta Neuropathologica*, **98**, 62–77

Di Santo, A. R. and Wagner, J. G. (1972). Pharmacokinetics of highly ionized drugs. II: Methylene blue — absorption metabolism, and excretion in man and dog after oral administration. *Journal of Pharmaceutical Sciences*, **61**, 1086–90

Dickson, D. W., Crystal, H., Mattiace, L. A., *et al.* (1989). Diffuse Lewy body disease: light and electron microscopic immunohistochemistry of senile plaques. *Acta Neuropathologica*, **78**, 572–84

Dickson, D. W., Ruan, D., Crystal, H., *et al.* (1991). Hippocampal degeneration differentiates diffuse Lewy body disease (DLBD) from Alzheimer's disease: light and electron microscopic immunocytochemistry of CA2–3 neurites specific to DLBD. *Neurology*, **41**, 1402–9

Dobson, C. B. and Itzhaki, R. F. (1999). Herpes simplex virus type 1 and Alzheimer's disease. *Neurobiology of Aging*, **20**, 457–65

Dobson, C. M. (1999). Protein misfolding, evolution and disease. *Trends in Biochememical Science*, **24**, 329–32

Doll, R. (1993). Review: Alzheimer's disease and environmental aluminium. *Age and Aging*, **22**, 138–53

Drewes, G., Lichtenberg-Kraag, B., Döring, F., *et al.* (1992). Mitogen activated protein (MAP) kinase transforms tau protein into an Alzheimer-like state. *EMBO Journal*, **11**, 2131–8

Drewes, G., Trinczek, B., Illenberger, S., *et al.* (1995). Microtubule-associated protein/microtubule affinity-regulating kinase (p110mark). A novel protein kinase that regulates tau-microtubule interactions and dynamic instability by phosphorylation of the Alzheimer-specific site serine 262. *Journal of Biological Chemistry*, **270**, 7679–88

Drubin, D. G., Feinstein, S. C., Shooter, E. M., and Kirschner, M. W. (1985). Nerve growth factor-induced neurite outgrowth in PC12 cells involves the coordinate induction of microtubule assembly and assembly-promoting factors. *Journal of Cell Biology*, **101**, 1799–807

D'Souza, I., Poorkaj, P., Hong, M., *et al.* (1999). Missense and silent tau gene mutations cause frontotemporal dementia with parkinsonism-chromosome 17 type, by affecting multiple alternative RNA splicing regulatory elements. *Proceedings of the National Academy of Science (USA)*, **96**, 5598–603

Dudek, S. M. and Johnson, G. V. W. (1993). Transglutaminase catalyzes the formation of sodium dodecyl sulfate-insoluble, Alz-50-reactive polymers of tau. *Journal of Neurochemistry*, 61, 1159–62

Duff, K., Eckman, C., Zehr, C., *et al.* (1996). Increased amyloid-β42(43) in brains of mice expressing mutant presenilin 1. *Nature*, **383**, 710–13

Dumanchin, C., Camuzat, A., Campion, D., *et al.* (1998). Segregation of a missense mutation in the microtubule-associated protein tau gene with frontotemporal dementia and parkinsonism. *Human Molecular Genetics*, 7, 1825–9

Duyckaerts, C., Brion, J-P., Hauw, J-J., and Flament-Durand, J. (1987). Quantitative asssessment of the density of neurofibrillary tangles and senile plaques in senile dementia of the Alzheimer type. Comparison of immunocytochemistry with a specific antibody and Bodian's protargol method. *Acta Neuropathologica*, **73**, 167–70

Duyckaerts, C., Bennecib, M., Grignon, Y., *et al.* (1997). Modeling the relation between neurofibrillary tangles and intellectual status. *Neurobiology of Aging*, **18**, 267–73

Ebneth, A., Godemann, R., Stamer, K., *et al.* (1998). Overexpression of tau protein inhibits kinesin-dependent trafficking of vesicles, mitochondria, and endoplasmic reticulum: Implications for Alzheimer's disease. *Journal of Cell Biology*, **143**, 777–94

Eikelenboom, P., Zhan, S-S., Van Gool, W. A., and Allsop, D. (1994). Inflammatory mechanisms in Alzheimer's disease. *Trends in Pharmacological Sciences*, **15**, 447–50

Elbaum, D., Brzyska, M., Bacia, A., and Alkon, D. L. (2000). Implication of novel biochemical property of β-amyloid. *Biochemical and Biophysical Research Communications*, **267**, 733–8

Engelender, S., Kaminsky, Z., Guo, X., *et al.* (1999). Synphilin-1 associates with α-synuclein and promotes the formation of cytosolic inclusions. *Nature Genetics*, **22**, 110–14

Exley C., PNC, Kelly S. M., and Birchall J. D. (1993). An interaction of β-amyloid with aluminium in vitro. *FEBS Letters*, **324**, 293–5

Ezquerra, M., Pastor, P., Valldeoriola, F., *et al.* (1999). Identification of a novel polymorphism in the promoter region of the tau gene highly associated to progressive supranuclear palsy in humans. *Neuroscience Letters*, **275**, 183–6

Farrer, L. A., Cupples, L. A., Haines, J. L., *et al.* (1997). Effects of age, sex, and ethnicity on the association between apolipoprotein E genotype and Alzheimer disease: a meta-analysis. *Journal of the American Medical Association*, **278**, 1349–56

Felgner, H., Frank, R., Biernat, J., *et al.* (1998). Domains of neuronal microtubule-associated proteins and flexural rigidity of microtubules. *Journal of Cell Biology*, **138**, 1067–75

Fergusson, J., Landon, M., Lowe, J., *et al.* (2000). Neurofibrillary tangles in progressive supranuclear palsy brains exhibit immunoreactivity to frameshift mutant ubiquitin-B protein. *Neuroscience Letters*, **279**, 69–72

Finch, C. E. and Cohen, D. M. (1997). Aging, metabolism, and Alzheimer disease: review and hypotheses. *Experimental Neurology*, **143**, 82–102

Flanagan, L. A., Cunningham, C. C., Chen, J., *et al.* (1997). The structure of divalent cation-induced aggregates of PIP2 and their alteration by gelsolin and tau. *Biophysical Journal*, **73**, 1440–7

Foster, N. L., Wilhemsen, K., Sima, A. A. F., *et al.* (1997). Frontotemporal dementia and parkinsonism linked to chromosome 17: a consensus conference. *Annals of Neurology*, **41**, 706–15

Fowler, C. J. (1998). The role of the phosphoinositide signalling system in the pathogenesis of sporadic Alzheimer's disease: a hypothesis. *Brain Research Reviews*, **25**, 373–80

Frappier, T., Liang, N. S., Brown, K., *et al.* (1999). Abnormal microtubule packing in processes of SF9 cells expressing the FTDP-17 V337M tau mutation. *FEBS Letters*, **455**, 262–6

Friedhoff, P., Schneider, A., Mandelkow, E-M., and Mandelkow, E. (1998*a*). Rapid assembly of Alzheimer-like paired helical filaments from microtubule-associated protein tau monitored by fluorescence in solution. *Biochemistry*, **37**, 10223–30

Friedhoff, P., von Bergen, M., Mandelkow, E-M., *et al.* (1998*b*). A nucleated assembly of Alzheimer paired helical filaments *Proceedings of the National Academy of Science (USA)*, **95**, 15712–17

Frisoni, G. B., Laakso, M. P., Beltramello, A., *et al.* (1999). Hippocampal and entorhinal cortex atrophy in frontotemporal dementia and Alzheimer's disease. *Neurology*, **52**, 91–100

Froelich, S., Houlden, H., Rizzu, P., *et al.* (1999). Construction of a detailed physical and transcript map of the FTDP-17 candidate region on chromosome 17q21. *Genomics*, **60**, 129–36

Galasko, D., Chang, L., Motter, R., *et al.* (1998). High cerebrospinal fluid tau and low amyloid β42 levels in the clinical diagnosis of Alzheimer disease and relation to apolipoprotein E genotype. *Archives of Neurology*, **55**, 937–45

Galvin, J. E., Uryu, K., Lee, V.M.-Y., and Trojanowski, J. Q. (1999). Axon pathology in Parkinson's disease and Lewy body dementia hippocampus contains α-, β-, and γ-synuclein. *Proceedings of the National Academy of Science (USA)*, **96**, 13450–5

Games, D., Adams, D., Allessandrini, R., *et al.* (1995). Alzheimer-type neuropathology in transgenic mice overexpressing V717F β-amyloid precursor protein. *Nature*, **373**, 523–7

Gao, Q. S., Memmott, J., Lafyatis, R., *et al.* (2000). Complex regulation of tau exon 10, whose miss-plicing causes frontotemporal dementia. *Journal of Neurochemistry*, **74**, 490–500

Garcia de Ancos, J., Correas, I., and Avila, J. (1993). Differences in microtubule binding and self-association abilities of bovine brain tau isoforms. *Journal of Biological Chemistry*, **268**, 7976–82

Geller, L. N. and Potter, H. (1999). Chromosome missegregation and trisomy 21 mosaicism in Alzheimer's disease. *Neurobiology of Disease*, **6**, 167–79

Gertz, H-J., Xuereb, J. H., Huppert, F. A., *et al.* (1996). The relationship between clinical dementia and neuropathological stageing (Braak) in a very elderly community sample. *European Archives of Psychiatry and Clinical Neuroscience*, **246**, 132–6

Gertz, H-J., Xuereb, J, Huppert, F., *et al.* (1998). Examination of the validity of the hierarchical model of neuropathological stageing in normal ageing and Alzheimer's disease. *Acta Neuropathologica*, **95**, 154–8

Geula, C., Wu, C-K., Saroff, D., *et al.* (1998). Ageing renders the brain vulnerable to amyloid β-protein neurotoxicity. *Nature Medicine*, **4**, 827–34

Ghetti, B., Piccardo, P., Spillantini, M. G., *et al.* (1996). Vascular variant of prion protein cerebral amyloidosis with τ-positive neurofibrillary tangles, the phenotype of the stop codon 145 mutation in *PRNP*. *Proceedings of the National Academy of Science (USA)*, **93**, 744–8

Giaccone, G., Pedrotti, B., Migheli, A., *et al.* (1996). βAPP and tau interaction, a possible link between amyloid and neurofibrillary tangles in Alzheimer's disease. *American Journal of Pathology*, **148**, 79–87

Giannakopoulos, P., Hof, P. R., Fiannakopoulos, A.-S., *et al.* (1995). Regional distribution of neurofibrillary tangles and senile plaques in the cerebral cortex of very old patients. *Archives of Neurology*, **52**, 1150–9

Giannakopoulos, P., Hof, P. R., Michel, J.-P., *et al.* (1997). Cerebral cortex pathology in ageing and Alzheimer's disease: a quantitative survey of large hospital-based geriatric and psychiatric cohorts. *Brain Research Reviews*, **25**, 217–45

Giannakopoulos, P. M. D., Gold, G., Hof, P. R., *et al.* (1998). Pathologic correlates of apraxia in Alzheimer disease. *Archives of Neurology*, **55**, 689–95

Giasson, B. I., Uryu, K., Trojanowski, J. Q., and Lee, V. M. Y. (1999). Mutant and wild type human α-synucleins assemble into elongated filaments with distinct morphologies *in vitro*. *Journal of Biological Chemistry*, **274**, 7619–22

Gilman, A. G., Goodman, L. S., and Gilman, A. (1980). In *The pharmacological basis of therapeutics* (ed. L. S. Goodman and A. G. Gilman), pp. 980. Macmillan Publishing Co., New York

Goedert, M. (1999). Filamentous nerve cell inclusions in neurodegenerative diseases, tauopathies and alpha-synucleinopathies. *Philosophical Transactions of the Royal Society, London Series B — Biological Sciences*, **354**, 1101–18

Goedert, M., Wischik, C. M., Crowther, R. A., *et al.* (1988). Cloning and sequencing of the cDNA encoding a core protein of the paired helical filament of Alzheimer disease: identification as the microtubule-associated protein tau. *Proceedings of the National Academy of Science (USA)*, **85**, 4051–5

Goedert, M., Spillantini, M. G., Jakes, R., *et al.* (1989*a*). Multiple isoforms of human microtubule-associated protein tau: sequences and localization in neurofibrillary tangles of Alzheimer's disease. *Neuron*, **3**, 519–526

Goedert, M., Spillantini, M. G., Potier, M. C., *et al.* (1989*b*). Cloning and sequencing of the cDNA encoding an isoform of microtubule-associated protein tau containing four tandem repeats: differential expressing of tau protein mRNAs in human brain. *EMBO Journal*, **8**, 393–9

Goedert, M., Cohen, E. S., Jakes, R., and Cohen, P. (1992*a*). p42 map kinase phosphorylation sites in microtubule-associated protein tau are dephosphorylated by protein phosphatase 2A1. *FEBS Letters*, **312**, 95–9

Goedert, M., Spillantini, M. G., Cairns, N. J., and Crowther, R. A. (1992*b*). Tau proteins of Alzheimer paired helical filaments: abnormal phosphorylation of all six brain isoforms. *Neuron*, **8**, 159–68

Goedert, M., Spillantini, M. G., and Crowther, R. A. (1992*c*). Cloning of big tau microtubule-associated protein characteristic of the peripheral nervous system. *Proceedings of the National Academy of Science (USA)*, **89**, 1983–7

Goedert, M., Jakes, R., Crowther, R. A., *et al.* (1993). The abnormal phosphorylation of tau protein at Ser-202 in Alzheimer's disease recapitulates phosphorylation during development. *Proceedings of the National Academy of Science (USA)*, **90**, 5066–70

Goedert, M., Jakes, R., Qi, Z., *et al.* (1995). Protein phosphatase 2A is the major enzyme in brain that dephosphorylates t protein phosphorylated by proline-directed protein kinases or cyclic AMP-dependent protein kinase. *Journal of Neurochemistry*, **65**, 2804–7

Goedert, M., Jakes, R., Spillantini, M. G., *et al.* (1996). Assembly of microtubule-associated protein tau into Alzheimer-like filaments induced by sulphated glycosaminoglycans. *Nature*, **383**, 550–3.

Goedert, M., Hasegawa, M., Jakes, R., *et al.* (1997*a*). Phosphorylation of microtubule-associated protein tau by stress-activated protein kinases. *FEBS Letters*, **409**, 57–62

Goedert, M., Trojanowski, J. Q., and Lee, V. M.-Y. (1997*b*). τ protein and the neurofibrillary pathology of Alzheimer's disease. In *Molecular mechanisms of dementia* (ed. W. Wasco, R. E. Tanzi), pp. 199–218. Humana Press, New Jersey

Goedert, M., Jakes, R., and Crowther, R. A. (1999). Effects of frontotemporal dementia FTDP-17 mutations on heparin-induced assembly of tau filaments. *FEBS Letters*, **450**, 306–11

Gómez-Isla, T., Price, J. L., McKell, D. W., Jr., *et al.* (1996). Profound loss of layer II entorhinal cortex neurons occurs in very mild Alzheimer's disease. *Journal of Neuroscience*, **16**, 4491–500

Gómez-Isla, T., Hollister, R., West, H., *et al.* (1997). Neuronal loss correlates with but exceeds neurofibrillary tangles in Alzheimer's disease. *Annals of Neurology*, **41**, 17–24

González, C., Farías, G., and Maccioni, R. B. (1998). Modification of tau to an Alzheimer's type protein interferes with its interaction with microtubules. *Cellular and Molecular Biology*, **44**, 1117–27

Götz, J., Probst, A., Spillantini, M. G., *et al.* (1995). Somatodendritic localization and hyperphosphorylation of tau protein in transgenic mice expressing the longest human brain tau isoform. *EMBO Journal*, **14**, 1304–13

Green, A. J. E., Harvey, R. J., Thompson, E. J., and Rossor, M. N. (1997). Increased S100β in the cerebrospinal fluid of patients with frontotemporal dementia. *Neuroscience Letters*, **235**, 5–8

Green, A. J. E., Harvey, R. J., Thompson, E. J., and Rossor, M. N. (1999). Increased tau in the cerebrospinal fluid of patients with frontotemporal dementia and Alzheimer's disease. *Neuroscience Letters*, **259**, 133–135

Greenberg, S. G. and Davies, P. (1990). A preparation of Alzheimer paired helical filaments that displays distinct tau proteins by polyacrylamide gel electrophoresis. *Proceedings of the National Academy of Science (USA)*, **87**, 5827–31

Grover, A., Houlden, H., Baker, M., *et al.* (1999). 5' Splice site mutations in *tau* associated with the inherited dementia FTDP-17 affect a stem-loop structure that regulates alternative splicing of exon 10. *Journal of Biological Chemistry*, **274**, 15134–43

Guevara, J., Espinosa, B., Zenteno, E., *et al.* (1998). Altered glycosylation pattern of proteins in Alzheimer disease. *Journal of Neuropathology and Experimental Neurology* **57**, 905–14

Gunnersen, D. and Haley, B. (1992). Detection of glutamine synthetase in the cerebrospinal fluid of Alzheimer's diseased patients: a potential diagnostic biochemical marker. *Proceedings of the National Academy of Science (USA)*, **89**, 11949–53

Gustafson, L. (1987). Frontal lobe degeneration of non-Alzheimer type. II. Clinical picture and differential diagnosis. *Archives of Gerontology and Geriatrics*, **6**, 209–23

Gustke, N., Steiner, B., Mandelkow, E-M., *et al.* (1992). The Alzheimer-like phosphorylation of tau protein reduces microtubule binding and involves Ser-Pro and Thr-Pro motifs. *FEBS Letters*, **307**, 199–205

Guttmann, R. P., Erickson, A. C., and Johnson, G. V. W. (1995). Tau self-assocation: stabilization with a chemical cross-linker and modulation by phosphorylation and oxidation state. *Journal of Neurochemistry*, **64**, 1209–15

Guy, S. P., Jones, D., Mann, D. M. A., and Itzhaki, R. F. (1991). Human neuroblastoma cells treated with aluminium express an epitope associated with Alzheimer's disease neurofibrillary tangles. *Neuroscience Letters*, **121**, 166–8

Haass, C. and De Strooper, B. (1999). The presenilins in Alzheimer's disease — proteolysis holds the key. *Science*, **286**, 916–19

Hanger, D. P., Hughes, K., Woodgett, J. R., *et al.* (1992). Glycogen synthase kinase-3 induces Alzheimer's disease-like phosphorylation: generation of paired helical filament epitopes and neuronal localization of the kinase. *Neuroscience Letters*, **147**, 58–62

Hanger, D. P., Betts, J. C., Loviny, T. L. F., *et al.* (1998). New phosphorylation sites identified in hyperphosphorylated tau (paired helical filament-tau) from Alzheimer's disease brain using nanoelectrospray mass spectrometry. *Journal of Neurochemistry*, **71**, 2465–76

Hansen, L. A., Masliah, E., Galasko, D., and Terry, R. D. (1993). Plaque-only Alzheimer disease is usually the Lewy body variant, and vice versa. *Journal of Neuropathology and Experimental Neurology*, **52**, 648–54

Harada, A., Oguchi, K., Okabe, S., *et al.* (1994). Altered microtubule organization in small-calibre axons of mice lacking tau protein. *Nature*, **369**, 488–91

Hardy, J. (1997). Amyloid, the presenilins and Alzheimer's disease. *Trends in Neuroscience*, **20**, 154–9

Hardy, J., Mullan, M., Chartier-Harlin, M.-C., *et al.* (1991). Molecular classification of Alzheimer's disease. *Lancet*, **337**, 1342–3

Haroutunian, V., Purohit, D. P., Perl, D. P., *et al.* (1999). Neurofibrillary tangles in nondemented elderly subjects and mild Alzheimer's disease. *Archives of Neurology*, **56**, 713–18

Harrington, C. R. and Colaco, C. A. L. S. (1997). Glycation of tau protein: implications for the aetiopathogenesis of Alzheimer's disease. In *Microtubule-associated proteins, modifications in disease.* (ed. J. Avila, R. Brandt, and K. S. Kosik), pp. 125–152. Harwood Academic Publishers, Amsterdam.

Harrington, C. R. and Roth, M. (1997). Susceptibility genetics in the etiopathogenesis of Alzheimer's disease: role for potential confounding factors. *International Psychogeriatrics*, **9**, 229–44

Harrington, C. R., Edwards, P. C., and Wischik, C. M. (1990). Competitive ELISA for measurement of tau proteins in Alzheimer's disease. *Journal of Immunological Methods*, **134**, 261–71

Harrington, C. R., Mukaetova-Ladinska, E. B., Hills, R, *et al.* (1991). Measurement of distinct immunochemical presentations of tau protein in Alzheimer disease. *Proceedings of the National Academy of Science (USA)*, **91**, 5842–6

Harrington, C. R., Louwagie, J., Rossau, R., *et al.* (1994a). Influence of apolipoprotein E genotype on senile dementia of the Alzheimer and Lewy body types. Significance for etiological theories of Alzheimer's disease. *American Journal of Pathology*, **145**, 1472–84.

Harrington, C. R., Perry, R. H., Perry, E. K., *et al.* (1994*b*). Senile dementia of Lewy body type and Alzheimer type are biochemically distinct in terms of paired helical filaments and hyperphosphorylated tau protein. *Dementia*, 5, 215–28

Harrington, C. R., Wischik C. M., McArthur, F. K., *et al.* (1994*c*). Alzheimer's-disease-like changes in tau protein processing: association with aluminium accumulation in brains of renal dialysis patients. *Lancet*, 343, 993–7

Harris, K. A., Oyler, G. A., Doolittle, G. M., *et al.* (1993). Okadaic acid induces hyperphosphorylated forms of tau protein in human brain slices. *Annals of Neurology*, 33, 77–87

Hasegawa, M., Crowther, R. A., Jakes, R., and Goedert, M. (1997). Alzheimer-like changes in microtubule-associated protein tau induced by sulfated glycosaminoglycans: inhibition of microtubule binding, stimulation of phosphorylation, and filament assembly depend on the degree of sulfation. *Journal of Biological Chemistry*, 272, 33118–24

Hasegawa, M., Smith, M. J., and Goedert, M. (1998). Tau proteins with FTDP-17 mutations have a reduced ability to promote microtubule assembly. *FEBS Letters*, 437, 207–10

Hasegawa, M., Smith, M. J., Iijima, M., *et al.* (1999). FTDP-17 mutations N279K and S305N in tau produce increased splicing of exon 10. *FEBS Letters*, 443, 93–6

Hayes, B. K. and Hart, G. W. (1994). Novel forms of protein glycosylation. *Current Opinion in Structural Biology*, 4, 692–6

Hendriks, L., De Jonghe, C., Lubke, U., *et al.* (1998). Immunoreactivity of presenilin-1 and tau in Alzheimer's disease brain. *Experimental Neurology*, 149, 341–8

Henke, H. and Lang, W. (1983). Cholinergic enzymes in neocortex, hippocampus and basal forebrain of non-neurological and senile dementia of Alzheimer-type patients. *Brain Research*, 267, 281–91

Heutink, P., Stevens, M., Rizzu, P., *et al.* (1997). Hereditary frontotemporal dementia is linked to chromosome 17q21-q22: a genetic and clinicopathological study of three Dutch families. *Annals of Neurology*, 41, 150–9

Higgins, J. J., Litvan, I., Li, W., and Nee, L. E. (1998). Progressive supranuclear gaze palsy is in linkage disequilibrium with the τ and not the α-synuclein gene. *Neurology*, 50, 270–3

Higgins, J. J., Adler, R. L., and Loveless, J. M. (1999*a*). Mutational analysis of the tau gene in progressive supranuclear palsy. *Neurology*, 53, 1421–4

Higgins, J. J., Litvan, I., Nee, L. E., and Loveless, J. M. (1999*b*). A lack of the R406W tau mutation in progressive supranuclear palsy and corticobasal degeneration. *Neurology*, 52, 404–6

Hoffmann, R., Dawson, N. F., Wade, J. D., and Otvos, L., Jr. (1997). Oxidized and phosphorylated synthetic peptides corresponding to the second and third tubulin-binding repeats of the τ protein reveal structural features of paired helical filament assembly. *Journal of Peptide Research*, 50, 132–42

Hofman, A., Rocca, W. A., Brayne, C., *et al.* (1991). The prevalence of dementia in Europe: a collaborative study of 1980–1990 findings. *International Journal of Epidemiology*, 20, 736–48

Holzer, M., Holzapfel, H-P., Zedlick, D., *et al.* (1994). Abnormally phosphorylated tau protein in Alzheimer's disease: heterogeneity of individual regional distribution and relationship to clinical severity. *Neuroscience*, 63, 499–516

Hong, M., Chen, D. C. R., Klein, P. S., and Lee, V. M.-Y. (1997). Lithium reduces tau phosphorylation by inhibition of glycogen synthase kinase-3. *Journal of Biological Chemistry*, 272, 25326–32.

Hong, M., Zhukareva, V., Vogelsberg-Ragaglia, V., *et al.* (1998). Mutation-specific functional impairments in distinct tau isoforms of hereditary FTDP-17. *Science*, 282, 1914–17

Horiuchi, M., Chabry, J., and Caughey, B. (1999). Specific binding of normal prion protein to the scrapie form via a localized domain initiates its conversion to the protease-resistant state. *EMBO Journal*, 18, 3193–203

Houlden, H., Baker, M., Adamson, J., *et al.* (1999*a*). Frequency of tau mutations in three series of non-Alzheimer's degenerative dementia. *Annals of Neurology*, 46, 243–8

Houlden, H., Rizzu, P., Stevens, M., *et al.* (1999*b*). Apolipoprotein E genotype does not affect the age of onset of dementia in families with defined tau mutations. *Neuroscience Letters*, **260**, 193–5.

Howe, L. R., Leevers, S. J., Gomez, N., *et al.* (1992). Activation of the MAP kinase pathway by the protein-kinase Raf. *Cell*, **71**, 335–42

Hulstaert, F., Blennow, K., Ivanoiu, A., *et al.* (1999). Improved discrimination of AD patients using β-amyloid$_{(1-42)}$ and tau levels in CSF. *Neurology*, **52**, 1555–62

Hussain, I., Powell, D., Howlett, D. R., *et al.* (1999). Identification of a novel aspartic protease (Asp 2) as β-secretase. *Molecular and Cellular Neuroscience*, **14**, 419–27

Hutchin, T. and Cortopassi, G. (1995). A mitochondrial DNA clone is associated with increased risk for Alzheimer disease. *Proceedings of the National Academy of Science (USA)*, **92**, 6892–5.

Hutton, M., Lendon, C., Rizzu, P., *et al.* (1998). Association of missense and 5′-splice-site mutations in tau with the inherited dementia FTDP-17. *Nature*, **393**, 702–5

Hwang, S. C., Jhon, D-Y., Bae, Y. S., *et al.* (1996). Activation of phospholipase C-γ by the concerted action of tau proteins and arachidonic acid. *Journal of Biological Chemistry*, **271**, 18342–9

Ii, K., Ito, H., Tanaka, K., and Hirano, A. (1997). Immunocytochemical co-localization of the proteasome in ubiquitinated structures in neurodegenerative diseases and the elderly. *Journal of Neuropathology and Experimental Neurology*, **56**, 125–31

Iijima, M., Tabira, T., Poorkaj, P., *et al.* (1999). A distinct familial presenile dementia with a novel missense mutation in the tau gene. *NeuroReport*, **10**, 497–501

Ikegami, S., Harada, A., and Hirokawa, N. (2000). Muscle weakness, hyperactivity, and impairment in fear conditioning in tau-deficient mice. *Neuroscience Letters*, **279**, 129–32

Ingelson, M., Blomberg, M., Benedikz, E., *et al.* (1999). Tau immunoreactivity detected in human plasma, but no obvious increase in dementia. *Dementia and Geriatric Cognitive Disorders*, **10**, 442–5

Irving, N. G. and Miller, C. C. J. (1997). Tau phosphorylation in cells transfected with wild-type or an AD mutant Presenilin 1. *Neuroscience Letters*, **222**, 71–4

Ishiguro, K., Ohno, H., Arai, H., *et al.* (1999). Phosphorylated tau in human cerebrospinal fluid is a diagnostic marker for Alzheimer's disease. *Neuroscience Letters*, **270**, 91–4

Ishiguro, K., Takamatsu, M., Tomizawa, K., *et al.* (1992). Tau protein kinase I converts normal tau protein into A68-like component of paired helical filaments. *Journal of Biological Chemistry*, **267**, 10897–01

Ishihara, T., Hong, M., Zhang, B., *et al.* (1999). Age-dependent emergence and progression of a tauopathy in transgenic mice overexpressing the shortest human tau isoform. *Neuron*, **24**, 751–62

Isoe, K., Ji, Y., Urakami, K., *et al.* (1998). Genetic association of oestrogen receptor gene polymorphisms with Alzheimer's disease. *Alzheimer's Research*, **3**, 195–7

Isoe, K., Urakami, K., Shimomura, T., *et al.* (1996). Tau proteins in cerebrospinal fluid from patients with Alzheimer's disease: a longitudinal study. *Dementia*, **7**, 175–6

Itoh, T. J. and Hotani, H. (1998). Microtubule-stabilizing activity of microtubule-associated proteins (MAPs). is due to increase in frequency of rescue in dynamic instability: shortening length decreases with binding of MAPs onto microtubules. *Journal of Cell Biology*, **143**, 777–94

Iwata, N., Tsubuki, S., Takaki, S., *et al.* (2000). Identification of the major Aβ$_{1-42}$-degrading catabolic pathway in brain parenchyma: suppression leads to biochemical and pathological deposition. *Nature Medicine*, **6**, 143–50

Iwatsubo, T., Mann, D. M. A., Odaka, A., *et al.* (1995). Amyloid β protein (Aβ) deposition: Aβ42(43) precedes Aβ40 in Down syndrome. *Annals of Neurology*, **37**, 294–9

Jakes, R., Novak, M., Davison, M., and Wischik, C. M. (1991). Identification of 3- and 4-repeat tau isoforms within the PHF in Alzheimer's disease. *EMBO Journal*, **10**, 2725–9

Jakes, R., Spillantini, M. G., and Goedert, M. (1994). Identification of two distinct synucleins from human brain. *FEBS Letters*, **345**, 27–32

Jakowec, M. W., Petzinger, G. M., Sastry, S., *et al.* (1998). The native form of α-synuclein is not found in the cerebrospinal fluid of patients with Parkinson's disease or normal controls. *Neuroscience Letters*, **253**, 13–16

James, N. D., Davis, D. R., Sindon, J., *et al.* (1996). Neurodegenerative changes including altered tau phosphorylation and neurofilament immunoreactivity in mice transgenic for the serine/threonine kinase Mos. *Neurobiology of Aging*, **17**, 235–41

Jameson, L., Frey, T., Zeeberg, B., *et al.* (1980). Inhibition of microtubule assembly by phosphorylation of microtubule-associated proteins. *Biochemistry*, **19**, 2472–9

Janciauskiene, S., Carlemalm, E., and Eriksson, S. (1995). In vitro amyloid fibril formation from α_1-antitrypsin. *Biological Chemistry Hoppe-Seyler*, **376**, 103–9

Jarrett, J. T., Berger, E. P., and Lansbury, J. P. T. (1993). The carboxy terminus of the β-amyloid protein is critical for the seeding of amyloid formation, implications for the pathogenesis of Alzheimer's disease. *Biochemistry*, **32**, 4693–7

Jenkins, S. M. and Johnson, G. V. W. (1998). Tau complexes with phospholipase C-τ *in situ*. *NeuroReport*, **9**, 67–71

Jensen, M., Schroder, J., Blomberg, M., *et al.* (1999). Cerebrospinal fluid Aβ42 is increased early in sporadic Alzheimer's disease and declines with disease progression. *Annals of Neurology*, **45**, 504–11

Jicha, G. A., Bowser, R., Kazam, I. G., and Davies, P. (1997). Alz-50 and MC-1, a new monoclonal antibody raised to paired helical filaments, recognize conformational epitopes on recombinant tau. *Journal of Neuroscience Research*, **48**, 128–32

Jicha, G. A., Rockwood, J. M., Berenfeld, B., *et al.* (1999). Altered conformation of recombinant frontotemporal dementia-17 mutant tau proteins. *Neuroscience Letters*, **260**, 153–6

Johnson, G. V. W., Cox, T. M., Lockhart, J. P., *et al.* (1997*a*). Transglutaminase activity is increased in Alzheimer's disease brain. *Brain Research*, **751**, 323–9

Johnson, G. V. W. and Jenkins, S. M. (1996). Tau protein in normal and Alzheimer's disease brain. *Alzheimer's Disease Review*, **1**, 38–54.

Johnson, G. V. W., Seubert, P., Cox, T. M., *et al.* (1997*b*). The τ protein in human cerebrospinal fluid in Alzheimer's disease consists of proteolytically derived fragments. *Journal of Neurochemistry*, **68**, 430–3

Julliams, A., Vanderhoeven, I., Kuhn, S., *et al.* (1999). No influence of presenilin 1 I143T and G384A mutations on endogenous tau phosphorylation in human and mouse neuroblastoma cells. *Neuroscience Letters*, **269**, 83–6

Juva, K., Verkkoniemi, A., Viramo, P., *et al.* (2000). APOE ε4 does not predict mortality, cognitive decline, or dementia in the oldest old. *Neurology*, **54**, 412–15

Kaech, S., Ludin, B., and Matus, A. (1996). Cytoskeletal plasticity in cells expressing neuronal microtubule microtubule-associated proteins. *Neuron*, **17**, 1189–99

Kakizuka, A. (1998). Protein precipitation: a common aetiology in neurodegenerative disorders? *Trends in Genetics*. **14**, 396–402

Kamboh, M. I., Sanghera, D. K., Ferrell, R. E., and DeKosky, S. T. (1995). APOE*4-associated Alzheimer's disease risk is modified by a1-antichymotrypsin polymorphism. *Nature Genetics*, **10**, 486–8

Kampers, T., Friedhoff, P., Biernat, J., *et al.* (1996). RNA stimulates aggregation of microtubule-associated protein tau into Alzheimer-like paired helical filaments. *FEBS Letters*, **399**, 344–9

Kampers, T., Pangalos, M., Geerts, H., *et al.* (1999). Assembly of paired helical filaments from mouse tau: implications for the neurofibrillary pathology in transgenic mouse models for Alzheimer's disease. *FEBS Letters*, **451**, 39–44

Kanai, M., Matsubara, E., Isoe, K., *et al.* (1998). Longitudinal study of cerebrospinal fluid levels of tau, Aβ1–40: and Aβ1–42(43) in Alzheimer's disease: a study in Japan. *Annals of Neurology*, **44**, 17–26

Kanai, M., Shizuka, M., Urakami, K., *et al.* (1999). Apolipoprotein E4 accelerates dementia and increases cerebrospinal fluid tau levels in Alzheimer's disease. *Neuroscience Letters,* 267, 65–8

Katayama, T., Imaizumi, K., Sato, N., *et al.* (1999). Presenilin-1 mutations downregulate the signalling pathway of the unfolded-protein response. *Nature Cell Biology,* 1, 479–85

Kawahara, M., Muramoto, K., Kobayashi, K., and Kuroda, Y. (1992). Functional and morphological changes in cultured neurons of rat cerebral cortex induced by long-term application of aluminium. *Biochemical and Biophysical Research Communications,* 189, 1317–22

Kawahara, M., Muramoto, K., Kobayashi, K., *et al.* (1994). Aluminium promotes the aggregation of Alzheimer's b-protein in vitro. *Biochemical and Biophysical Research Communications,* 198, 531–5

Kehoe, P. G., Russ, C., McIlroy, S., and Owen, M. J. (1999). Variation in *DCP1*, encoding *ACE*, is associated with susceptibility to Alzheimer disease. *Nature Genetics,* 21, 71–2

Kelly, J. W. (1998). The alternative conformations of amyloidogenic proteins and their multi-step assembly pathways. *Current Opinion in Structural Biology,* 8, 101–6

Kenessey, A., Yen, S-H., Liu, W-K., *et al.* (1995). Detection of D-aspartate in tau proteins associated with Alzheimer paired helical filaments. *Brain Research,* 675, 183–9

Kennard, M. L., Feldman, H., Yamada, T., and Jefferies, W. A. (1996). Serum levels of the iron binding protein p97 are elevated in Alzheimer's disease. *Nature Medicine,* 2, 1230–5

Khachaturian, Z. S. (1995). Diagnosis of Alzheimer's disease. *Archives of Neurology,* 42, 1097–1105.

Kidd, M. (1963). Paired helical filaments in electron microscopy in Alzheimer's disease. *Nature,* 197, 192–3

Kim, S-H., Wang, R., Gordon, D. J,. *et al.* (1999). Furin mediates enhanced production of fibrillogenic ABri peptides in familial British dementia. *Nature Neuroscience,* 2, 984–8

Kimura, T., Takamatsu, J., Ikeda, K., *et al.* (1996). Accumulation of advanced glycation end products of the Maillard reaction with age in human hippocampal neurons. *Neuroscience Letters,* 208, 53–6

Kimura, T., Takamatsu, J., Miyata, T., *et al.* (1998). Localization of identified advanced glycation end-product structures, N^{ε}-(carboxymethyl)lysine and pentosidine, in age-related inclusions in human brains. *Pathology International,* 48, 575–9

King, M. E., Ahuja, V., Binder, L. I., and Kuret, J. (1999). Ligand dependent tau filament formation: implications for Alzheimer's disease progression. *Biochemistry,* 38, 14851–9

Klatzo, I., Wisniewski, H., and Streicher, E. (1965). Experimental production of neurofibrillary degeneration. 1. Light microscopic observation. *Journal of Neuropathology and Experimental Neurology,* 24, 187–99

Klymkowsky, M. W. (1999). Weaving a tangled web: the interconnected cytoskeleton. *Nature Cell Biology,* 1, E121-E123

Ko, L. W., Ko, E. C., Nacharaju, P., *et al.* (1999). An immunochemical study on tau glycation in paired helical filaments. *Brain Research,* 830, 301–13

Koo, E. H., Lansbury, J. P. T., and Kelly, J. W. (1999). Amyloid diseases: abnormal protein aggregation in neurodegeneration. *Proceedings of the National Academy of Science (USA),* 96, 9989–90

Kosaka, K., Yoshimura, M., Ikeda, K., and Budka, H. (1984). Diffuse type of Lewy body disease: progressive dementia with abundant cortical lewy bodies and senile changes of various degree — a new disease? *Clinical Neuropathology,* 3, 185–92

Ksiezak-Reding, H., Yang, G., Simon, M., and Wall, J. S. (1998). Assembled tau filaments from native paired helical filaments as determined by scanning transmission electron microscopy (STEM). *Brain Research,* 814, 86–98

Kumar, A., Schapira, M. B., Grady, C. L., *et al.* (1995). Anatomic, metabolic, neuropsychological, and molecular genetic studies of three pairs of identical twins discordant for dementia of the Alzheimer's type. *Archives of Neurology,* 48, 160–8

Kwei, S.L., Clement, A., Faissner, A., and Brandt, R. (1998). Differential interactions of MAP2, tau and MAP5 during axiogenesis in culture. *NeuroReport*, **9**, 1035–40

Kwok, J. B. J., Li, Q-X., Hallupp, M., *et al.* (2000). Novel Leu273Pro amyloid precursor protein mutation increases amyloid β42(43) peptide levels and induces apoptosis. *Annals of Neurology*, **47**, 249–53

Lai, R. Y. K., Gertz, H-J. Wischik, D. J, *et al.* (1995). Examination of phosphorylated tau protein as a PHF-precursor at early stage Alzheimer's disease. *Neurobiology of Aging*, **16**, 433–45

Lang, E., Szendrei, G. I., Elekes, I., *et al.* (1992*a*). Reversible β-pleated sheet formation of a phospho-rylated synthetic τ peptide. *Biochemical and Biophysical Research Communications*, **182**, 63–9.

Lang, E., Szendrei, G. I., Lee, V. M.-Y., and Otvos, L. Jr. (1992*b*). Immunological and conformational characterization of a phosphorylated immunodominant epitope on the paired helical filaments found in Alzheimer's disease. *Biochemical and Biophysical Research Communications*, **187**, 783–90

Lange-Carter, C. A., Pleiman, C. M., Gardner, A. M., *et al.* (1993). A divergence in the MAP kinase regulatory network defined by MEK kinase and Raf. *Science*, **260**, 315–19

Lansbury, J. P. T. (1999). Evolution of amyloid: what normal protein folding may tell us about fibrillo-genesis and disease. *Proceedings of the National Academy of Science (USA)*, **96**, 3342–4

Lanska, D. J., Currier, R. D., Cohen, M., *et al.* (1994). Familial progressive subcortical gliosis. *Neurology*, **44**, 1633–43

Ledesma, M. D., Correas, I., Avila, J., and Diaz-Nido, J. (1992). Implication of brain cdc2 and MAP2 kinases in the phosphorylation of tau protein in Alzheimer's disease. *FEBS Letters*, **308**, 218–24

Ledesma, M. D., Bonay, P., Colaco, C., and Avila, J. (1994). Analysis of microtubule-associated protein tau glycation in paired helical filaments. *Journal of Biological Chemistry*, **269**, 21614–19

Ledesma, M. D., Bonay, P., and Avila, J. (1995). β-Protein from Alzheimer's disease patients is glycated at its tubulin-binding domain. *Journal of Neurochemistry*, **65**, 1658–64

Ledesma, M. D., Medina, M., and Avila, J. (1996). The in vitro formation of recombinant τ polymers. Effect of phosphorylation and glycation. *Molecular and Chemical Neuropathology*, **27**, 249–58

Ledesma, M. D., Pérez, M., Colaco, C., and Avila, J. (1998). Tau glycation is involved in aggregation of the protein but not in the formation of filaments. *Molecular and Cellular Biochemistry*, **44**, 1111–16

Lee, V. M-Y., Balin, B. J., Otvos, L. J., Jr., and Trojanowski, J. Q. (1991). A68: a major subunit of paired helical filaments and derivatized forms of normal tau. *Science*, **251**, 675–78

Lee, J. M., Zemaitaitis, M. O., Zainelli, G. M., and Muma, N. (1999). Transglutaminase-induced crosslinking of tau protein in progressive supranuclear palsy (PSP). *Journal of Neuropathology and Experimental Neurology*, **58**, 547 [Abstract]

Lehmann, D. J., Johnston, C., and Smith, A. D. (1997). Synergy between the genes for butyryl-cholinesterase K variant and apolipoprotein E4 in late-onset confirmed Alzheimer's disease. *Human Molecular Genetics*, **6**, 1933–6

Lemere, C. A., Lopera, F., Kosik, K. S., *et al.* (1996). The E280A presenilin 1 Alzheimer mutation pro-duces increased Aβ42 deposition and severe cerebellar pathology. *Nature Medicine*, **2**, 1146–50

Lendon, C. L., Lynch, T., Norton, J., *et al.* (1998). Hereditary dysphasic disinhibition dementia. A frontotemporal dementia linked to 17q21–22. *Neurology*, **50**, 1546–55

Leterrier, J-F., Linden, M., and Nelson, B. D. (1990). How do microtubules interact in vitro with purified subcellular organelles? *Biochemical Journal*, **269**, 556–8

Levitan, D., and Greenwald, I. (1995). Facilitation of *lin-12*-mediated signalling by *sel-12*, a *Caenorhabolitis elegans* S182 Alzheimer's disease gene. *Nature*, **377**, 351–4

Levy-Lahad, E., Wasco, W., Poorkaj, P., *et al.* (1995). Candidate gene for the chromosome 1 familial Alzheimer's disease locus. *Science*, **269**, 973–7

Li, J. J., Surini, M., Catsicas, S., *et al.* (1995). Age-dependent accumulation of advanced glycosylation end products in human neurons. *Neurobiology of Aging*, **16**, 69–76

Li, T., Holmes, C., Sham, P. C., *et al.* (1997). Allelic functional variation of serotonin transporter expression is a susceptibility factor for late onset Alzheimer's disease. *NeuroReport*, 8, 683–6

Li, Y. M., and Dickson, D. W. (1997). Enhanced binding of advanced glycation end products (AGE). by the ApoE4 isoform links the mechanism of plaque deposition in Alzheimer's disease. *Neuroscience Letters*, 226, 155–8

Lichtenberg-Kraag, B., Mandelkow, E.-M., Biernat, J., *et al.* (1992). Phosphorylation-dependent epitopes of neurofilament antibodies on tau protein and relationship with Alzheimer tau. *Proceedings of the National Academy of Science (USA)*, 89, 5384–8

Lilius, L., Fabre, S. F., Basun, H., *et al.* (1999). Tau gene polymorphisms and apolipoprotein E 4 may interact to increase risk for Alzheimer's disease. *Neuroscience Letters*, 277, 29–32

Linden, M. and Karlsson, G. (1996). Identification of porin as a binding site for MAP2. *Biochemical and Biophysical Research Communications*, 218, 833–836

Lindwall, G. and Cole, R. D. (1984). Phosphorylation affects the ability of tau protein to promote microtubule assembly. *Journal of Biological Chemistry*, 259, 5301–5

Lippa, C. F., Fujiwara, H., Mann, D. M. A., *et al.* (1998). Lewy bodies contain altered α-synuclein in brains of many familial Alzheimer's disease patients with mutations in presenilin and amyloid precursor protein genes. *American Journal of Pathology*, 153, 1365–70

Lippa, C. F., Ozawa, K., Mann, D. M. A., *et al.* (1999). Deposition of β-amyloid subtypes 40 and 42 differentiates dementia with Lewy bodies from Alzheimer disease. *Archives of Neurology*, 56, 1111–18

Litersky, J. M. and Johnson, G. V. W. (1992). Phosphorylation by cAMP-dependent protein kinase inhibits the degradation of tau by calpain. *Journal of Biological Chemistry*, 267, 1563–8

Loftus, S. K., Morris, J. A., Carstea, E. D., *et al.* (1997). Murine model of Niemann-Pick C disease: mutation in a cholesterol homeostasis gene. *Science*, 277, 232–5

Lomas, D. A., Evans, D. L., Finch, J. T., and Carrell, R. W. (1992). The mechanism of Z α1-antitrypsin accumulation in the liver. *Nature*, 357, 605–7

Love, S., Bridges, L. R., and Case, C. P. (1995). Neurofibrillary tangles in Niemann-Pick disease type C. *Brain*, 118, 119–29

Loveland, K. L., Herszfeld, D., Chu, B., *et al.* (1999). Novel low molecular weight microtubule-associated protein-2 isoforms contain a functional nuclear localization sequence. *Journal of Biological Chemistry*, 274, 19261–8

Lovestone, S. and Anderton, B. H. (1992). Cytoskeletal abnormalities in Alzheimer's disease. *Current Opinion in Neurology and Neurosurgery*, 5, 883–8

Lovestone, S. and Reynolds, C. H. (1997). The phosphorylation of tau: a critical stage in neurodevelopment and neurodegenerative processes. *Neuroscience*, 78, 309–24

Lovestone, S., Reynolds, C. H., Latimer, D., *et al.* (1994). Alzheimer's disease-like phosphorylation of the microtubule-associated protein tau by glycogen synthase kinase-3 in transfected mammalian cells. *Current Biology*, 4, 1077–86

Lovestone, S., Hartley, C. L., Pearce, J., and Anderton, B. H. (1996). Phosphorylation of tau by glycogen synthase kinase-3β in intact mammalian cells: the effects on the organization and stability of microtubules. *Neuroscience*, 73, 1145–57

Lowe, J. (1998). Establishing a pathological diagnosis in degenerative dementias. *Brain Pathology*, 8, 403–6

Lu, P-J., Wulf, G., Zhou, X. Z., (1999). The prolyl isomerase Pin1 restores the function of Alzheimer-associated phosphorylated tau protein. *Nature*, 399, 784–8

Lu, Q. and Wood, J. G. (1993). Functional studies of Alzheimer's disease tau protein. *Journal of Neuroscience*, 13, 508–15

McGeer, P. L., and McGeer, E. G. (1995). The inflammatory response system of brain: implications for therapy of Alzheimer and other neurodegenerative diseases. *Brain Research Reviews*, 21, 195–218

McKee, A. C., Kosik, K. S., and Kowall, N. W. (1991). Neuritic pathology and dementia in Alzheimer's disease. *Annals of Neurology*, 30, 156–65

McKeith, I. G., Galasko, D., Kosaka, K., Perry, E. K., Dickson, D. W., *et al.* (1996). Consensus guide-lines for the clinical and pathologic diagnosis of dementia with Lewy bodies (DLB): report of the consortium on DLB international workshop. *Neurology*, 47, 1113–24.

McKeith, I. G., Perry, E. K., and Perry, R. H. The Consortium on Dementia with Lewy Bodies (1999). Report of the second dementia with Lewy body international workshop. Diagnosis and treatment. *Neurology*, 53, 902–5

Mahley, R. W. and Huang, Y. D. (1999). Apolipoprotein E: from atherosclerosis to Alzheimer's disease and beyond. *Current Opinion in Lipidology*, 10, 207–17

Mandelkow, E.-M., Drewes, G., Biernat, J., *et al.* (1992). Glycogen synthase kinase-3 and the Alzheimer-like state of microtubule-associated protein tau. *FEBS Letters*, 314, 315–21

Mann, D. M. A. and South, P. W. (1993). The topographic distribution of brain atrophy in frontal lobe dementia. *Acta Neuropathologica*, 85, 334–340

Mann, D. M. A., South, P. W., Snowdon, J. S., and Neary, D. (1993). Dementia of frontal lobe type: neuropathology and immunohistochemistry. *Journal of Neurology, Neurosurgery and Psychiatry*, 56, 605–14

Mantyh, P. W., Ghilardi, J. R., Rogers, S., *et al.* (1993). Aluminium, iron, and zinc ions promote aggre-gation of phyridogical concentrations of β-amyloid peptide. *Journal of Neurochemistry*, 61, 1171–4

Martínez, M., Fernández, E., Frank, A., *et al.* (1999). Increased cerebrospinal fluid cAMP levels in Alzheimer's disease. *Brain Research*, 846, 265–7

Matsumara, N., Yamazaki, T., and Ihara, Y. (1999). Stable expression in Chinese hamster ovary cells of mutated tau genes causing frontotemporal dementia and parkinsonism linked to chromosome 17 (FTDP-17). *American Journal of Pathology*, 154, 1649–56

Maruyama, H., Toji, H., Harrington, C. R., *et al.* (2000). Lack of an association of oestrogen receptor α gene polymorphisms and transcriptional activity with Alzheimer disease. *Archives of Neurology*, 57, 236–40

Matsuo, E. S., Shin, R-W., Billingsley, M. L., *et al.* (1994). Biopsy-derived adult human brain tau is phosphorylated at many of the same sites as Alzheimer's disease paired helical filament tau. *Neuron*, 13, 989–1002

Mattson, M. P., and Guo, Q. (1997). Cell and molecular neurobiology of presenilins: a role for the endoplasmic reticulum in the pathogenesis of Alzheimer's disease. *Journal of Neuroscience Research*, 50, 505–13

Mawal-Dewan, M., Sen, P. C., Abdel-Ghany, M., Shalloway, D., and Racker, E. (1992). Phosphorylation of tau protein by purified p34cdc28 and a related protein kinase from neurofilaments. *Journal of Biological Chemistry*, 267, 19705–9

Mehta, P. D., Patrick, B. A., Dalton, A. J., *et al.* (1999). Increased levels of tau-like protein in patients with Down syndrome. *Neuroscience Letters*, 275, 159–62

Mehta, P. D., Pirttila, T., Mehta, S. P., *et al.* (2000). Plasma and cerebrospinal fluid levels of amyloid β proteins 1–40 and 1–42 in Alzheimer disease. *Neurology*, 54, 100–5

Mena, R., Wischik, C. M., Novak, M., *et al.* (1991). A progressive deposition of paired helical filaments (PHF) in the brain characterizes the evolution of dementia in Alzheimer's disease. An immunocy-tochemical study with a monoclonal antibody against the PHF core. *Journal of Neuropathology and Experimental Neurology*, 50, 474–90

Mena, R., Edwards, P., Pérez-Olvera, O., and Wischik, C. M. (1995). Monitoring pathological assem-bly of tau and β-amyloid proteins in Alzheimer's disease. *Acta Neuropathologica*, 89, 50–6

Mena, R., Edwards, P. C., Harrington, C. R., *et al.* (1996). Stageing the pathological assembly of truncated tau protein into paired helical filaments in Alzheimer's disease. *Acta Neuropathologica*, **91**, 633–41

Mertens, S., Craxton, M., and Goedert, M. (1997). SAP kinase-3, a new member of the family of mammalian stress-activated protein kinases. *FEBS Letters*, **383**, 273–6

Mesco, E. R., Kachen, C., and Timiras, P. S. (1991). Effects of aluminum on tau proteins in human neuroblastoma cells. *Molecular and Chemical Neuropathology*, **14**, 199–212

Miller, C. C. J., Brion, J-P., Calvert, R., *et al.* (1986). Alzheimer's paired helical filaments share epitopes with neurofilament sidearms. *EMBO Journal*, **5**, 269–76

Miller, B. L., Ikonte, C., Ponton, M., *et al.* (1997). A study of the Lund-Manchester research criteria for frontotemporal dementia: clinical and single-photon emission CT correlations. *Neurology*, **48**, 937–42

Molina, L., Touchon, J., Herpé, M., *et al.* (1999). Tau and apo E in CSF: potential aid for discriminating Alzheimer's disease from other dementias. *NeuroReport*, **10**, 3491–5

Montejo de Garcini, E., Serrano, L., and Avila, J. (1986). Self assembly of microtubule associated protein tau into filaments resembling those found in Alzheimer's disease. *Biochemical and Biophysical Research Communications*, **141**, 790–6

Montoya, S. E., Aston, C. E., DeKosky, S. T., *et al.* (1998). Bleomycin hydrolase is associated with risk of sporadic Alzheimer's disease. *Nature Genetics*, **18**, 211–12

Mori, H., Kondo, J., and Ihara, Y. (1987). Ubiquitin is a component of paired helical filaments in Alzheimer's disease. *Science*, **235**, 1641–4

Mori, H., Hosoda, K., Matsubara, E., *et al.* (1995). Tau in cerebrospinal fluids: establishment of the sandwich ELISA with antibody specific to the repeat sequence in tau. *Neuroscience Letters*, **186**, 181–3

Morishima-Kawashima, M., Hasegawa, M., Takio, K., *et al.* (1993). Ubiquitin is conjugated with amino-terminally processed tau in paired helical filaments. *Neuron*, **10**, 1151–60

Morishima-Kawashima, M., Hasegawa, M., Takio, T, *et al.* (1995*a*). Hyperphosphorylation of tau in PHF. *Neurobiology of Aging*, **16**, 365–80

Morishima-Kawashima, M., Hasegawa, M., Tario, K., *et al.* (1995*b*). Proline-directed and non-proline-directed phosphorylation of PHF-tau. *Journal of Biological Chemistry*, **270**, 823–9

Morsch, R., Simon, W., and Coleman, P. D. (1999). Neurons may live for decades with neurofibrillary tangles. *Journal of Neuropathology and Experimental Neurology*, **58**, 188–97

Motter, R., Vigo-Pelfrey, C., Kholodenko, D., *et al.* (1995). Reduction of β-amyloid peptide42 in the cerebrospinal fluid with Alzheimer's disease. *Annals of Neurology*, **38**, 643–8

Mountjoy, C. Q., Rossor, M. N., Iversen, L. L., and Roth, M. (1984). Correlation of cortical cholinergic and GABA deficits with quantitative neuropathological findings in senile dementia. *Brain*, **107**, 507–18

Mukaetova-Ladinska, E. B., Harrington, C. R., Hills, R., *et al.* (1992). Regional distribution of paired helical filaments and normal tau proteins in ageing and in Alzheimer's disease with and without occipital lobe involvement. *Dementia*, **3**, 61–9

Mukaetova-Ladinska, E. B., Harrington, C. R., Roth, M., and Wischik, C. M. (1993). Biochemical and anatomical redistribution of tau protein in Alzheimer's disease. *American Journal of Pathology*, **143**, 565–78

Mukaetova-Ladinska, E. B., Harrington, C. R., Roth, M., and Wischik, C. M. (1996). Alterations in tau potein metabolism during normal aging. *Dementia*, **7**, 95–103

Muller, T. (1992). Light-microscopic demonstration of methylene blue accumulation sites in mouse brain after supravital staining. *Acta Anatomica*, **144**, 39–44

Münch, G., Taneli, Y., Schraven, E., *et al.* (1994). The cognition-enhancing drug tenilsetam is an inhibitor of protein crosslinking by advanced glycosylation. *Journal of Neural Transmission*, [Parkinson's disease Section.] **8**, 193–208

Münch, G., Thome, J., Foley, P., *et al.* (1997). Advanced glycation end products in ageing and Alzheimer's disease. *Brain Research Reviews*, 23, 134–43

Münch, G., Cunningham, A. M., Riederer, P., and Braak, E. (1998). Advanced glycation endproducts are associated with Hirano bodies in Alzheimer's disease. *Brain Research*, 796, 307–10

Muñoz-Montano, J. R., Moreno, F. J., Avila, J., and DiazNido, J. (1999). Downregulation of glycogen synthase kinase-3 β (GSK-3 β) protein expression during neuroblastoma IMR-32 cell differentiation. *Journal of Neuroscience Research*, 55, 278–85

Munroe, W. A., Southwick, P. C., Chang, L., *et al.* (1995). Tau protein in cerebrospinal fluid as an aid in the diagnosis of Alzheimer's disease. *Annals of Clinical and Laboratory Science*, 25, 207–17

Murakami, N., Oyama, F., Gu, Y., *et al.* (1998). Accumulation of tau in autophagic vacuoles in chloroquine myopathy. *Journal of Neuropathology and Experimental Neurology*, 57, 664–73

Murayama, H., Shin, R-W., Higuchi, J., *et al.* (1999). Interaction of aluminum with PHFτ in Alzheimer's disease neurofibrillary degeneration evidenced by desferrioxamine-assisted chelating autoclave method. *American Journal of Pathology*, 155, 877–85

Murrell, J. R., Koller, D., Foroud, T., *et al.* (1997). Familial multiple-system tauopathy with presenile dementia is localized to chromosome 17. *American Journal of Human Genetics*, 61, 1131–8

Murrell, J. R., Spillantini, M. G., Zolo, P., *et al.* (1999). Tau gene mutation G389R causes a tauopathy with abundant Pick body-like inclusions and axonal deposits. *Journal of Neuropathology and Experimental Neurology*, 58, 1207–26

Nacharaju, P., Ko, L-W., and Yen, S-H. C. (1997). Characterization of in vitro glycation sites of tau. *Journal of Neurochemistry*, 69, 1709–19

Nacharaju, P., Lewis, J., Easson, C., *et al.* (1999). Accelerated filament formation from tau protein with specific FTDP-17 missense mutations. *FEBS Letters*, 447, 195–9

Nagy, Z., Esiri, M. M., Jobst, K. A., *et al.* (1995). Relative roles of plaques and tangles in the dementia of Alzheimer's disease: correlations using three sets of neuropathological criteria. *Dementia*, 6, 21–31

Nalbantoglu, J., Gilfix, B. M., Bertrand, P., *et al.* (1994). Predictive value of apolipoprotein E genotyping in Alzheimer's disease: results of an autopsy series and an analysis of several combined studies. *Annals of Neurology*, 36, 889–95

Nathan, B. P., Bellosta, C., Sanan, D. A., *et al.* (1994). Differential effects of apolipoproteins E3 and E4 on neuronal growth in vitro. *Science*, 264, 850–2

Naylor, G. J (1986). A two-year double-blind crossover trial of the prophylactic effect of methylene blue in manic-depressive psychosis. *Biological Psychiatry*, 21, 915–20

Naylor, G. J., Smith, A. H. W., and Connelly, P. (1987). A controlled trial of methylene blue in severe depressive psychosis. *Biological Psychiatry*, 22, 657–9

Nebreda, A. R. and Hunt, T. (1993). The c-Mos protooncogene protein-kinase turns on and maintains the activity ofMAP kinase, but not Mpf, in cell-free extracts of Xenopus oocytes and eggs. *EMBO Journal*, 12, 1979–86

Neill, D., Curran, M. D., Middleton, D., *et al.* (1999). Risk for Alzheimer's disease in older late-onset cases is associated with HLA-DRB1*03. *Neuroscience Letters*, 275, 137–40

Nelson, P. T. and Saper, C. B. (1995). Ultrastructure of neurofibrillary tangles in the cerebral cortex of sheep. *Neurobiology of Aging*, 16, 315–23

Nelson, P. T., Greenberg, S. G., and Saper, C. B. (1994). Neurofibrillary tangles in the cerebral cortex of sheep. *Neuroscience Letters*, 170, 187–90

Neupert, W. (1997). Protein import into mitochondria. *Annual Review of Biochemistry*, 66, 863–917

Nicoll J. A. R., and Roberts, G. W., and Grahem, D. I. (1995). Apolipoprotein E ε4 allele is associated with deposition of amyloid β-protein following head injury. *Nature Medicine*, 1, 135–7

Nitsch, R. M., Rebeck, G. W., Deng, M., *et al.* (1995). Cerebrospinal fluid levels of amyloid β-protein in Alzheimer's disease: inverse correlation with severity of dementia and effect of apolipoprotein E genotype. *Annals of Neurology*, **37**, 512–18

Novak, M., Jakes, R., Edwards, P. C., *et al.* (1991). Difference between the tau protein of Alzheimer paired helical filament core and normal tau revealed by epitope analysis of mAbs 423 and 7. 51. *Proceedings of the National Academy of Science (USA)*, **88**, 5837–41

Novak, M., Kabat, J., and Wischik, C. M. (1993). Molecular characterization of the minimal protease resistant tau unit of the Alzheimer's disease paired helical filament. *EMBO Journal*, **12**, 365–70

Okamura, N., Arai, H., Higuchi, M., *et al.* (1999). Cerebrospinal fluid levels of amyloid β-peptide$_{1-42}$, but not tau have positive correlation with brain glucose metabolism in humans. *Neuroscience Letters*, **273**, 203–7

Okuizumi, K., Onodera, O., Namba, Y., *et al.* (1995). Genetic association of the very low low density lipoprotein (VLDL) receptor gene with sporadic Alzheimer's disease. *Nature Genetics*, **11**, 207–9

Oliva, R., Tolosa, E., Ezquerra, M., *et al.* (1998). Significant changes in the tau A0 and A3 alleles in progressive supranuclear palsy and improved genotyping by silver detection. *Annals of Neurology*, **55**, 1122–4

Ordway, J. M., Tallaksen-Greene, S., Gutekunst, C-A., *et al.* (1997). Ectopically expressed CAG repeats cause intranuclear inclusions and a progressive late onset neurological phenotype in the mouse. *Cell*, **91**, 753–63

Ott, A., Slooter, A. J. C., Hofman, A., *et al.* (1998). Smoking and risk of dementia and Alzheimer's disease in a population-based cohort study; the Rotterdam Study. *Lancet*, **351**, 1840–3

Otto, M., Wiltfang, J., Tumani, H., *et al.* (1997). Elevated levels of tau protein in cerebrospinal fluid of patients with Creutzfeldt-Jakob disease. *Neuroscience Letters*, **225**, 210–12

Palmer, D. N., Martinus, R. D., Cooper, S. M., *et al.* (1989). Ovine ceroid lipofuscinosis. The major lipopigment protein and the lipid-binding subunit of mitochondrial ATP synthase have the same NH_2-terminal sequence. *Journal of Biological Chemistry*, **264**, 5736–40

Papasozomenos, S. C. and Su, Y. (1991). Altered phosphorylation of tau protein in heat-shocked rats and patients with Alzheimer's disease. *Proceedings of the National Academy of Science (USA)*, **88**, 4543–7

Pastor, P., Ezquerra, M., Muñoz, E., *et al.* (2000). Significant association between the tau gene A0/A0 genotype and Parkinson's disease. *Annals of Neurology*, **47**, 242–5

Patrick, G. N., Zukerberg,. L, Nikolic, M., *et al.* (1999). Conversion of p35 to p25 deregulates Cdk5 activity and promotes neurodegeneration. *Nature*, **402**, 615–22

Paudel, H. K. and Li, W. (1999). Heparin-induced conformational change in microtubule-associated protein tau as detected by chemical cross-linking and phosphopeptide mapping. *Journal of Biological Chemistry*, **274**, 8029–38

Payami, H., Schellenberg, G. D., Zareparsi, S., *et al.* (1997). Evidence for association of HLA-A2 allele with onset age of Alzheimer's disease. *Neurology*, **49**, 512–18

Percy, M. E. (1993). Peripheral biological markers or predictive tests for Alzheimer disease in the general population and in Down syndrome. In *Alzheimer disease, Down syndrome, and their relationship*, (ed. J. M. Berg, H. Karlinsky, and A. J. Holland), pp. 199–223. Oxford University Press.

Pérez, M., Valpuesta, J. M., Medina, M., *et al.* (1996). Polymerization of τ into filaments in the presence of heparin: the minimal sequence required for τ–τ interaction. *Journal of Neurochemistry*, **67**, 1183–90

Pericak-Vance, M. A., Bass, M. P., Yamaoka, L. H., *et al.* (1997). Complete genomic screen in late-onset familial Alzheimer disease: evidence for a new locus on chromosome 12. *Journal of the American Medical Assocociation*, **278**, 1237–41

Perl, D. P. and Brody, A. R. (1980). Alzheimer's disease: X-ray spectrometric evidence of aluminum accumulation in neurofibrillary tangle-bearing neurones. *Science*, **208**, 297–9

Perl, D. P., Purohit, P., Kakulas, B. A., and Hof, P. R. (1999). Changes in the neuropathologic features of parkinsonism-dementia complex of Guam (PDC), cases from the 1960s compared to current cases. *Journal of Neuropathology and Experimental Neurology*, **58**, 515

Perry, E. K., Gibson, P. H., Blessed, G., *et al.* (1978). Correlation of cholinergic abnormalities with senile plaques and mental test scores in senile dementia. *British Medical Journal*, **2**, 1457–9

Perry, E. K., Blessed, G., Tomlinson, B. E., *et al.* (1981). Neurochemical activities in human temporal lobe related to ageing and Alzheimer-type changes. *Neurobiology of Aging*, **2**, 251–6

Perry, G., Friedman, R., Shaw, G., and Chau, V. (1987). Ubiquitin is detected in neurofibrillary tangles and senile plaque neurites of Alzheimer disease brains. *Proceedings of the National Academy of Science (USA)*, **84**, 3033–6

Perry, R. H., Irving, D., Blessed, G., *et al.* (1990). Senile dementia of the Lewy body type. A clinically and neuropathologically distinct form of Lewy body dementia in the elderly. *Journal of the Neurological Sciences*, **95**, 119–39

Perry, R., McKeith, I., and Perry, E., ed. (1996). *Dementia with Lewy bodies. Clinical, pathological, and treatment issues*. Cambridge University Press

Perutz, M. F., Johnson, T., Suzuki, M., and Finch, J. T. (1994). Glutamine repeats as polar zippers: their possible role in inherited neurodegenerative disorders. *Proceedings of the National Academy of Science (USA)*, **91**, 5355–8

Petersen, R. B., Tabaton, M., Chen, S. G., *et al.* (1995). Familial progressive subcortical gliosis: presence of prions and linkage to chromosome 17. *Neurology*, **45**, 1062–7.

Pick, A. (1892). Über die Beziehungen der senilen Hirnatrophie zur Aphasia. *Prager. Med. Wochenschr.*, **17**, 165–7

Pirttilä, T., Koivisto, K., Mehta, P. D., *et al.* (1998). Longitudinal study of cerebrospinal fluid amyloid proteins and apolipoprotein E in patients with probable Alzheimer's disease. *Neuroscience Letters*, **249**, 21–4

Polymeropoulos, M. H., Lavedan, C., Leroy, E., *et al.* (1997). Mutation in the α-synuclein gene identified in families with Parkinson's disease. *Science*, **276**, 2045–7

Poorkaj, P., Bird, T. D., Wijsman, E., *et al.* (1998). Tau is a candidate gene for chromosome 17 frontotemporal dementia. *Annals of Neurology*, **43**, 815–25

Post, K., Pitschke, M., Schäfer, O., *et al.* (1998). Rapid acquisition of β-sheet structure in the prion protein prior to multimer formation. *Biological Chemistry*, **379**, 1307–17

Poulter, L., Barratt, D., Scott, C. W., and Caputo, C. B. (1993). Locations and immunoreactivities of phosphorylation sites on bovine and porcine tau proteins and a PHF-tau fragment. *Journal of Biological Chemistry*, **268**, 9636–44

Price, D. L., Sisodia, S. S., and Borchelt, D. R. (1998). Genetic neurodegenerative diseases: the human illness and transgenic models. *Science*, **282**, 1079–83

Price, J. L., Davis, P. B., Morris, J. C., and White, D. L. (1991). The distribution of tangles, plaques and related immunohistochemical markers in healthy ageing and Alzheimer's disease. *Neurobiology of Aging*, **12**, 295–312

Prusiner, S. B., Scott, M. R., DeArmond, S. J., and Cohen, F. E. (1998). Prion protein biology. *Cell*, **93**, 337–48

Pryer, N. K., Walker, R. A., Skeen, V. P., *et al.* (1992). Brain microtubule-associated proteins modulate microtubule dynamic instability *in vitro*: real-time observations using video microscopy. *Journal of Cell Science*, **103**, 965–76

Raby, C. A., Morganti-Kossmann, M. C., Kossmann, T., *et al.* (1998). Traumatic brain injury increases β-amyloid peptide 1–42 in cerebrospinal fluid. *Journal of Neurochemistry*, **71**, 2505–9

Ransmayr, G., Cervera, P., Hirsch, E. C., *et al.* (1992). Alzheimer's disease: is the decrease of the cholinergic innervation of the hippocampus related to intrinsic hippocampal pathology? *Neuroscience*, 47, 843–51

Reinikainen, K. J., Riekkinen, P. J., Paljarvi, L., *et al.* (1988). Cholinergic deficit in Alzheimer's disease: A study based on CSF and autopsy data. *Neurochemical Research*, 13, 135–46

Rendon, A., Jung, D., and Jancsik, V. (1990). Interactions of microtubules and microtubule-associated proteins (MAPs) with rat brain mitochondria. *Biochemical Journal*, 269, 555–6

Resch, J. F., Lehr, G. S., and Wischik, C. M. (1991). Design and synthesis of a potential affinity/cleaving reagent for beta-pleated sheet protein structures. *Biorganic and Medicinal Chemistry Letters*, 1, 519–22

Reynolds, C. H., Utton, M. A., Gibb, G. M., *et al.* (1997). Stress-activated protein kinase/c-jun N-terminal kinase phosphorylates τ protein. *Journal of Neurochemistry*, 68, 1736–44

Riemenschneider, M., Buch, K., Schmolke, M., *et al.* (1997). Diagnosis of Alzheimer's disease with cerebrospinal fluid tau protein and aspartate aminotransferase. *Lancet*, 350, 784

Rizzu, P., Van Swieten, J. C., Joose, M., *et al.* (1999). High prevalence of mutations in the microtubule-associated protein tau in a population study of frontotemporal dementia in the Netherlands. *American Journal of Human Genetics*, 64, 414–21

Roberts, G. W., Allsop, D., and Bruton, C. (1990). The occult aftermath of boxing. *Journal of Neurology, Neurosurgery and Psychiatry*, 53, 373–8

Roberts, G. W., Gentleman, S. M., Lynch, A., and Graham, D. I. (1991). βA4 amyloid protein deposition in brain after head trauma. *Lancet*, 338, 1422–3

Roder, H. M. and Ingram, V. M. (1991). Two novel kinases phosphorylate tau and the KSP site of heavy neurofilament subunits in high stoichiometric ratios. *Journal of Neuroscience*, 11, 3325–43

Roertgen, K. E., Parisi, J. E., Clark, H. B., *et al.* (1996). Aβ-associated cerebral angiopathy and senile plaques with neurofibrillary tangles and cerebral hemorrhage in an aged wolverine (*Gulo gulo*). *Neurobiology of Aging*, 17, 243–7

Rogaev, E. I., Sherrington, R., Rogaeva, E. A., *et al.* (1995). Familial Alzheimer's disease in kindreds with missense mutations in a gene on chromosome 1 related to the Alzheimer's disease type 3 gene. *Nature*, 376, 775–8

Roks, G., Dermaut, B., Heutink, P., *et al.* (1999). Mutation screening of the tau gene in patients with early-onset Alzheimer's disease. *Neuroscience Letters*, 277, 137–9

Rossor, M., Fahrenkrug, J., Emson, P., *et al.* (1980). Reduced cortical choline acetyltransferase activity in senile dementia of Alzheimer type is not accompanied by changes in vasoactive intestinal polypeptide. *Brain Research*, 201, 249–53

Rossor, M. N., Garrett, N. J., Johnson, A. L., *et al.* (1982). A post-mortem study of the cholinergic and GABA systems in senile dementia. *Brain*, 105, 313–30

Royston, M. C., Rothwell, N. J., and Roberts, G. W. (1992). Alzheimer's disease: pathology to potential treatments? *Trends in Pharmacological Science*, 13, 131–3

Ruben, G. C., Iqbal, K., Grundke-Iqbal, I., and Johnson, JE., Jr. (1993). The organization of the microtubule associated protein tau in Alzheimer paired helical filaments. *Brain Research*, 602, 1–13

Rubenstein, R., Kascsak, R. J., Merz, P. A., *et al.* (1986). Paired helical filaments associated with Alzheimer's disease are readily soluble structures. *Brain Research*, 372, 80–8

Ruiz, P. J. G., and Gulliksen, L. (1999). Did Don Quixote have Lewy body disease? *Journal of the Royal Society of Medicine*, 92, 200–1

Sadot, E., Gurwitz, D., Barg, J., *et al.* (1996). Activation of m1 muscarinic acetylcholine receptor regulates τ phosphorylation in transfected PC12 cells. *Journal of Neurochemistry*, 66, 877–80

Saitoh, T., Xia, Y., Chen, X., *et al.* (1995). The CYP2D6B mutant allele is overrepresented in the Lewy body variant of Alzheimer's disease. *Annals of Neurology*, 37, 110–12

Salehi, A., Ravid, R., Gonatas, N. K., and Swaab, D. F. (1995). Decreased activity of hippocampal neurons in Alzheimer's disease is not related to the presence of neurofibrillary tangles. *Journal of Neuropathology and Experimental Neurology*, 54, 704–9

Sasaki, N., Fukatsu, R., Tsuzuki., K, *et al.* (1998). Advanced glycation end products in Alzheimer's disease and other neurodegenerative diseases. *American Journal of Pathology*, 153, 1149–55

Sato-Harada, R., Okabe, S., Umeyama, T., *et al.* (1996). Microtubule-associated proteins regulate microtubule function as the track for intracellular membrane organelle transports. *Cell Structure and Function*, 21, 283–95

Saudou, F., Finkbeiner, S., Devys, D., and Greenberg, M. E. (1998). Huntingtin acts in the nucleus to induce apoptosis but death does not correlate with the formation of intranuclear inclusions. *Cell*, 95, 55–66

Schenk, D., Barbour, R., Dunn, W., *et al.* (1999). Immunization with amyloid-beta attenuates Alzheimer disease-like pathology in the PDAPP mouse. *Nature*, 400, 173–7

Scheuner, D., Eckman, C., Jensen, M., *et al.* (1996). Secreted amyloid β-protein similar to that in the senile plaques of Alzheimer's disease is increased *in vivo* by the presenilin 1 and 2 and APP mutations linked to familial Alzheimer's disease. *Nature Medicine*, 2, 864–70

Schneider, A., Biernat, J., von Bergen, M., *et al.* (1999). Phosphorylation that detaches tau protein from microtubules (Ser262, Ser214). also protects it against aggregation into Alzheimer paired helical filaments. *Biochemistry*, 38, 3549–58

Schultz, C., Dehgani, F., Hubbard, G. B., *et al.* (2000). Filamentous tau pathology in nerve cells, astrocytes, and oligodendrocytes of aged baboons. *Journal of Neuropathology and Experimental Neurology*, 59, 39–52

Schweers, O., Schönbrunn-Hanebeck, E., Marx, A., and Mandelkow, E. (1994). Structural studies of tau protein and Alzheimer paired helical filaments show no evidence for β structure. *Journal of Biological Chemistry*, 269, 24290–7

Schweers, O., Mandelkow, E.-M., Biernat, J., and Mandelkow, E. (1995). Oxidation of cysteine-322 in the repeat domain of microtubule-associated protein τ controls the *in vitro* assembly of paired helical filaments. *Proceedings of the National Academy of Science (USA)*, 92, 8463–7

Scott, C. W., Fieles, A., Sygowski, L. A., and Caputo, C. B. (1993). Aggregation of tau protein by aluminum. *Brain Research*, 628, 77–84

Seidl, R., Greber, S., Schuller, E., *et al.* (1997). Evidence against oxidative DNA damage in Down syndrome. *Neuroscience Letters*, 235, 137–140

Selkoe, D. J. (1998). The cell biology β-amyloid precursor protein and presenilin in Alzheimer's disease. *Trends in Cell Biology*, 8, 447–53

Selkoe, D. J. (1999). Translating cell biology into therapeutic advances in Alzheimer's disease. *Nature*, 399, A23-A31

Sergeant, N., David, J-P., Goedert, M., *et al.* (1997). Two-dimensional characterization of paired helical filament-tau from Alzheimer's disease: demonstration of an additional 74-kDa component and age-related biochemical modifications. *Journal of Neurochemistry*, 69, 834–44

Sergeant, N., Wattez, A., and Delacourte, A. (1999). Neurofibrillary degeneration in progressive supranuclear palsy and corticobasal degeneration: tau pathologies with exclusively "exon 10" isoforms. *Journal of Neurochemistry*, 72, 1243–9

Seubert, P., Mawal-Dewan, M., Barbour, R., *et al.* (1995*a*). Detection of phosphorylated Ser262 in fetal tau, adult tau, and paired helical filament tau. *Journal of Biological Chemistry*, 270, 18917–22

Seubert, P., Vigo-Pelfrey, C., Esch, F., *et al.* (1995*b*). Isolation and quantification of soluble Alzheimer's β-peptide from biological fluids. *Nature*, 359, 325–7

Sherrington, R., Rogaev, E. I,. Liang, Y., *et al.* (1995). Cloning of a gene bearing missense mutations in early-onset familial Alzheimer's disease. *Nature*, 375, 754–60

Shin, R-W., Lee, V. M-Y., and Trojanowski, J. Q. (1994). Aluminum modifies the properties of Alzheimer's disease PHFτ proteins in vivo and in vitro. *Journal of Neuroscience*, 14, 7221–33

Shoji, M., Matsubara, E., Kanai, M., *et al.* (1998). Combination assay of CSF tau, Aβ1–40 and Aβ1–42(43). as a biochemical marker of Alzheimer's disease. *Journal of the Neurological Sciences*, 158, 134–40

Sima, A. A. F., Defendini, R., Keohane, C., *et al.* (1996). The neuropathology of chromosome 17-linked dementia. *Annals of Neurology*, 39, 734–43

Sims, T. J., Bailey, A., J., Harrington, C. R., and Wischik, C. M. (1996). Glycation-induced cross-linking of amyloid β protein and τ-protein: relevance to Alzheimer's disease. *International Journal of Experimental Pathology*, 77, A21

Skoog, I., Vanmechelen, E., Andreasen, L. A., *et al.* (1995). A population-based study of tau protein and ubiquitin in cerebrospinal fluid in 85-year-olds: relation to severity of dementia and cerebral atrophy, but not to the apolipoprotein E4 allele. *Neurodegeneration*, 4, 433–42

Smith, M. A., Kutty, R. K., Richey, P. L., *et al.* (1994*a*). Heme oxygenase-1 is associated with the neurofibrillary pathology of Alzheimer's disease. *American Journal of Pathology*, 145, 42–47

Smith, M. A., Taneda, S., Richey, P. L., *et al.* (1994*b*). Advanced Maillard reaction end products are associated with Alzheimer disease pathology. *Proceedings of the National Academy of Science (USA)*, 91, 5710–14

Smith, M. A., Sayre, L. M., Monnier, V. M., and Perry, G. (1995). Radical AGEing in Alzheimer's disease. *Trends in Neuroscience*, 18, 172–6

Spillantini, M. G., Schmidt, M. L., Lee, V. M-Y., *et al.* (1997). a-Synuclein in Lewy bodies. *Nature*, 388, 839–40

Spillantini, M. G., Crowther, R. A., Kamphorst, W., *et al.* (1998*a*). Tau pathology in two Dutch families with mutations in the microtubule-binding region of tau. *American Journal of Pathology*, 153, 1359–63

Spillantini, M. G., Murrell, J. L., Goedert, M., *et al.* (1998*b*). Mutation in the tau gene in familial multiple system tauopathy with presenile dementia. *Proceedings of the National Academy of Science (USA)*, 95, 7737–41

Spittaels, K., Van den Haute, C., Van Dorpe, J., *et al.* (1999). Animal model prominent axonopathy in the brain and spinal cord of transgenic mice overexpressing four-repeat human tau protein. *American Journal of Pathology*, 155, 2153–65

Stahl, N., Baldwin, M. A., Burlingame, A. L., and Prusiner, S. B. (1990). Identification of glycoinositol phospholipid linked and truncated forms of the scrapie prion protein. *Biochemistry*, 29, 8879–84

Sternberger, L. A., and Sternberger, N. H. (1983). Monoclonal antibodies distinguish phosphorylated and nonphosphorylated forms of neurofilaments in situ. *Proceedings of the National Academy of Science (USA)*, 80, 6126–30

Sternberger, N. H., Sternberger, L. A., and Ulrich, J. (1985). Aberrant neurofilament phosphorylation in Alzheimer's disease. *Proceedings of the National Academy of Science (USA)*, 82, 4274–6

Stevens, M., van Duijn, C. M,. Kamphorst, W., *et al.* (1998). Familial aggregation in frontotemporal dementia. *Neurology*, 50, 1541–5

Stewart, R. and Lioklitsa, D. (1999). Type 2 diabetes mellitus, cognitive impairment and dementia. *Diabetes Medicine*, 16, 93–112

Strittmatter, W. J., Saunders, A. M., Schmechel, D., *et al.* (1993). Apolipoprotein E: high avidity binding to β-amyloid and increased frequency of type 4 allele in late-onset familial Alzheimer disease. *Proceedings of the National Academy of Science (USA)*, 90, 1977–81

Strittmatter, W. J., Weisgraber, K. H., Goedert, M., *et al.* (1994). Hypothesis: microtubule instability and paired helical filament formation in the Alzheimer disease brain are related to apolipoprotein E genotype. *Experimental Neurology*, 125, 163–71

Sturchler-Pierrat, C., Abramowski, D., Duke, M., *et al.* (1997). Two amyloid precursor protein transgenic models with Alzheimer disease-like pathology. *Proceedings of the National Academy of Science (USA)*, **93**, 13287–92

Sumi, S. M., Bird, T. D., Nochlin, D., and Raskind, M. A. (1992). Familial presenile dementia with psychosis associated with cortical neurofibrillary tangles and degeneration of the amygdala. *Neurology*, **42**, 120–7

Sunderland, T., Wolozin, B., Galasko, D., *et al.* (1999). Longitudinal stability of CSF tau levels in Alzheimer patients. *Biological Psychiatry*, **46**, 750–5

Suzuki, N., Iwatsubo, T., Odaka, A., *et al.* (1994). High tissue content of soluble β1–40 is linked to cerebral amyloid angiopathy. *American Journal of Pathology*, **145**, 452–60

Suzuki, K., Parker, C. C., Pentchev, P. G., *et al.* (1995). Neurofibrillary tangles in Niemann-Pick disease type C. *Acta Neuropathologica*, **89**, 227–38

Tabaton, M., Perry, G., Smith, M., *et al.* (1997). Is amyloid β-protein glycated in Alzheimer's disease? *NeuroReport*, **8**, 907–9

Takahashi, M., Tsujioka, Y., Yamada, T., *et al.* (1999a). Glycosylation of microtubule-associated protein tau in Alzheimer's disease brain. *Acta Neuropathologica*, **97**, 635–41

Takahashi, Y., Ueno, A., and Mihara, H. (1999b). Optimization of hydrophobic domains in peptides that undergo transformation from α-helix to β-fibril. *Bioorganic and Medicinal Chemistry*, **7**, 177–85

Takashima, A., Noguchi, K., Sato, K., *et al.* (1993). Tau protein kinase I is essential for amyloid b-protein induced neurotoxicity. *Proceedings of the National Academy of Science (USA)*, **90**, 7789–93

Takashima, A., Murayama, M., Murayama, O., *et al.* (1998). Presenilin 1 associates with glycogen synthase kinase-3β and its substrate tau. *Proceedings of the National Academy of Science (USA)*, **95**, 9637–41

Takeda, A., Yasuda, T., Miyata, T., *et al.* (1998). Advanced glycation end products co-localized with astrocytes and microglial cells in Alzheimer's disease brain. *Acta Neuropathologica*, **95**, 555–8

Tamaoka, A., Fraser, P. E., Ishii, K., *et al.* (1998). Amyloid-β-protein isoforms in brain of subjects with PS1-linked, βAPP-linked and sporadic Alzheimer disease. *Molecular Brain Research*, **56**, 178–85

Tamaoka, A., Sekijima, Y., Matsuno, S., *et al.* (1999). Amyloid β protein species in cerebrospinal fluid and in brain from patients with Down syndrome. *Annals of Neurology*, **46**, 933

Tanzi, R. E., Kovacs, D. M., Kim, T-W., *et al.* (1996). The gene defects responsible for familial Alzheimer's disease. *Neurobiology of Disease*, **3**, 159–68

Tato, R. E., Frank, A., and Hernanz, A. (1995). Tau protein concentrations in cerebrospinal fluid of patients with dementia of the Alzheimer type. *Journal of Neurology, Neurosurgery and Psychiatry*, **59**, 280–3

Terry, R. D. and Peña, C. (1965). Experimental production of neurofibrillary degeneration. 2. Electron microscopy, phosphatase histochemistry and electron probe analysis. *Journal of Neuropathology and Experimental Neurology*, **24**, 200–10

Terry, R. D., Masliah, E., Salmon, D. P., *et al.* (1991). Physical basis of cognitive alterations in Alzheimer's disease: synapse loss is the major correlate of cognitive impairment. *Annals of Neurology*, **30**, 572–80

The Lund and Manchester Groups (1994). Clinical and neuropathological criteria for frontotemporal dementia. *Journal of Neurology, Neurosurgery and Psychiatry*, **57**, 416–18

The Ronald and Nancy Reagen Research Institute of The Alzheimer's Association and The National Institute on Ageing Working Group (1998). Concensus report of the Working Group on: 'Molecular and Biochemical Markers of Alzheimer's Disease'. *Neurobiology of Aging*, **19**, 109–16

Theuring, F., Thunecke, M., Kosciessa, U., and Turner, J. (1997). Transgenic animals as models for neurodegenerative diseases in humans. *Trends in Biotechnology*, **15**, 320–5

Thunecke, M., Bodewitz, G., Kosciessa, U., *et al.* (2000). Motor deficits in transgenic mice expressing human tau cDNA constructs., unpublished.

Tint, I., Slaughter, T., Fischer, I., and Black, M. M. (1998). Acute inactivation of tau has no effect on dynamics of microtubules in growing axons of cultured sympathetic neurons. *Journal of Neuroscience*, 18, 8660–73

Tohgi, H., Utsugisawa, K., Nagane, Y., *et al.* (1999). The methylation status of cytosines in a τ gene promoter region alters with age to downregulate transcriptional activity in human cerebral cortex. *Neuroscience Letters*, 275, 89–92

Tomidokoro, Y., Ishiguro, K., Igeta, Y., *et al.* (1999). Carboxyl-terminal fragments of presenilin-1 are closely related to cytoskeletal abnormalities in Alzheimer's brains. *Biochemical and Biophysical Research Communications*, 256, 512–18

Tortorella, M. D., Burn, T. C., Pratta, M. A., *et al.* (2000). Purification and cloning of aggrecanase-1: a member of the ADAMTS family of proteins. *Science*, 284, 1664–6

Tran, P. B. and Miller, R. J. (1999). Aggregates in neurodegenerative disease: crowds and power? *Trends in Neuroscience*, 22, 194–7

Trinczek, B., Biernat, J., Baumann, K., *et al.* (1995). Domains of tau protein, differential phosphorylation, and dynamic instability of microtubules. *Molecular Biology of the Cell*, 6, 1887–902

Trinczek, B., Ebneth, A., and Mandelkow, E. (1999). Tau regulates the attachment/detachment but not the speed of motors in microtubule-dependent transport of single vesicles and organelles. *Journal of Cell Science*, 112, 2355–67

Troncoso, J. C., Costello, A., Watson, A. L., Jr., and Johnson, G. V. W. (1993). In vitro polymerization of oxidized tau into filaments. *Brain Research*, 613, 313–16

Tumani, H., Shen, G. Q., Peter, J. B., and Bruck, W. (1999). Glutamine synthetase in cerebrospinal fluid, serum, and brain — A diagnostic marker for Alzheimer disease? *Archives of Neurology*, 56, 1241–6

Urakami, K., Mori, M., Wada, K., *et al.* (1999). A comparison of tau protein in cerebrospinal fluid between corticobasal degeneration and progressive supranuclear palsy. *Neuroscience Letters*, 259, 127–9

Uterman, G. (1994). The apolipoprotein E connection. *Current Biology*, 4, 362–5

van Duinen, S. G., Lammers, G-J., Maat-Schieman, M. L. C., and Roos, R. A. C. (1999). Numerous and widespread α-synuclein-negative Lewy bodies in an asymptomatic patient. *Acta Neuropathologica*, 97, 533–9

Van Hoesen, G. W., and Damasio, A. R. (1990). Neural correlates of cognitive impairment in Alzheimer's disease. In *Handbook of Physiology. The Nervous System.* pp. 871–98. Vol. V, Waverly Press, Baltimore

van Leeuwen, F. W., Burbach, J. P. H., and Hol, E. M. (1998a). Mutation in RNA: a first example of misreading in Alzheimer's disease. *Trends in Neuroscience*, 21, 331–5

van Leeuwen, F. W., de Kleijn, D. P. V., van den Hurk, H. H., *et al.* (1998b). Frameshift mutants of β amyloid precursor protein and ubiquitin-B in Alzheimer's and Down patients. *Science*, 279, 242–7

van Rossum, D. and Hanisch, U. K. (1999). Cytoskeletal dynamics in dendritic spines: direct modulation by glutamate receptors? *Trends in Neuroscience*, 22, 290–5

Vandermeeren, M., Mercken, M., Vanmechelen, E., *et al.* (1993). Detection of τ proteins in normal and Alzheimer's disease cerebrospinal fluid with a sensitive sandwich enzyme-linked immunosorbent assay. *Journal of Neurochemistry*, 61, 1828–34

Vanmechelen, E. (1998). Tau protein in the diagnosis of old-age dementia. *Archives of Gerontology and Geriatrics*, 27, 519–24

Varani, L., Hasegawa, M., Spillantini, M. G., *et al.* (1999). Structure of tau exon 10 splicing regulatory element RNA and destabilization by mutations of frontotemporal dementia and parkinsonism linked to chromosome 17. *Proceedings of the National Academy of Science (USA)*, 96, 8229–34

Vassar, R., Bennett, B. D., Babu-Khan, S., *et al.* (1999). β-Secretase cleavage of Alzheimer's amyloid precursor protein by the transmembrane aspartic protease BACE. *Science*, **286**, 735–41

Vidal, R., Frangione, B., Rostagno, A., *et al.* (1999). A stop-codon mutation in the *BRI* gene associated with familial British dementia. *Nature*, **399**, 776–81

Vigo-Pelfrey, C., Seubert, C., Barbour, R., *et al.* (1995). Elevation of microtubule-associated protein tau in the cerebrospinal fluid of patients with Alzheimer's disease. *Neurology*, **45**, 788–93

Vincent, I., Rosado, M., Kim, E., and Davies, P. (1994). Increased production of paired helical filament epitopes in cell culture system reduces the turnover of τ. *Journal of Neurochemistry*, **62**, 715–23

Vincent, I., Jicha, G., Rosado, M., and Dickson, D. W. (1997). Aberrant expression of mitotic cdc2/cyclin B1 kinase in degenerating neurons of Alzheimer's disease brain. *Journal of Neuroscience*, **17**, 3588–98

Vincent, I., Zheng, J. H., Dickson, D. W., *et al.* (1998). Mitotic phosphoepitopes precede paired helical filaments in Alzheimer's disease. *Neurobiology of Aging*, **19**, 287–96

Vitek, M. P., Bhattacharya, K., Glendenning, J. M., *et al.* (1994). Advanced glycation end products contribute to amyloidosis in Alzheimer's disease. *Proceedings of the National Academy of Science (USA)*, **91**, 4766–70

Vito, P., Lacaná, E., and D'Adamio, L. (1996). Interfering with apoptosis: Ca^{2+}-binding protein ALG-2 and Alzheimer's disease gene *ALG-3*. *Science*, **271**, 521–5

Vulliet, R., Halloran, S. M., Braun, R. K., *et al.* (1992). Proline-directed phosphorylation of human tau protein. *Journal of Biological Chemistry*, **267**, 22570–4

Wagner, U., Utton, M., Gallo, J-M., and Miller, C. C. J. (1996). Cellular phosphorylation of tau by GSK-3β influences tau binding to microtubules and microtubule organisation. *Journal of Cell Science*, **109**, 1537–43.

Walker, L. C. (1997). Animal models of cerebral β-amyloid angiopathy. *Brain Research Reviews*, **25**, 70–84

Wallace, D. C. (1994). Mitochondrial DNA sequence variation in human evolution and disease. *Proceedings of the National Academy of Science (USA)*, **91**, 8739–46

Wang, J.-Z., Gong, C.-X., Zaidi, T., Grundke-Iqbal, I., and Iqbal, K. (1995). Dephosphorylation of Alzheimer paired helical filaments by protein phosphatase-2A and -2B. *Journal of Biological Chemistry*, **270**, 4854–60

Wang, J-Z., Grundke-Iqbal, I., and Iqbal, K. (1996). Glycosylation of microtubule-associated protein tau: an abnormal posttranslational modification in Alzheimer's disease. *Nature Medicine*, **2**, 871–5

Weber, K, Schmahl, W, and Münch, G (1998). Distribution of advanced glycation end products in the cerebellar neurons of dogs. *Brain Research*, **791**, 11–17

White, III. C. L., Tripp, P., Eagen, K. P., *et al.* (1995). Quantification of synapse density in Alzheimer disease neocortex using a two-site enzyme-linked immunosorbent assay (ELISA) and antibodies to synaptophysin. *Journal of Neuropathology and Experimental Neurology*, **54**, 430-[Abstract]

Wijker, M., Wszolek, Z. K., Wolters, E. C. H., *et al.* (1996). Localization of the gene for rapidly progressive autosomal dominant parkinsonism and dementia with pallido-ponto-nigral degeneration to chromosome 17q21. *Human Molecular Genetics*, **5**, 151–4

Wilcock, G. K. and Esiri, M. M. (1982). Plaques, tangles and dementia, a quantitative study. *Journal of the Neurological Sciences*, **56**, 407–17

Wilcock, G. K., Esiri, M. M., Bowen, D. M., and Smith, C. C. T. (1982). Alzheimer's disease. Correlation of cortical choline acetyltransferase activity with the severity of dementia and histological abnormalities. *Journal of the Neurological Sciences*, **57**, 407–17

Wilhelmsen, K. C. (1997). Frontotemporal dementia is on the MAPτ. *Annals of Neurology*, **41**, 139–40

Wilhelmsen, K. C., Lynch, T., Pavlou, E., *et al.* (1994). Localization of disinhibition-dementia-parkinsonism-amyotrophy complex to 17q21–22. *American Journal of Humuman Genetics*, 55, 1159–65

Wille, H., Drewes, G., Biernat, J., *et al.* (1992). Alzheimer-like paired helical filaments and antiparallel dimers formed from microtubule-associated protein tau *in vitro*. *Journal of Cell Biology*, 118, 573–84

Wilson, D. M., and Binder, L. I. (1995). Polymerization of microtubule-associated protein tau under near-physiological conditions. *Journal of Biological Chemistry*, 270, 24306–14

Wischik, C. M. (1989). Cell biology of the Alzheimer tangle. *Current Opinion in Cell Biology*, 1, 115–22

Wischik, C. M., Crowther, R. A., Stewart, M., and Roth, M. (1985). Subunit structure of paired helical filaments in Alzheimer's disease. *Journal of Cell Biology*, 100, 1905–12

Wischik, C. M., Novak, M., Edwards, P. C., *et al.* (1988*a*). Structural characterization of the core of the paired helical filament of Alzheimer disease. *Proceedings of the National Academy of Science (USA)*, 85, 4884–8

Wischik, C. M., Novak, M., Thøgersen, H. C., *et al.* (1988*b*). Isolation of a fragment of tau derived from the core of the paired helical filament of Alzheimer's disease. *Proceedings of the National Academy of Science (USA)*, 85, 4506–10

Wischik, C. M., Edwards, P. C., Lai, R. Y. K., *et al.* (1995*a*). Quantitative analysis of tau protein in paired helical filament preparations: implications for the role of tau protein phosphorylation in PHF assembly in Alzheimer's disease. *Neurobiology of Aging*, 16, 409–31

Wischik, C. M., Harrington, C. R., and Mena, R (1995*b*). Molecular determinants of paired helical filament assembly and its therapeutic implications in Alzheimer's disease. *International Review of Psychiatry*, 7, 299–338

Wischik, C. M., Lai, R., Harrington C. R., *et al.* (1995c). Structure, biochemistry and molecular pathogenesis of paired helical filaments in Alzheimer's disease. In *Pathobiology of Alzheimer's disease* (ed. A. Goate and F. Ashall) pp. 9–39. Academic Press, London.

Wischik, C. M., Edwards, P. C., Lai, R. Y. K. *et al.* (1996). Selective inhibition of Alzheimer disease-like tau aggregation by phenothiazines. *Proceedings of the National Academy of Science (USA)*, 93, 11213–18

Wischik, C. M., Lai, R. Y. K., and Harrington, C. R. (1997). Modelling prion-like processing of tau protein in Alzheimer's disease for pharmaceutical development. In *Microtubule-Associated Proteins: Modifications in Disease* (ed. J. Avila, R. Brandt, and K. S. Kosik). pp. 185–241. Harwood Academic Publishers, Amsterdam.

Wisniewski, H. M., Maslinska, D., Kitaguchi, T., *et al.* (1990). Topographic heterogeneity of amyloid β-protein epitopes with various forms of ceroid lipofuscinoses, suggesting defective processing of amyloid precursor protein. *Acta Neuropathologica*, 80, 26–34

Wisniewski, T., Aucuouturier, P., Soto, C., and Frangione, B. (1998). The prionoses and other conformational disorders. *Amyloid: International Journal of Experimental Clinical Investigation*, 5, 212–24

Wolfe, M. S., De Los Angeles, J., Miller, D. D., *et al.* (1999*a*). Are presenilins intramembrane-cleaving proteases? Implications for the molecular mechanism of Alzheimer's disease. *Biochemistry*, 38, 11223–30

Wolfe, M. S., Xia, W., Ostaszewski, B. L., *et al.* (1999*b*). Two transmembrane aspartates in presenilin-1 required for presenilin endoproteolysis and γ-secretase activity. *Nature*, 398, 513–17

Wolozin, B. L., Pruchnicki, A., Dickson, D. W., and Davies, P. (1986). A neuronal antigen in the brains of Alzheimer patients. *Science*, 232, 648–50

Xia, Y., De Silva, H. A. R., Rosi, B. L., *et al.* (1996). Genetic studies in Alzheimer's disease with an NACP/α-synuclein polymorphism. *Annals of Neurology*, 40, 207–15

Xu, W., Liu,. L, Emson, P., *et al.* (2000). The CCTTT polymorphism in the *NOS2A* gene is associated with dementia with Lewy bodies. *NeuroReport,* 11, 297–9

Yamamoto, H., Saitoh, Y., Yasugawa, S., and Miyamoto, E. (1990). Dephosphorylation of τ factor by protein phosphatase 2A in synaptosomal cytosol fractions, and inhibition by aluminium. *Journal of Neurochemistry,* 55, 683–90

Yamamoto, H., Hasegawa, M., Ono, T., *et al.* (1995). Dephosphorylation of fetal-tau and paired helical filaments-tau by protein phosphatases 1 and 2A and calcineurin. *Journal of Biochemistry,* 118, 1224–31

Yamaoka, L. H., Welsh-Bohmer, K. A., Hulette, C. M., *et al.* (1996). Linkage of frontotemporal dementia to chromosome 17: clinical and neuropathological characterization of phenotype. *American Journal of Human Genetics,* 59, 1306–12

Yan, S-D., Chen, X., Schmidt, A-M., *et al.* (1994). Glycated tau protein in Alzheimer disease: a mechanism for induction of oxidant stress. *Proceedings of the National Academy of Science (USA),* 91, 7787–91

Yan, S. D., Yan, S. F., Chen, X., *et al.* (1995). Non-enzymatically glycated tau in Alzheimer's disease induces neuronal oxidant stress resulting in cytokine gene expression and release of amyloid β-peptide. *Nature Medicine,* 1, 693–699

Yanagawa, H., Chung, S-H., Ogawa, Y., *et al.* (1998). Protein anatomy: C-tail region of human tau protein as a crucial element in Alzheimer's paired helical filament formation *in vitro. Biochemistry* 37, 1979–88

Yang, L. S. and Ksiezak-Reding, H. (1998). Ubiquitin immunoreactivity of paired helical filaments differs in Alzheimer's disease and corticobasal degeneration. *Acta Neuropathologica,* 96, 520–6

Yang, L.-S. and Ksiezak-Reding, H. (1999). Ca^{2+} and Mg^{2+} selectively induces aggregates of PHF-tau but not normal human tau. *Journal of Neuroscience Research,* 55, 36–43

Yang, S.-D., Yu, J.-S., Shia, S.-G., and Huang, J.-J. (1994). Protein kinase F_A/glycogen synthase kinase-3a after heparin potentiation phosphorylates τ on sites abnormally phosphorylated in Alzheimer's disease brain. *Journal of Neurochemistry,* 63, 1416–25

Yasuda, M., Kawamata, T., Komure, O., *et al.* (1999). A mutation in the microtubule-associated protein tau in pallido-nigro-luysian degeneration. *Neurology,* 53, 864–8

Zemlan, F. P., Rosenberg, W. S., Luebbe, P. A., *et al.* (1999). Quantification of axonal damage in traumatic brain injury: affinity purification and characterization of cerebrospinal fluid tau proteins. *Journal of Neurochemistry,* 72, 741–50

Zheng, C. F. and Guan, K. L. (1993). Properies of MEKS, the kinases that phosphorylate and activate the extracellular signal-regulated kinases. *Journal of Biological Chemistry,* 268, 23933–9

Zheng-Fischhöfer, Q., Biernat, J., Mandelkow, E-M., *et al.* (1998). Sequential phosphorylation of tau by glycogen synthase kinase-3β and protein kinase A at Thr212 and Ser214 generates the Alzheimer-specific epitope of antibody AT100 and requires a paired-helical-filament-like conformation. *European Journal of Biochemistry,* 252, 542–52

Zubenko, G. S., Moossy, J., Martinez, A. J., *et al.* (1989). A brain regional analysis of morphologic and cholinergic abnormalities in Alzheimer's disease. *Archives of Neurology,* 46, 634–8

Chapter 6

Apolipoprotein E as a risk factor for Alzheimer's disease

Ann M. Saunders

6.1 Introduction

Molecular and epidemiological studies suggest that Alzheimer's disease (AD) has multiple aetiologies. Mutations in three known genes, the amyloid precursor protein (*APP*) and pre-senilin 1 (*PS1*) and *PS2* genes, nearly always cause the disease (Goate *et al.* 1991; Levy-Lahad *et al.* 1995; Sherrington *et al.* 1995). These genetic defects are very rare, occurring in fewer than 2% of all cases (Farrer *et al.* 1997). Apolipoprotein E (*APOE*: gene; apoE:protein) is a fourth genetic factor involved in the development of AD. Unlike the three causative genes, *APOE* is a susceptibility locus that accounts for approximately half of late-onset AD (Roses *et al.* 1995). The remarkable progress during the past six years in understanding the suscep-tibility genetics of *APOE* and AD and the influence of a common polymorphism of the gene on recovery from acute brain stress is documented in this chapter. While the role of apoE as a plasma lipid-transport molecule has been well studied over the past two decades, the normal functions of apoE in the central nervous system and its role in the aetiology of AD have not been identified. Hypotheses and supporting data on the role of apoE in AD will be discussed. (Sequence information for apoE is available in Appendix 4).

6.2 Background of Apolipoprotein E

ApoE is a lipid transport molecule that is a constituent of liver-synthesized very low density lipoproteins (VLDL) and a subclass of high density lipoproteins (HDL) (Weisgraber 1994). VLDL transports triglycerides from the liver to all tissues except brain, and HDL redistrib-utes cholesterol among cells. The protein is also a major constituent of chylomicrons, which are synthesized in the intestine and transport dietary cholesterol and triglycerides. ApoE mediates the cellular uptake of lipid complexes through the low density lipoprotein (LDL)-receptor and other related receptors (Krieger and Herz 1994). Located on the long arm of human chromosome 19, *APOE* is within an apolipoprotein gene family and has three common alleles, designated ε2, ε 3 and ε 4. These genetic variations result in amino acid substitutions (arginine or cysteine) at positions 112 and 158 of the protein (Zannis *et al.* 1993). In most Caucasian populations, *APOE* ε 3/3 is the most common genotype and ε 3 is the most common allele; ε 4 and ε 2 are considered variants. *APOE*ε 2/2 is the most common genotype associated with type III hyperlipoproteinemia, and the apoE2 protein is defective in LDL-receptor binding. ApoE4 has normal LDL-receptor binding, but is associated with elevated plasma cholesterol and LDL levels (Weisgraber 1994).

The largest amount of *APOE* mRNA is found in the liver. The second largest concentration, approximately one-third the level seen in liver, is in the brain. Other sites of production include spleen, lung, adrenal, ovary, kidney, and muscle (Blue *et al.* 1983; Driscoll and Getz 1984; Elshourbagy *et al.* 1985; Lin *et al.* 1986). Brain apoE is synthesized locally, not by the liver, as shown in liver transplant patients (Linton *et al.* 1991) and is the main apolipoprotein in cerebrospinal fluid (CSF). Interesting models involving the storage and redistribution of cholesterol following peripheral (Ignatius *et al.* 1986, 1987; Boyles *et al.* 1989) and central nervous system (CNS) (Poirier *et al.* 1991, 1993*a*) injury were proposed about a decade ago. Other functions of apoE in the nervous system, unrelated to lipid transport, have also been proposed. These include the possibility of it acting as a neurotrophic factor or modulator of neurotrophin activity (Nathan *et al.* 1995; Gutman *et al.* 1997; Puttfarcken *et al.* 1997), an antioxidant (Miyata and Smith 1996), and a mediator of immune responses (Macy *et al.* 1983; Mistry *et al.* 1995; Mazzone, 1996). The most popular hypotheses concern amyloid plaques and neurofibrillary tangles (NFT), the two pathological hallmarks of AD. In these hypotheses, apoE is thought to have an effect on amyloid deposition (Schmechel *et al.* 1993; Strittmatter *et al.* 1993*b,c*; Wisniewski and Frangione 1992) or in the stabilization of microtubules (Roses 1994; Strittmatter *et al.* 1994*b*).

6.3 Apolipoprotein E as a susceptibility gene for Alzheimer's disease

6.3.1 Identification of apolipoprotein E as a candidate gene

Pericak-Vance and colleagues (1991) were the first to apply the Affected Pedigree Member (APM) analysis to late-onset AD (Weeks and Lange 1988). This method has the advantage of including family members other than affected siblings, such as cousins and aunts. APM analysis rapidly screens for statistically significant variations of polymorphic alleles in the general population, and allows for the identification of a relatively large physical region of linkage without clear outer boundaries. With the APM analysis, Duke Univeristy Medical Center linked late-onset, familial AD (FAD) to a region consisting approximately 0.2% of the genome on chromosome 19 (Pericak-Vance *et al.* 1991). At that time, we initiated a large effort in cloning, mapping, and testing a variety of candidates including two nerve growth factor subunits, a family of serine proteases and DNA repair enzymes. *APOE* ranked very low on our list of candidate genes on chromosome 19 to test since far more alluring aetiologic scenarios could be generated for nearly every other nearby gene.

In an independent series of biochemical experiments, we identified a CSF protein, apoE, that bound to immobilized amyloid beta-peptide (Aβ), a fragment of the *APP* gene and one of the peptides found in AD senile plaques (Strittmatter *et al.* 1993*a*). It was difficult to imagine a role for a serum cholesterol-transport protein in the aetiology of AD, but we knew that *APOE* was in the middle of the chromosome 19-linkage region. Our next step was to look for an association between familial, late-onset AD and any of the commonly expressed alleles. Soon after we initiated the analyses, two timely reports on the detection of apoE in each of the specific amyloids formed by distinct proteins in several diseases were published (Namba *et al.* 1991; Wisniewski and Frangione 1992).

Table 6.1 Apolipoprotein E genotype and allele distributions of 83 affected family members in 30 Duke AD pedigrees (FAD) and 91 unrelated grandparents from the Center d'Etude Polymorphism (CEPH). The ε 4 allele frequencies on this patient and control series were originally reported by Strittmatter et al. (1993a).

	FAD	CEPH
	%	%
APOE **genotype**		
[ε] **2/2**	0	1
[ε] **2/3**	0	11
[ε] **2/4**	3	8
[ε] **3/3**	20	57
[ε] **3/4**	57	21
[ε] **4/4**	20	2
APOE **allele**		
[ε] **2**	0.04	0.10
[ε] **3**	0.44	0.73
[ε] **4**	0.52	0.16

When association of the three common *APOE* alleles with AD was examined in late-onset AD pedigrees, we found that the *APOE* ε 4 allele frequency was 52%, compared to 16% for age-matched controls (Strittmatter *et al.* 1993*c*). Table 6.1 shows the distribution of the *APOE* alleles and genotypes in our first analysis of 1 affected member from each of 30 AD pedigrees. We then looked at a series of sporadic 176 AD cases that had both clinical diagnoses and pathological confirmation (Saunders *et al.* 1993*b*). The ε 4 allele frequency in this sporadic series of autopsy cases was 40%, a finding that was significantly different from controls. Several other patient series were quickly examined, including the first affected twin in a collaborative study, a prospectively ascertained clinical series of 80 consecutive patients with possible/probable AD attending the Bryan Memory Disorders Clinic with control spouses, and a series of patients randomly selected from early-onset pedigrees (Saunders *et al.* 1993*a*). In both of the late-onset AD groups, the ε 4 allele frequency was elevated to 40% and 41% respectively. The early-onset families, however, did not show an ε 4 association.

The *APOE4* association with AD was rapidly and widely confirmed throughout the world in patients with familial and sporadic late-onset AD (Anwar *et al.* 1993; Borgaonkar *et al.* 1993; Houlden *et al.* 1993; Noguchi *et al.* 1993; Poirier *et al.* 1993*b*; Rebeck *et al.* 1993; Ueki *et al.* 1993). The ε 4 allele is also associated with sporadic early-onset AD (Chartier-Harlin *et al.* 1994; Nalbantoglu *et al.* 1994; Okuizumi *et al.* 1994; van Duijn *et al.* 1994) and with early-onset AD families without presenilin or APP mutations (Houlden *et al.* 1998). These multiple confirmations established the ε 4 allele as the most important genetic marker for risk for disease identified so far, accounting for approximately 50% of the genetic component of AD (Roses *et al.* 1995). The variability of the world-wide data depends on the control ε 4 allele frequency in each population and the ascertainment biases for collecting AD and control cases; however, the associations with AD are consistent. For example, the control ε *4* allele frequency in Japan is less than 9% in several series, but the AD ε *4* allele frequency is greater than 24% (Noguchi *et al.* 1993; Ueki *et al.* 1993; Dai *et al.* 1994; Kawamata *et al.* 1994). One of the first epidemiological studies on *APOE* and AD published involved a population in Finland where the *APOE* ε *4* allele frequency in the general population is quite high at 22% (Kuusisto *et al.* 1994). However, age-matched controls for the AD cases in the population had an allele frequency of only 16.5%. It was thought that the high incidence of fatal myocardial infarction, which the ε *4* allele also serves as a risk factor, contributed to the attrition of many ε *4* bearers before the age of risk for AD. The association of *APOE* ε *4* and AD in African-Americans (Hendrie *et al.* 1995; Maestre *et al.* 1995; Tang *et al.* 1998) and Hispanics (Tang *et al.* 1998) remains controversial and may be absent in a sample of Nigerian AD cases and controls (Osuntokun *et al.* 1995).

6.3.2 Genetics of apolipoprotein E in Alzheimer's disease

In 1993, we reported that individuals inheriting two copies of the ε *4* allele have an increased risk and earlier age of onset than individuals with one ε *4* allele. Likewise, individuals with one ε *4* allele have a greater risk and earlier onset of disease than those with no ε *4* alleles (Corder *et al.* 1993). These data demonstrated that the effect of *APOE* ε *4* on risk and age of onset is dose-related and not as an autosomal dominant trait. This finding has been confirmed in numerous studies in the past six years (Anwar *et al.* 1993; Brousseau *et al.* 1994; Kuusisto *et al.* 1994; Mahieux *et al.* 1994; Tsai *et al.* 1994; Maestre *et al.* 1995; Kukull *et al.* 1996; Myers *et al.* 1996; Bickeboller *et al.* 1997). The rarer *APOE* ε *2* allele is under-represented in AD, and it appears to reduce the risk and delay the onset of disease. First shown in a series containing more than 700 familial and sporadic AD patients (Corder *et al.* 1994), the finding was observed in several other studies (Benjamin *et al.* 1994; Smith *et al.* 1994; Sorbi *et al.* 1994; Talbot *et al.* 1994; West *et al.* 1994; Kukull *et al.* 1996; Bickeboller *et al.* 1997; Farrer *et al.* 1997). This effect is strongest with the ε *2/3* genotype; the influence of the very rare ε *2/2* genotype on AD risk could not be discerned even in a very large meta-analysis (Farrer *et al.* 1997). The effect of the most commonly inherited allele, ε *3*, on risk and age of onset falls between ε *4* and ε *2*.

On the basis of *APOE* genotype alone, there is more than a two-decade difference in the age of onset (Corder *et al.* 1993). The mean age of onset of individuals with a ε *4/4* genotype is younger than 70 years while the mean age of onset for the *APOE* ε *2/3* genotype is older than 90 years. The *APOE* ε *3/4* genotype represents approximately 21% of the population and has a distribution of age of onset between *APOE* ε *4/4* and *APOE3/3*, with a mean age of onset in the early to mid-70s. There also appears to be an interaction of *APOE* genotypes with the age of onset in families with early-onset AD due to mutations in *APP*. Patients with an *APP* mutation and an *APOE* ε *4* allele have earlier ages of onset. In contrast, there are asymptomatic individuals with an *APP* mutation and an *APOE* ε *2/3* genotype who are at least one standard deviation older than the mean age of onset in the pedigree *APP* (St George-Hyslop *et al.* 1994; Nacmias *et al.* 1995; Rogaev *et al.* 1995). A similar interaction may exist with the *PS2* gene (Nochlin *et al.* 1998). *APOE* genotypes do not influence the age of onset in early-onset families with mutations in the *PS1* gene (Brice *et al.* 1996; Fox *et al.* 1997; Lendon *et al.* 1997; Houlden *et al.* 1998).

6.3.3 Association of apolipoprotein E and dementia with Lewy bodies

Recent neuropathological studies estimate that 15–25% of elderly demented patients have Lewy bodies, a classic pathological hallmark of Parkinson's disease, in their brain stem and cortex. These patients may represent the most common pathologic subgroup of pure AD (McKeith *et al.* 1996). Clinically, diagnosis of dementia with Lewy bodies (DLB) can be discriminated from AD and other dementias by fluctuation in cognitive function, persistent visual hallucinations and spontaneous motor features of parkinsonism (McKeith *et al.* 1996). At autopsy, AD pathology is frequently present, usually as diffuse or neuritic plaques, with NFT being much less common.

In a survey of reports on the association of *APOE ε 4* and DLB, the levels of association range from very high, paralleling the data with AD, to none. The basis of these discrepant data appears to be the criteria employed to create patient series. In multiple reports clearly stating that the study subjects have AD with concomitant Parkinson's disease pathology (Lewy bodies), there is a statistically significant association of the *APOE4* allele with the disease (Galasko *et al.* 1994; Gearing *et al.* 1995*a*; Kalaria and Premkumar 1995; Helisalmi *et al.* 1996; Kawanishi *et al.* 1996; Olichney *et al.* 1996). There has also been a reported effect of the ε 4 allele on age of onset in men (Gearing *et al.* 1995*a*). These data support the notion that DLB is a subclass of AD, not of Parkinson's disease, with perhaps a second genetic polymorphism influencing the appearance of the Lewy bodies. The association data become less clear when selection criteria are versions of 'Parkinson's disease with concomitant AD lesions', with no discrimination as to which patients have enough plaques to meet the pathological criteria for an AD diagnosis, or 'Lewy body disease'.

Despite the confusion in the Lewy body literature, studies have demonstrated that there is no association between *APOE ε 4* and risk for either pure Parkinson's disease or Parkinson's disease with dementia (not of the AD-type) (Harrington *et al.* 1994; Rubinsztein *et al.* 1994; Ibarreta *et al.* 1995; Koller *et al.* 1995; Martinoli *et al.* 1995; Morris *et al.* 1996; Whitehead *et al.* 1996; The French Parkinson's Disease Genetics Study Group 1997). One study reported a modest influence of *APOE4* on the age of onset in sporadic Parkinson's disease (Zareparsi *et al.* 1997).

6.3.4 **Apolipoprotein E4 and recovery from acute brain stresses**

In addition to the role of *APOE* as an important susceptibility gene for AD, additional data implicate *APOE* in recovery from several types of acute brain stress (Tardiff *et al.* 1994; Alberts *et al.* 1995; Mayeux *et al.* 1995; Newman *et al.* 1995; Nicoll *et al.* 1995; Roses and Saunders 1995; Sorbi *et al.* 1995; Jordan *et al.* 1997; McCarron *et al.* 1998). Whether the same mechanism that leads to an increased risk and an earlier onset of AD is involved in poorer recovery from acute brain stresses is a matter of lively debate. The first suggestion that *APOE ε 4* was involved in the recovery of brain injury was published in 1995 (Nicoll *et al.* 1995). In the report, Nicoll and colleagues studied head trauma patients who were comatose and died within a 30 day period after injury. They identified a much higher ε 4 allele frequency in patients who died with increased amyloid deposited in their brains than in patients who died without increased amyloid deposition. We examined their data and were surprised to note that the average age of the amyloid-bearing patients was over 50 years, more than two decades older than the non-amyloid bearing patients (Roses and Saunders 1995). We proposed an alternative hypothesis to their data that head trauma patients without an ε4 allele had more efficient recovery from their injury. The younger patient group may reflect the general population with more head injuries. Similar *APOE* allele-specific effects on recovery from post-traumatic coma have also been reported (Sorbi *et al.* 1995).

On the basis of our analysis of the head trauma data, we looked at other syndromes of severe brain stress. We ascertained a consecutive series of intracerebral haemorrhage patients entering Duke University Medical Center (Alberts *et al.* 1995). There was a statistically significant difference in mortality between the group of patients with an ε *4* allele and those with the ε *2/3* or ε *3/3* genotypes. Patients with an ε *4* allele had a much higher mortality (68% *vs.* 19%). If patients with an ε *4* allele survived through their initial haemorrhage, their functional recovery was generally poor compared to the ε *4*-negative patients who had an almost normal functional recovery. These observations on recovery after intracerebral haemorrhage were recently supported by an independent study in Glasgow (McCarron *et al.* 1998). There is also suggestive evidence that cognitive impairment in stroke patients is associated with the *APOE* ε *4* allele (Basun *et al.* 1996; Slooter *et al.* 1997). Mayeux and colleagues examined the association between *APOE* genotypes and head trauma (Mayeux *et al.* 1995), basing their study on an earlier suggestion that head injury was a risk factor for AD (Roberts *et al.* 1994). They reported a ten-fold increase in the risk of AD associated with the combination of an ε *4* allele and history of traumatic brain injury, compared to a two-fold increase in risk with *APOE4* alone. Head injury in the absence of an ε *4* allele did not increase risk for the disease. Their data imply a synergistic relationship between the ε *4* allele and head trauma that increases the risk of AD. A recent preliminary examination of *APOE* genotypes and dementia pugilistica suggests that the *APOE* ε *4* allele is associated with increased severity of neurological deficits in boxers with chronic traumatic brain injury as the result of their profession (Jordan *et al.* 1997).

There are also provocative data suggesting that ε *4*-bearing cardiopulmonary bypass patients do not recover some neuropsychological parameters as well as patients without an ε *4* allele (Tardiff *et al.* 1994; Newman *et al.* 1995). Patients coming to the Duke University Medical Center for elective cardiopulmonary bypass surgery were neuropsychologically tested both before and several times after surgery. Nearly all patients exhibited cognitive deficits immediately following surgery; however, recovery of normal cognition was still significantly impaired in ε *4*-bearing patients several months after the procedure.

These clinical observations are further substantiated by recent studies performed in our Center on an experimental mouse model of focal ischaemia and reperfusion (Laskowitz *et al.* 1997; Sheng *et al.* 1998). *APOE*-deficient mice were subjected to a 60- or 90-minute episode of middle cerebral artery filament occlusion and allowed to recover for 24 hours. With 60 minutes of ischaemia, the *APOE*-deficient mice had significantly larger cortical infarcts compared to wild-type mice and all mice survived. After 90 minutes of ischaemia, mortality in the *APOE*-deficient mice was 40% versus 0% in the wild-type mice. As an extension, we then examined transgenic mice constructed with the human *APOE* ε *3* and *APOE* ε *4* genes under the control of the natural human promoter and tissue expression elements (Sheng *et al.* 1998). Infarct volumes were smaller in the *APOE* ε *3* transgenic animals, similar to those seen earlier in wild-type mice, compared to the *APOE* ε *4* transgenic mice. Numerous studies have demonstrated an upregulation of apoE expression following ischaemic insult in mice and gerbils, suggesting that it is involved in the post-ischaemic response (Hall *et al.* 1995; Kida *et al.* 1995; Ali *et al.* 1996; Horsburgh and Nicoll 1996; Ishimaru *et al.* 1996; Oostveen *et al.* 1998).

6.4 Apolipoprotein E and aetiology of Alzheimer's disease

In the past six years, the genetics of *APOE* as a major susceptibility gene have been well documented. Elucidation of the protein's normal functions in the CNS and how the apoE4 protein influences metabolism to increase the risk of disease are now required. Before 1993, there were only a few studies of apoE metabolism in the adult CNS (Roses 1995). It was known that mRNA for *APOE* was expressed primarily in astrocytes and not observed in neurons (Diedrich *et al.* 1991) and that the expression of *APOE* mRNA was increased as a response to brain injury (Poirier *et al.* 1991) and also in AD and Creutzfeld-Jacob disease (Namba *et al.* 1991). ApoE was the primary apolipoprotein observed in the CNS (Elshourbagy *et al.* 1985), but there were no experimental data on the role of apoE in lipid transport or metabolism in the brain.

Since in 1993 the literature on apoE in the brain was sparse, we decided to conduct a general survey on the location of apoE in the brains of AD patients and controls. It was immediately noted that apoE immunoreactivity was present in amyloid plaques, blood vessels, NFT, and a subset of neurons that did not contain NFT (Namba *et al.* 1991; Schmechel *et al.* 1993). With the initial genetic and immunochemical data in hand, we began several lines of experimentation that included *in vitro* binding studies of apoE iso-forms to Aβ, APP, and tau, and immunocytochemical studies to determine if there were isoform-specific differences in the intensity, location, or size of plaques and tangles. A third line of inquiry concentrated on the more basic issue of apoE localization within neurons. According to the literature, it was not supposed to be there, but in our first publication on *APOE* and AD, we included a photomicrograph showing apoE immunoreactivity in tangle-free neurons (Strittmatter *et al.* 1993*b*).

Today, the neurobiology of apoE is a new and rapidly developing area, and the interaction of apoE with the major microscopic markers of AD, plaques, and tangles, has generated considerable experimental activity. Most extracellular models, for the apoE isoform-specific effects in AD, concern the role of apoE in Aβ deposition while intracellular models focus on the function of apoE in intraneuronal metabolism, with particular regard to modifying cytoskeletal stability (see Fig. 6.1). Although the extracellular role of apoE in amyloidgenesis is by far the most popular hypothesis, interest in the function of apoE in microtubular stability may increase with the recents reports of tau mutations in the chromosome 17 fron-totemporal dementias (Clark *et al.* 1998; Dumanchin *et al.* 1998; Poorkaj *et al.* 1998; Spillantini *et al.* 1998*a, b*). Brain apoE, synthesized by astrocytes and microglia, may enter neurons by binding to the LDL-receptor related protein (LRP) or other LDL- and related VLDL-receptor mechanisms (Rebeck *et al.* 1993; Krieger and Herz 1994; Weisgraber *et al.* 1994). Ultrastructural studies have clearly demonstrated human apoE immunoreactivity in the cytoplasm of neurons, frequently associated with the outer membranes of mitochondria and peroxisomes (Han *et al.* 1994*a*). An intraneuronal source of apoE was recently demon-strated using *in situ* hybridization (Xu *et al.* 1998). These experiments showed low levels of human *APOE* mRNA in select cortical neurons. *APOE* mRNA has also been detected in human neuronal cell lines using reverse-transcription polymerase chain reactions (Dupont-Wallois *et al.* 1997).

6.4.1 Apolipoprotein E and amyloid

Extreme variations of Aβ deposition were commonly observed in different patients and in non-demented individuals meeting the pathological criteria for AD. Comparisons of Aβ immunoreactivity had demonstrated large variations in the density and size of plaques between patients (Katzman *et al.* 1988; Price *et al.* 1991; Terry *et al.* 1991; Arriagada *et al.* 1992; Hyman *et al.* 1993). With the genetic association of *APOE* with AD, the amyloid

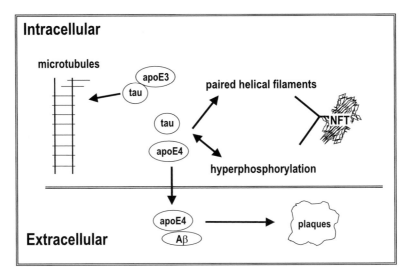

Fig. 6.1 Schematic representation of two of the more popular hypotheses on the role of apoE4 in the aetiology of AD. In the intracellular model, apoE4 may not bind tau as well as apoE3 (or apoE2). Over time, a bias toward microtubule destabilization and the formations of neurofibrillary tangles (NFT) may occur in individuals with an *APOE ε4* allele. In the extracellular model, apoE4 may bind to Aβ more readily than apoE3 and facilitate the deposition of amyloid in the plaques. The end result of both models is eventual neuronal cell death.

burden could be re-examined by comparing patients with defined *APOE* genotypes. The amyloid burden could be correlated with *APOE* genotype in samples paired for disease and duration (Schmechel *et al.* 1993). It is important to incorporate survival in the analysis of Aβ deposition. At first glance, the increased Aβ burden in a homozygous *APOE4* patient with a younger age of onset would seem to support a theory of more rapid pathogenesis based on Aβ toxicity. Our genetic data clearly demonstrate that survival (duration of the disease after onset) is related to the age of onset, not to the inheritance of the *APOE ε 4* allele (Corder *et al.* 1995). Despite the fact that *APOE ε 4* homozygous patients have a greater amyloid burden earlier, their survival is not affected by the Aβ load because they live as long as *APOE ε 3* homozygous patients with the same age of onset. Thus, Aβ deposition is a consequence of the disease expressed as a function of *APOE* genotype and time. Several studies have confirmed the increased amyloid deposition in ε 4-bearing individuals, both with and without AD (Berr *et al.* 1994; Gearing *et al.* 1995*b*; Polvikoski *et al.* 1995; Marz *et al.* 1996; Mukaetova-Ladinska *et al.* 1997; McNamara *et al.* 1998). The increased deposition of amyloid has been attributed to either selective increases in the amount of Aβ1–40 rather than Aβ1–42 (Gearing *et al.* 1996; Ishii *et al.* 1997; Mann *et al.* 1997) or to nonselective increases in both peptides (McNamara *et al.* 1998).

Perhaps one of the most striking pieces of evidence that apoE plays a role in amyloid deposition is the observation that a lack of apoE dramatically reduced Aβ deposition in a transgenic model of AD (Bales *et al.* 1997). To investigate the role of apoE on the amyloid deposition, *APOE*-deficient mice were crossed with transgenic mice over-expressing a human mutant *APP* gene. In six month old mice homozygous for the APP mutation transgene and the wild-type mouse *APOE* gene, the cerebral cortex and hippocampus had numerous large amyloid deposits. In contrast, six month old mice homozygous for the *APP* gene but lacking the wild-type mouse *APOE* gene had no amyloid deposits. These data support an important role for apoE in facilitating Aβ deposition *in vivo*.

In vitro assays have consistently demonstrated apoE binding to the Aβ peptide; however, the isoform specificity is clearly dependent on the source and state of the apoE protein. The nature of apoE in the brain is not yet known, but the discrepancies in data underscore the importance of subtle difference in apoE conformation in its activity. The initial report on the association of *APOE* with AD included data showing that CSF apoE avidly binds synthetic Aβ *in vitro* (Strittmatter *et al.* 1993*b*). A follow-up study demonstrated both purified human apoE3 and apoE4 formed complexes with synthetic Aβ peptide (Strittmatter *et al.* 1993*c*). Complex formation between apoE4 and Aβ occurred in minutes; whereas binding to apoE3 required hours (Strittmatter *et al.* 1993*c*). Subsequent studies by other laboratories have different data depending on the molecular nature of the apoE protein. Both unpurified apoE3 isoform in conditioned media from transfected cells and human VLDL isolated from an *APOE ε 3* homozygote bind Aβ with much greater avidity than apoE4 (LaDu *et al.* 1994, 1995, 1997, Yang *et al.* 1997). Nascent apoE isoforms expressed in transfected baby hamster kidney cells form complexes with Aβ in the order of apoE2>apoE3>>apoE4 (Haas *et al.* 1997). No isoform-specific differences in Aβ binding were observed when apoE isoforms were produced in *E. coli* (Chan *et al.* 1996); another group reported that they could not detect Aβ/recombinant apoE4 complexes even after 4 days of incubation (Yang *et al.* 1997). Two recent reports have data suggesting that the apoE found within plaques is different, possibly degraded, when compared to apoE from serum (Aizawa *et al.* 1997; Yamada *et al.* 1997).

Evidence for a direct apoE/Aβ interaction lead several research teams to investigate the effect of apoE isoforms on fibrillogenesis. The first reports demonstrated that apoE4 in particular promoted spontaneous Aβ fibril formation. (Sanan *et al.* 1994; Wisniewski *et al.* 1994; Castano *et al.* 1995). Sanan and colleagues demonstrated that both the apoE3 and apoE4 isoforms interact with Aβ1–40 peptides to produce novel monofibrils (Sanan *et al.* 1994). This interaction is greatly influenced by the conformational state of the Aβ peptide used, with apoE preferentially binding to Aβ peptides with a beta-sheet conformation (Golabek *et al.* 1996).

6.4.2 Apolipoprotein E and microtubule-associated proteins

The immunoreactivity of apoE antibodies with NFT inside neurons is as striking as the immunoreactivity with amyloid deposits in plaques and blood vessels (Namba *et al.* 1991; Schmechel *et al.* 1993; Han *et al.* 1994*b*). The staining of tangles implied an intraneuronal role for apoE. We proposed a hypothesis that involves the differential interaction of apoE3 (and apoE2) compared to apoE4 with microtubule-associated proteins (MAP) (Strittmatter *et al.* 1994*b*). ApoE2 and apoE3 may sequester or protect tau so that the formation of paired helical filaments (PHF) and associated hyperphosphorylation of tau near the soma are fractionally slowed during ageing. There is a remarkable *in vitro* difference in the binding of apoE4 and apoE3 to tau. ApoE3 binds to the microtubule-binding domains of tau over a wide range of pH values and concentrations, but does not bind to apoE4 (Strittmatter *et al.* 1994*a, b*). Like tubulin, neither apoE3 nor apoE4 complexes with tau that has been hyperphosphorylated *in vitro* by incubation with a crude rat brain extract (Huang *et al.* 1995). Studies using fragments of apoE and tau have demonstrated which regions of each molecule are critical for complex formation (Strittmatter *et al.* 1994*b*). Tau binds to the LDL-receptor binding domain of apoE3, and apoE3 binds to the microtubule-binding repeat region of tau, the same region that appears to promote self-assembly of tau into PHF. The effect of phosphorylation of domain I of the microtubule-binding repeat region of tau is to abolish the ability of apoE3 to bind to it (Huang *et al.* 1995). This domain contains the only phosphorylation site in the microtubule-binding region.

Since the dendritic microtubule-associated protein MAP2c also affects microtubule assembly and stability, we examined the interactions between apoE isoforms and MAP2c (Huang *et al.* 1994). Like tau, MAP2c contains a highly conserved microtubule-binding repeat region. Recombinant MAP2c binds to apoE3 but does not bind to apoE4. Since apoE3 binds to the microtubule-binding region of tau and both tau and MAP2c contain similar microtubule-binding domains, apoE3 may also bind the microtubule binding domain of MAP2c.

The association of apoE3 and apoE4 with other cytoskeletal proteins has also been examined using gel shift and overlay assays (Fleming *et al.* 1996). In the gel shift assay, apoE3 formed SDS-stable complexes with the longest and shortest isoforms of recombinant tau and the 160-kDa neurofilament protein. ApoE4 did not bind any of these proteins in this assay. ApoE2 did not bind the longest isoform of tau and only weakly associated with the shortest form. The gel shift assay only reveals the strongest protein–protein interactions that remain after electrophoresis in the presence of SDS. The association of apoE3 and apoE4 with the longest isoform of tau, actin and tubulin was further examined in an overlay assay with known amounts of the cytoskeletal proteins slot-blotted onto nitrocellulose and incubated with either isoform. In this assay, both apoE isoforms bound the longest tau isoform and tubulin equally well. In contrast, apoE3 bound actin with a significantly greater affinity than did apoE4. These results indicate that apoE isoforms interact with cytoskeletal proteins with at least two different affinities. The more avid interaction results in the formation of SDS-stable complexes and occurs almost exclusively with apoE3, whereas lower avidity binding of apoE and other cytoskeletal proteins, measured with the overlay assay, is observed with both isoforms. How these different *in vitro* associations for apoE3 and apoE4 with cytoskeletal proteins contribute to the differential functions of apoE within the cell are not known. A recent study using a biologically active synthetic peptide derived from the LDL-receptor binding domain of apoE suggests that apoE affects the phosphorylation of tau. This effect may occur through the modulation of several calcium-associated signal transduction pathways that increase the activity of certain protein phosphatases which in turn dephosphorylate tau (Wang *et al.* 1998).

Two lines of evidence support the theory that apoE is involved in the stabilization of the microtubular system. The inhibitory effect of exogenous apoE4 on neurite outgrowth in neuroblastoma cells is associated with microtubule depolymerization (Nathan *et al.* 1995). Cells treated with apoE4 showed fewer microtubules and a greatly reduced ratio of depolymerized to monomeric tubulin than did cells treated with apoE3. The effect of apoE4 on depolymerization of microtubules was shown by biochemical, immunocytochemical, and ultrastructural studies.

A second line of evidence is more controversial and perhaps a reflection of how unidentified environmental factors may influence the *APOE*-deficient mouse's phenotype. Masliah and colleagues have shown that apoE-deficient mice display a relatively dramatic age-dependent disruption of the synaptic and dendritic organization of the neocortex and limbic system, suggesting that apoE might be involved in maintaining the synapto-dendritic complex by preserving the stability of the microtubular cytoskeleton (Masliah *et al.* 1995). The apoE-deficient mice showed decreased immunoreactivity with antibodies against MAP2 and neurofilaments, as well as vacuolization and disruption of the dendritic cytoskeleton at the ultrastructural level. Immunocytochemical evalution showed a significant decrease and redistribution of α and β tubulin, but not of kinesin. A recent study by Anderson and colleagues (1998) and our own unpublished observations do not find consistent significant changes in these mice. Studies looking at the phosphorylation of tau (Genis *et al.* 1995; Mercken and Brion, 1995) or cognitive function (Gordon *et al.* 1996; Masliah *et al.* 1997; Oitzl *et al.* 1997; Anderson *et al.* 1998; Zhou *et al.* 1998) in the *APOE*-deficient mouse also vary by laboratory. Relatively minor variances in diet, housing, etc. may have a significant effect on the brain stress response of the *APOE*-deficient mouse.

Over time, a bias towards destabilization of microtubules and the formation of tangles may occur in individuals who inherit *APOE*4 alleles. The interaction of apoE2 and apoE3 with tau may regulate the function and metabolism of tau. This regulation would not be present in individuals who make only the apoE4 protein or would be reduced in heterozygous individuals, leading to a shorter functional life span of neurons.

6.5 **Conclusions**

Remarkable progress has been made since 1993 in understanding the genetics of the *APOE* alleles in both the risk and age of onset of AD, and related studies are strongly indicating that the *APOE ε 4* allele influences a person's outcome following a variety of acute brain insults. In striking contrast, very little is known about how a small change in a small protein (one amino acid in a 299 amino acid protein) can lead to disease onset distributions varying over two decades. The data implicating apoE in metabolism associated with AD are only beginning to be examined experimentally in many laboratories. We know that apoE can bind Aβ, tau, lipid particles, LDL- and related receptors and other proteins. Which of these phenomena, if any, are relevant to the expression of AD remains to be determined. The two most popular hypotheses concern the role of apoE isoforms in amyloid plaque deposition and NFT formation. There are, of course, several other pathogenic hypotheses involving apoE that can be generated and tested. Critical roles for apoE in neuronal metabolism may involve cation transport, membrane trafficking, lipid metabolism, intracellular APP metabolism, or cellular responses to inflammation. As more biologists enter the rapidly growing field of apoE neurobiology, these and other hypotheses will be tested, adding relevant new data to the pathogenic mechanisms of AD and other neurodegenerative diseases.

References

Aizawa, Y., Fukatsu, R., Takamaru, Y., *et al.* (1997). Amino-terminus truncated apolipoprotein E is the major species in amyloid deposits in Alzheimer's disease-affected brains: A possible role for apolipoprotein E in Alzheimer's disease. *Brain Research*, **768**, 208–14.

Alberts, M. J., Graffagnino, C., McClenny, C., (1995). ApoE genotype and survival from intracerebral haemorrhage. *Lancet*, **346**, 575.

Ali, S. M., Dunn, E., Oostveen, J. A., (1996). Induction of apolipoprotein E mRNA in the hippocampus of the gerbil after transient global ischaemia. *Molecular Brain Research,* **38**, 37–44.

Anderson, R., Barnes, J. C., Bliss, T. V., *et al.* (1998) Behavioural, physiological and morphological analysis of a line of apolipoprotein E knockout mouse. *Neuroscience*, **85**, 93–110.

Anwar, N., Lovestone ,S., Cheetham, M.E., *et al.* (1993). Apolipoprotein E-epsilon4 allele and Alzheimer's disease. *Lancet*, **342**, 1308–10.

Arriagada, P. V., Growdon, J. H., Hedley, W. E., and Hyman, B. T. (1992). Neurofibrillary tangles but not senile plaques parallel duration and severity of Alzheimer's disease. *Neurology*, **42**, 631–9.

Bales, K. R., Verina, T., Dodel, R. C., *et al.* (1997). Lack of apolipoprotein E dramatically reduces amyloid beta-peptide deposition *Nature Genetics*, **17**, 263–4.

Basun, H., Corder, E. H., Guo, Z., *et al.* (1996). Apolipoprotein E polymorphism and stroke in a population sample aged 75 years or more. *Stroke*, **27**, 1310–15.

Benjamin R., Leake A., McArthur F.K., *et al.* (1994). Protective effect of apoE epsilon2 in Alzheimer's disease. *Lancet*, **344**, 473.

Berr, C., Hauw, J. J., Delaere, P., *et al.* (1994). Apolipoprotein E allele epsilon4 is linked to increased deposition of the amyloid beta-peptide (A-beta) in cases with or without Alzheimer's disease. *Neuroscience Letters*, **178**, 221–4.

Bickeboller, H., Campion, D., Brice, A., *et al.* (1997). Apolipoprotein E and Alzheimer disease: Genotype-specific risks by age and sex. *American Journal of Human Genetics*, **60**, 439–46.

Blue, M. L., Williams, D. L., Zucker, S., *et al.* (1983). Apolipoprotein-E synthesis in human-kidney, adrenal-gland, and liver. *Proceedings of the National Academy of Science (USA)*, **80**, 283–7.

Borgaonkar, D. S., Schmidt, L. C., Martin, S. E., *et al.* (1993). Linkage of late-onset Alzheimer's disease with apolipoprotein E. *Lancet*, **342**, 625.

Boyles, J. K., Zoellner, C. D., Anderson, L. J., *et al.* (1989). A role for apolipoprotein E, apolipoprotein A-I, and low density lipoprotein receptors in cholesterol transport during regeneration and remyelination of the rat sciatic nerve. *Journal of Clinical Investigation*, **83**, 1015–31.

Brice, A., Tardieu, S., Didierjean, O., *et al.* (1996). Apolipoprotein E genotype does not affect age at onset in patients with chromosome 14 encoded Alzheimer's disease. *Journal of Medical Genetics*, **33**, 174–5.

Brousseau, T., Legrain, S., Berr, C., *et al.* (1994). Confirmation of the epsilon4 allele of the apolipoprotein E gene as a risk factor for late-onset Alzheimer's disease. *Neurology*, **44**, 342–4.

Castano, E. M., Prelli, F., Pras, M., and Frangione, B. (1995). Apolipoprotein E carboxyl-terminal fragments are complexed to amyloids A and L: Implications for amyloidogenesis and Alzheimer's disease. *Journal of Biological Chemistry*, **270**, 17610–15.

Chan, W., Fornwald, J., Brawner, M., and Wetzel, R. (1996). Native complex formation between apolipoprotein E isoforms and the Alzheimer's disease peptide Abeta. *Biochemistry*, **35**, 7123–30.

Chartier-Harlin, M. C., Parfitt, M., Legrain, S., *et al.* (1994). Apolipoprotein E, epsilon4 allele as a major risk factor for sporadic early and late-onset forms of Alzheimer's disease: Analysis of the 19q13.2 chromosome. *Human Molecular Genetics*, **3**, 569–74.

Clark, L. N., Poorkaj, P., Wszolek, Z., *et al.* (1998). Pathogenic implications of mutations in the tau gene in pallido-ponto-nigral degeneration and related neurodegenerative disorders linked to chromosome 17. *Proceedings of the National Academy of Science (USA)*, **95**, 13103–7.

Corder, E. H., Saunders, A. M., Strittmatter, W. J., *et al.* (1993). Gene dose of apolipoprotein E type 4 allele and the risk of Alzheimer's disease in late onset families. *Science*, **261**, 921–3.

Corder, E. H., Saunders, A. M., Risch, N. J., *et al.* (1994). Protective effect of apolipoprotein E type 2 allele for late onset Alzheimer disease. *Nature Genetics*, **7**, 180–4.

Corder, E. H., Saunders, A. M., Strittmatter, W. J., *et al.* (1995). Apolipoprotein E, survival in Alzheimer's disease patients, and the competing risks of death and Alzheimer's disease. *Neurology*, **45**, 1323–8.

Dai, X. Y., Nanko, S., Hattori, M., *et al.* (1994). Association of apolipoprotein E4 with sporadic Alzheimer's disease is more pronounced in early onset type. *Neuroscience Letters,* 175, 74–6.

Diedrich, J. F., Minnigan, H., Carp, R. I., *et al.* (1991). Neuropathological changes in scrapie and Alzheimer's disease are associated with increased expression of apolipoprotein E and cathepsin D in astrocytes. *Journal of Virology,* 65, 4759–68.

Driscoll, D. M., and Getz, G. S. (1984). Extrahepatic synthesis of apolipoprotein E. *Journal of Lipid Research,* 25, 1368–79.

Dumanchin, C., Camuzat, A., Campion, D., *et al.* (1998). Segregation of a missense mutation in the microtubule-associated protein tau gene with familial frontotemporal dementia and parkinsonism. *Human Molecular Genetics,* 7, 1825–9.

Dupont-Wallois, L., Soulie, C., Sergeant, N., *et al.* (1997). ApoE synthesis in human neuroblastoma cells. *Neurobiology of Disease,* 4, 356–64.

Elshourbagy, N. A., Liao, W. S., Mahley, R. W., and Taylor, J. M. (1985). Apolipoprotein E mRNA is abundant in the brain and adrenals, as well as in the liver, and is present in other peripheral tissues of rats and marmosets. *Proceedings of the National Academy of Science (USA),* 82, 203–7.

Farrer, L. A., Cupples, L. A., Haines, J. L., *et al.* (1997). Effects of age, sex, and ethnicity on the association between apolipoprotein E genotype and Alzheimer disease: A meta-analysis. *Journal of the American Medical Association,* 278, 1349–56.

Fleming, L. M., Weisgraber, K. H., Strittmatter, W. J., *et al.* (1996). Differential binding of apolipoprotein E isoforms to tau and other cytoskeletal proteins. *Experimental Neurology,* 138, 252–60.

Fox, N. C., Kennedy, A. M., Harvey, R. J., *et al.* (1997). Clinicopathological features of familial Alzheimer's disease associated with the M139V mutation in the presenilin 1 gene. Pedigree but not mutation specific age at onset provides evidence for a further genetic factor. *Brain,* 120, 491–501.

Galasko, D., Saitoh, T., Xia, Y., *et al.* (1994). The apolipoprotein E allele epsilon4 is overrepresented in patients with the Lewy body variant of Alzheimer's disease. *Neurology,* 44, 1950–1.

Gearing, M., Mirra, S. S., Hedreen, J. C., *et al.* (1995a). The consortium to establish a registry for Alzheimer's disease (CERAD). Part X. Neuropathology confirmation of the clinical diagnosis of Alzheimer's disease. *Neurology,* 45, 461–6.

Gearing, M., Schneider, J. A., Robbins, R. S., *et al.* (1995b). Regional variation in the distribution of apolipoprotein E and Abeta in Alzheimer's disease. *Journal of Neuropathology and Experimental Neurology,* 54, 833–41.

Gearing, M., Mori, H., and Mirra, S. S. (1996). Abeta-peptide length and apolipoprotein E genotype in Alzheimer's disease. *Annals of Neurology,* 39, 395–9.

Genis, I., Gordon, I., Sehayek, E., and Michaelson, D. M. (1995). Phosphorylation of tau in apolipoprotein E-deficient mice. *Neuroscience Letters,* 199, 5–8.

Goate, A., Chartier-Harlin, M. C., Mullan, M., *et al.* (1991). Segregation of a missense mutation in the amyloid precursor protein gene with familial Alzheimer's disease. *Nature,* 349, 704–6.

Golabek, A. A., Soto, C., Vogel, T., and Wisniewski, T. (1996). The interaction between apolipoprotein E and Alzheimer's amyloid beta- peptide is dependent on beta-peptide conformation. *Journal of Biological Chemistry,* 271, 10602–6.

Gordon, I., Genis, I., Grauer, E., *et al.* (1996). Biochemical and cognitive studies of apolipoprotein-E-deficient mice. *Molecular & Chemical Neuropathology,* 28, 97–103.

Gutman, C. R., Strittmatter, W. J., Weisgraber, K. H., and Matthew, W. D. (1997). Apolipoprotein E binds to and potentiates the biological activity of ciliary neurotrophic factor. *Journal of Neuroscience,* 17, 6114–21.

Haas, C., Cazorla, P., Miguel, C. D., *et al.* (1997). Apolipoprotein E forms stable complexes with recombinant Alzheimer's disease beta-amyloid precursor protein. *Biochemical Journal,* 325, 169–75.

Hall, E.D., Oostveen, J. A., Dunn, E., and Carter, D. B. (1995). Increased amyloid protein precursor and apolipoprotein E immunoreactivity in the selectively vulnerable hippocampus following transient forebrain ischaemia in gerbils. *Experimental Neurology*, 135, 17–27.

Han, S. H., Einstein, G., Weisgraber, K. H., *et al.* (1994*a*). Apolipoprotein E is localized to the cytoplasm of human cortical neurons: A light and electron microscopic study. *Journal of Neuropathology and Experimental Neurology*, 53, 535–44.

Han, S. H., Hulette, C., Saunders, A. M., *et al.* (1994*b*). Apolipoprotein E is present in hippocampal neurons without neurofibrillary tangles in Alzheimer's disease and in age-matched controls. *Experimental Neurology*, 128, 13–26.

Harrington, C. R., Louwagie, J., Rossau, R., *et al.* (1994). Influence of apolipoprotein E genotype on senile dementia of the Alzheimer and Lewy body types: Significance for aetiological theories of Alzheimer's disease. *American Journal of Pathology*, 145, 1472–84.

Helisalmi, S., Linnaranta, K., Lehtovirta, M., *et al.* (1996). Apolipoprotein E polymorphism in patients with different neurodegenerative disorders. *Neuroscience Letters*, 205, 61–4.

Hendrie, H. C., Hall, K. S., Hui, S., *et al.* (1995). Apolipoprotein E genotypes and Alzheimer's disease in a community study of elderly African Americans. *Annals of Neurology*, 37, 118–20.

Horsburgh, K. and Nicoll, J.A. (1996). Selective alterations in the cellular distribution of apolipoprotein E immunoreactivity following transient cerebral ischaemia in the rat. *Neuropathology and Applied Neurobiology*, 22, 342–9.

Houlden, H., Crook, R., Backhovens, H., *et al.* (1998). ApoE genotype is a risk factor in nonpresenilin early-onset Alzheimer's disease families. *American Journal of Medical Genetics*, 81, 117–21.

Houlden, H., Crook, R., Duff, K., *et al.* (1993). Confirmation that the apolipoprotein e4 allele is associated with late-onset, familial alzheimers-disease *Neurodegeneration*, 2, 283–6.

Huang, D. Y., Goedert, M., Jakes, R., *et al.* (1994). Isoform-specific interactions of apolipoprotein E with the microtubule-associated protein MAP2c: Implications for Alzheimer's disease. *Neuroscience Letters,* 182, 55–8.

Huang, D. Y., Weisgraber, K. H., Goedert, M., *et al.* (1995). ApoE3 binding to tau tandem repeat I is abolished by tau serine262 phosphorylation. *Neuroscience Letters*, 192, 209–12.

Hyman, B. T., Marzloff, K., and Arriagada, P. V. (1993). The lack of accumulation of senile plaques or amyloid burden in Alzheimer's disease suggests a dynamic balance between amyloid deposition and resolution. *Journal of Neuropathology and Experimental Neurology*, 52, 594–600.

Ibarreta, D., Gomez-Isla, T., Portera-Sanchez, A., *et al.* (1995). Apolipoprotein E genotype in Spanish patients of Alzheimer's or Parkinson's disease. *Journal of Neurolological Science*, 134, 146–9.

Ignatius, M. J., Gebicke, H. P., Skene, J. H., *et al.* (1986). Expression of apolipoprotein E during nerve degeneration and regeneration. *Proceedings of the National Academy of Science (USA)*, 83, 1125–9.

Ignatius, M. J., Shooter, E. M., Pitas, R E., and Mahley, R.W. (1987). Lipoprotein uptake by neuronal growth cones *in vitro*. *Science* , 236, 959–62

Ishii, K., Tamaoka, A., Mizusawa, H., *et al.* (1997). Aβ1–40 but not Aβ1–42 levels in cortex correlate with apolipoprotein E epsilon4 allele dosage in sporadic Alzheimer's disease. *Brain Research*, 748, 250–2.

Ishimaru, H., Ishikawa, K., Ohe, Y., *et al.* (1996). Cystatin C and apolipoprotein E immunoreactivities in CA1 neurons in ischaemic gerbil hippocampus. *Brain Research*, 709, 155–62.

Jordan, B. D., Relkin, N. R., Ravdin, L. D., *et al.* (1997). Apolipoprotein E epsilon4 associated with chronic traumatic brain injury in boxing. *Journal of the American Medical Association*, 278, 136–40.

Kalaria, R. N. and Premkumar, D. R. (1995). Apolipoprotein E genotype and cerebral amyloid angiopathy. *Lancet*, 346, 1424.

Katzman, R., Terry, R., DeTeresa, R., *et al.* (1988). Clinical, pathological, and neurochemical changes in dementia: A subgroup with preserved mental status and numerous neocortical plaques. *Annals of Neurology,* 23, 138–44.

Kawamata, J., Tanaka, S., Shimohama, S., *et al.* (1994). Apolipoprotein E polymorphism in Japanese patients with Alzheimer's disease or vascular dementia. *Journal Neurology, Neurosurgery and Psychiatry,* 57, 1414–16.

Kawanishi, C., Suzuki, K., Odawara, T., *et al.* (1996). Neuropathological evaluation and apolipoprotein E gene polymorphism analysis in diffuse Lewy body disease. *Journal of the Neurological Sciences,* 136, 140–2.

Kida, E., Pluta, R., Lossinsky, A. S., *et al.* (1995). Complete cerebral ischaemia with short-term survival in rat induced by cardiac arrest. II. Extracellular and intracellular accumulation of apolipoproteins E and J in the brain. *Brain Research,* 674, 341–6.

Koller, W. C., Glatt, S. L., Hubble, J. P., *et al.* (1995). Apolipoprotein E genotypes in Parkinson's disease with and without dementia. *Annals of Neurology,* 37, 242–5.

Krieger, M. and Herz, J. (1994). Structures and functions of multiligand lipoprotein receptors: Macrophage scavenger receptors and LDL receptor-related protein (LRP). *Annual Reviews in Biochemistry,* 63, 601–37.

Kukull, W. A., Schellenberg, G. D., Bowen, J. D., *et al.* (1996). Apolipoprotein E in Alzheimer's disease risk and case detection: A case-control study. *Journal of Clinical Epidemiology,* 49, 1143–8.

Kuusisto, J., Koivisto, K., Kervinen, K., *et al.* (1994). Association of apolipoprotein E phenotypes with late onset Alzheimer's disease: Population based study. *British Medical Journal,* 309, 636–8.

LaDu, M. J., Falduto, M. T., Manelli, A. M., *et al.* (1994). Isoform-specific binding of apolipoprotein E to beta-amyloid. *Journal of Biological Chemistry,* 269, 23403–6.

LaDu, M. J., Pederson, T. M., Frail, D. E., *et al.* (1995). Purification of apolipoprotein E attenuates isoform-specific binding to beta-amyloid. *Journal of Biological Chemistry,* 270, 9039–42.

LaDu, M. J., Lukens, J. R., Reardon, C. A., and Getz, G. S. (1997). Association of human, rat, and rabbit apolipoprotein E with beta-amyloid. *Journal of Neuroscience Research,* 49, 9–18.

Laskowitz, D. T., Sheng, H., Bart, R. D., *et al.* (1997). Apolipoprotein E-deficient mice have increased susceptibility to focal cerebral ischaemia. *Journal of Cerebral Blood Flow Metabolism,* 17, 753–8.

Lendon, C. L., Martinez, A., Behrens, I. M., *et al.* (1997). E280A PS-1 mutation causes Alzheimer's disease but age of onset is not modified by ApoE alleles. *Human Mutation,* 10, 186–95.

Levy-Lahad, E., Wijsman, E. M., Nemens, E., *et al.* (1995). A familial Alzheimer's disease locus on chromosome I. *Science,* 269, 970–3.

Lin, C. T., Xu, Y. F., Wu, J. Y., and Chan, L. (1986). Immunoreactive apolipoprotein-E is a widely distributed cellular protein — Immunohistochemical localization of apolipoprotein-E in baboon tissues. *Journal of Clinical Investigation,* 78, 947–58.

Linton, M. F., Gish, R., Hubl, S. T., *et al.* (1991). Phenotypes of apolipoprotein B and apolipoprotein E after liver transplantation. *Journal of Clinical Investigation,* 88, 270–81.

McCarron, M. O., Muir, K. W., Weir, C. J., *et al.* (1998). The apolipoprotein E epsilon4 allele and outcome in cerebrovascular disease. *Stroke,* 29, 1882–7.

McKeith, I. G., Galasko, D., Kosaka, K., *et al.* (1996). Consensus guidelines for the clinical and pathologic diagnosis of dementia with Lewy bodies (DLB): Report of the consortium on DLB international workshop. *Neurology,* 47, 1113–24.

McNamara, M. J., Gomez-Isla, T., and Hyman, B. T. (1998). Apolipoprotein E genotype and deposits of Abeta40 and Abeta42 in Alzheimer disease. *Archives of Neurology,* 55, 1001–4.

Macy, M., Okano, Y., Cardin, A. D., *et al.* (1983). Suppression of lymphocyte activation by plasma lipoproteins. *Cancer Research,* 43, 2496s-02s.

Maestre, G., Ottman, R., Stern, Y., *et al.* (1995). Apolipoprotein E and Alzheimer's disease: Ethnic variation in genotypic risks. *Annals of Neurology*, 37, 254–9.

Mahieux, F., Couderc, R., Moulignier, A., *et al.* (1994). Apolipoprotein E4: Phenotype in patients with Alzheimer's disease. *Annals of Neurology*, 35, 506–7.

Mann, D. M., Iwatsubo, T., Pickering-Brown, S. M., *et al.* (1997). Preferential deposition of amyloid beta protein (Abeta) in the form Abeta40 in Alzheimer's disease is associated with a gene dosage effect of the apolipoprotein E E4 allele. *Neuroscience Letters*, 221, 81–4.

Martinoli, M. G., Trojanowski, J. Q., Schmidt, M. L., *et al.* (1995). Association of apolipoprotein epsilon4 allele and neuropathologic findings in patients with dementia. *Acta Neuropathologica*, 90, 239–43.

Marz, W., Scharnagl, H., Kirca, M., *et al.* (1996). Apolipoprotein E polymorphism is associated with both senile plaque load and Alzheimer-type neurofibrillary tangle formation. *Annals of NY Academy of Science*, 777, 276–80.

Masliah, E., Mallory, M., Ge, N., *et al.* (1995). Neurodegeneration in the central nervous system of apoE-deficient mice. *Experimental Neurology*, 136, 107–22.

Masliah, E., Samuel, W., Veinbergs, I., *et al.* (1997). Neurodegeneration and cognitive impairment in apoE-deficient mice is ameliorated by infusion of recombinant apoE. *Brain Research*, 751, 307–14.

Mayeux, R., Ottman, R., Maestre, G., *et al.* (1995). Synergistic effects of traumatic head injury and apolipoprotein-epsilon4 in patients with Alzheimer's disease. *Neurology*, 45, 555–7.

Mazzone, T. (1996). Apolipoprotein E secretion by macrophages: Its potential physiological functions. *Current Opinion in Lipidology*, 7, 303–7.

Mercken, L. and Brion, J. P. (1995). Phosphorylation of tau protein is not affected in mice lacking apolipoprotein E. *Neuroreport*, 6, 2381–4.

Mistry, M. J., Clay, M. A., Kelly, M. E., *et al.* (1995). Apolipoprotein E restricts interleukin-dependent T lymphocyte proliferation at the G1(A)/G1(B) boundary. *Cell Immunology*, 160, 14–23.

Miyata, M. and Smith, J. D. (1996). Apolipoprotein E allele-specific antioxidant activity and effects on cytotoxicity by oxidative insults and beta-amyloid peptides. *Nature Genetics*, 14, 55–61.

Morris, C. M., Massey, H. M., Benjamin, R., *et al.* (1996). Molecular biology of APO E alleles in Alzheimer's and non-Alzheimer's dementias. *Journal of Neural Transmission Supplement*, 47, 205–18.

Mukaetova-Ladinska, E. B., Harrington, C. R., Roth, M., and Wischik, C. M. (1997). Presence of the apolipoprotein E type epsilon4 allele is not associated with neurofibrillary pathology or biochemical changes to tau protein. *Dementis and Geriatric Cognitive Disorders*, 8, 288–95.

Myers, R. H., Schaefer, E. J., Wilson, P. W. F., *et al.* (1996). Apolipoprotein E epsilon4 association with dementia in a population-based study: The Framingham study. *Neurology*, 46, 673–7.

Nacmias, B., Latorraca, S., Piersanti, P., *et al.* (1995). ApoE genotype and familial Alzheimer's disease: A possible influence on age of onset in APP717 Val /Ile mutate. *Neuroscience Letters*, 183, 1–3.

Nalbantoglu, J., Gilfix, B. M., Bertrand, P., *et al.* (1994). Predictive value of apolipoprotein E genotyping in Alzheimer's disease: Results of an autopsy series and an analysis of several combined studies. *Annals of Neurology*, 36, 889–95.

Namba, Y., Tomonaga, M., Kawasaki, H., *et al.* (1991). Apolipoprotein E immunoreactivity in cerebral amyloid deposits and neurofibrillary tangles in Alzheimer's disease and kuru plaque amyloid in Creutzfeldt-Jakob disease. *Brain Research*, 541, 163–6.

Nathan, B. P., Chang, K. C., Bellosta, S., *et al.* (1995). The inhibitory effect of apolipoprotein E4 on neurite outgrowth is associated with microtubule depolymerization. *Journal of Biological Chemistry*, 270, 19791–9.

Newman, M. F., Croughwell, N. D., Blumenthal, J. A., *et al.* (1995). Predictors of cognitive decline after cardiac operation. *Annals of Thoracic Surgery*, 59, 1326–30.

Nicoll, J. A., Roberts, G. W., and Graham, D. I. (1995). Apolipoprotein E epsilon4 allele is associated with deposition of amyloid beta- protein following head injury. *Nature Medicine,* 1, 135–7.

Nochlin, D., Bird, T. D., Nemens, E. J., *et al.* (1998). Amyloid angiopathy in a Volga German family with Alzheimer's disease and a presenilin-2 mutation (N141I). *Annals of Neurology,* 43, 131–5.

Noguchi, S., Murakami, K., and Yamada, N. *et al.* (1993). Apolipoprotein E genotype and Alzheimer's disease. *Lancet,* 342, 737.

Oitzl, M. S., Mulder, M., Lucassen, P. J., *et al.* (1997). Severe learning deficits in apolipoprotein E-knockout mice in a water maze task. *Brain Research,* 752, 189–96.

Okuizumi, K., Onodera, O., Tanaka, H., *et al.* (1994). ApoE-epsilon4 and early-onset Alzheimer's. *Nature Genetics,* 7, 10–11.

Olichney, J. M., Hansen, L. A., Galasko, D., *et al.* (1996). The apolipoprotein E epsilon4 allele is associated with increased neuritic plaques and cerebral amyloid angiopathy in Alzheimer's disease and Lewy body variant. *Neurology,* 47, 190–6.

Oostveen, J. A., Dunn, E., Carter, D. B., and Hall, E. D. (1998). Neuroprotective efficacy and mechanisms of novel pyrrolopyrimidine lipid peroxidation inhibitors in the gerbil forebrain ischaemia model. *Journal of Cerebral Blood Flow Metabolism,* 18, 539–47.

Osuntokun, B. O., Sahota, A., Ogunniyi, A. O., *et al.* (1995). Lack of an association between apolipoprotein E epsilon and Alzheimer's disease in elderly Nigerians. *Annals of Neurology,* 38, 463–5.

Pericak-Vance, M. A., Bebout, J. L., Gaskell, P. J., *et al.* (1991). Linkage studies in familial Alzheimer disease: Evidence for chromosome 19 linkage. *American Journal of Human Genetics,* 48, 1034–50.

Poirier, J., Baccichet, A., Dea, D., and Gauthier, S. (1993*a*). Cholesterol synthesis and lipoprotein reuptake during synaptic remodelling in hippocampus in adult rats. *Neuroscience,* 55, 81–90.

Poirier, J., Davignon, J., Bouthillier, D., *et al.* (1993*b*). Apolipoprotein E polymorphism and Alzheimer's disease. *Lancet,* 342, 697–9.

Poirier, J., Hess, M., May, P. C., and Finch, C. E. (1991). Astrocytic apolipoprotein E mRNA and GFAP mRNA in hippocampus after entorhinal cortex lesioning. *Molecular Brain Research,* 11, 97–106.

Polvikoski, T., Sulkava, R., Haltia, M., *et al.* (1995). Apolipoprotein E, dementia, and cortical deposition of beta-amyloid protein. *New England Journal of Medicine,* 333, 1242–7.

Poorkaj, P., Bird, T. D., Wijsman, E., *et al.* (1998).Tau is a candidate gene for chromosome 17 frontotemporal dementia. *Annals of Neurology,* 43, 815–25.

Price, D. L., Davis, P. B., Morris, J. C., and White, D. L. (1991). The distribution of tangles, plaques and related immunohistochemical markers in healthy ageing and Alzheimer's disease. *Neurobiology of Ageing,* 12, 295–312.

Puttfarcken, P. S., Manelli, A. M., Falduto, M. T., *et al.* (1997). Effect of apolipoprotein E on neurite outgrowth and beta-amyloid-induced toxicity in developing rat primary hippocampal cultures. *Journal of Neurochemistry,* 68, 760–9.

Rebeck, G. W., Reiter, J. S., Strickland, D. K., and Hyman, B. T. (1993). Apolipoprotein E in sporadic Alzheimer's disease: Allelic variation and receptor interactions. *Neuron,* 11, 575–80.

Roberts, G. W., Gentleman, S. M., Lynch, A., *et al.* (1994). Beta amyloid protein deposition in the brain after severe head injury: Implications for the pathogenesis of Alzheimer's disease. *Journal of Neurology, Neurosurgery and Psychiatry,* 57, 419–25.

Rogaev, E., Sherrington, R., Rogaeva, E., *et al.* (1995).Familial Alzheimer's disease in kindreds with missense mutations in a gene on chromosome 1 related to the Alzheimer's disease type 3 gene. *Nature,* 376, 600–2.

Roses, A. D. (1994). Apolipoprotein E affects the rate of Alzheimer disease expression: beta- Amyloid burden is a secondary consequence dependent on *APOE* genotype and duration of disease. *Journal of Neuropathology and Experimental Neurology,* 53, 429–37.

Roses, A. D. (1995). On the metabolism of apolipoprotein E and the Alzheimer diseases. *Experimental Neurology*, 132, 149–56.

Roses, A. D., Devlin, B., Conneally, P. M., *et al.* (1995). Measuring the genetic contribution of apoE in late-onset Alzheimer-disease *American Journal of Human Genetics*, 57, ssp1163

Roses, A. D. and Saunders, A. M. (1995). Head injury, amyloid beta and Alzheimer's disease. *Nature Medicine*, 1, 603–4.

Rubinsztein, D. C., Hanlon, C. S., Irving, R. M., *et al.* (1994). Apo E genotypes in multiple sclerosis, Parkinson's disease, schwannomas and late-onset Alzheimer's disease. *Molecular & Cellular Probes.* 8, 519–25

Sanan, D. A., Weisgraber, K. H., Russell, S. J., *et al.* (1994). Apolipoprotein E associates with beta amyloid peptide of Alzheimer's disease to form novel monofibrils. Isoform ApoE4 associates more efficiently than ApoE. *Journal of Clinical Investigation.* 94, 860–9.

Saunders, A. M., Schmader, K., Breitner, J. C., *et al.* (1993a). Apolipoprotein E epsilon4 allele distributions in late-onset Alzheimer's disease and in other amyloid-forming disease. *Lancet,* 342, 710–11.

Saunders, A. M., Strittmatter, W. J., Schmechel, D., *et al.* (1993b). Association of apolipoprotein E allele epsilon4 with late-onset familial and sporadic Alzheimer's disease. *Neurology,* 43, 1467–72.

Schmechel, D. E., Saunders, A. M., Strittmatter, W. J., *et al.* (1993). Increased amyloid beta-peptide deposition in cerebral cortex as a consequence of apolipoprotein E genotype in late-onset Alzheimer disease. *Proceedings of the National Academy of Science (USA)*, 90, 9649–53.

Sheng, H., Laskowitz, D. T., Bennett, E., *et al.* (1998). Apolipoprotein E isoform-specific differences in outcome from focal ischaemia in transgenic mice. *Journal of Cerebral Blood Flow Metabolism,* 18, 361–6.

Sherrington, R., Rogaev, E. I., Liang, Y., *et al.* (1995). Cloning of a gene bearing missense mutations in early-onset familial Alzheimer's disease. *Nature,* 375, 754–60.

Slooter, A. J., Tang, M. X., van Duijn, C. M., *et al.* (1997). Apolipoprotein E epsilon4 and the risk of dementia with stroke: A population- based investigation. *Journal of the American Medical Association,* 277, 818–21.

Smith, A. D., Johnston, C., Sim, E., *et al.* (1994) . Protective effect of apoE epsilon-2 in Alzheimers-disease. *Lancet,* 344, 473–4

Sorbi, S., Nacmias, B., Forleo, P., *et al.* (1994). ApoE allele frequencies in Italian sporadic and familial Alzheimer's disease. *Neuroscience Letters,* 177, 100–2.

Sorbi, S., Nacmias, N., Piacentini, S., *et al.* (1995). ApoE as a prognostic factor for post-traumatic coma. *Nature Medicine.* 1, 852.

Spillantini, M. G., Crowther, R. A., Kamphorst, W., *et al.* (1998a). Tau pathology in two Dutch families with mutations in the microtubule- binding region of tau. *American Journal of Pathology,* 153, 1359–63.

Spillantini, M. G., Murrell, J. R., Goedert, M., *et al.* (1998b). Mutation in the tau gene in familial multiple system tauopathy with presenile dementia. *Proceedings of the National Academy of Science (USA),* 95, 7737–41.

St George-Hyslop, P., Crapper McLachlan, D., Tsuda, T., *et al.* (1994). Alzheimer's disease and possible gene interaction. *Science,* 263, 537.

Strittmatter, W. J., Huang, D. Y., Bhasin, R., *et al.* (1993a). Avid binding of beta amyloid peptide to its own precursor. *Experimental Neurology,* 122, 327–34.

Strittmatter, W. J., Saunders, A. M., Schmechel, D., *et al.* (1993b). Apolipoprotein-E — high-avidity binding to beta-amyloid and increased frequency of type-4 allele in late-onset familial Alzheimer-disease. *Proceedings of the National Academy of Science (USA)*, 90, 1977–81.

Strittmatter, W. J., Weisgraber, K. H., Goedert, M., *et al.* (1993*c*). Binding of human apolipoprotein E to synthetic amyloid beta peptide: Isoform-specific effects and implications for late-onset Alzheimer disease. *Proceedings of the National Academy of Science (USA)*, **90**, 8098–102.

Strittmatter, W. J., Saunders, A. M., Goedert, M., *et al.* (1994*a*). Isoform-specific interactions of apolipoprotein E with microtubule- associated protein tau: Implications for Alzheimer disease. *Proceedings of the National Academy of Science (USA)*, **91**, 11183–6.

Strittmatter, W. J., Weisgraber, K. H., Goedert, M., *et al.* (1994*b*). Hypothesis: Microtubule instability and paired helical filament formation in the Alzheimer disease brain are related to apolipoprotein E genotype. *Experimental Neurology*, **125**, 163–71.

Talbot, C., Lendon, C., Craddock, N., *et al.* (1994). Protection against Alzheimer's disease with apoE epsilon2. *Lancet*, **343**, 1432–3.

Tang, M. X., Stern, Y., Marder, K., *et al.* (1998). The *APOE*-epsilon4 allele and the risk of Alzheimer disease among African Americans, whites, and Hispanics. *Journal of the American Medical Association*, **279**, 751–5.

Tardiff, B., Newman, M., Saunders, A., *et al.* (1994). Apolipoprotein-E allele frequency in patients with cognitive deficits following cardiopulmonary bypass. *Circulation*, **90**, I-201.

Terry, R. D., Masliah, E., Salmon, D. P., *et al.* (1991). Physical basis of cognitive alterations in Alzheimer's disease: Synapse loss is the major correlate of cognitive impairment. *Annals of Neurology*, **30**, 572–80.

The French Parkinson's Disease Genetics Study Group (1997). Apolipoprotein E genotype in familial Parkinson's disease. *Journal of Neurology Neurosurgery and Psychiatry*, **63**, 394–5.

Tsai, M. S., Tangalos, E. G., Petersen, R. C., *et al.* (1994). Apolipoprotein E: Risk factor for Alzheimer disease. *American Journal of Human Genetics*, **54**, 643–9.

Ueki, A., Kawano, M., Namba, Y., *et al.* (1993). A high frequency of apolipoprotein E4 isoprotein in Japanese patients with late-onset nonfamilial Alzheimer's disease. *Neuroscience Letters*, **163**, 166–8.

van Duijn, C. M., de Knijff, P., Cruts, M., *et al.* (1994). Apolipoprotein E4 allele in a population-based study of early-onset Alzheimer's disease. *Nature Genetics*, **7**, 74–8.

Wang, X., Luebbe, P., Gruenstein, E., and Zemlan, F. (1998). Apolipoprotein E (ApoE) peptide regulates tau phosphorylation via two different signalling pathways. *Journal of Neuroscience Research*, **51**, 658–65.

Weeks, D. E. and Lange, K. (1988). The affected-pedigree-member method of linkage analysis. *American Journal of Human Genetics*, **42**, 315–26.

Weisgraber, K. H. (1994). Apolipoprotein E: structure–function relationships. *Advances in Protein Chemistry*, **45**, 249–302.

West, H. L., Rebeck, G. W., and Hyman, B. T. (1994). Frequency of the apolipoprotein E epsilon2 allele is diminished in sporadic Alzheimer disease. *Neuroscience Letters*, **175**, 46–8.

Whitehead, A. S., Bertrandy, S., Finnan, F., *et al.* (1996). Frequency of the apolipoprotein E epsilon4 allele in a case-control study of early onset Parkinson's disease. *Journal of Neurology, Neurosurgery and Psychiatry*, **61**, 347–51.

Wisniewski, T. and Frangione, B. (1992). Apolipoprotein E: A pathological chaperone protein in patients with cerebral and systemic amyloid. *Neuroscience Letters*, **135**, 235–8.

Wisniewski, T., Castano, E. M., Golabek, A., *et al.* (1994). Acceleration of Alzheimer's fibril formation by apolipoprotein E *in vitro*. *American Journal of Pathology*, **145**, 1030–5.

Xu, P. T., Gilbert, J. R., Qiu, H. L., *et al.* (1998). Regionally specific neuronal expression of human *APOE* gene in transgenic mice. *Neuroscience Letters*, **246**, 65–8.

Yamada, T., Wakabayashi, K., Kakihara, T., *et al.* (1997). Further characterization of a monoclonal antibody recognizing apolipoprotein E peptides in amyloid deposits. *Annals of Clinical Laboratory Science*, **27**, 276–81.

Yang, D. S., Smith, J. D., Zhou, Z., *et al.* (1997). Characterization of the binding of amyloid-beta peptide to cell culture- derived native apolipoprotein E2, E3, and E4 isoforms and to isoforms from human plasma. *Journal of Neurochemistry,* **68**, 721–5.

Zannis, V. I., Kardassis, D., and Zanni, E. E. (1993). Genetic mutations affecting human lipoproteins, their receptors, and their enzymes. *Advances in Human Genetics,* **21**, 145–319.

Zareparsi, S., Kaye, J., Camicioli, R., *et al.* (1997). Modulation of the age at onset of Parkinson's disease by apolipoprotein E genotypes. *Annals of Neurology,* **42**, 655–8.

Zhou, Y., Elkins, P. D., Howell, L. A., *et al.* (1998). Apolipoprotein-E deficiency results in an altered stress responsiveness in addition to an impaired spatial memory in young mice. *Brain Research,* **788**, 151–9.

Chapter 7

The presenilins

Martin Citron

7.1 **The presenilin genes**

Studies on the pathology of Alzheimer's disease (AD) brains have implicated tau and Aβ (and therefore APP) as important in the pathogenesis of AD. As a significant number of AD cases are genetic in aetiology, there has been an intense search for loci and 'causative' gene defects in AD. It was soon noted that mutations in the *APP* gene account for only a small portion of all early-onset familial AD cases and that there must be other loci on chromosome 1 and 14, the latter accounting for most early-onset cases. Using positional cloning, the chromosome 14 gene 'presenilin 1' (*PS1*) was identified first (Sherrington *et al.* 1995), the chromosome 1 gene 'presenilin 2' (*PS2*) shortly thereafter (Levy-Lahad *et al.* 1995; Rogaev *et al.* 1995).

Both genes encode novel transmembrane proteins that have 67% amino acid identity. Two regions of nonhomology are the N-terminus and the large hydrophilic loop. The presenilins belong to a family of genes with high interspecies conservation. The human proteins are almost identical with the rat counterparts and show high similarity with the C. elegans homologs *sel-12* and *spe-4* (Levitan and Greenwald 1995; Sherrington *et al.* 1995). A drosophila presenilin homologue showing 53% identity to PS1 and PS2 has also been identified (Hong and Koo 1997). *PS1* comprises 12 exons and covers *c.* 75 kb, but the open reading frame spans only exons 3–12 (approximately 24 kb) (Clark *et al.* 1995; Cruts *et al.* 1996). *PS2* is encoded by 10 exons and is less than 90 kb in size. Most intron/exon boundaries are located at equivalent positions in both genes (Rogaev *et al.* 1995; Prihar *et al.* 1996; Sherrington *et al.* 1996). The intronic sequences immediately flanking the exons are not similar indicating that the presenilin genes are not the result of a recent gene duplication (Levy-Lahad *et al.* 1996). Northern blot analysis demonstrates two messages for PS1 at approximately 2.7 and 7.5 kb (Sherrington *et al.* 1995) and two for PS2 at 2.3 and 2.6 kb (Levy-Lahad *et al.* 1995, Rogaev *et al.* 1995). Despite the great degree of homology between the presenilins, the pattern of alternative splicing in the two genes is less conserved. In *PS2*, exons 3 and 4 can be spliced out, whereas a similar event is not observed in *PS1*. The splicing of exon 8 in *PS2* has been observed in all tissues, but the equivalent splice event for *PS1* occurs only in leukocytes (Rogaev *et al.* 1995; Sherrington *et al.* 1995). An additional PS1 transcript lacking four amino acids (VRSQ) at the 3' end of exon 3 has also been reported (Clark *et al.* 1995). The significance of the spliced transcripts is currently unclear. Northern Blot analysis showed that both PS1 and PS2 are expressed in most tissues, for example heart, liver, pancreas, spleen, kidney, testis, and brain (Rogaev *et al.* 1995; Sherrington *et al.* 1995). *In situ* hybridization in brain demonstrated that the expression patterns for PS1 and PS2 messages were similar and both were primarily detected in neurons (Kovacs *et al.* 1996). These findings suggest that presenilin mutations exert their effect in neurons. Presenilin message is found in brain regions that are affected as well as in those that are relatively spared in AD. While PS1 expression is somewhat higher in affected brain regions, the PS1 expression pattern in human is not sufficient to account for selective vulnerability in AD brain (Lee *et al.* 1996; Page *et al.* 1996).

7.1.1 The presenilin mutations

The PS1 gene was identified as the chromosome 14 FAD locus by a positional cloning approach in which cDNA sequences from affected pedigree members were analysed for mutations. The first study reported 5 missense mutations cosegregating with the disease in 5 different pedigrees (Sherrington *et al.* 1995). This initial discovery prompted a search for additional *PS1* mutations. So far more than 40 missense mutations, and the deletion of exon 9 (ΔE9) (Perez-Tur *et al.* 1995; Crook *et al.* 1998) resulting in one case from a splice-site mutation (Perez-Tur *et al.* 1995), are known to segregate with the disease in at least 70 families of various ethnic origins. Many of the reported FAD mutations in *PS1* occur in single kindreds only. Thus there is a very high probability that families with early onset FAD will have additional *PS1* mutations. Most of the mutated residues are clustered around the conserved transmembrane domains, but some are in other parts of the protein as well (Fig. 7.1). All, except one (Yasuda *et al.* 1999), occur at positions conserved between the human presenilin proteins. Interestingly, no nonsense or frameshift mutations in PS1 have been demonstrated to cosegregate with AD. This suggests that either haploinsufficiency is lethal or that all the other mutations exert their effect by gain of function. The first of these two alternatives can be ruled out based on knock out experiments (see below). *PS1* mutations are dominant and cause typical AD with high penetrance. Age of disease onset varies between the third and fifth decades. Thus, *PS1* mutations cause the most aggressive known form of AD. Interestingly, apolipoprotein E (*APOE*) genotype has no effect on the phenotype of *PS1* mutations (Van Broeckhoven *et al.* 1994). Only three mutations in PS2, N141I, M239V, and R62H have been found to cause AD (Fig. 7.1). These mutations have a greater variability in penetrance with a wide range of onset age (Sherrington *et al.* 1996).

7.2 The presenilin proteins

7.2.1 Properties of the presenilin proteins

The cDNA sequence of the presenilin proteins immediately suggests that they are novel polytopic transmembrane proteins. The exact number of transmembrane regions has been subject to debate and 6, 7, and 8 transmembrane domains have been suggested (Sherrington *et al.* 1995; Doan *et al.* 1996; Lehman *et al.* 1997). While a definitive solution of this problem requires structural information which is currently not available, experimental data for PS1 indicate that the N-and C-terminal domains and the long hydrophilic stretch between transmembrane 6 and 7 are oriented towards the cytoplasm (Doan *et al.* 1996). These results have led to the currently generally favoured model (Fig. 7.1).

As soon as the first presenilin antibodies became available, everybody in the field began to search for the predicted full length presenilin proteins. These products were indeed detected

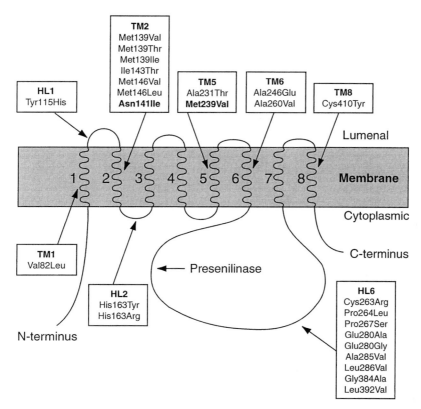

Fig. 7.1 Schematic diagram (not to scale) of PS1, showing the 8 transmembrane model with the N-terminus, the large hydrophilic loop and the C-terminus all on the cytoplasmic side. PS2 is supposed to have the same structure. The presenilinase cleavage site is indicated by an arrow. Boxes show some of the many PS1 mutations and their positions in the molecule. PS2 mutations are indicated in bold.

upon overexpression of presenilin cDNA in transfected cells (Kovacs *et al.* 1996). Endogenous PS1 (Thinakaran *et al.* 1996; Podlisny *et al.* 1997) and PS2 (Kim *et al.* 1997, Tomita *et al.* 1997) could not be detected at the predicted size on gels. However, proteolytic aminoterminal fragments (NTF) of about 30 kDa and carboxyterminal fragments (CTF) of about 20 kDa were readily found in brain, other tissues and nontransfected cells (Thinakaran *et al.* 1996; Podlisny *et al.* 1997). Using a pulse-chase paradigm, a precursor product relationship between the short-lived full length protein, only detectable upon over-expression in transfected cells, and the stable proteolytic fragments was established and the main proteolytic cleavage site of PS1 was determined (Podlisny *et al.* 1997). The protease(s) cleaving presenilin have not been identified yet. This cleavage site is deleted in the *PS1* ΔE9 mutant (Perez-Tur *et al.* 1995) which therefore accumulates as holoprotein (Thinakaran *et al.* 1996). Overexpression of PS1 holoprotein in transfected cells or transgenic mice does not lead to a dramatic increase in the amount of proteolytic fragments. Only a minor portion of overexpressed PS1 and PS2 is processed into proteolytic fragments. These accumulate to saturable levels at 1:1 stoichiometry. Furthermore, overexpression of human PS1 in mouse cells leads to replacement of the endogenous mouse fragments by the human counterparts (Thinakaran *et al.* 1996). Likewise, human PS2 can replace mouse PS1 and even the human *PS1* ΔE9 mutant, which cannot undergo the regular endoproteolytic cleavage, replaces the murine PS1 derivatives, indicating that endoproteolytic processing is not obligatory for replacement (Thinakaran *et al.* 1997). As noted above, overexpressed wild-type PS1 has a short half life, but the proteolytic fragments are long lived. This immediately suggests the existence of different degradation pathways for the full-length protein and the proteolytic fragments. The PS1 ΔE9 mutant is also long lived, which suggests that endoproteolytic cleavage and stability are not linked. Rather, full length PS1 is first stabilized and then subsequently turned over into the NTF and CTF. These fragments represent the mature and functional form of wild-type PS1 (Ratovitsky *et al.* 1997). Additional evidence in favour of this model comes from the direct observation of both PS1 fragments occurring in a tightly bound non-covalent complex in glycerol velocity gradients. The complex presumably contains stabilizing cofactors. Upon overexpression, unclipped wild-type PS1 sediments at lower weight than the fragment complex; in contrast the PS1 ΔE9 deletion mutant sediments at a molecular weight similar to that observed for the fragments. These data suggest that this mutant forms a complex similar to the endogenous fragments (Capell *et al.* 1998), whereas the full-length precursor is degraded rapidly. The stability to degradation is dependent on complex formation, not on cleavage *per se* — uncomplexed NTF and CTF are rapidly degraded by the proteasome (Steiner *et al.* 1998) but the ΔE9 molecule which is not cleaved, but complexed, is stable (Capell *et al.* 1998). Fig.7.2 summarizes this current understanding of presenilin metabolism.

Initial immunolocalization studies of presenilins in transfected cells have demonstrated a predominant endoplasmic reticulum and Golgi distribution (Kovacs *et al.* 1996; Walter *et al.* 1996; De Strooper *et al.* 1997). The localization pattern is similar regardless of whether the antibodies are generated to either N- or C-terminal epitopes. However, these studies could not distinguish the full-length presenilin molecules from the stable fragments. A subcellular fractionation study of stably transfected cells has demonstrated that full-length PS1 and PS2 are located mainly in the endoplasmic reticulum (ER) (where the proteolytic cleavage takes place), while NTF and CTF are located principally in the Golgi (Zhang *et al.* 1998*a*).

7.3 **The biological function of presenilins**

Despite intense efforts the normal function of presenilins remains unclear. Therefore, the presenilins may serve as a warning example of the difficulties encountered during genomic study in attempting to interpret the function of new genes. Typically, one would overexpress or knock out the gene of interest and look for a phenotype. Overexpression of the wild type presenilin genes in transgenic mice has not been informative, because no phenotype was observed (Borchelt *et al.* 1996; Duff *et al.* 1996; Citron *et al.* 1997). Knockout mice of PS1 have been generated, but they die shortly after birth. PS1$^{-/-}$ embryos exhibited abnormal patterning of the axial skeleton and spinal ganglia due to defects in somite segmentation and differentiation. Expression of mRNA encoding Notch1 and Delta-like gene 1 (Dll1), a vertebrate Notch ligand, is markedly reduced in the presomitic mesoderm of PS1$^{-/-}$ embryos compared to controls. Apparently, PS1 is critical for the spatiotemporal expression

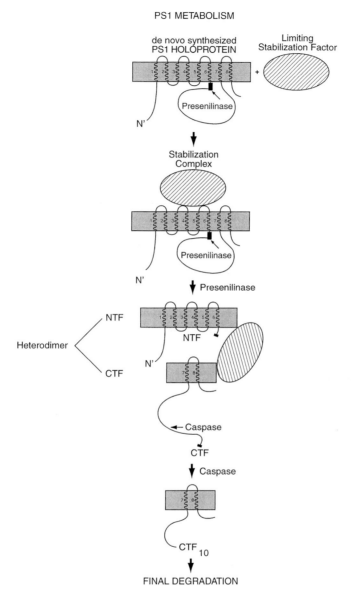

Fig. 7.2 Schematic summary of PS1 processing pathways. Newly synthesized PS1 holoprotein forms a stable complex with a limiting cellular factor. All PS1 molecules that cannot form the stabilization complex (overexpressed PS1 or PS1 fragments) are rapidly degraded. The unidentified presenilinase cleaves full length PS1 when it is in the stabilization complex. The resulting NTF-CTF presenilin heterodimer (complexed to other cellular proteins) represents the mature form of PS1. Presumably this complex rather than the uncleaved holoprotein is responsible for the biological and pathological functions of PS. The 20 kDa CTF can be cleaved by caspases to generate the alternative CTF_{10}. This cleavage is not required for the activity of presenilins in amyloidogenesis and Notch signalling (Brockhaus *et al.* 1998).

of Notch1 and Dll1(Wong *et al.* 1997). Another independent study also demonstrated the requirement of PS1 for proper formation of the axial skeleton, normal neurogenesis, and neuronal survival in the embryo (Shen *et al.* 1997). Although these data demonstrate that PS1 is essential for mouse embryonic development, the function of PS1 in the adult animal remains unknown. A surprising insight into the function of presenilin came when brain cultures were generated from PS1$^{-/-}$ embryos and analysed for changes in APP processing: a dramatic reduction in γ-secretase cleavage after both the 40th and the 42nd amino acid of Aβ, leading to an 80% reduction in Aβ40 and Aβ1–42 production, was observed. Thus, PS1 appears to facilitate a proteolytic activity that cleaves the integral membrane domain of APP (De Strooper *et al.* 1998). An extension of these studies demonstrated that the processing defect is not specific for APP but is also observed for the C-terminal fragments of other molecules, for example APLP1. In addition, the maturation of TrkB and BDNF-inducible autophosphorylation are compromised. Thus, PS1 may play an essential role in modulating trafficking and metabolism of some membrane and secretory proteins in neurons (Naruse *et al.* 1998). The limited information available from the knockout studies has been complemented by work in *C. elegans*. The *sel-12* presenilin homolog in *C. elegans* was identified as a suppressor of the egg-laying defect caused by constitutive activation of *lin-12*, a Notch receptor family member (Levitan and Greenwald 1995). The egg-laying defect of mutant *sel-12* can be rescued by human PS1 and PS2 (Levitan *et al.* 1996). This *sel-12* rescue assay is the only assay for presenilin function currently available and showed that the endoproteolytic cleavage is dispensable for presenilin function, because the ΔE9 mutant which is not cleaved (see above) can rescue (Levitan *et al.* 1996; Baumeister *et al.* 1997). In this assay the C-terminal domain of PS1 including transmembrane 7 is dispensable, but the large loop between transmembrane 6 and 7 is not (Baumeister *et al.* 1997).

Evidence has been presented to suggest that PS2 is a pro-apoptotic factor: A piece of PS2 cDNA in the antisense orientation was found to rescue a T cell hybridoma from Fas-induced apoptosis (Vito *et al.* 1996). Overexpression of PS2 in NGF differentiated PC12 cells enhances apoptosis upon NGF withdrawal, and this effect can be inhibited by overexpressing a PS2 antisense RNA (Wolozin *et al.* 1996). However, neuronal loss has so far not been observed in any transgenic mouse line overexpressing PS. Thus, overexpression of PS2 in transiently transfected cells may have artifactually caused apoptosis. There is still considerable controversy over the contribution — if any — of apoptosis to AD pathology.

An obvious approach towards understanding presenilin function is to identify binding proteins and thereby assign presenilin to interesting metabolic pathways. Numerous binding proteins have been identified, Table 7.1 lists the major binding proteins identified so far. One could imagine binding proteins needed for the normal function of presenilin which are not involved in generating the AD pathology when presenilin is mutated and other proteins that are intimately involved in causing the mutant effects. The main problem is validation of the binding proteins in the absence of functional presenilin assays. Most of the suggested candidates were identified using the yeast two hybrid system and were identified as binding to the large loop between transmembrane 6 and 7. Some of the candidates show also co-immunoprecipitation with presenilin at least under some experimental conditions. Further functional validation is generally not available. This article is restricted to the discussion of one presenilin binding protein which is thought to be involved in the pathogenic process and has therefore received more attention than the others.

Table 7.1 Presenilin binding proteins. Two publications claim differential effects of wild type vs. mutant presenilin on β-catenin. Zhang et al. (1998b) claim that PS1 stabilizes β-catenin and that PS1 mutants as well as PS1 knockout show reduced stabilization which causes increased neuronal apoptosis. Nishimura et al. (1999) claim that both PS1 and PS2 mutations, but not PS1 knockout cause defective intracellular trafficking, but not destabilization of β-catenin.

Name of protein	Interacts with aa	Experimental evidence	Comments	Reference
(1) Glycogen synthase	PS1 250–298 kinase-3β & tau	colp	differential binding to wild type vs. mutant PS1 claimed	Takashima et al. 1998
(2) μ-calpain	PS2 298–352	Y2H, colp		Shinozaki et al. 1998
(3) ABP280 and aFH1	PS1 263–411	Y2H, colp, colocalization		Zhang et al. 1998c
(4) Calsenilin	PS2 409–448	Y2H, colp, colocalization	overexpression of calsenilin increases levels of alternate PS2 CTF	Buxbaum et al. 1998
(5) Δ-catenin	PS1 263–407	Y2H, colp		Zhou et al. 1997
(6) β-catenin	PS1 NTF/ CTF complex	glycerol gradient, colp	no binding to PS2 under the same conditions	Yu et al. 1998
	PS1 CTF	colp	no binding to PS2 under same conditions, binding to PS1 NTF only when NTF complexed to CTF	Tesco et al. 1998
	PS1 NTF and CTF	colp		Zhang et al. 1998b

Abbreviations: co-immunoprecipitation (colp); C-terminal fragment (CTF); N-terminal fragment (NTF); yeast two-hybrid (Y2H).

The obvious first candidate for investigation is APP: the presenilin knockout data discussed above implicate wild type PS1 in APP processing, the presenilin mutant effects discussed below indicate a specific role of mutant PS1 and PS2 in APP processing and Aβ is assumed to be critically involved in all forms of AD. Indeed, a study using massive transient coexpression of APP and PS2 in COS cells has provided evidence for a PS2-APP interaction (Weidemann *et al.* 1997). Another more controlled study in which stably transfected cells with varying APP and presenilin expression levels were used, also suggests interaction between APP and PS1 and PS2 in cells. However, APP has not been detected in the presenilin NTF-CTF complex isolated from glycerol velocity gradients (Capell *et al.* 1998). A second detailed study using crosslinking, coimmunoprecipitation and testing of various cell lines and multiple antibodies could not confirm PS-APP interaction. The authors argue that this is not simply a detection problem: if only 1% of total brain APP interacted with PS, the entire presenilin pool would be complexed with APP (Thinakaran *et al.* 1998).

7.4 **Presenilins in Alzheimer's disease**

In contrast to the questions and controversies about the biological functions of presenilins, a pathological pathway by which presenilin mutations cause Alzheimer's disease has become almost universally accepted, even though the mechanistic details are not clear: presenilin mutations increase Aβ1–42 generation. The first data in support of this idea were accumulated even before the presenilin genes had been cloned and were known to everyone in the field long before the landmark paper was published. It was shown that fibroblasts and plasma of *PS1* and *PS2* mutation carriers had significantly increased Aβ1–42 (but not Aβ1–40 or cellular APP) levels compared to wild type controls. Most interestingly, the results were obtained by sampling human mutation carriers, excluding the possibility that the data were just the result of overexpression artefacts or other manipulations of a transgenic system (Scheuner *et al.* 1996). These results were confirmed in a neuropathological study on brains of *PS1* FAD patients. Using quantitative image analysis four brains of patients with the *PS1* E280A mutation were compared with brains of 12 sporadic AD patients. The *PS1* mutant brains exhibited a significant increase in the Aβ1–42, but not Aβ1–40, burden (Lemere *et al.* 1996). A variety of studies have used overexpression of mutant presenilin genes in transfected cell lines and/or transgenic mice. The first study showed that mice overexpressing mutant but not wild type PS1 show increased Aβ1–42 brain levels (Duff *et al.* 1996). These findings were confirmed and extended to transfected cell lines (Borchelt *et al.* 1996). A third independent study found the same effect for both PS2 mutations. Most importantly, it was rigorously demonstrated that the presenilin mutants, but not the presenilin wild type molecules specifically affect Aβ1–42 generation: Aβ1–40, secreted APP (sAPPα and sAPPβ) and cellular full-length APP were unaffected. The effect was independent of the presenilin expression level and found for all presenilin mutations analysed in the study. In transfected cells the *PS2* mutations had a similar effect on Aβ1–42 levels as the *PS1* mutations (Citron *et al.* 1997). However, the weaker effect of the *PS2* mutations *in vivo* could result from expression level differences. Since 1997 the Aβ1–42 effect has been replicated in numerous cell lines and with a large number of different presenilin mutations.

The extent of Aβ1–42 increase conferred by a specific *PS1* mutation *in vitro* might inversely correlate with the age of disease onset *in vivo*. However, this is apparently not the case (Citron *et al.* 1998; Mehta *et al.* 1998). Even within one family in which all members carry the same mutation, the age of disease onset was found to vary significantly, indicating that other genetic (or epigenetic?) factors have an influence on the pathogenic process (Lopera *et al.* 1997). The Aβ1–42 effects of presenilin mutations and the Swedish APP mutation which enhances β-secretase cleavage (Citron *et al.* 1992) are additive. As a result, transgenic mice overexpressing the Swedish mutant variant of APP show elevated brain Aβ1–42 levels and accelerated Aβ deposition compared to mice expressing only the Swedish APP mutant (Borchelt *et al.* 1997; Holcomb *et al.* 1998). Likewise, the Aβ1–42 effects of PS1 mutations and the APP717 mutation which elevates specifically Aβ1–42 (Suzuki *et al.* 1994) are additive *in vitro* (Citron *et al.* 1998).

The Aβ1–42 increase observed upon expression of mutant presenilin in a wild type background suggests that the presenilin mutations cause a gain rather than a loss of function. However, it has been shown that several *PS1* mutations rescue a *sel-12* mutation less effectively than the wild type variant. At first glance, this finding is more consistent with a loss of function model, but on the other hand, the ΔE9 mutation which has a strong Aβ1–42 effect (Citron *et al.* 1998), shows good *sel-12* rescue (Levitan *et al.* 1996; Baumeister *et al.* 1997). Thus, the Aβ1–42 increase observed in mammalian cells and loss of *sel-12* rescue activity do not correlate. Conclusive data in support of the gain of function model for the presenilin mutations have come from two studies in which transgenic mice expressing wild-type human PS1 or a mutant variant were tested for rescue of PS1$^{-/-}$ embryonic lethality. These studies argue strongly for gain of function, because they demonstrate that (i) the mutant and the wild-type variant rescue to similar degrees; (ii) a 50% PS1 reduction in PS1$^{\pm}$ mice did not cause an Aβ1–42 increase; (iii) expression of human mutant PS1 on murine PS1 null background is sufficient to elevate Aβ1–42 levels (Davis *et al.* 1998; Qian *et al.* 1998). After the *sel-12* rescue assay the 'Aβ1–42 increase test' has recently become the second functional assay to characterize structure-(dys)function relationships in the presenilin proteins. A presenilin mutant protein conferring increased Aβ1–42 production upon transfection is modified by site directed mutagenesis, transfected and the Aβ1–42 effect is compared with that of the original presenilin mutant. Using this assay one can dissect functional domains of the presenilin proteins. Two recent publications have used this approach to demonstrate that overexpression of a mutant NTF of PS1 (Citron *et al.* 1998) or PS2 (Tomita *et al.* 1998) is not sufficient to cause the Aβ1–42 effect. Instead, overexpression of the holoprotein is required. An even more intriguing result is the recent finding that the entire loop domain of PS1 is dispensable for the Aβ1–42 effect (amino acids 305–372 were deleted; G. Thinakaran, personal communication). This immediately implies that all loop binding proteins (the vast majority of all proposed presenilin binding candidates including β-catenin) are irrelevant for the Aβ1–42 effect (and therefore presumably the pathogenic process). Similar approaches will soon allow the definition of the minimal pathogenic region of presenilin. This will lead to a better understanding of how presenilin mutations cause the specific Aβ1–42 increase.

7.5 Questions and conclusions

(1) What is the role of wild type presenilin in the adult animal? The normal biological function of the presenilins remains unclear. The standard functionation approaches of making knockouts and transgenics have not yet led to a precise picture of the role of

presenilin in the adult brain, but conditional knockouts will be very useful in answering the question. PS1 seems to be a critical cofactor in γ-secretase cleavage of APP. The only functional assay for presenilin activity is complementation of an egg-laying defect in *C. elegans.*

(2) Which of the many presenilin binding protein candidates are really important? In the absence of good assays for presenilin function this question is difficult to address. One might want to focus on candidates that could be involved in the pathogenic process. Such candidates could bind differently to wild type versus mutant presenilin and should not bind to presenilin regions which are dispensable for the Aβ1–42 effect.

(3) How do presenilin mutations cause FAD? Although the mechanistic details have yet to be elucidated, it has been rigorously demonstrated that presenilin mutations linked to FAD consistently and specifically increase Aβ1–42 production, most likely by a gain of function mechanism. Thus, by increasing Aβ1–42 production, presenilin mutants initiate the β-amyloid cascade. Up to now studies suggesting alternative pathogenesis models, such as enhanced apoptosis due to presenilin mutations, have either not been extended to include several mutations and/or have not been reproducible by other groups.

(4) Is anything fundamentally different between the effects of APP mutations and presenilin mutations? At first glance, there appears to be no difference. However, the fact that presenilin pathology is not modulated by *APOE* genotype (in contrast to APP mutant cases) remains puzzling and needs to be explained.

(5) Could presenilin be a therapeutic target? The knockout data suggest that eliminating PS1 would dramatically reduce Aβ production. One could therefore screen for presenilin function inhibitors and hope to indirectly reduce Aβ production. Whether such a strategy is superior to direct inhibition of secretase enzymes remains to be seen. The immediate obstacle for such a screen is the absence of a functional assay for PS1.

Acknowledgements

I would like to thank Drs G. Thinakaran and C. Haass for sharing unpublished data.

Editor's note added in proof — recent data

ⅼ Putative identification of γ-secretase

Four recent reports, all presented in the same issue of *Nature* (DeStrooper *et al.* 1999; Struhl and Greenwald 1999; Wolfe *et al.* 1999*b*; Ye *et al.* 1999), provide strong evidence that PS1 is directly involved in γ-secretase activity and may even be γ-secretase itself. See Appendix VI for a more complete description of these four papers.

ⅼⅼ PS2 knockout mouse

Bart DeStrooper and colleagues describe the phenotype of the PS2 knockout mouse and also the PS1/PS2 double homozygous knockout mouse (Herreman *et al.* 1999). Previously it was reported that a PS1 knockout results in premature death (Shen *et al.* 1997; Wong *et al.* 1997). The PS2 knockout however, was largely unaffected except for mild pulmonary fibrosis. Microscopic examination of the brain and other organs revealed no abnormalities in tissue structure, but from age 3 months onwards animals displayed thickening of alveoli walls and haemorrhaging. APP processing was not altered and no obvious changes in apoptotic processes. By contrast the double homozygous PS1/PS2 knockout is more affected even than the PS1 knockout, indicating that PS2 also has some involvement in Notch processing.

References

Baumeister, R., Leimer, U., Zweckbronner, I., *et al.* (1997). Human presenilin-1, but not familial Alzheimer's disease (FAD) mutants, facilitate *Caenorhabditis elegans* Notch signalling independently of proteolytic processing. *Genes Function,* 1, 149–59.

Borchelt, D. R., Thinakaran, G., Eckman, C. B., *et al.* (1996). Familial Alzheimer's disease-linked presenilin 1 variants elevate As1–42/1–40 ratio *in vitro* and *in vivo. Neuron,* 17, 1005–13.

Borchelt, D. R., Ratovitski, T., van Lare, J., *et al.* (1997). Accelerated amyloid deposition in the brains of transgenic mice coexpressing mutant presenilin 1 and amyloid precursor proteins. *Neuron,* 19, 939–45.

Brockhaus, M., Grünberg, J., Röhrig, S., *et al.* (1998) Caspase-mediated cleavage is not required for the activity of presenilins in amyloidogenesis and NOTCH signaling. *Neuroreport,* 9, 1481–6.

Buxbaum, J.D., Choi, E.K., Luo, Y.X., *et al.* (1998). Calsenilin: A calcium-binding protein that interacts with the presenilins and regulates the levels of a presenilin fragment. *Nature Medicine,* 4, 1177–81.

Capell, A., Grünberg, J., Pesold, B., *et al.* (1998). The proteolytic fragments of the Alzheimer's disease-associated presenilin-1 from heterodimers and occur as a 100–150-kDa molecular mass complex. *Journal of Biological Chemistry,* 273, 3205–11.

Citron, M., Oltersdorf, T., Haass, C., *et al.* (1992). Mutation of the β-amyloid precursor protein in familial Alzheimer's disease increases β-protein production. *Nature,* 360, 672–4.

Citron, M., Westaway, D., Xia, W., *et al.* (1997). Mutant presenilins of Alzheimer's disease increase production of 42-residue amyloid β-protein in both transfected cells and transgenic mice. *Nature Medicine,* 3, 67–72.

Citron, M., Eckman, C. B., Diehl, T. S., *et al.* (1998). Additive effects of PS1 and APP mutations on secretion of the 42-residue amyloid β-protein. *Neurobiology of Disease,* 5, 107–16.

Clark, R. F. and Alzheimer's Disease Collaborative Research Group (1995). The structure of the presenilin 1 (S182) gene and identification of six novel mutations in early onset AD families. *Nature Genetics,* 11, 219–22.

Cruts, M., Hendriks, L., and Van Broeckhoven, C. (1996). The presenilin genes: a new gene family involved in Alzheimer's disease pathology. *Human Molecular Genetics,* 5, 1449–55.

Davis, J. A., Naruse, S., Chen, H., *et al.* (1998). An Alzheimer's disease-linked PS1 variant rescues the developmental abnormalities of PS1-deficient embryos. *Neuron,* 20, 603–9.

De Strooper, B., Beullens, M., Contreras, B., *et al.* (1997) Phosphorylation, subcellular localization and membrane orientation of the Alzheimer's disease associated presenilins. *Journal of Biological Chemistry,* 272, 3590–8.

De Strooper, B., Saftig, P., Craessaerts, K., *et al.* (1998). Deficiency of presenilin-1 inhibits the normal cleavage of amyloid precursor protein. *Nature,* 391, 387–91.

De Strooper, B., Annaert, W., Cupers, P., *et al.* (1999). A presenilin-1-dependent gamma-secretase-like protease mediates release of Notch intracellular domain. Nature, 398, 518–22.

Doan, A., Thinakaran, G., Borchelt, D. R., *et al.* (1996). Protein topology of presenilin 1. *Neuron,* 17, 1023–30.

Duff, K., Eckman, C., Zehr, C., *et al.* (1996). Increased amyloid-β42(43) in brains of mice expressing mutant presenilin 1. *Nature,* 383, 710–13.

Herreman, A., Hartmann, D., Annaert, W., *et al.* (1999). Presenilin 2 deficiency causes a mild pulmonary phenotype and no changes in amyloid precursor protein processing but enhances the embryonic lethal phenotype of presenilin 1 deficiency. *Proceedings of the National Academy of Science (USA)*, **96**, 11872–7.

Holcomb, L., Gordon, M. N., McGowan, E., *et al.* (1998). Accelerated Alzheimer-type phenotype in transgenic mice carrying both mutant amyloid precursor protein and presenilin 1 transgenes. *Nature Medicine*, **4**, 97–100.

Hong, C. S. and Koo, E. H. (1997). Isolation and characterization of Drosophila presenilin homolog. *Neuroreport*, **3**, 665–8.

Kim, T. W., Pettingell, W. H., Hallmark, O. G., *et al.* (1997). Endoproteolytic cleavage and proteasomal degradation of presenilin 2 in transfected cells. *Journal of Biological Chemistry*, **272**, 11006–10.

Kovacs, D. M., Fausett, H. J., Page, K. J., *et al.* (1996). Alzheimer-associated presenilins 1 and 2: neuronal expression in brain and localization to intracellular membranes in mammalian cells. *Nature Medicine*, **2**, 224–9.

Lee, M. K., Slunt, H. H., Martin, L. J., *et al.* (1996). Expression of presenilin 1 and 2 (PS1 and PS2) in human and murine tissues. *Journal of Neuroscience*, **16**, 7513–25.

Lehman, S., Chiesa, R., and Harris, D. A. (1997). Evidence for a six-transmembrane domain structure of presenilin 1. *Journal of Biological Chemistry*, **272**, 12047–51.

Lemere, C. A., Lopera, F., Kosik, K. S., *et al.* (1996). The E280A presenilin 1 mutation leads to a distinct Alzheimer's disease phenotype: increased $A\beta_{42}$ deposition and severe cerebellar pathology. *Nature Medicine*, **2**, 1146–50.

Levitan, D. and Greenwald, I. (1995). Facilitation of *lin-12* -mediated signalling by *sel-12*, a *Caenorhabditis elegans* S182 Alzheimer's disease gene. *Nature*, **377**, 351–4.

Levitan, D., Doyle, T. G., Brousseau, D., *et al.* (1996). Assessment of normal and mutant human presenilin function in *Caenorhabditis elegans*. *Proceedings of the National Academy of Science (USA)*, **93**, 14940–4.

Levy-Lahad, E., Wasco, W., Poorkaj, P., *et al.* (1995). Candidate gene for the chromosome 1 familial Alzheimer's disease locus. *Science*, **269**, 973–7.

Levy-Lahad, E., Poorkaj, P., Wang, K., *et al.* (1996). Genomic structure and expression of STM2, the chromosome 1 familial Alzheimer's disease gene. *Genomics*, **34**, 198–204.

Lopera, F., Ardilla, A., Martinez, A., *et al.* (1997). Clinical features of early-onset Alzheimer disease in a large kindred with an E280A presenilin-1 mutation. *Journal of the American Medical Association*, **277**, 793–9.

Mehta, N. D., Refolo, L. M., Eckman, C., *et al.* (1998). Increased Aβ42(43) from cell lines expressing presenilin 1 mutations. *Annals of Neurology*, **43**, 256–8.

Naruse, S., Thinakaran, G., Luo, J. J., *et al.* (1998). Effects of PS1 deficiency on membrane protein trafficking in neurons. *Neuron*, **21**, 1213–21.

Nishimura, M., Yu, G., Levesque, G., *et al.* (1999). Presenilin mutations associated with Alzheimer disease cause defective intracellular trafficking of beta-catenin, a component of the presenilin protein complex. *Nature Medicine*, **5**, 164–9.

Page, K., Hollister, R., Tanzi, R. E., and Hyman, B. T. (1996). In situ hybridization analysis of presenilin 1 mRNA in Alzheimer disease and in lesioned rat brain. *Proceedings of the National Academy of Science (USA)*, **93**, 14020–4.

Perez-Tur, J., Froehlich, S., Prihar, G., *et al.* (1995). A mutation in Alzheimer's disease destroying a splice acceptor site in the presenilin-1 gene. *Neuroreport*, **7**, 297–301.

Podlisny, M. B., Citron, M., Amarante, P., *et al.* (1997). Presenilin proteins undergo heterogeneous endoproteolysis between Thr291 and Ala299 and occur as stable N- and C-terminal fragments in normal and Alzheimer brain tissue. *Neurobiology of Disease*, **3**, 325–37.

Prihar, G., Fuldner, R. A., Perez-Tur, J., *et al.* (1996). Structure and alternative splicing of the presenilin-2 gene. *Neuroreport,* 7, 1680–4.

Qian, S., Jiang, P., Guan, X. M., *et al.* (1998). Mutant human presenilin 1 protects presenilin 1 null mouse against embryonic lethality and elevates Aβ1–42/43 expression. *Neuron,* 20, 611–17.

Ratovitsky, T., Slunt, H. H., Thinakaran, G., *et al.* (1997). Endoproteolytic processing and stabilization of wild-type and mutant presenilin. *Journal of Biological Chemistry,* 272, 24536–41.

Rogaev, E. I., Sherrington, R., Rogaeva, E. A., *et al.* (1995). Familial Alzheimer's disease in kindreds with missense mutations in a gene on chromosome 1 related to the Alzheimer's disease type 3 gene. *Nature,* 376, 775–8.

Scheuner, D., Eckman, C., Jensen, M., *et al.* (1996). Secreted amyloid β-protein similar to that in the senile plaques of Alzheimer's disease is increased in vivo by the presenilin 1 and 2 and APP mutations linked to familial Alzheimer's disease. *Nature Medicine,* 2, 864–70.

Shen, J., Bronson, R. T., Chen, D. F., *et al.* (1997). Skeletal and CNS defects in presenilin-1-deficient mice. *Cell,* 89, 629–39.

Sherrington, R., Rogaev, E. I., Liang, Y., *et al.* (1995). Cloning of a novel gene bearing missense mutations in early onset familial Alzheimer disease. *Nature,* 375, 754–60.

Sherrington, R., Froelich, S., Sorbi, S., *et al.* (1996). Alzheimer's disease associated with mutations in presenilin-2 are rare and variably penetrant. *Human Molecular Genetics,* 5, 985–8.

Shinozaki, K., Maruyama, K., Kume, H., *et al.* (1998). The presenilin 2 loop domain interacts with the mu-calpain C- terminal region. *International Journal of Molecular Medicine,* 1:797–9.

Steiner, H., Capell, A., Pesold, B., *et al.* (1998). Expression of Alzheimer's disease-associated presenilin-1 is controlled by proteolytic degradation and complex formation. *Journal of Biological Chemistry,* 273, 15309–15312

Struhl, G. and Greenwald, I. (1999). Presenilin is required for activity and nuclear access of Notch in Drosophila. *Nature,* 398, 522–5.

Suzuki, N., Cheung, T. T., Cai, X.-D., *et al.* (1994). An increased percentage of long amyloid β protein secreted by familial amyloid β protein precursor (βAPP717) mutants. *Science,* 264, 1336–40.

Takashima, A, Murayama, M, Murayama, O, *et al.* (1998). Presenilin 1 associates with glycogen synthase kinase-3 beta and its substrate tau. *Proceedings of the National Academy of Sciences (USA),* 95, 9637–41.

Tesco, G., Kim, T.W., Diehlmann, A., *et al.* (1998). Abrogation of the presenilin 1 beta-catenin interaction and preservation of the heterodimeric presenilin 1 complex following caspase activation. *Journal of Biological Chemistry,* 273, 33909- 14.

Thinakaran, G., Borchelt, D. R., Lee, M. K., *et al.* (1996). Endoproteolysis of presenilin 1 and accumulation of processed derviatives *in vivo. Neuron,* 17, 181–90.

Thinakaran, G., Harris, C. L., Ratovitski, T., *et al.* (1997). Evidence that levels of presenilins (PS1 and PS2) are coordinately regulated by competition for limiting cellular factors. *Journal of Biological Chemistry,* 272, 28415–22.

Thinakaran, G., Regard, J. B., Bouton, C. M. L., *et al.* (1998). Stable association of presenilin derivatives and absence of presenilin interactions with APP. *Neurobiology of Disease,* 4, 438–53.

Tomita, T., Maruyama, K., Saido, T. C., *et al.* (1997). The presenilin 2 mutation (N141I) linked to familial Alzheimer disease (Volga German families) increases the secretion of amyloid β protein ending at the 42nd (or 43rd) residue. *Proceedings of the National Academy of Science (USA),* 94, 2025–30.

Tomita, T., Tokuhiro, S., Hashimoto, T., *et al.* (1998). Molecular dissection of domains in mutant presenilin 2 that mediate overproduction of amyloidogenic forms of amyloid β peptides. *Journal of Biological Chemistry,* 273, 21153–60.

Van Broeckhoven, C., Backhoven, H., Cruts, M., *et al.* (1994). ApoE genotype does not modulate age of onset in families with chromosome 14 encoded Alzheimer's disease. *Neuroscience Letters,* 169, 179–80.

Vito, P., Lacana, E., and D'Adamio, L. (1996). Interfering with apoptosis: Ca^{2+}-binding protein ALG-2 and Alzheimer's disease gene ALG-3. *Science*, 271, 521–5.

Walter, J., Capell, A., Grünberg, J., *et al.* (1996). The Alzheimer's disease-associated presenilins are differentially phosphorylated proteins located predominantly within the endoplasmic reticulum. *Molecular Medicine*, 2, 673–91.

Weidemann, A., Paliga, K., Dürrwang, U., *et al.* (1997). Formation of stable complexes between two Alzheimer's disease gene products: presenilin-2 and β-amyloid precursor protein. *Nature Medicine*, 3, 328–32.

Wolfe, M.S., Xia, W.M., Ostaszewski, B.L., *et al.* (1999). Two transmembrane aspartates in presenilin-1 required for presenilin endoproteolysis and gamma-secretase activity. *Nature*, 398, 513–17.

Wolozin, B., Iwasaki, K., Vito, P., *et al.* (1996). Requirement of the familial Alzheimer's disease gene PS-2 for apoptosis. *Science*, 274, 1710–1713.

Wong, P. C., Zheng, H., Chen, H., *et al.* (1997). Presenilin 1 is required for Notch1 and Dll1 expression in the paraxial mesoderm. *Nature*, 387, 288–92.

Yasuda, M., Maeda, K., Hashimoto, M., *et al.* (1999). A pedigree with a novel presenilin 1 mutation at a residue that is not conserved in presenilin 2. *Archives of Neurology*, 56, 65–9.

Ye, Y.H., Lukinova, N., Fortini, M.E. (1999). Neurogenic phenotypes and altered Notch processing in *Drosophila* Presenilin mutants. *Nature*, 398, 525–9.

Yu, G., Chen, F.S., Levesque, G., *et al.* (1998). The presenilin 1 protein is a component of a high molecular weight intracellular complex that contains beta-catenin. *Journal of Biological Chemistry*, 273, 16470–5.

Zhang, J., Kang, D. E., Xia, W., *et al.* (1998*a*). Subcellular distribution and turnover of presenilins in transfected cells. *Journal of Biological Chemistry*, 273, 12436–42.

Zhang, Z.H., Hartmann, H., Do, V.M., *et al.* (1998*b*). Destabilization of beta-catenin by mutations in presenilin-1 potentiates neuronal apoptosis. *Nature*, 395, 698–702.

Zhang, W.J., Han, S.W., McKeel, D.W., *et al.* (1998*c*). Interaction of presenilins with the filamin family of actin- binding proteins. *Journal of Neuroscience*, 18, 914–22.

Zhou, J.H., Liyanage, U., Medina, M., H *et al.* (1997) Presenilin 1 interaction in the brain with a novel member of the Armadillo family. *Neuroreport*, 8, 2085–90.

Chapter 8

Transgenic models of Alzheimer's disease neuropathology

Karen Duff

8.1 Introduction

Patients with Alzheimer's disease (AD) have a characteristic neuropathology which is associated with neurodegeneration and cognitive impairment. At post mortem, the disease is characterized by the presence in the brain of extra-cellular plaques composed mainly of a deposited protein fragment called beta amyloid (Aβ), and intracellular neurofibrillary tangles (NFT) composed of an abnormal form of the tau protein. The brain shows degeneration, especially in neurons involved in the cholinergic system, which is thought to underlie the cognitive problems that give rise to dementia. The development of plaques and tangles, neurodegeneration, cholinergic dysfunction, and cognitive impairment therefore appear to be linked, but it is not clear how degeneration is initiated and why some areas of the brain are more sensitive to degeneration than others.

To address these questions, scientists have looked to animal models. These fall into several categories including aged animals, lesioned animals, and genetically engineered animals.

Aged animals: Aged animals ranging from rodents, cats, dogs, polar bears, and monkeys have been examined for AD related pathologic and behavioural changes (Cummings *et al.* 1996; Tekirian *et al.* 1996; Gearing *et al.* 1997; Geula *et al.* 1998). Rodents do not develop any of the hallmark features of AD upon ageing, but cats and higher animals do show some accumulation of amyloid (diffuse and/or compact). Only polar bears appear to show neurofibrillary pathology (Tekirian *et al.* 1996). As most of the animal models need to age for many years, they are not realistic model animals for extensive research purposes. More recently, aged monkeys injected with fibrillar beta-amyloid were shown to undergo neurodegeneration, making these animals more informative models of AD than non-injected animals.

Lesioned animals: Most of the lesioned animals have been generated to study the effect of cholinergic deficit on cognitive function, and its restoration by drug therapy (reviewed by Smith 1988; Muir *et al.* 1993; Myhrer 1993; Wenk 1993; Muir 1997). Unfortunately, several of the drugs that restore deficits in lesioned animals, do not ameliorate cognitive impairment in AD patients and although useful in the study of neurochemistry, these animals have had little use in drug development for AD.

Genetically engineered animals: Since the identification of pathogenic mutations in several genes, researchers have attempted to genetically engineer rodents to model AD. Because of their short generation time and low cost, transgenic rodents have been studied extensively. The following article describes the rationale, usefulness and drawbacks of this model system.

8.2 Genetic analysis suggests a unifying mechanism in AD aetiology

There are four well-recognized risk factors in human AD: genetic lesions, Down syndrome, environmental insult (such as head injury), and old age. The genetic forms were the first to be studied and have given us great insight into some of the causes of AD. In 1991, John Hardy and his colleagues used linkage analysis to demonstrate that a mutation at codon 717 of the amyloid precursor protein (*APP*) gene caused classic, early onset familial AD in a small number of families (Goate *et al.* 1991). Since then, several other mutations have been identified in *APP*; two in the same codon (Murrell *et al.* 1991, Chartier-Harlin *et al.* 1991), one in the adjacent codon (Eckman *et al.* 1997), and a double mutation at codons 670 and 671 (Mullan *et al.* 1992). Although the *APP* mutations only account for a total of 5% of early onset cases (less than 1% of the total number of AD cases), they were the first indication that APP may be the culprit in AD. Several groups have subsequently identified AD causing mutations in genes other than *APP*. Mutations in the presenilin 1 (*PS1*) gene on chromosome 14 (Sherrington *et al.* 1995) account for most of the early onset cases of familial AD (FAD), whereas mutations in the closely related presenilin 2 (*PS2*) gene on chromosome 1 are associated with late onset AD (Levy-Lahad *et al.* 1995) (see Cruts *et al.* 1996 for review). Most of the familial cases of late onset AD, however, are caused by a polymorphism in the apolipoprotein E (*APOE*) gene on chromosome 19 where it seems that certain allelic combinations of the apoE protein are particular risky for AD (Corder *et al.* 1993, 1994).

Researchers first focused their attention on the APP protein for three simple reasons; mutations in the *APP* gene are known to cause AD, an extra copy of the *APP* gene due to trisomy 21 is linked to AD in Down syndrome, and the Aβ region of APP makes up the core of the AD amyloid plaque. The *APP* gene is located on chromosome 21 and is expressed as several alternatively spliced transcripts, the most abundant of which encode proteins of 770, 751, and 695 amino acids (Yoshikai *et al.* 1991). The precursor protein undergoes a complex series of post-translational processing events that release the bulk of the protein into the extra-cellular space. Events at the C terminal can generate a range of fragments including the potentially amyloidogenic beta amyloid fragment. This peptide exists in several forms but the most abundant is 40 amino acids long and is known as Aβ1–40. A less abundant species is 42 (or 43) amino acids long and has been designated Aβ1–42(43).

Under certain conditions both types of Aβ have the potential to form insoluble, fibrillar, beta pleated strands of amyloid that are deposited in specific regions of the brain. *In vitro* studies on synthetic Aβ have shown that this tendency to fibrillarize increases when hydrophobic residues are included at the carboxy terminal (that is extending the molecule from Aβ1–40 to Aβ1–42(43); Jarrett *et al.* 1993). Cells transfected with an APP cDNA containing the double mutation at codons 670 and 671 have been shown to produce an approximate six-fold increase in Aβ fragments compared to cells transfected with a non mutant gene (Citron *et al.* 1992; Cai *et al.* 1993). The 716 and 717 mutations on the other hand do not lead to an increase in the amount of Aβ but lead to an increase in the amount of the

Aβ1–42(43) form relative to Aβ1–40 (Suzuki *et al.* 1994; Eckman *et al.* 1997). Mutations in the *APP* gene are not the only influencing factor on APP processing however. Researchers have found that the level of Aβ1–42(43) is elevated relative to Aβ1–40 in fibroblasts isolated from AD patients known to carry mutations in the *PS1* gene (Scheuner *et al.* 1996). Thus in individuals with APP or PS mutations, AD may be caused by perturbations in APP metabolism and elevation of the Aβ1–42(43) form of Aβ may be the critical pathogenic event. Although we now know that the causes of AD are heterogeneous, the phenotype is remarkably consistent, with amyloid plaques and NFT being the main pathognomic features. The relative contributions of amyloid plaques and NFT to AD dementia have been contested since the pathology of the disease was first described in 1904. However, AD causing genetic lesions in different genes all influence Aβ accumulation. This simple fact continues to convince many that Aβ is at the root of disease aetiology with tau possibly having an indirect, secondary role.

8.3 Genetically engineered models: history of the field

The race to generate an animal model for AD began in 1991 when the first APP mutation was discovered. Since then, several different approaches have been undertaken to produce a mouse model with the hallmarks of AD; plaques, tangles, neurodegeneration, and cognitive deficits. These approaches fall into three main categories: cDNA over-expression models, whole gene over-expression models, and gene targeted models. Although several models have now been created (Games *et al.* 1995; Borchelt *et al.* 1996; Duff *et al.* 1996; Hsiao *et al.* 1996; Nalbantoglu *et al.* 1997; Sturchler-Pierrat *et al.* 1997; Citron *et al.* 1997), a mouse with all features of the phenotype, including amyloid accumulation, tangle formation, cell loss, and cognitive impairment has not yet been generated.

8.4 APP transgenic mice

Four transgenic APP lines have been described which show some of the pathology (essentially, neuritic plaques) of AD. The most robust of these include the Athena/Exemplar mouse (PDAPP) (Games *et al.* 1995), the Hsiao mouse (Tg2576) (Hsiao *et al.* 1996), and the Novartis mouse (Sturchler-Pierrat *et al.* 1997). The PDAPP mouse uses an *APP* mini-gene containing the *APP* I717F mutation with expression driven by the Platelet-derived growth factor (PDGF) promoter. The Hsiao mouse uses an *APP*695 cDNA with the K/M670/1N/L mutation, driven by the human prion promoter, whereas the Novartis mouse uses an *APP*751 K/M670/1N/L construct under the control of a thy-1 promoter. These mice produce high levels of total Aβ (in excess of 20 pm/g wet weight tissue) and all develop amyloid deposits in the cortex and hippocampus between 6 months and 1 year of age. None develop tangles or PHF, although some abnormally phosphorylated tau immunoreactivity is seen in the vicinity of the deposits (Sturchler-Pierrat 1997), which is reminiscent of early stage PHF formation in the humans. One interpretation is that Aβ accumulation and/or deposition initiates tau pathology in both mice and humans, but in mice, physiological differences or differences between mouse and human Tau isofoms or representivity precludes the formation of AD type tauopathy. The two mice with the highest amyloid load (PDAPP and Tg2576) do not show extensive cell loss (Irizarry *et al.* 1997*a, b.*) but claims of cell loss in the Novartis mouse have been made. The Tg2576 mouse has been reported to show behavioural abnormalities suggestive of age related hippocampal dysfunction (Hsiao *et al.*

1996) but the PDAPP mouse has been shown to be cognitively impaired from a young age, with no further impairment developing with increased age and amyloid burden (Justice and Motter 1997). It therefore seems that these mice are reliable models of amyloid deposition, but cannot yet be considered to be models for human AD.

8.5 Presenilin transgenic mice

Although the functions of the presenilins are not understood, the identification of two *C. elegans* isologues of PS1 (reviewed in Haass 1997) have provided some clues. The first isologue is *spe-4*. Mutations in this gene disrupt spermatogenesis through disruption of protein trafficking in the Golgi. The second isologue is *sel-12*: mutations in which produce an egg-laying defect, probably through disruption of the Notch signalling pathway. A functional relationship between *sel-12* and *PS1* is illustrated by the observation that *PS1* can rescue *sel-12* mutant *C. elegans* (reviewed in Haass 1997), and further support for a role of the PS in Notch signalling comes from the observation that PS1 knockout mice show developmental abnormalities similar to those seen in mice in which components of the Notch system have been knocked out (Conlon *et al.* 1995; Wong *et al.* 1997). A role for the presenilins (particularly PS2) in apoptosis has also been proposed (Vito *et al.* 1996; Wolozin *et al.* 1996).

Presenilin biology has been examined *in vivo* through the creation of transgenic mice. Mice from different labs (Borchelt *et al.* 1996; Duff *et al.* 1996; Citron *et al.* 1997) differ in the promoter and strain of mice used but were similar in achieving high levels of protein production (1–3 fold over endogenous) in neuronal regions of the brain. Full length PS1 (at 46 kDa) was only seen in mice producing large amounts of human protein as expected from studies of transfected cells that show that the protein is rapidly turned over (Thinakaran *et al.* 1996). The holoprotein undergoes endoproteolytic cleavage in a highly regulated manner, generating terminal derivatives that accumulate to saturable levels at a 1:1 stoichiometry (Thinakaram *et al.* 1996). This was also seen in the mouse brain where the transgene derived protein was processed correctly into 18 kDa N terminal and 28 kDa C terminal fragments. The human fragments have slightly retarded mobility on a gel compared to the endogenous mouse PS1 derivatives and when the levels of both mouse and human derivatives were compared directly, the presence of the human protein led to diminished accumulation of the mouse PS1 fragments (Lee *et al.* 1997). Both transgenic mice and transfected cells overexpressing an exon 9 deletion (ΔE9) cDNA do not show cleavage of the mutant protein; however, the mice still show a reduction in the amount of mouse PS1 fragments (Lee *et al.* 1997). The reason for diminution in the mouse cleavage products is as yet unclear. Perhaps the most interesting observation so far is that the fragments derived from mutant PS1 accumulate to a greater degree than fragments from wild type PS1 (Lee *et al.* 1997). Moreover, the uncleaved ΔE9 mutant cDNA also accumulates to a greater degree than the fragments derived from wild type human PS1 (Lee *et al.* 1997). These observations together suggest that the mutations in PS1 somehow affect the protein's metabolism but how that relates to the pathogenesis of AD remains to be seen.

Perhaps the greatest insight into how mutations in PS1 might cause AD has come from the analysis of Aβ levels in mice overexpressing mutant and wild type *PS1* transgenes. A report by Scheuner *et al.* (1996) on Aβ levels in fibroblasts from AD patients with *PS1* mutations first indicated a link between PS1 and APP processing. Descriptions of the same effect in mouse brain tissue in all three sets of PS1 transgenic mice have now been published. The first report (Duff *et al.* 1996) examined the levels of mouse Aβ1–40 and 1–42(43) using a sandwich enzyme linked immunoreactive assay (ELISA) system. The two subsequent reports (Borchelt *et al.* 1996; Citron *et al.* 1996) examined the level of human Aβ derived from a mutant human *APP* transgene that had been crossed into the PS1 mice. All three reports showed similar results: overexpressing mutant PS1 in the brains of transgenic mice led to the elevation of Aβ1–42, but not Aβ1–40. This effect was a direct result of the mutation and not overexpression of the human protein as the overexpression of wild-type PS1 did not have any significant effect on Aβ levels. The physiological significance of the specific elevation of Aβ1–42(43) appears to be the observation that AD patients with *PS1* mutations show plaques composed primarily of Aβ1–42(43) (Mann *et al.* 1996). The fact that AD causing mutations in *APP* and *PS1* both lead to an elevation in Aβ strongly suggests that this event is a significant and possibly crucial mechanism underlying the aetiology of AD.

The mice are currently undergoing intensive analysis in several labs for any changes in behaviour , electrophysiology, pathology, and biochemistry but the results are likely to be subtle, especially if the AD phenotype in PS1 linked cases is related solely to Aβ levels and not to a defect in the PS1 protein itself. So far, the only other phenotype identified in the PS1 mutant mice has been a disruption in intracellular calcium levels (Barrow *et al.* submitted for publication), but although of relevance to AD, the disruption does not lead to obvious neurotoxicity resulting in cell death. Mice have been examined for AD related changes in histopathology, but no obvious changes have been observed. Recently, the elevation of Aβ1–42 specifically in PS2 mutant mice has been reported which agrees with published reports for PS2 transfected cells (Tomita *et al.* 1997). There are no reports of targeted (knock-in) mutant PS1/2 mice although they are currently under construction in several labs.

8.6 Tau transgenic mice

One of the deficits of the current AD transgenic models is the lack of tau pathology. In humans, tau pathology takes the form of intracellular tangles of an abnormally phosphorylated form of the tau protein, which associates into paired helical filaments (PHF). Both amyloid plaques and tau tangles are pathognomic features of human AD, and their relative contribution to the disease has long been disputed. The identification of AD-causing mutations in APP in 1991 added weight to the amyloid based hypothesis of pathogenesis, which assumes that tau abnormalities are a secondary lesion that form in response to amyloid accumulation. On careful examination, transgenic mice with extensive amyloid deposition have been shown to develop tau abnormalities, in the form of elevated hyper-phosphorylayed tau immunoreactivity around deposits (Sturchler-Pierrat *et al.* 1997). Some disruption of tau may occur in response to amyloid accumulation, but it does not progress to resemble human tauopathy. The idea that a species barrier prevents this progression has recently been reinforced by data from the Yankner group (Geula *et al.* 1998) suggesting that primates and rodents differ in their response to injected amyloid not only in terms of neurodegeneration, but also in the accumulation of abnormal tau around the injected amyloid. Whether the monkeys used in the study develop PHF or tangles has not yet been determined.

Several models have aimed to examine whether tau alone, and hyperphosphorylated tau especially, has the capacity to undergo pathogenic change. Transgenic mice that overexpress one of the isoforms of human tau (tau40, which contains four microtubule binding repeats), show some hyperphosphorylation but do not show any overt signs of neurodegeneration (Gotz *et al.* 1995). Mice that overexpress tau phosphorylating agents such as glycogen synthase kinase 3β (GSK-3β), have been created and do not show overt pathology, although the assessment of the mice has been confounded by an early lethality phenotype (C. Miller, personal communication).

Recently, the identification of mutations in tau that cause frontal temporal lobe dementia (FTDP-17) has placed tau back in the spotlight as a possible primary candidate for neurodegeneration (reviewed in Hardy *et al.* 1998). So far, genetic analysis has not linked tau mutations directly to AD, but tau dysfunction may still have a significant role to play in the disease, if not in its initiation, then in its progression. Several transgenic mice expressing different forms of the tau gene are currently underway to model the FTDP-17 diseases, which might also have utility in the modelling of AD.

8.7 Beyond amyloid: secondary phenotypes in amyloid depositing mice

Although there is good evidence that Aβ accumulation contributes to AD pathogenesis, it seems likely that AD is a multi-step disease, with several parts of the phenotype contributing to disease progression. This can be most clearly seen in AD patients with a huge amyloid burden who do not show signs of cognitive impairment (Snowdon *et al.* 1997), and in transgenic animals that have accumulated amyloid but do not show cell loss (Irizarry 1997*a*, *b*). In an attempt to examine how the cell responds to an environment of elevated and deposited amyloid, amyloid depositing mice have been examined for signs of cell disturbance such as tau phosphorylation (Sturchler-Pierrat *et al.* 1997), cholinergic system dysfunction, (Wong *et al.* unpublished data), oxidative damage (Smith *et al.* 1998), inflammatory/immune response (Frautschy *et al.* 1998), and morphological changes at the electron microscope level (Masliah *et al.* 1996) Although these secondary phenotypes do not lead to neurodegeneration in the mice, the effects in humans may be more detrimental, and possible therapeutics could therefore include inflamatories and antioxidants.

8.8 Modulating and enhancing the phenotype: transgenic crosses

One of the great advantages of transgenic animals is that different mice can be mated together so that the effect of transgene interaction on the disease phenotype can be observed. This type of cross has been reported by two labs, using different lines of mutant APP and mutant PS1 mice (Borchelt *et al.* 1997; Holcomb *et al.* 1998). In the cross performed by Borchelt and colleagues, an APP mouse that develops amyloid deposits at 18 months was crossed with a mutant PS1 line. The doubly transgenic PS/APP progeny develop visible amyloid deposits at nine months of age. In the cross performed by Holcomb *et al.* (1998) a mutant APP transgenic line, Tg2576 (Hsiao *et al.* 1996) and a mutant PS1 line, PDPS1 (Duff *et al.* 1996) were crossed. The Tg2576 line has been shown to develop Aβ deposits in the brain between 9 and 12 months of age, and deposition is temporally linked to Aβ elevation. The PDPS1 line shows an approximately 1.5 fold elevation of Aβ1–42(43) from birth. When these two animals are mated together, Aβ-containing deposits are observed in the cortex and hippocampus of doubly transgenic progeny as early as 12 weeks of age (Holcomb *et al.* 1998). It would appear therefore, that marginal increases in Aβ1–42(43) levels, evoked by the *PS1* mutant transgene, can accelerate the deposition process by several months (see Fig. 8.1). As the mice have a severe Aβ pathology for an

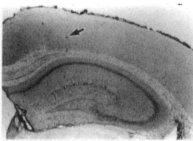

P/A 3m

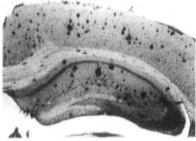

P/A 6m

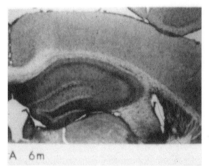

A 6m

Fig. 8.1 Brain sections from a PS/APP mouse at 3 months, at 6 months, and an APP singly transgenic littermate also at 6 months. Sections were stained with an antibody that recognizes human Aβ. Amyloid deposition is greatly accelerated in the doubly transgenic animal compared to the singly transgenic APP animal, and reproducible deposition is first visible at 10–12 weeks.

extended time relative to singly transgenic APP mice, other features of the disease such as tau abnormalities or major cell loss may become apparent as the animals age. If the lack of extensive tauopathy in the transgenic mice is due to differences between mouse and human tau, then it is possible that human tau isoforms introduced into the elevated amyloid environment of APP over-expressing mice might provide the substrate required for more severe tauopathy to develop. Crosses to tau over-expressing mice are currently underway.

Two other transgenic crosses have also given some insight into the process of pathology development in AD. Mucke and colleagues performed a cross between PDAPP and a line of mice over-expressing TGFβ and also showed an acceleration of deposition, especially in the vasculature (Wyss-Coray *et al.* 1997). Bales and colleagues crossed PDAPP to an apoE knockout line and showed that when apoE is removed from the brain environment, amyloid deposition is greatly retarded (Bales *et al.* 1997). As *APOE* genotype influences AD age of onset (Corder *et al.* 1993; 1994), it is possible that apoE isoforms differentially influence Aβ accumulation, thereby modulating the risk of developing AD. Conversely, apoE also appears to associate with tau (Strittmater *et al.* 1994) but the biochemical implications have not been well addressed.

8.9 Future directions

Disease modelling aims to generate an animal that recreates a human disease both for scientific investigation and as a model system in which to test therapeutic agents designed to alleviate, or inhibit the disease in humans. Attempts to model the disease have focused on recreating the pathology of AD in the hope that neurodegeneration and cognitive impairment will follow. Although extensive amyloid accumulation has now been achieved in the mice, the mice do not undergo extensive degeneration, although some subtle cell loss has been reported in two of the transgenic mouse lines (Nalbantoglu *et al.* 1997; Sturchler-Pierrat *et al.* 1997). It is early days in the analysis of the various mouse lines and the extent to which the phenotype of human AD has been recreated remains to be seen. However, if Aβ accumulation is central to the disease, then mouse models such as the *PS/APP* double transgenic will be useful for the testing of compounds designed to modulate Aβ levels.

Editor's note added in proof — recent data

PS2 knockout mouse

Bart DeStrooper and colleagues describe the phenotype of the PS2 knockout mouse and also the PS1/PS2 double homozygous knockout mouse (Herreman *et al.* 1999). This is described in further detail at the end of Chapter 7.

References

Bales, K. R., Verina, T., Dodel, R. C., *et al.* (1997). Lack of apolipoprotein E dramatically reduces amyloid beta-peptide deposition. *Nature Genetics*, 3, 263–4.

Borchelt, D. R., Thinakaran, G., Eckman, C. B., *et al.* (1996). Familial Alzheimer's disease-linked presenilin 1 variants elevate Aβ1–42/1–40 ratio *in vitro* and *in vivo*. *Neuron*, 5, 1005–13.

Borchelt, D. R., Ratovitski, T., van Lare, J., *et al.* (1997). Accelerated amyloid deposition in the brains of transgenic mice co-expressing mutant presenilin 1 and amyloid precursor proteins. *Neuron*, 4, 939–45.

Cai, X. D., Golde, T. E., and Younkin, S. G. (1993). Excess amyloid β production is released from a mutant amyloid β protein precursor linked to familiar Alzheimer's disease. *Science*, 259, 514–16.

Chartier-Harlin, M. C., Crawford, F., Houlden, H., *et al.* (1991) Early onset Alzheimer's disease caused by a mutation at codon 717 of the β- amyloid precursor protein gene. *Nature*, 353, 844–6.

Citron, M., Oltersdorf, T., Haass, C., *et al.* (1992) Mutation of the β-amyloid precursor protein in familial Alzheimer's disease increases b-protein production. *Nature*, 360, 672–4.

Citron, M., Westaway, D., Xia, W., *et al.* (1997) Mutant presenilins of Alzheimer's disease increase production of 42-residue amyloid beta-protein in both transfected cells and transgenic mice. *Nature Medicine*, 3, 67–72.

Conlon, R. A., Reaume, A. G., and Rossant, J. (1995). Notch1 is required for the coordinate segmentation of somites. *Development*, 121, 1533–45.

Corder, E., Saunders, A., Strittmatter, W., *et al.* (1993) Gene dose of apolipoprotein E type 4 allele and the risk of Alzheimer's disease in late onset families. *Science*, **261**, 921–3.

Corder, E. H., Saunders, A. M., Risch, N. J., *et al.* (1994). Protective effect of apolipoprotein E type 2 allele for late onset Alzheimer disease. *Nature Genetics*, **7**, 180–4.

Cruts, M., Hendriks, L., and Van Broeckhoven, C. (1996). The presenilin genes, a new gene family involved in Alzheimer's disease pathology. *Human Molecular Genetics*, **5**, 1449–55.

Cummings, B. J., Head, E., Ruehl, W., *et al.* (1996). The canine as an animal model of human ageing and dementia. *Neurobiology of Ageing*, **17**, 259–68.

Cummings, B. J., Satou, T., Head, E., *et al.* (1996). Diffuse plaques contain C-terminal A beta 42 and not A beta 40, evidence from cats and dogs. *Neurobiology of Ageing*, **17**, 653–9.

Duff, K., Eckman, C., Zehr, C., *et al.* (1996). Increased amyloid-β42(43) in brains of mice expressing mutant presenilin 1. *Nature*, **383**, 710–13.

Eckman, C. B., Mehta, N. D., Crook, R., *et al.* (1997). A new pathogenic mutation in the APP gene (I716V) increases the relative proportion of A-beta 42(43). *Human Molecular Genetics*, **12**, 2087–9.

Frautschy, S. A., Yang, F., Irrizarry, M., *et al.* (1998) Microglial response to amyloid plaques in APPsw transgenic mice. *American Journal of Pathology*, **152**, 307–17.

Games, D., Adams, D., Alessandrini, R., *et al.* (1995) Alzheimer-type neuropathology in transgenic mice over-expressing the V717F β-amyloid precursor protein. *Nature*, **373**, 523–7.

Gearing, M., Tigges, J., Mori, H., and Mirra, S. S. (1997). beta-Amyloid (A beta) deposition in the brains of aged orangutans. *Neurobiology of Ageing*, **18**, 139–46.

Geula, C., Wu, C. K., Saroff, D., *et al.* (1998) Ageing renders the brain vulnerable to amyloid beta-protein neurotoxicity. *Nature Medicine*, **4**, 827–31.

Goate, A., Chartier-Harlin, M. C., Mullan, M., *et al.* (1991). Segregation of a missense mutation in the amyloid precursor protein gene with familial Alzheimer's disease. *Nature*, **349**, 704–6.

Gotz, J., Probst, A., Spillantini, M. G., *et al.* (1995). Somatodendritic localization and hyperphosphorylation of tau protein in transgenic mice expressing the longest human brain tau isoform. *European Molecular Organisation Journal*, **14**, 1304–131.

Haass, C. (1997). Presenilins, genes for life and death. *Neuron*, **18**, 687–90.

Hardy, J. (1997). Amyloid, the presenilins and Alzheimer's disease. *Trends in Neuroscience*, **20**, 154–9.

Hardy, J., Duff, K., Gwinn-Hardy, K., *et al.* (1998). Genetic dissection of Alzheimer's disease and related dementia's, amyloid and its relationship to tau. *Nature Neuroscience*, **1**(5) p. 355–8.

Herreman, A., Hartmann, D., Annaert, W., *et al.* (1999). Presenilin 2 deficiency causes a mild pulmonary phenotype and no changes in amyloid precursor protein processing but enhances the embryonic lethal phenotype of presenilin 1 deficiency. *Proceedings of the National Academy of Science (USA)*, **96**, 11872–7.

Holcomb, L., Gordon, M. N., McGowan, E., *et al.* (1998). Accelerated Alzheimer-type phenotype in transgenic mice carrying both mutant amyloid precursor protein and presenilin 1 transgenes. *Nature Medicine*, **1**, 97–100.

Hsiao, K., Chapman, P., Nilsen, S., *et al.* (1996). Correlative memory deficits, Aβ elevation, and amyloid plaques in transgenic mice. *Science*, **274**, 99–102.

Irizarry, M. C., McNamara, M., Fedorchak, K., *et al.* (1997a). APPsw transgenic mice develop age-related A-beta deposits and neuropil abnormalities, but no neuronal loss in CA1. *Journal of Neuropathology and Experimental Neurology*, **9**, 965–73.

Irizarry, M. C., Soriano, F., McNamara, M., *et al.* (1997b). A-beta deposition is associated with neuropil changes, but not with overt neuronal loss in the human amyloid precursor protein V717F (PDAPP) transgenic mouse. *Journal of Neuroscience*, **17**, 7053–9.

Jarrett, J., Berger, E., and Lansbury, P. (1993). The carboxy terminus of β-amyloid protein is critical for the seeding of amyloid formation, implications for the pathogenesis of Alzheimer's disease. *Biochemistry*, **32**, 4693.

Justice, A. and Motter, R. (1997). Behavioural characterisation of PDAPP transgenic Alzheimer mice. Abs 636. 6, *Society for Neurosciences*, New Orleans.

Lee, M. K., Borchelt, D. R., Kim, G., *et al.* (1997). Hyperaccumulation of FAD-linked presenilin 1 variants *in vivo. Nature Medicine*, 3, 756–60.

Levy-Lahad, E., Wijsman, E. M., Nemens, E., *et al.* (1995). Candidate gene for the chromosome 1 familial Alzheimer's disease locus. *Science*, 269, 973–7.

Mann, D. M., Iwatsubo, T., Cairns, N. J., *et al.* (1996). Amyloid-β protein (Aβ) deposition in chromosome 14-linked Alzheimer's disease, predominance of Aβ42(43). *Annals of Neurology*, 40, 149–56.

Masliah, E., Sisk, A., Mallory, M., *et al.* (1996). Comparison of neurodegenerative pathology in transgenic mice overexpressing V717F beta-amyloid precursor protein and Alzheimer's disease. *Journal of Neuroscience*, 16, 5795–811.

Muir, J. L. (1997). Acetylcholine, ageing, and Alzheimer's disease. *Pharmacology and Biochemical Behaviour*, 56, 687–96.

Muir, J. L., Page, K. J., Sirinathsinghji, D. J., *et al.* (1993). Excitotoxic lesions of basal forebrain cholinergic neurons, effects on learning, memory and attention. *Behavioural Brain Research*, 57, 123–31.

Mullan, M. Crawford, F., Axelman, K., *et al.* (1992). A pathogenic mutation for probable Alzheimer's disease in the APP gene at the N-terminus of beta-amyloid. *Nature Genetics*, 1, 345–7.

Murrell, J. Farlow, M., Ghetti, B., and Benson, M. D. (1991). A mutation in the amyloid precursor protein associated with hereditary Alzheimer's disease. *Science*, 254, 97–9.

Myhrer, T. (1993). Animal models of Alzheimer's disease, glutamatergic denervation as an alternative approach to cholinergic denervation. *Neuroscience Biobehaviour Reviews*, 17, 195–202.

Nalbantoglu, J., Tirado-Santiago, G., Lahsaini, A., *et al.* (1997). Impaired learning and LTP in mice expressing the carboxy terminus of the Alzheimer amyloid precursor protein. *Nature*, 387, 500–5.

Scheuner, D., Eckman, C., Jensen, M., *et al.* (1996). The amyloid β-protein deposited in the senile plaques of Alzheimer's disease is increased *in vivo* by the presenilin 1 and 2 and APP mutations linked to familial Alzheimer's disease. *Nature Medicine*, 2, 864–70.

Sherrington, R., Rogaev, E. I., Liang, Y., *et al.* (1995). Cloning of a gene bearing missense mutations in early-onset familial Alzheimer's disease. *Nature*, 375, 754–60.

Smith, G. (1988). Animal models of Alzheimer's disease, experimental cholinergic denervation. *Brain Research*, 472, 103–18.

Smith, M. A., Hirai, K., Hsiao, K., *et al.* (1998). Amyloid-beta deposition in Alzheimer transgenic mice is associated with oxidative stress. *Journal of Neurochemistry*, 70, 2212–5.

Snowdon, D. A., Greiner, L. H., Mortimer, J. A., *et al.* (1997). Brain infarction and the clinical expression of Alzheimer disease. The Nun Study. *Journal of American Medical Association*, 277, 813–17.

Strittmatter, W. J., Saunders, A. M., Goedert, M., *et al.* (1994). Isoform-specific interactions of apolipoprotein E with microtubule-associated protein tau,implications for Alzheimer disease. *Proceedings of the National Academy of Science (USA)*, 91, 11183–6.

Sturchler-Pierrat, C., Abramowski, D., Duke, M., *et al.* (1997). Two amyloid precursor protein transgenic mouse models with Alzheimer disease-like pathology. *Proceedings of the National Academy of Science (USA)*, 94, 13287–92.

Suzuki, N., Cheung, T., Cai, X-D., *et al.* (1994). An increased percentage of long amyloid β protein secreted by familial amyloid β protein precursor (βAPP717) mutants. *Science*, 264, 1336–40.

Tekirian, T. L., Cole, G. M., Russell, M. J., *et al.* (1996). Carboxy terminal of beta-amyloid deposits in aged human, canine, and polar bear brains. *Neurobiology of Ageing*,17, 249–57.

Thinakaran, G., Borchelt, D. R., Lee, M. K., *et al.* (1996). Endoproteolysis of presenilin-1 and accumulation of processed derivatives *in vivo. Neuron*, 17, 181–90.

Tomita, T., Maruyama, K., Saido, T. C., *et al.* (1997). The presenilin 2 mutation (N141I) linked to familial Alzheimer disease (Volga German families) increases the secretion of amyloid β protein ending at the 42nd (or 43rd) residue. *Proceedings of the National Academy of Science (USA)*, **94**, 2025–30.

Vito, P., Lacana, E., and D'Adamio, L. (1996). Interfering with apoptosis, Ca($^{2+}$)-binding protein ALG-2 and Alzheimer's disease gene ALG-3. *Science*, **271**, 521–5.

Weidemann, A., Paliga, K., Durrwang, U., *et al.* (1997). Formation of stable complexes between two Alzheimer's disease gene products, presenilin-2 and b-amyloid precursor protein. *Nature Medicine*, **3**, 328–32.

Wenk, G. L. (1993). A primate model of Alzheimer's disease. *Behavioural Brain Research*, **57**, 117–22.

Wolozin, B., Iwasaki, K., Vito, P., *et al.* (1996). Participation of presenilin 2 in apoptosis, enhanced basal activity conferred by an Alzheimer Mutation. *Science*, **274**, 1710–13.

Wong, P. C., Zheng, H., Chen, H., *et al.* (1997). Presenilin 1 is required for Notch1 and DII1 expression in the paraxial mesoderm. *Nature*, **387**, 288–92.

Wyss-Coray, T., Masliah, E., Mallory, M., *et al.* (1997). Amyloidogenic role of cytokine TGF-beta1 in transgenic mice and in Alzheimer's disease. *Nature*, **389**, 603–6.

Yoshikai, S., Sasaki, H., Doh-ura, K., *et al.* (1991). Genomic organization of the human-amyloid beta-protein precursor gene. *Gene*, **102**, 291–2.

Chapter 9

Cellular targets of amyloid beta peptide: potential roles in neuronal cell stress and toxicity

Shi Du Yan, Alex Roher, Claudio Soto, Futwan Al-Mohanna, Kate Collison, Ann Marie Schmidt and David Stern

9.1 Introduction: cellular cofactors and Aβ-induced cellular dysfunction

Extracellular accumulations of amyloid in neuritic plaques, composed predominately of amyloid-beta peptide (Aβ), and intracellular neurofibrillary tangles (NFT), composed largely of hyperphosphorylated paired helical filament (PHF) tau, are pathognomonic features of Alzheimer's disease (AD) (Goedert 1993; Haass and Selkoe 1994; Kosik 1994; Trojanowski and Lee 1994; Yankner 1996). With time, these lesions increase in number and volume, concomitant with neuronal toxicity and death (Yankner *et al.* 1990; Goedert 1993; Haass and Selkoe 1994; Kosik 1994; Trojanowski 1994; Cummings and Cotman 1995; Yankner 1996; Funato *et al.* 1998). While amyloidogenic peptides are condensed into copious fibrillar deposits in the middle-to-late stages of AD, the relationship of such lesions to mechanisms of early cellular dysfunction is undefined. The densely packed deposits of Aβ found at the centre of neuritic plaques may have a protective function by sequestering toxic amyloid from cellular elements. Our studies have sought to identify mechanisms through which Aβ might effect changes in cellular properties at an early time, prior to the end-stage pathologicalal picture of neuritic plaques and NFT. The subject of this chapter is the elucidation of cellular cofactors, one a cell surface receptor, receptor for advanced glycation endproducts (RAGE) and the other an intracellular enzyme, amyloid β peptide binding protein alcohol dehydrogenase (ABAD), which target and potentiate cellular perturbation at low levels of Aβ.

9.2 RAGE — a receptor for advanced glycation endproducts and amyloid beta-peptide

In AD, it is widely accepted that later in the course of the disease, when Aβ fibrils are abundant, nonspecific interactions of such fibrils with the cell surface may be frequent and disruptive for cellular functions (Yankner *et al.* 1990; Behl *et al.* 1994; Hensley *et al.* 1994; Younkin, 1994; Cotman and Anderson 1995; Mattson 1995) (Plate 4). Aβ can destabilize plasma membranes (Pollard *et al.* 1995), causing changes in ionic homoeostasis, and could trigger cell death by several mechanisms. However, earlier in the course of the disease, when Aβ fibrils are present at lower levels and Aβ is, presumably, present principally in oligomeric soluble forms, higher affinity interactions with cell surface molecules are more likely to be relevant (Plate 4). An important requirement for any such ligand-receptor interaction involving Aβ is the role of chronicity. In many Biological systems, exposure of cells to high concentrations of ligands results in down-regulation of receptors, as exemplified by the low density lipoprotein (LDL) receptor (Herz and Willnow 1995). However, an Aβ binding site/receptor might be expected to have quite different properties; in view of the sustained presence of Aβ in brain parenchyma and vasculature, and the long times over which neuronal dysfunction occurs, cellular acceptor sites for Aβ might be expected to display prolonged expression on the cell surface, and even to be upregulated by ligand.

RAGE is a member of the immunoglobulin superfamily of cell surface molecules with greatest homology to the neural cell adhesion molecule (NCAM) and muc18 (Neeper *et al.* 1992; Schmidt *et al.* 1992; Schmidt *et al.* 1994). The extracellular domain comprises three immunoglobulin-like regions, including one N-terminal 'V'-type domain, followed by two 'C'-type domains. The remainder of the molecule is made up of a single transmembrane spanning domain and a short cytosolic tail at the C-terminus. The latter region displays greatest homology to the B-cell activation marker CD20. RAGE was first identified during our search for cellular binding sites for advanced glycation endproducts (AGE). More recently, we have found that RAGE is also a receptor for Aβ (Yan 1996; Shi *et al.* 1997), thus providing the basis for our hypothesis concerning the role of RAGE as a cellular cofactor in Aβ-induced cell stress (see below). Our studies in neurodegenerative disorders began because of the possible relevance of AGE ligands of RAGE to cellular injury in AD. Advanced glycation endproducts form over extended times as a result of glycoxidation of free amino groups on protein and lipid substrates (Ruderman *et al.* 1992; Brownlee 1995; Schmidt *et al.* 1995; Smith *et al.* 1995; King and Brownlee 1996). Certain amino groups are more likely sites for glycoxidation, as when amino groups are juxtaposed (such as an N-terminal lysine) or when there is a proximal imidazole group (Shapiro *et al.* 1980; Sell and Monnier 1989; Ruderman *et al.* 1992; Shilton *et al.* 1993). AGE modification of proteins/lipids is also critically dependent on the half-life of the substrate in tissues, as well as concomitant hyperglycaemia and an oxidant tissue microenvironment. Both PHF tau and Aβ are potential substrates for glycoxidation in view of their accumulation in brain parenchyma over years (Smith *et al.* 1994; Vitek *et al.* 1994; Yan *et al.* 1994, 1995). Tau is especially susceptible to AGE modification because of its high lysine content and its presence within the cell where aldose phosphates are more potent for protein modification, compared with aldoses present extracellularly. Immunohistochemical (Fig. 9.1) and biochemical studies (Fig. 9.2) demon-

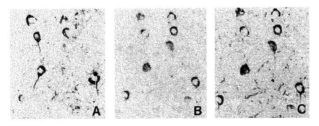

Fig. 9.1 Immunostaining of adjacent sections from AD-affected temporal lobe with antibody to tau-1 (A,C) and AGE (B). Magnification: × 100 (adapted from Yan *et al.* 1994).

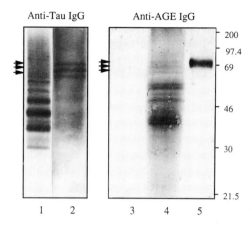

Anti-Tau IgG   Anti-AGE IgG

Fig. 9.2 Immunoblotting of PHF tau preparations with anti-tau-1 IgG (lane 2) and anti-AGE IgG (lane 4). Lanes 1 and 3 show immunoblotting of normal tau prepared from brain samples from age-matched normal individuals with anti-tau-1 IgG and anti-AGE IgG, respectively. Lane 5 shows immunoblotting of AGE albumin with anti-IgG. Migration of simultaneously run molecular weight standards is shown on the far right (adapted from Yan *et al.* 1994).

strated the presence of AGE epitopes colocalized with NFT, due, in part, to AGE-modification of PHF tau (Yan *et al.* 1994,1995). When tau was subjected to glycation *in vitro*, higher molecular weight forms were observed (Yan *et al.* 1994) and generation of oxygen free radicals occurred (Fig. 9.3; Yan *et al.* 1995). Thus, formation of AGE-modified tau could result in intermolecular crosslinking (a property of AGE) and the generation of adducts capable of elaborating intracellular reactive oxygen intermediates. Studies are underway in several laboratories to determine which AGE are most abundant in AD brain, and to assess the time course of their formation in relation to appearance of NFT and other pathological changes. AGE-modification of tau, at whatever stage it occurs, has the potential to increase neuronal stress by promoting the insolubility and toxicity of PHF tau. Thus, it is not a prin-

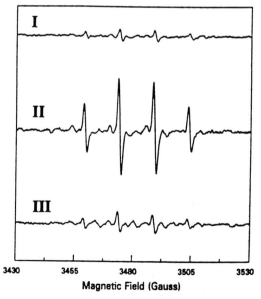

Magnetic Field (Gauss)

Fig. 9.3 Generation of reactive oxygen intermediates by AGE-recombinant tau by electron paramagnetic resonance (EPR) spin trapping measurement of free radical generation in the presence of DMPO (5,5-dimethyl-1-pyrroline-N-oxide; 50 mM): I, buffer alone; II, AGE-tau (100 µg/ml); and, III, AGE-tau (100 µg/ml) + superoxide dismutase (100 U/ml); (Adapted from Yan *et al.* 1995).

cipal factor underlying formation of PHF tau, but AGE adducts can enhance the pathogenicity of PHF thereby promoting their ability to disturb cellular homoeostasis.

Although tau was identified as a target for glycoxidation, we were especially interested in events outside the cell, in view of the accumulations of extracellular Aβ which are well-known as a hallmark of AD. Studies from Mike Vitek's laboratory demonstrated glycoxidation of Aβ, and suggested that AGE-modified Aβ might enhance aggregation of soluble Aβ, thereby accelerating formation of Aβ macromolecular assemblies (Vitek *et al.* 1994). We were intrigued by this observation, and began experiments to determine whether AGE-modified Aβ would bind to RAGE. However, we promptly encountered a technical problem; most preparations of glycated Aβ made by our laboratory *in vitro*, by incubating synthetic Aβ with high concentrations of glucose, ribose, or their respective aldose phosphates for varying times, irreversibly precipitated. Furthermore and unexpectedly, nonglycated Aβ, employed as a control for AGE-modified Aβ, bound to RAGE. These results coincided with other investigations underway in the laboratory in which we identified a 50–55 kDa polypeptide in lung extract which bound Aβ and turned out to be identical to RAGE, based on N-terminal sequence analysis (Yan *et al.* 1996). Although initially these results were quite surprising, since AGE-modified structures would appear to share little in common with a synthetic peptide capable of assembling into β-sheet fibril structures, we have subsequently identified other nonglycated ligands of RAGE. These include amphoterin, a molecule highly expressed during development (Hori *et al.* 1995), and EN-RAGE, a calgranulin-like molecule with properties of a proinflammatory cytokine (Hofmann *et al.* 1998). The binding of synthetic Aβ1–40 and Aβ1–42 to RAGE was dose-dependent, with K_d in the 70–100 nM range (Yan *et al.* 1996); the binding affinity of RAGE for Aβ in β-sheet conformation appeared somewhat higher than for preparations predominately in random conformation. As Aβ assembles into multiple macromolecular structures, it is not surprising that several different cell surface binding sites capable of interacting with this amyloidogenic peptide have been described in addition to RAGE. These other sites include the type A macrophage scavenger receptor, the p75 component of the neurotrophin receptor, the serpin-enzyme complex receptor, and the integrin $\alpha_5\beta_1$ (Boland *et al.* 1995; 1996; El Khoury *et al.* 1996; Yaar *et al.* 1997; Matter *et al.* 1998). Increased expression of megalin/gp330 (a lipoprotein receptor that serves as an acceptor site for apoE) (LaFerla *et al.* 1997) in neurons that display intracellular apoE and Aβ, as well as evidence of DNA fragmentation, suggest that uptake of apoE/Aβ complex via this receptor system may load cells with intracellular Aβ in a relatively stable complex that promotes toxicity, and, eventually, apoptosis (LaFerla *et al.* 1997). The list of cellular binding sites for Aβ is certain to lengthen as the interaction of Aβ with other cell surface structures is tested. For example, interaction of Aβ with the receptor for tumour necrosis factor-alpha (TNFα) has been proposed (Shen *et al.* 1998).

The potential relevance of RAGE in AD was emphasized by immunohistological examination of brain samples harvested from patients; expression of the receptor was increased in neurons, microglia and cells of the vessel wall (endothelium and vascular smooth muscle) contiguous to deposits of Aβ (Plate 5) (Yan *et al.* 1996). Increased expression of RAGE in AD brain was confirmed by *in situ* hybridization, compared with age-matched controls (Plate 5). The apparent juxtaposition of ligand and receptor suggested possible sustained receptor activation, as well as ligand-mediated upregulation of receptor expression. Subsequent analysis of the RAGE promoter has demonstrated the presence of two functional NF-κβ sites which participate in ligand-induced enhancement of RAGE expression

(Li and Schmidt 1997). Once it was evident that RAGE was present in AD brain, the key issue was to determine if RAGE participated in detoxification of Aβ, or, if it might contribute to the pathogenicity of Aβ, thereby promoting cellular perturbation. The serpin-enzyme complex receptor and $\alpha_5\beta_1$ integrin have been shown to bind Aβ selectively in the random conformation (Boland *et al.* 1995; 1996; Matter *et al.* 1998), suggesting a possible role in relation to the low levels of nonfibrillar Aβ present throughout life, and in regulating concentrations of soluble Aβ present in the extracellular space. The type A macrophage scavenger receptor is well-known for its capacity to support the internalization and disposal of lipoproteins modified by oxidation and/or glycation (Krieger and Herz 1994). Cellular uptake studies of soluble Aβ, comparing RAGE and the scavenger receptor, are consistent with the notion that the scavenger receptor is more effective for endocytosis (Mackic *et al.* 1998). In contrast, RAGE appears to have properties of a potent signal transduction receptor for Aβ: engagement of RAGE by Aβ results in activation of the MAP kinase pathway, resulting in sustained nuclear translocation of NF-κβ and induction of the expression of key target genes (Yan *et al.* 1997a). Although further studies must be performed to elucidate details of this pathway, the broad outline provides a mechanism for induction of haem oxygenase type I, Interleukin 6 (IL-6), and macrophage-colony stimulating factor (M-CSF) in a microenvironment rich in Aβ. Each of these markers of cellular activation has been observed in AD brain.

The relevance of such RAGE-dependent mechanisms to the pathogenesis of neuronal injury and lesion formation in AD is illustrated by our recent data concerning M-CSF (Yan *et al.* 1997a). In terms of macrophage function, M-CSF has a dual role promoting macrophage growth, migration, differentiation, and survival, as well as causing cell activation with increased expression of apoE and the scavenger receptor (type A). In contrast, neurons do not express c-fms, the receptor for M-CSF, and, thus, do not respond to M-CSF in a receptor-dependent manner. Binding of Aβ to neuroblastoma cells resulted in increased expression of M-CSF transcripts and protein due mainly to Aβ engagement of RAGE, as it was blocked by anti-RAGE IgG (Fig. 9.4A) (Yan *et al.* 1997a). Aβ-RAGE-mediated induction of M-CSF was closely correlated with activation of NF-κβ in neuroblastoma cells; anti-RAGE IgG blocked in parallel NF-κβ activation (Fig. 9.4B) and M-CSF expression. Promoter-reporter constructs spanning the NF-κβ DNA binding motif in the M-CSF gene showed increased expression of the reporter following transient transfection into neuroblastoma cells in the presence of Aβ. Anti-RAGE IgG and a soluble truncated form of the receptor blocked expression of the reporter gene. These data underscore the potential importance of Aβ-RAGE-dependent activation of NF-κβ in the induction of M-CSF in AD.

Consistent with the relevance of these findings to AD, immunohistological studies of AD brain showed increased levels of M-CSF in neurons and microglia, compared with control samples from age-matched apparently normal individuals (Plate 6). In addition, M-CSF antigen was increased in CSF samples from patients with AD compared with age-matched controls (Shi *et al.* 1997). Evidence of M-CSF was most striking in proximity to deposits of Aβ, suggesting the following possible sequence of events: Aβ binding to neuronal RAGE elicits M-CSF production, which draws in microglia through its chemotactic properties. Once present in the vicinity of Aβ, microglial RAGE promotes further M-CSF expression establishing an autocrine mechanism whereby M-CSF increases microglial survival and proliferation even in the toxic Aβ-rich environment. Furthermore, M-CSF increases

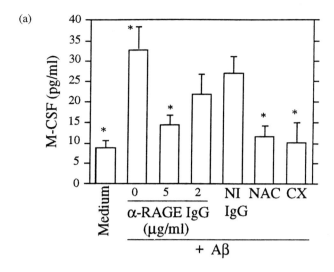

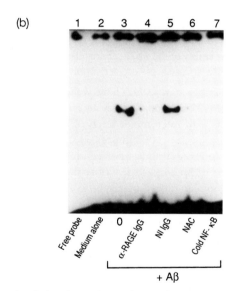

Fig. 9.4 Macrophage-colony stimulating factor (M-CSF) expression by neuroblastoma cells: role of RAGE. (A): neuroblastoma cells were exposed to Aβ1–40; 1 μM for 8 hrs at 37°C alone or in the presence of anti (α)-RAGE IgG, nonimmune (NI) IgG, N-acetylcysteine (NAC) or cyclo-heximide (CX). Release of M-CSF antigen was quantitated by ELISA. * denotes $p<0.05$. (B): electrophoretic mobility shift assay with ^{32}P-labelled NF-kβ probe on nuclear extracts from neuroblastoma cells incubated for 6 hr at 37°C in medium alone (lane 1) or medium supplemented with Aβ1–40; 1 μM alone (lane 2) or Aβ + αRAGE IgG (lane 3), Aβ + nonimmune (NI) IgG (lane 4) or Aβ + NAC (lane 5). Where indicated, a 100-fold molar excess of unlabelled NF-kβ probe was added to nuclear extracts from neuroblastoma cells exposed to Aβ (lane 6); (Adapted from Yan et al. 1997a).

microglial expression of the scavenger receptor and apoE, as well as other indices of macrophage activation. Since the neuron cannot respond to M-CSF, although it undertakes an active role in M-CSF synthesis, and, thus, the recruitment of microglia, the neuron does not benefit from the survival-promoting properties of M-CSF. Rather, the neuron is subject to the combined deleterious effects of Aβ and products of increased numbers of activated microglia (Plate 7). Although there may be several pathways leading to increased expression of M-CSF in AD brain, our data suggest that Aβ engagement of RAGE is one mechanism triggering synthesis of these growth factors/cytokines.

Prior to this work, the concept of cellular receptors mediating Aβ toxicity had not been proposed since the suggested involvement of tachykinin receptors (Yankner *et al.* 1990) was discounted (Shearman 1996). There may be several reasons for the lack of emphasis on identification of cell surface binding sites transmitting cellular stress in an Aβ-rich environment:

(1) Aβ is noxious to a broad spectrum of cell types. Until recently many toxicity studies were made using the Aβ25–35 peptide at concentrations ranging from 10–50 μM (Pike *et al.* 1993; Cotman and Anderson 1995; Mattson 1995; Mattson and Goodman 1995; Mark *et al.* 1996; Cribbs *et al.* 1997). However, the Biological significance of the Aβ25–35 is unclear since this peptide is neither present in the amyloid deposits nor generated *in vivo* (Seubert *et al.* 1992; Rocher *et al.* 1993; Vigo-Pelfrey *et al.* 1993; Wang *et al.* 1996). Moreover, the rapid induction of cell death at micromolar levels is most probably due to the indiscriminate ability of the Aβ25–35 to perturb membranes rather than to the specific induction of cellular stress i.e. NF-κβ activation and expression of M-CSF.

(2) Experiments by Cribbs *et al.* (1997) have shown that all-D- and all-L- enantiomers of Aβ1–42 and Aβ25–35 are equally toxic to cultured hippocampal neurons. However, these experiments used micromolar levels of peptides and evaluated only loss of cell viability, not more specific induction of cell stress responses which do not lead to cell death within the time constraints reported in their experiments. At the high levels of L- or D-enantiomers of Aβ employed (Cribbs *et al.* 1997) receptor-dependent processes, seen in the nanomolar range, are likely to have been overwhelmed by nonspecific effects.

(3) A recent report from the laboratory of Schubert (Liu *et al.* 1997) suggested that certain subclones of PC12 cells, which do not express RAGE, when treated with micromolar quantities of Aβ25–35 showed signs of toxicity. Again, unspecific membrane disturbances at the micromolar level may account for this toxicity. At these higher levels of Aβ, the neuronal stress-promoting properties of RAGE are overwhelmed by receptor-independent mechanisms. Furthermore, certain clones of PC12 cells, as well as other cultured cell lines, may not have the capacity to express RAGE. Additional specific mechanisms are likely to mediate Aβ toxicity over a range of amyloid peptide concentrations. In contrast, we demonstrate that in those PC12 cell lines expressing RAGE (Yan *et al.* 1997a; 1998) the Aβ1–40 at nanomolar concentrations has the ability of binding this receptor resulting in the activation of NF-κβ. An increased expression of RAGE has also been observed in primary cultures of rat cortical neurons (Hori *et al.* 1995) and in the AD brain (Yan *et al.* 1997a). However, in terms of primary cultures of rat cortical neurons (Hori *et al.* 1995) or AD brain (Yan *et al.* 1996), evidence of RAGE expression has been clearly demonstrated.

The receptor-dependent concept for promotion of cell stress in response to Aβ has important features likely to underlie, in part, *in vivo* findings. For example, the biological effects of lower concentrations of Aβ would be magnified, inducing neuronal dysfunction, and also triggering probable cytoprotective mechanisms, such as induction of haem oxygenase type I. Thus, analysis of receptor-dependent mechanisms of Aβ-mediated cellular perturbation requires the ability to sensitively detect the presence of the receptor, its ability to signal, and altered cellular function(s) consequent to ligand engagement. The probable importance of receptors for Aβ in AD is exemplified by an analogy to the blood coagulation mechanism (Davie *et al.* 1991; Esmon 1993). Cellular cofactors are critical for function of the procoagulant mechanism under physiological conditions, which require triggering of coagulation in the presence of low concentrations of reactants and multiple inhibitors. However, *in vitro*, when high levels of particular reactants can be added in the absence of cellular cofactors and inhibitors, individual reactions can be analysed and high velocities of the reactions can be attained. Results in the latter artificial system provide, at best, a very rough simulation of the *in vivo* situation. A corollary to the proposed involvement of Aβ receptors in the pathogenesis of neuronal injury in AD is that early in the course of this disorder, before irreversible cellular events occur, inhibition of Aβ-cell surface interactions could be neuroprotective, and, potentially, therapeutic. However, to be completely convincing, this hypothesis must await development of appropriate transgenic animal models that imitate the pathophysiology of AD. Mice overexpressing RAGE and/or the scavenger receptor, along with other susceptibility factors, such as presenilins or β-amyloid precursor protein (APP) mutants, may represent excellent candidates for such models.

9.3 ABAD — an intracellular target of amyloid beta-peptide

Evidence pointing to increased production of Aβ in culture and in brains of transgenic mice overexpressing presenilins, or mutations in APP, associated with early onset familial Alzheimer's disease (FAD), have highlighted a role for Aβ in the pathogenesis of neurodegeneration (Haass and Selkoe 1994; Kosik 1994; Dewji and Singer 1996; Haass 1996; Tanzi *et al.* 1996; Yankner 1996; Hardy 1997). Processing of APP may occur by several pathways (Haass and Selkoe 1994). Although initially it was thought that secreted Aβ was predominately formed in lysosomal-endosomal compartments or on the cell surface, recent studies have indicated a contribution of the endoplasmic reticulum (ER), also a site for localization of presenilins (Kovacs *et al.* 1996), in the generation of amyloidogenic peptide, especially Aβ1–42 (Cook *et al.* 1997; Hartmann *et al.* 1997; Tienari *et al.* 1997; Wild-Bode *et al.* 1997; Xu *et al.* 1997). The juxtaposition of presenilin and APP in the same subcellular organelle suggested that the earliest stages of cellular stress due to generation of Aβ1–42 might occur in this cellular compartment. Using the yeast two-hybrid system, we identified a polypeptide, ERAB, found in ER and in mitochondria which specifically binds Aβ. This molecule was named ERAB, or ER-associated Aβ binding protein, as it was originally localized within the ER (Yan *et al.* 1997*a*). In view of its recently elucidated properties as a generalized alcohol dehydrogenase capable of magnifying cell stress in response to Aβ, we have renamed it ABAD or amyloid β -peptide binding protein alcohol dehydrogenase (Kobayashi *et al.* 1996; Furuta *et al.* 1997; Yan *et al.* 1997*b*; 1998; He *et al.* 1998). ABAD is a single-chain polypeptide of Mr ≈27 kDa which assembles into tetramers and is an intracellular enzyme (Kobayashi *et al.* 1996; Furuta *et al.* 1997; He *et al.* 1998; Yan *et al.* 1998).

The observations that ABAD is expressed at increased levels in AD brain, that it binds Aβ, and that it potentiates Aβ toxicity led us to explore its properties in detail.

Analysis of brain tissue harvested from apparently normal individuals over a range of ages has shown a steady rise in levels of ABAD with increasing age. With superimposed AD, ABAD expression is further enhanced, especially in proximity to Aβ deposits (Plate 8) (Yan *et al.* 1997*a*). *In situ* hybridization confirmed the strongly increased expression of ABAD in AD brain, compared with age-matched controls (Plate 9). The presumed enzymatic properties of ABAD suggested roles in metabolic homoeostasis, in addition to its potential contribution to the pathogenesis of cellular dysfunction in AD. ABAD functions as a reversible, NAD/NADH-dependent β -hydroxyacyl Coenzyme A dehydrogenase participating in the β-fatty acid oxidation pathway (Kobayashi *et al.* 1996; Furuta *et al.* 1997; He *et al.* 1998; Yan *et al.* 1998), and as a generalized alcohol dehydrogenase using diverse substrates from linear alcohols (e.g. ethanol, propanol, butanol, pentanol, octanol, and decanol) to steroids (such as oestradiol) (Yan *et al.* 1998). This property of ABAD to catabolize reduction/oxidation of such a range of structures is probably relevant to its role(s) in metabolism, as well as to its altered properties following interaction with Aβ. As might be expected for an enzyme with such broad functions relevant to energy homoeostasis and alcohol metabolism, ABAD is distributed widely in normal tissues. Transcripts of ABAD are most abundant in heart, liver, and skeletal muscle (Yan *et al.* 1997*b*). Within cells, ABAD is found principally in two locales, the ER and mitochondria. Whereas certain cells show more ABAD in mitochondria, others show a greater predominance of ABAD associated with ER. For example, in transfected HeLa cells ABAD is especially noted in the ER (Plate 10). Dual fluorescence confocal microscopy colocalized ABAD (red fluorescence; Plate 10A) and the ER marker protein, disulphide isomerase (green fluorescence Plate 10B) resulting in yellow fluorescence (Plate 10C) (Yan *et al.* 1997*b*).

Our attention was drawn to ABAD because of its ability to potentiate cell stress and cytotoxicity in an Aβ-rich microenvironment. Blockade of endogenous ABAD in neuroblastoma cells ameliorated Aβ-induced suppression of the reduction of 3-(4,5-dimethylthiazol-2-yl)-2,5-diphenyl tetrazolium bromide (MTT) and diminished Aβ-induced DNA fragmentation (Yan *et al.* 1997*b*). Introduction of liposome-F(ab')$_2$ complexes, the latter prepared from blocking anti-ABAD IgG, into neuroblastoma cells prevented the appearance of cytosolic histone-associated DNA fragments (Fig. 9.5A). In contrast, similar studies with nonimmune F(ab')$_2$-liposomes or liposomes alone did not display a protective effect, and high levels of DNA fragmentation were observed. A more physiological system for assessing the impact of Aβ–ABAD interactions within intact cells is cotransfection with a mutant form of APP and wild-type ABAD (Yan *et al.* 1998). For these studies, we used the London APP mutant (V717G) because of its reported generation of high levels of Aβ1–42 within the ER. COS cells cotransfected with expression plasmids for wild-type ABAD and mutant APP(V717G) demonstrated prominent DNA fragmentation (Fig. 9.5B) compared with cultures overexpressing either ABAD or mutant APP alone, or those exposed only to lipofectamine. These results strongly supported the hypothesis that ABAD could promote cell stress in response to increased levels of Aβ. Because of the broad enzymatic properties of ABAD, we reasoned that its enzymatic activity might contribute to Aβ-mediated cytotoxicity. The putative active site of ABAD was subjected to site-directed mutagenesis with two key residues, tyrosine (168) and lysine (172), both replaced by glycine (Yan *et al.* 1998). Expression of this mutant form of ABAD in *E. coli* resulted in the isolation of an ≈27 kDa polypeptide with identical mobility on SDS-PAGE and N-terminal sequence compared with wild-type ABAD. Mutant ABAD also shared the Aβ binding properties of the natural molecule with virtually indistinguishable K$_d$s in ligand binding studies. In contrast to native

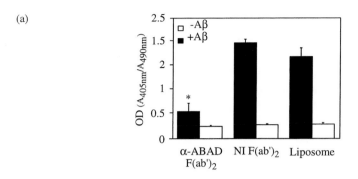

(a)

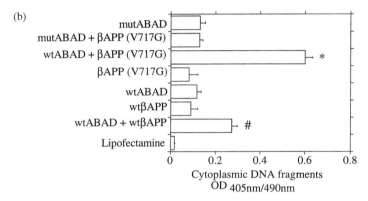

(b)

Fig. 9.5 The role of ABAD as a cellular cofactor for Ab-induced cell stress. A: neuroblastoma cells were incubated with anti (α)-ABAD F(ab')₂/liposome complex, nonimmune (NI) F(ab')₂/liposome complex, or liposomes alone for 24 hr, then cultures were exposed to Aβ (1–42; 2.5 μM) for a further 24 hr, and DNA fragmentation was assessed by ELISA for cytoplasmic histone-associated DNA fragments. B: cotransfection of COS cells to overexpress ABAD and βAPP(V717G): effect on DNA fragmentation. COS cells were transfected/cotransfected with plasmids resulting in overexpression of the indicated protein (wild-type [wt] ABAD or mutationally-inactivated [mut] ABAD [Y168G/K172G] and/or βAPP[V717G]) or with lipofectamine alone. At the far left, the transfected gene product(s) are indicated. After 48 hr, samples were harvested for ELISA for DNA fragmentation as in (A). (Adapted from Yan *et al.* 1997b and Yan *et al.* 1998) *P<0.01, #P<0.05.

ABAD, the mutant molecule was devoid of enzymatic activity as a β-hydroxyacyl-Coenzyme A dehydrogenase or as an alcohol dehydrogenase. Expression of mutant ABAD in COS and neuroblastoma cells demonstrated its localization in ER and mitochondria, as with the wild-type molecule. Thus, mutationally-inactivated ABAD was an ideal reagent for testing the effect of intrinsic enzymatic activity on potentiation of Aβ-induced cell stress. Cotransfection studies with mutant ABAD and mutant APP(V717G) demonstrated virtually no increase in DNA fragmentation compared with studies utilizing wild-type ABAD and mutant APP (Fig. 9.5B). These experiments emphasized the importance of ABAD enzymatic activity in ABAD-mediated induction of cell stress.

To assess mechanisms underlying ABAD potentiation of Aβ-induced cytotoxicity, the direct interaction of ABAD and Aβ were considered (Yan *et al.* 1998). Radioligand binding studies were performed with ^{125}I-labelled ABAD and Aβ immobilized on microtitre plates. Using either Aβ1–40 or Aβ1–42, dose-dependent and saturable binding of ^{125}I-ABAD was observed with a K_d of about 35–60 nM. Binding appeared to be specific, as other peptides with the potential to form β-sheet structures, such as prion protein-derived peptide (residues 109–141) or human amylin in random conformation, showed no binding (Yan *et al.* 1997*b*). In addition, Aβ–ABAD interaction was mediated by the N-terminal, hydrophilic portion of the amyloid peptide, as Aβ1–20 bound to ABAD whereas Aβ25–35 was inactive in this regard. The results of these radioligand binding studies, displaying saturable binding of ABAD to Aβ in the nanomolar range, led us to re-evaluate ABAD enzymatic activity in the presence of a range of amyloid peptide concentrations. Levels of Aβ which occupied ABAD binding sites (20–400 nM) had virtually no effect on ABAD activity based on ABAD-dependent reduction of S-acetoacyl-Coenzyme A and oxidation of β-oestradiol or octanol. At higher concentrations of Aβ, suppression of ABAD enzymatic activity was observed, with K_is of about 1.6–3.5 µM (Yan *et al.* 1998). Thus, concentrations of Aβ that suppressed ABAD activity were about an order of magnitude higher than those that result in the binding of Aβ to ABAD. Since only low levels of Aβ are expected to be present within cells (that is in the nanomolar range), these data suggested that Aβ was likely to modulate properties of ABAD other than inhibition of its enzymatic activity. To test this hypothesis, we had to demonstrate whether ABAD and Aβ might interact in intact cells. Aβ is assumed to be present only within membrane-bound compartments in the cell (for example within the lumen of the ER) whereas ABAD is in the cytosol. Pilot co-immunoprecipitation and crosslinking studies with ^{125}I-Aβ added to cultures and cells expressing ABAD have, thus far, demonstrated the presence of ^{125}I-Aβ-ABAD complex (Yan *et al.* 1997*b*). These observations provide support for the possibility that a direct interaction of ABAD and the amyloid peptide can occur within intact cells. However, further studies will be required to definitively prove formation of ABAD-Aβ complex in live cells. A critical reagent in this regard will be a mutant form of ABAD with diminished capacity to bind Aβ. Properties of this mutant form of ABAD, especially in terms of its promotion of Aβ-induced cytotoxicity, will be essential for determining whether direct interaction of ABAD and Aβ contributes to cell stress.

The likely presence of Aβ-ABAD complex in cells suggested the importance of considering altered properties of this entity relevant to potentiation of Aβ cytotoxicity in a cellular context. First, an Aβ-rich environment appears to promote translocation of ABAD in certain cells; in the presence of Aβ, ABAD transfers, in part, from the ER to an association with the plasma membrane (Yan *et al.* 1997*b*, 1998). Second, we considered whether ABAD-Aβ complex might support the generation of reactive aldehydes, some of which, such as 4-hydroxynonenal, have been ascribed cytotoxic properties (Mattson 1995; Mark *et al.* 1996). Cotransfection of COS cells with plasmids causing overexpression of ABAD and mutant APP(V717G) resulted in the generation of maldondialdehyde and 4-hydroxynonenal epitopes, compared with cells overexpressing ABAD or mutant APP alone (Fig. 9.6). The possible relevance of these findings to AD is emphasized by the detection of malondialdehyde and 4-hydroxynonenal adducts, as well as other oxidation-related epitopes, in affected areas of AD brain (Mattson 1995; Mark *et al.* 1996; Smith *et al.* 1996; Pappolla *et al.* 1998). Further studies are under way to determine the mechanism(s) through which ABAD and/or

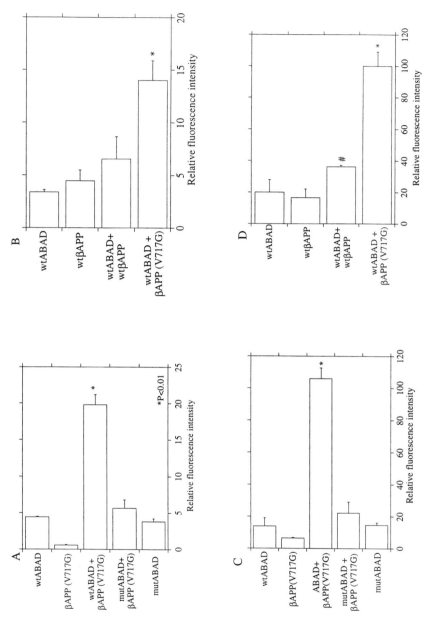

Fig. 9.6 Expression of malondialdehyde (MDA) and 4-hydroxynonenal (HNE) epitopes in COS cells expressing wt or mut ABAD (see legend to Fig. 5B) with or without APP(V717G). COS cells were transiently transfected with pcDNA3/wtABAD or pcDNA3/mut ABAD(Y168G/K172G) either alone or in the presence of pAdlox/APP(V717G). Cultures were fixed and stained with antibodies to MDA and ABAD, or HNE and ABAD. Quantitative analysis of images was performed with NIH image. Relative fluorescence intensity (arbitrary units) is shown in COS cell cultures transfected with the indicated constructs. Each bar is labelled with the gene products overexpressed by transfection (adapted from Yan *et al.* 1998).

ABAD-Aβ complex leads to the generation of reactive aldehydes. Cotransfection experiments with mutant APP(V717G) in which mutationally-inactivated ABAD replaced wild-type ABAD resulted in no formation of malondialdehyde or 4-hydroxynonenal (Yan *et al.* 1998). Thus, ABAD enzymatic activity is essential for generation of these reactive aldehydes. The next important step in our analysis of ABAD-Aβ-mediated production of reactive aldehydes will be to determine the role of Aβ binding to ABAD for generation of malondialdehyde and hydroxynonenal. One possibility is that ABAD-Aβ complex subtly changes substrate preference for ABAD among the range of alcohols within a cell. Alternatively, the ABAD-Aβ complex might trigger formation of reactive oxygen intermediates causing formation of reactive aldehydes by a quite distinct mechanism. Finally, the possibility of an indirect mechanism not requiring ABAD to directly interact with Aβ must be considered. Aβ might change the nature/abundance of alcohol substrates present within the cell, and ABAD then oxidizes these new alcohol species resulting in formation of malondialdehyde and 4-hydroxynonenal adducts.

Thus ABAD might be an important intracellular cofactor in Aβ-induced cytotoxicity. However, our results raise many unexpected questions. By what mechanism does Aβ gain access to ABAD? Although Aβ-induced destabilization of membranes may be involved, further studies will be required to demonstrate if and how Aβ-ABAD interaction allows the peptide to cross Biological membranes. Alternatively, Aβ and ABAD may not interact directly, but Aβ may change the intracellular milieu to facilitate ABADs participation in enzymatic reactions leading to formation of toxic products. Also, it will be essential to extend our studies of ABAD to determine if blocking ABAD in a range of cell types, and, especially, *in vivo*, prevents Aβ-mediated cell stress eventuating in cytotoxicity. The potential of Aβ to modulate properties of an intracellular target, an enzyme that participates in cellular homoeostasis, may identify early cellular events signalling trouble within neurons at a time when intervention might reverse early functional perturbations. It is important to note that other neurotoxic species also interact with intracellular enzymes fundamental in cellular metabolism as illustrated by binding of huntingtin and other proteins containing polyglutamine domains to glyceraldehyde-3-phosphate dehydrogenase (DiFiglia *et al.* 1997; Lunkes and Mandel 1997; Paulson and Fishbeck 1997; Skinner *et al.* 1997).

9.4 The role of cellular cofactors in Aβ-induced cell stress and neurotoxicity

There is much still unknown about the pathogenesis and even pathological manifestations of sporadic AD. This is exemplified by the very recent recognition of distinct hitherto unsuspected extracellular proteinaceous deposits of ≈100 kDa polypeptide in AD with monoclonal antibodies to plaque-derived substances (Schmidt *et al.* 1997). The identification and characterization of specific cellular targets of Aβ, such as RAGE, scavenger receptor, megalin/gp330, the p75 component of the neurotrophin receptor, and ABAD, provides a context for considering early cellular perturbations due to Aβ, both in relation to cell surface binding sites/receptors, and intracellular targets, and may provide new insights into molecular mechanisms and future therapeutic approaches. These cellular cofactors for Aβ-induced cell stress are probably distinct from those which initially trigger the development of AD. The cellular cofactors related to Aβ cytotoxicity can be considered progression factors propagating cellular dysfunction in an Aβ-rich environment, rather than acting as the key factor(s) which cause the change in the cellular environment leading to accumulation and/or overproduction of particular forms of Aβ probably important in the cause of AD. None the less, cellular factors are likely to have an essential role in the ultimate neuronal cytotoxicity of Aβ, by propagating an ascending cycle of cellular dysfunction. Aβ-induced cellular perturbation occurs over a wide range of amyloid peptide concentrations and probably exerts its effects by different mechanisms at these different levels of Aβ. At higher concentrations of Aβ, the involvement of specific cell-associated targets of Aβ (such as RAGE and ABAD) would be minimal, as increased levels of Aβ directly destabilize membranes resulting in changes in calcium flux and generation of reactive oxygen species. However, at the lower concentrations of Aβ likely to be present early in AD, cellular cofactors may have a central role in targeting the effects of Aβ to particular cells and manifesting changes in cellular properties. Although the mechanisms underlying the effects of such cellular cofactors can be productively studied in vitro, more important results will come from in vivo studies. Transgenic models of AD-type pathology have shown Aβ deposition, but less striking cellular changes, especially in terms of neurotoxicity (Carlson *et al.* 1997). Thus, development of doubly transgenic mice overexpressing a mutant form of APP, to achieve an Aβ-rich microenvironment, along with targeted overexpression of a cellular cofactor, such as RAGE or ABAD in neurons (and/or astroglia and cells of the vessel wall), may provide important insights into the pathogenesis of chronic cellular perturbation in AD. Though it will take some time to carry out and analyse the results of such experiments, a possible role for cellular cofactors in AD opens a new facet in the biology of the cellular effects of Aβ which is likely to be a critical addition to the 'amyloid hypothesis'.

Acknowledgements

Drs Gabriel Godman and Giuseppe Andres (Department of Pathology) provided invaluable suggestions during planning and preparation of the manuscript.

References

Behl, C., Davis, J., Lesley, R., and Schubert, D. (1994). Hydrogen peroxide mediates amyloid-β toxicity. *Cell*, 77, 817–27.

Boland, K., Manias, K., and Perlmutter, D. (1995). Specificity in recognition of amyloid beta-peptide by the serpin-enzyme complex receptor in hepatoma cells and neuronal cells. *Journal of Biological Chemistry*, 270, 28022–8.

Boland, K., Behrens, M., Choi, D., *et al.* (1996). The serpin-enzyme complex receptor recognizes soluble, nontoxic amyloid-beta peptide but not aggregated, cytotoxic amyloid-beta peptide. *Journal of Biological Chemistry*, 271, 18032–44.

Brownlee, M. (1995). Advanced glycosylation in diabetes and aging. *Annual Reviews in Medicine*, 46, 223–34.

Carlson, G., Borchelt, D., Dake, A., *et al.* (1997). Genetic modification of the phenotypes produced by amyloid precursor protein overexpression in transgenic mice. *Human Molecular Genetics*, 6, 1951–9.

Cook, D., Forman, M., Sung, J., *et al.* (1997). Alzheimer's amyloid-beta (1–42) is generated in the endoplasmic reticulum/intermediate compartment of NT2N cells. *Nature Medicine*, 3, 1021–3.

Cotman, C., and Anderson, A. (1995). A potential role for apoptosis in neurodegeneration and Alzheimer's disease. *Molecular Neurobiology*, 10, 19–45.

Cribbs, D., Pike, C., Weinstein, S., *et al.* (1997). All-D-enantiomers of beta-amyloid exhibit similar Biological properties to all-L-beta-amyloids. *Journal of Biological Chemistry*, **272**, 7431–6.

Cummings, B. and Cotman, C. (1995). Image analysis of beta-amyloid load in Alzheimer's disease and relation to dementia severity. *Lancet*, **346**, 449–53.

Davie, E., Fujikawa, K. and Kisiel, W. (1991). The coagulation cascade, initiation, maintenance, and regulation. *Biochemistry*, **30**, 10363–70.

Dewji, N. and Singer, S. (1996). Genetic clues to Alzheimer's disease. *Science*, 271, 159–60.

DiFiglia, M., Sapp, E., Chase, K., *et al.* (1997). Aggregation of huntingtin in neuronal intranuclear inclusions and dystrophic neurites in brain. *Science*, **277**, 1990–3.

El Khoury, J., Hickman, S., Thomas, C., *et al.* (1996). Scavenger receptor-mediated adhesion of microglia to β-amyloid fibrils. *Nature*, **382**, 716–19.

Esmon, C. (1993). Cell-mediated events that control blood coagulation and vascular injury *Annual Reviews in Cell Biology*, **9**, 1–26.

Funato, H., Yoshimura, M., Kusui, K., *et al.* (1998). Quantitation of amyloid beta-protein in the cortex during aging and in Alzheimer's disease. *American Journal of Pathology*, **152**, 1633–40.

Furuta, S., Kobayashi, A., Miyazawa, S., and Hashimoto, T. (1997). Cloning and expression of cDNA for a newly identified iszyme of bovine liver 3-hydroxyacyl-CoA dehydrogenase and its import into mitochondria. *Biochimica et Biophysica Acta*, **1350**, 317–24.

Goedert, M. (1993). Tau protein and the neurofibrillary pathology of Alzheimer's disease. *Trends in Neuroscience*, **16**, 460–5.

Haass, C. (1996). Presenile because of presenilin, the presenilin genes and early onset Alzheimer's disease. *Current Opinions in Neurology*, **9**, 254–9.

Haass, C and Selkoe, D. (1994). Cellular processing of β -amyloid precursor protein and the genesis of amyloid β-peptide. *Cell*, **75**, 1039–42.

Hardy, J. (1997). Amyloid, the presenilins and Alzheimer's disease. *Trends in Neuroscience*, **20**, 154–9.

Hartmann, T, Bieger, S., Bruhl, B., *et al.* (1997). Distinct sites of intracellular production for Alzheimer's disease amyloid-beta 40/42 amyloid peptides *NatureMedicine*, **3**, 1016–1020.

He, X-Y., Schulz, H., and Yang, S-Y. (1998). A human brain L-3-hydroxyacyl-coenzyme A dehydrogenase is identical to amyloid beta-peptide-binding protein involved in Alzheimer's disease. *Journal of Biological Chemistry*, **273**, 10741–6.

Hensley, K., Carney, J., Mattson, M., *et al.* (1994). A model for β-amyloid aggregation and neurotoxicity based on free radical generation by the peptide, relevance to Alzheimer disease. *Proceedings of the National Academy of Sciences (USA)*, **91**, 3270–4.

Herz, J. and Willnow, T. (1995). Lipoprotein and receptor interactions *in vivo*. *Current Opinions in Lipidology*, **6**, 97–103.

Hofmann, M., Drury, S., Fu, C., *et al.* (1999). RAGE mediates a novel proinflammatory axis: the cell surface receptor for S100/calgranulin polypeptides. *Cell*, **97**, 889–901.

Hori, O., Brett, J., Nagashima, M., *et al.* (1995). RAGE is a cellular binding site for amphoterin, mediation of neurite outgrowth and co-expression of RAGE and amphoterin in the developing nervous system. *Journal of Biological Chemistry*, **270**, 25752–61.

King, G. and Brownlee, M. (1996). The cellular and molecular mechanisms of diabetic complications. *Endocrinology and Metabolism Clinics of North America*, **25**, 255–70.

Kobayashi, A., Jiang, L., and Hashimoto, T. (1996) Two mitochondrial 3-hydroxyacyl-CoA dehydrogenases in bovine liver. *Journal of Biochemistry*, **119**, 775–82.

Kosik, K. (1994). Alzheimer's disease sphinx, a riddle with plaques and tangles. *Journal of Cell Biology*, **127**, 1501–4.

Kovacs, D., Fausett, H., Page, K., *et al.* (1996). Alzheimer-associated presenilins 1 and 2, neuronal expression in brain and localization to intracellular membranes in mammalian. *Nature Medicine*, 2, 224–9.

Krieger, M. and Herz, J. (1994). Structures and functions of multiligand lipoprotein receptors, macrophage scavenger receptors and LDL receptor-related protein. *Annual Reviews in Biochemistry*, 63, 601–37.

LaFerla, F., Troncoso, J., Strickland, D., *et al.* (1997). Neuronal cell death in Alzheimer's disease correlates with apoE uptake and intracellular amyloid-beta stabilization. *Journal of Clinical Investigation*, 100, 310–20.

Li, J. and Schmidt, A-M. (1997). Characterization and functional analysis of the promoter of RAGE. *Journal of Biological Chemistry*, 272, 16498–506.

Liu, Y., Dargusch, R., and Schubert, D. (1997). Beta amyloid toxicity does not require RAGE protein. *Biochemical and Biophysical Research Communications*, 237, 37–40.

Lunkes, A. and Mandel, J-L. (1997). Polyglutamines, nuclear inclusions and neurodegeneration. *Nature Medicine*, 3, 998–9.

Mackic, J., Stins, M., McComb, J., *et al.* (1998). Human blood-brain barrier receptors for Alzheimer's amyloid beta peptide 1–40. *Journal of Clinical Investigation*, 102, 734–43.

Mark, R., Blanc, E., and Mattson, M. (1996). Amyloid beta-peptide and oxidative cellular injury in Alzheimer's disease. *Molecular Neurobiology*, 12, 915–24.

Matter, M., Zhang, Z., Nordstadt, C., and Ruoslahti, E. (1998). The alpha-5 beta-1 integrin receptor binds the Alzheimer disease amyloid-beta protein and mediates its internalization. *Keystone Symposium Proceedings*, X5, 101. (Abstract).

Mattson, M. (1995). Free radicals and disruption of neuronal ion homoeostasis in Alzheimer's disease, a role for amyloid beta-peptide? *Neurobiology of Aging*, 16, 679–82.

Mattson, M. and Goodman, Y. (1995). Different amyloidogenic peptides share a similar mechanism of neurotoxicity involving reactive oxygen species and calcium. *Brain Research*, 676, 219–24.

Neeper, M., Schmidt, A.M., Brett, J., *et al.* (1992). Cloning and expression of RAGE, a cell surface receptor for advanced glycosylation end products of proteins. *Journal of Biological Chemistry*, 267, 14998–5004.

Pappolla, M., Chyan, Y-J., Omar, R., *et al.* (1998). Evidence of oxidative stress and *in vivo* neurotoxicity of beta-amyloid in a transgenic mouse model of Alzheimer's disease. *American Journal of Patholology*, 152, 871–7.

Paulson, H. and Fishbeck, K. (1997). Trinucleotide repeats in neurogenetic disorders. *Annual Reviews in Neuroscience*, 19, 79–107.

Pike, C., Burdick, D., Walencewicz, A., *et al.* (1993). Neurodegeneration induced by β-amyloid peptides *in vitro*, the role of peptide assembly state. *Neuroscience*, 13, 1676–87.

Pollard, H., Arispe, N., and Rojas, E. (1995). Ion channel hypothesis for Alzheimer amyloid peptide neurotoxicity. *Cellular Molecular Neurobiology*, 15, 513–26.

Rocher, A.E., Lowenson, J.D., Clarke, S., *et al.* (1993) Structural alterations in the peptide backbone of β-amyloid core protein may account for its deposition and stability in Alzheimer's disease. *Journal of Biological Chemistry*, 268, 3072–83.

Ruderman, N., Williamson, J., and Brownlee, M. (1992). Glucose and diabetic vascular disease. *Federation of American Societies for Experimental Biology (FASEB) Journal*, 6, 2905–14.

Schmidt, A.-M., Yan, S.-D., and Stern, D. M. (1995). The dark side of glucose. *Nature Medicine*, 1, 1002–4.

Schmidt, A.M., Vianna, M., Gerlach, M., *et al.* (1992). Isolation and characterization of binding proteins for advanced glycosylation endproducts from lung tissue which are present on the endothelial cell surface. *Journal of Biological Chemistry*, **267**, 14987–97.

Schmidt, A.M., Hori, O., Brett, J., *et al.* (1994). Cellular receptors for AGEs. *Arteriosclererosis and Thrombosis*, **14**, 1521–8.

Schmidt, M.-L., Lee, V., Forman, M., *et al.* (1997). Monoclonal antibodies to a 100-kD protein reveal abundant amyloid-beta-negative plaques throughout gray matter of Alzheimer's disease brain. *American Journal of Patholology*, **151**, 69–80.

Sell, D. and Monnier, V.M. (1989). Structure elucidation of senescence cross-link from human extracellular matrix, implication of pentoses in the aging process. *Journal of Biological Chemistry*, **264**, 21597–602.

Seubert, P., Vigo-Pelfrey, C., Esch, F., *et al.* (1992). Isolation and quantification of soluble Alzheimer's beta-peptide from Biological fluids. *Nature*, **359**, 325–7.

Shapiro, R., McManus, M., Zalut, C., and Bunn, F. (1980). Sites of nonenzymatic glycosylation of human hemoglobin. *American Journal of Biological Chemistry*, **255**, 3120–7.

Shearman, M. (1996). Cellular MTT reduction distinguishes the mechanism of action of beta-amyloid from that of tachykinin receptor peptides. *Neuropeptides*, **30**, 125–32.

Shen, Y., Yang, L-B., Lue, L-F., and Rogers, J. (1998). p55 and p75 TNF receptor subtypes bind amyloid beta-peptide and are differentially expressed in the Alzheimer's brain. *Neurobiology of Aging*, **19**, S45, 188. (Abstract).

Shilton, B., Campbell, R., and Walton, D. (1993). Site specificity of glycation of horse liver alcohol dehydrogenase. *European Journal of Biochemistry*, **215**, 567–72.

Skinner, P., Koshy, B., Cummings, C., *et al.* (1997). Ataxin-1 with an expanded glutamine tract alters nuclear matrix-associated structures. *Nature*, **389**, 971–4.

Smith, M. A., Taneda, S., Richey, P., *et al.* (1994). Advanced Maillard reaction end products are associated with Alzheimer disease pathology. *Proceedings of the National Academy of Sciences (USA)*, **91**, 5710–14.

Smith, M., Sayre, L., Monnier, V., and Perry, G. (1995). Radical AGEing in Alzheimer's disease. *Trends in Neuroscience*, **18**, 172–6.

Smith, M., Perry, G., Richey, P., *et al.* (1996). Oxidative damage in Alzheimer's. *Nature*, **382**, 120–1.

Tanzi, R., Kovacs, D., Kim, T., *et al.* (1996). The gene defects responsible for familial Alzheimer's disease. *Neurobiology of Disease*, **3**, 159–69.

Tienari, P., Ida, N., Ikonen, E., *et al.* (1997). Intracellular and secreted Alzheimer beta-peptide species are generated by distinct mechanisms in cultured hippocampal neurons. *Proceedings of the National Academy of Sciences (USA)*, **94**, 4125–30.

Trojanowski, J. and Lee, V. (1994). Paired helical filament tau in Alzheimer's disease, the kinase connection. *American Journal of Pathology*, **144**, 449–53.

Vigo-Pelfrey, C., Lee, D., Keim, P., *et al.* (1993). Characterization of beta-amyloid peptide from human cerebrospinal fluid. *Journal of Neurochemistry*, **61**, 1965–8.

Vitek, M., Bhattacharya, K., Vlassara, H., *et al.* (1994). AGEs contribute to amyloidosis in Alzheimer's disease. *Proceedings of the National Academy of Sciences USA*, **91**, 4766–70.

Wang, R., Sweeney, D., Gandy, S.E., and Sisodia, S.S. (1996). The profile of souble amyloid β protein in cultured cell media. Detection and quantification of amyloid b protein and variants by immunoprecipitation-mass spectrometry. *Journal of Biological Chemistry*, **271**, 31894–902.

Wild-Bode, C., Yamazaki, T., Capeil, A., *et al.* (1997). Intracellular generation and accumulation of amyloid beta-peptide terminating at amino acid 42. *Journal of Biological Chemistry*, **272**, 16085–8.

Xu, H., Sweeney, D., Wang, R., *et al.* (1997). Generation of Alzheimer beta-amyloid protein in the trans-Golgi network in the apparent absence of vesicle formation. *Proceedings of the National Academy of Sciences (USA)*, **94**, 3748–52.

Yaar, M., Zhai, S., Pilch, P., *et al.* (1997). Binding of beta-amyloid to the p75 neurotrophin receptor induces apoptosis. *Journal of Clinical Investigation*, **100**, 2333–40.

Yan, S.D., Chen, X., Schmidt, A.M., *et al.* (1994) Glycated tau protein in Alzheimer disease, a mechanism for induction of oxidant stress *Proceedings of the National Academy of Sciences (USA)*, **91**, 7787–91.

Yan, S.D., Yan, S.F., Chen, X., *et al.* (1995) Nonenzymatically glucated tau in Alzheimer's disease induces neuronal oxidant stress resulting in cytokine gene expression and release of amyloid-beta peptide. *Nature Medicine*, **1**, 693–9.

Yan, S.-D., Chen, X., Chen, M., *et al.* (1996). RAGE and amyloid-β peptide neurotoxicity in Alzheimer's disease. *Nature*, **382**, 685–91.

Yan, S.-D., Zhu, H., Fu, J., *et al.* (1997*a*). Amyloid beta-peptide-RAGE interaction elicits neuronal expression of M-CSF, a proinflammatory pathway in Alzheimer's disease. *Proceedings of the National Academy of Sciences (USA)*, **94**, 5296–301.

Yan, S.D., Fu, J., Soto, C., *et al.* (1997*b*). An intracellular protein that bind amyloid-beta peptide and mediates neurotoxicity in Alzheimer's disease. *Nature*, **389**, 689–95.

Yan, S.D., Stern, D., Kane, M., *et al.* (1998). RAGE — A beta interactions in the pathophysiology of Alzheimer's disease. *Restorative Neurology and Neuroscience*, **12**, 167–73.

Yan, S-D., Shi, Y., Zhu, A., *et al.* (1999). Role of ERAB/L-3-hydroxyacyl-Coenzyme A dehydrogenase type II activity in amyloid beta-peptide-induced cytotoxicity. *Journal of Biological Chemistry*, **274**, 2145–56.

Yankner, B. (1996). Mechanisms of neuronal degeneration in Alzheimer's disease. *Neuron*, **16**, 921–32.

Yankner, B., Duffy, L., and Kirschner, D. (1990). Neurotrophic and neurotoxic effects of amyloid-β protein, reversal by tachykinin neuropeptides. *Science*, **250**, 279–82.

Younkin, S. (1994). Evidence that amyloid beta-peptide is the real culprit in Alzheimer's disease. *Annals of Neurology*, **37**, 287–8.

Zhu, A., Zhu, H., Zhu, Y., *et al.* (1998) RAGE interaction with amyloid beta-peptide fibrils activates signal transduction mechanisms and results in apoptosis, activation of MAP kinases and nuclear translocation of NF-κβ. *Society for Neuroscience*, **I**, p228, (Abstract).

Chapter 10

Reflections on Alzheimer's disease as a specific neurotransmitter disorder

Peter Davies

10.1 Introduction

More than 20 years ago, stimulated by work of Hornykiewicz and colleagues on Parkinson's disease (Hornykiewicz 1973), several groups set out to investigate the status of specific neurotransmitter systems in the brains of patients with Alzheimer's disease (AD). At that time, AD was generally considered to be a rare, presenile dementia, with diffuse degeneration of the cerebral cortex and certain deeper structures. The idea that there would be specificity to the degeneration in terms of the neurotransmitter systems affected was not popular, but a series of papers appeared that suggested preferential involvement of cholinergic neurons (Bowen *et al.* 1976; Davies and Maloney 1976; Perry *et al.* 1977*a*). These papers, and several more that followed, stimulated an enormous upsurge of interest in AD, especially in the idea that this disease could be treated with agents that were designed to improve cholinergic transmission. This enormous field has been reviewed recently by Ladner and Lee (1998); however, it seems worth re-examining the issue of transmitter specificity in the light of more recent neuroanatomical studies of AD, especially studies of the progression of the disease. Research on a disease like AD does not always progress in an entirely logical or predictable fashion, and my own thinking has evolved partly on the basis of the technology available, and partly on the basis of more prosaic constraints.

10.2 Cholinergic markers in Alzheimer's disease

There is no doubt that comparisons of brains of patients dying with AD with those of non-demented patients reveals huge deficits in the activities of the marker enzymes, choline acetyltransferase (ChAT) and acetyl cholinesterase (AchE) in the cerebral cortex, as well as less marked losses in regions including the basal ganglia and even in the cerebellum (Davies 1979). Such deficits, as well as reductions in potassium-stimulated acetylcholine release, have also been reported to be found in samples of tissue removed from living patients by brain biopsy (Sims *et al.* 1982). Examination of markers of GABA, dopamine, noradrenalin, and serotonin neurons yielded less consistent evidence for deficits (Bowen *et al.* 1976; Perry *et al.* 1977*b*; Davies 1979b; Cross *et al.* 1984), and this led to the notion of selective vulnerability of cholinergic neurons in AD. At the time of these initial reports, the anatomy of the cholinergic system in higher mammals was not well known, and as soon as this was at least partially clear (Johnston *et al.* 1979; Lehmann *et al.* 1980), evidence for loss of cholinergic neurons in the AD brain was quickly published (Whitehouse *et al.* 1981). At this time there were two main concerns: first, to try to develop therapies to restore cholinergic transmission, and second, to attempt to explain the selective vulnerability of the basal forebrain cholinergic neurons.

The 'cholinergic hypothesis' (Smith and Swash 1978; Bartus *et al.* 1982) of AD became very popular in the sense that a huge amount of energy was expended to develop drugs to treat the cholinergic deficiency in AD, and this cannot be regarded as entirely wasted effort. In the United States, the only compounds approved by the Food and Drug Administration (FDA) for the treatment of the cognitive deficits in AD patients are two cholinesterase inhibitors (as of early 1999). Since the FDA demands evidence of efficacy prior to approval of a drug, and the review process is rigorous, it is evident that patients experience some benefits from treatment with these agents. A great deal of work is still going on in this field, and it is expected that other cholinesterase inhibitors and perhaps cholinergic agonists will be approved in the near future. How much benefit to patients is possible through this approach is not yet clear, but from the vantage point of one who was involved in the early work in this area, the thought that even a few patients and families experience some relief is very gratifying.

The issue of selective vulnerability of cholinergic neurons was always difficult to reconcile with the pathology of AD, once the anatomy of the cholinergic system became clear. The widespread occurrence of neurofibrillary tangles (NFT) and neuronal loss in the cerebral cortex made it obvious that the vulnerability was only relatively selective. It became increasingly clear that many of the neurons containing NFT in the cortex used glutamate as the neurotransmitter, although there were no reliable markers for glutamatergic neurons that could be used in human autopsy tissues. There are few, if any, cholinergic neurons in the cortex of higher mammals (Struble *et al.* 1986). Several groups attempted to use neuropeptide concentrations as markers of the status of cortical neurons, and decreases in somatostatin and corticotropin releasing factor (CRF) were reported (Davies *et al.* 1980; McKinney *et al.* 1982). Vasoactive intestinal peptide and cholecystokinin octapeptide were shown to be present in numerous cortical neurons, but concentrations of these peptides did not appear to be reduced in the AD brain (Perry *et al.* 1981). Although the effects of AD were not completely without specificity, several cortical neuronal types were affected, in addition to the basal forebrain cholinergic neurons (Perry *et al.* 1987; Bierer *et al.* 1995).

10.3 Pathogenesis of the cholinergic deficit

The question that increasingly occupied my attention was the nature of the factors that resulted in the dysfunction and death of the cholinergic neurons. These neurons were very sensitive to the AD process, and the marker enzymes, ChAT and AchE, offered simple and sensitive means to monitor the status of these cells. Were there features of these neurons that might be identified as conferring sensitivity to degeneration in AD? In the early 1980s, little was known about the receptors present on basal forebrain cholinergic neurons, or about the distinctive patterns of gene expression (aside from ChAT and AchE) in these cells. To attempt to develop new probes for unique features of these cells, 'shotgun' experiments were undertaken, with the aim of producing monoclonal antibodies that would specifically label such neurons. Mice were immunized with basal forebrain tissue crudely dissected from normal and AD brains, and the antibodies generated (several thousand of them) were screened for differential reactivity. Specific probes for basal forebrain cholinergic neurons were not produced, but a small group of antibodies were discovered that reacted much more strongly with AD tissue than with tissues from controls, and one of these antibodies, designated Alz50, appeared to be a unique new reagent.

From the time of the first publication in 1986 (Wolozin et al. 1986), to the present, Alz50 has been a very popular reagent for studies of AD. This antibody reacts with neurons undergoing the neurofibrillary degeneration characteristic of this disease, but reacts with much more than just the NFT. The original publications with this antibody emphasized the fact that both neurons and their processes are stained, and the antibody has been used to trace neuronal pathways involved in AD (Hyman et al. 1988a). Alz50 also appeared to be able to label neurons early in the course of the degenerative process: some of those stained appearing to be normal by morphologic criteria. Basal forebrain cholinergic neurons were stained too, but many of the more severe AD cases coming to autopsy had few of these cells remaining, and hence little staining in this brain region. Ben Wolozin, Brad Hyman, and their colleagues (Wolozin and Davies 1987; Hyman et al. 1988b) studies in the hippocampus first suggested that vulnerable neurons, not yet obviously engaged in degenerative processes, could be identified with Alz50. My lab became very interested in this marker of early neuronal pathology, and especially in attempting to identify the biochemical events that were involved in its appearance in cells.

10.4 Tau biochemistry

When Alz50 was first produced, the biology of NFT formation was poorly understood. The prevailing thinking was that tangles were highly insoluble, abnormal structures that formed in the perikarya of neurons. There was evidence for the presence of tau and perhaps neurofilament proteins in the tangle, but polyclonal and monoclonal antibodies to tangles had been produced that did not cross react with normal brain proteins (for example see Ihara et al. 1983). This seemed to suggest that unique proteins might also be present in the tangle, or that normal brain proteins were very highly modified in the formation of these extraordinarily insoluble structures. The near-heroic efforts of Wischik, Ihara, and others (Crowther et al. 1989; Hasegawa et al. 1992) succeeded in sequencing small peptide fragments extracted from tangles, and these sequences were identified as coming from the microtubule binding regions of tau, and from the small protein, ubiquitin. The relationship of the Alz50 antigen to this insoluble tangle structure was unclear. Although Alz50 labelled some neurofibrillary tangles, but it did not react with either extracellular tangles in brain tissue, nor with tangles isolated by the then-popular techniques that involved harsh detergent extractions and, in some cases, protease digestion. On the other hand, Alz50 reacted with a small group of readily soluble proteins from the AD brain, which did not appear to be present in tissue from controls. No one, including the author, realized at that time that Alz50 was detecting conformational alterations of tau that appear to occur very early in the pathway that leads to tau incorporation into NFT (Jicha et al. 1997a). This discovery actually took more than 10 years of work, involving a number of different groups, and it is not my intention to review this controversial story here. In one sense, we had succeeded: a marker useful for the study of the early pathogenesis of AD had been produced, and this has been very widely used in AD research. As the role of tau in NFT formation became better known, it became possible to develop additional reagents to explore the biochemistry of neuronal degeneration in AD in more detail (for example Vincent *et al.* 1996; Jicha *et al.* 1997*b*).

10.5 **Early events in Alzheimer's disease**

Most of the work cited up to this point had been performed on autopsy brain tissue obtained from either normal individuals, or from patients dying after several years of suffering from AD. Clearly, much of this work involved examination of the biology of the end-stages of AD, and it was difficult to know how to separate consequences of the disease process from those events that were critically involved in the process. This is still a difficult issue. A critical insight in this area has come from the work of the Braaks (Braak and Braak 1991; Braak *et al.* 1993), who perhaps better than anyone else, appreciated the fact that AD 'spread' through the brains of affected individuals in a fairly predictable fashion. Prior to their publications, most of us would grade the severity of AD by the numbers of plaques and tangles present in a sampling of cortical regions: the more lesions, the more severe the disease. The Braaks proposed an alternative scheme, one that depends on the extent to which the disease involves different brain regions. In the published scheme, stages of AD are defined by the spread of AD from transentorhinal cortex, to the hippocampal formation, and then out to the neocortex. The severity of the disease is thus staged according to the extent to which it has spread out from the entorhinal cortex, to involve more and more regions of the hippocampus and neocortex, rather than by the number of lesions present in any given region. This staging scheme has been criticized because some odd cases occur in which the disease appears to follow a different pattern (for example cases in which the hippocampus is much less severely involved than the neocortex). However, these exceptions do not, in my view, detract from the enormous value of this staging scheme. It appears to provide a very objective way to identify cases, and regions of the brain in these cases, prior to the development of any detectable pathology. This would seem to be exactly what is required if identification of the very earliest pathogenic events is to be possible.

To illustrate this point, suppose we define a group of cases coming to autopsy as Braak stage 2, by the detection of NFT in the entorhinal cortex and hippocampal formation, with minimal pathology in the rest of the cortex. The assumption can be made that had these patients lived longer, most of them would have reached stage 3 or 4, in which tangles appear in the medial temporal and in the inferior parietal cortex. However, in our stage 2 cases, much of the neocortex is free of *visible* pathology, but may already contain the earliest bio-chemical changes that would have led to visible pathology had the patient survived. The occasional exceptions will not greatly influence the study results, as reasonable numbers of cases have to be examined, and it is also possible to check data against those obtained from stage 3 and 4 cases. The availability of an objective, reproducible staging system such as this also greatly facilitates the comparison of results from different groups of researchers (Nagy *et al.* 1997).

The Braaks original staging system used silver staining to define the 'spread' of pathology in the AD brain, and focused on the detection of neurofibrillary pathology, rather than amyloid deposits. They focused on the development and spread of *neuronal* pathology, rather than on the development of extracellular protein deposits. They have pointed out that there is both a temporal and a spatial mismatch between the neuronal pathology and amyloid deposits (Braak *et al.* 1989), something that others have also noted (Dickson *et al.*

1991; Davies 1994). This presents a real difficulty in trying to develop hypotheses concerning the relationship between amyloid deposition and neuronal degeneration. A debate at the 6th International Conference on Alzheimer's Disease (Amsterdam 1998) made it clear that many of the leading figures in the field recognize this problem. It seems likely that amyloid deposition *per se* will not prove to be the critical issue. This does not rule out potentially important roles for alterations in processing of the amyloid precursor protein (APP), amyloid formation within neurons (if it occurs in AD), or of any other currently unknown toxic form of soluble amyloid.

The staging system appears particularly useful in the involvement of specific neuronal systems in AD. However, similar neuroanatomically based studies could be performed using any marker: of amyloid deposits, of microglial activation, astrocytic reactivity, etc. A similar staging system using these other potential markers might prove very helpful to the particular sub-field of AD research. More recent studies from the Braaks and others (Braak *et al.* 1994) have begun to use antibodies such as Alz50 or AT8 (the latter recognizing phosphorylated serine 202 in tau) to define the progressive involvement of different neuronal systems by detection of specific molecular markers. The progression of AD pathology through the brain is the opposite of the order of myelination during development (Braak *et al.* 1998). Regions affected earliest by the neurodegeneration of AD are those that are among the last in which myelination takes place during development. It is amazing to remember that a very similar point was made in 1978 by the late Dr Norman Geschwind, following my presentation of a long list of brain regions arranged in ascending order of magnitude of cholinergic deficit (see discussion following Davies 1979a). Geschwind commented that the order was precisely the reverse of the order of myelination during development. However it is still difficult to see what such correlation might mean.

The most powerful aspect of the Braaks' work is perhaps the definition of a hierarchy of neuronal vulnerability in the AD brain, although this is not yet complete. We do not yet know where the ventral forebrain cholinergic neurons fit into this hierarchy: the anatomy of these neurons is complex, and it would require double-labelling studies to identify affected neurons as cholinergic. Such studies appear to be underway (Sassin *et al.* 1998). For the moment, my lab is focused on the CA2 region of the hippocampus, as this is a readily identified region in which the anatomic connections are well known. Our autopsy service provides a reasonable number of cases (4 or 5 per year) in which pathology is extensive in the entorhinal cortex and in the CA1 region, but in which the neocortex is largely unaffected. In such cases, studies of CA2 neurons, which are for the most part free of obvious pathology, allows the testing of hypotheses regarding early events in neuronal degeneration. Photographs of some of the cases we have used in these studies are shown in Fig. 10.1. These tissue sections are stained with the monoclonal antibody TG3, a very sensitive early marker of AD pathology (Vincent *et al.* 1996; Jicha *et al.* 1997b). All these cases have neuronal and neuritic plaque staining in the entorhinal cortex, and in the figure the staining of neurons and neuritic elements in CA1 can be seen. The cases labelled A, B, and C have relatively few neurons labelled by TG3. D is a section of hippocampus from a patient with relatively mild AD, as shown by the fact that neocortical pathology is present but very sparse. We would consider this case too advanced to be useful for hippocampal studies. Double labelling experiments using cases such as A–C can show whether a particular marker is expressed early in the course of the neurofibrillary degeneration. For example, using this kind of strategy, recent studies (Vincent *et al.* 1998) have identified activation of cdc2 in CA2 neurons presumably occurring prior to NFT formation in these cells. Similar studies could be performed using samples of association cortex from cases similar to that illustrated in D.

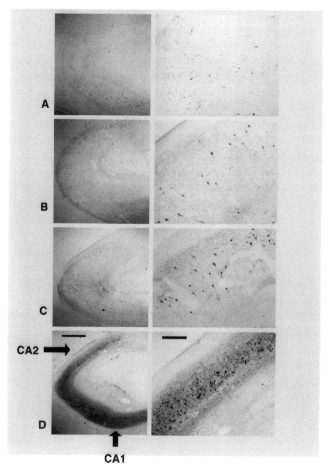

Fig. 10.1 Vibratome sections of the hippocampus from four cases selected by examination of neuropathology reports were stained with TG3. These reports stated that NFT were numerous in the entorhinal cortex, but that neocortical pathology was minimal or absent. None of these cases would meet neuropathological criteria for diagnosis of AD (Ball *et al.* 1997). In the left set of panels the hippocampal formation was photographed with a 2× objective (scale bar is 5 mm). The orientation of the sections is very similar, and the arrows on panel D show the positions of the CAI and CA2 regions, which are in the same relative positions in the panels above. On the right side, the CA2 region of each case is shown at slightly higher magnification (scale bar is 2.5 mm). Note how few pyramidal neurons are labelled in cases A and B.

10.6 **Conclusion**

Examination of the hierarchy of neuronal involvement in AD, as proposed by the Braaks, does not suggest obvious reasons why one group of neurons might degenerate more readily than another. There has yet to be a marriage between the neurotransmitter studies and the more classical neuroanatomical views of the problem. Many of the pyramidal cells of the hippocampus and of the neocortex, identified by the Braaks as degenerating early in AD, are glutamatergic, and yet the transmitter studies clearly indicate that a loss of cholinergic, somatostatin, and CRF neurons also occurs. A scheme such as that developed by the Braaks, but establishing a hierarchy of neuronal involvement in AD on the basis of neurotransmitter type would seem to be worth developing. One prediction that seems obvious is that glutamatergic pyramidal cells are among the earliest involved in AD, but we do not yet know when the ventral forebrain cholinergic neurons fall victim to the pathology, in relation to entorhinal cortex pyramidal cells. Deficits in glutamate release seem more likely to occur early in AD than excessive release and excitotoxicity. But the transmitter(s) used by the neuron may be irrelevant to its position in the hierarchy of degeneration?

Is it perhaps the nature of the neurotransmitter receptors that are important? Armstrong and his colleagues (Ikonomovic *et al.* 1997; Mizukami *et al.* 1997) are investigating the *loss* of specific transmitter receptors as marking vulnerable neurons in AD, and their data suggesting that the Glu R2/3 glutamate receptor is absent from hippocampal neurons undergoing the earliest stages of AD degeneration is intriguing. The strategy used by Ikonomovic *et al.* (1997) was similar to that described above and illustrated in the figure. However, in this study, *no* neurons were found to double label with the antibody to Glu R2/3 and MC1, another early marker of tau pathology. This suggested that the Glu R2/3 subunit was lost prior to the development of the degenerative changes. One would like to see this work extended to other brain regions, bearing in mind the order in which the resident neurons become involved in the pathology. It has always impressed me that the distribution of nicotinic acetylcholine receptors in the normal human brain as reported, particularly in the studies of the Perrys' is similar to that of neurons vulnerable to AD pathology (Perry *et al.* 1989). The same authors have shown quite extensive losses of this receptor class quite early in AD (Court *et al.* 1997), suggesting again that they may identify vulnerable cell populations. This issue would be well worth revisiting, comparing the distribution of nicotinic receptors with the spread of pathology as defined in the Braak scheme. Several more specific examples could be given, but it is hoped that the idea is clear enough. Is there in fact a hierarchy of loss of specific receptors which matches the hierarchy of degeneration outlined by the Braaks? Is there a particular neurotransmitter receptor with a distribution in brain such that receptor density can predict the position of that region in the degenerative cascade? This might be a fruitful way to look at old data, as well as a new conceptual framework for collection of new results.

Other parameters might be more important than the transmitter or receptor used by a group of neurons, perhaps the particular isoforms of microtubule associated proteins (MAP) that are expressed in each different neuronal type. There is little detailed information on this point, although there are apparently different tau isoforms expressed in the dentate granule cells of the hippocampus as compared to those in the pyramidal cells (Goedert *et al.* 1989), but much more detailed studies are clearly desirable. There may be as many as 32 different isoforms of MAP2 expressed in the central nervous system (Kalcheva *et al.* 1995; Shafit-Zagardo and Kalcheva 1998), and no studies as yet of possible links to vulnerability to AD. Recent work which attempts to link neurotransmitter deficits with the more classical features of AD pathology, for example those that have proposed that the metabolism of the amyloid precursor protein may be regulated by the cholinergic transmission (Davies *et al.* 1991; Wallace *et al.* 1991; Buxbaum *et al.* 1992), seem very worth while. Perhaps work of this type, which attempts to integrate information from different sub-fields of research on AD will ultimately provide the best way forward. For the present, it is difficult to develop models which account for the apparent specificity of AD in terms of transmitter system involvement *and* take account of neuroanatomical data on the distribution of neuronal pathology. Development and testing of such models will be important for moving beyond cholinergic therapy.

Acknowledgements

The author's work is supported by grants AG06803 and NIMH38623. Dennis W. Dickson, M.D. performed the neuropathology on the cases described, and his advice and friendship over many years are much appreciated.

References

Ball, M., Braak, H., and Coleman, P., *et al.* (1997). Consensus recommendations for the postmortem diagnosis of Alzheimer's — disease. *Neurobiology of Aging*, **18**, S1–S2.

Bartus, R., Dean, R., Beer, B., and Lippa, A. (1982). The cholinergic hypothesis of geriatric memory dysfunction. *Science*, **217**, 408–17.

Bierer, L. M., Haroutunian, V., Gabriel, S., *et al.* (1995). Neurochemical correlates of dementia severity in Alzheimer's disease: relative importance of the cholinergic deficits. *Journal of Neurochemistry*, **64**,749–60.

Bowen, D. M., Smith, C. B., White, P., and Davison, A. N. (1976) Neurotransmitter-related enzymes and indices of hypoxia in senile dementia and other abiotrophies. *Brain*, **99**, 459–96.

Braak, H. and Braak, E. (1991). Neuropathologic staging of Alzheimer-related changes. *Acta Neuropathologica*, **82**, 239–59.

Braak, H., Braak, E., Bohi, J., and Bratzke, H. (1998). Evolution of Alzheimer's disease related cortical lesions. *Journal of Neural Transmission Supplement*, **54**, 97–106.

Braak, H., Braak, E., Ohm, T., and Bohl, J. (1989). Alzheimer's disease: mismatch between amyloid plaques and neuritic plaques. *Neuroscience Letters*, **103**, 24–8.

Braak, H, Braak, E, and Bohl, J. (1993). Staging of Alzheimer-related cortical destruction. *European Neurology*, **33**, 403–8.

Braak, E., Braak, H., and Mandelkow, E. M. (1994). A sequence of cytoskeleton changes related to the formation of neurofibrillary tangles and neuropil threads. *Acta Neuropathologica*, **87**, 554–67.

Buxbaum, J. D., Oishi, M., Chen, H. I., *et al.* (1992). Cholinergic agonists and interleukin 1 regulate processing and secretion of the Alzheimer beta/A4 amyloid protein precursor. *Proceedings of the National Academy of Sciences (USA)*, **89**,10075–8.

Court, J. A., Lloyd, S., Johnson, M. *et. al* (1997). Nicotinic and muscarinic cholinergic receptor binding in the human hippocampal formation during development and aging. *Development Brain Research*, **101**, 93–105.

Cross, A. J., Crow, T. J., Johnson, J. A., *et al* (1984). Studies on neurotransmitter receptor systems in neocortex and hippocampus in senile dementia of the Alzheimer-type. *Journal of Neurological Science*, **64**, 109–17.

Crowther, T., Goedert, M., and Wischik, C. M. (1989). The repeat region of microtubule-associated protein tau forms part of the core of the paired helical filament of Alzheimer's disease. *Annals of Medicine*, **21**, 127–32.

Davies, P. (1979a) Biochemical changes in Alzheimer's disease — senile dementia: Neurotransmitters in senile dementia of the Alzheimer's type in *Congenital and Acquired Cognitive Disorders* (Ed R. Katzman.) Raven Press, New York pp 153–160 Research Publications: Association for Research in Nervous and Mental Disease. Volume 57.

Davies, P. (1979b). Neurotransmitter-related enzymes in senile dementia of the Alzheimer type. *Brain Research*, **171**, 319–27.

Davies, P. (1994). Neuronal abnormalities, not amyloid, are the cause of dementia in Alzheimer's Disease. in *Alzheimer's Disease*, (ed. Terry, R. D., R. Katzman, K. L. Bick) pp 327–34. Raven Press New York.

Davies, P. and Maloney, A. J. F. (1976). Selective loss of central cholinergic neurons in Alzheimer's disease. *Lancet;* II, l403.

Davies, P., Katzman, R., and Terry, R. D. (l980). Reduced somatostatin- like immunoreactivity in cerebral cortex from cases of Alzheimer disease and Alzheimer senile dementia. *Nature*, **288**, 279–80.

Davis, K. L., Santucci, A. C., and Haroutunian, V. (1991). Increased biosynthesis of Alzheimer amyloid precursor protein in the cerebral cortex of rats with lesions of the nucleus basalis of Meynert. *Molecular Brain Research*, **10**, 173–8.

Dickson, D. W., Crystal, H. A., Mattiace, L. A., *et al.* (1992). Identification of normal and pathological aging in prospectively studied nondemented elderly humans. *Neurobiology of Aging*, **13**, 179–89.

Goedert, M., Spillantini, M. G., Potier, M. C. *et. al.* (1989). Cloning and sequencing of the cDNA encoding an isoform of microtubule-associated protein tau containing four tandem repeats: differential expression of tau protein mRNA's in human brain. *European Molecular Biology Organisation Journal*, **8**, 393–399.

Hasegawa, M., Morishima-Kawashima, M., *et al.* (1992). Protein sequence and mass spectrometric analyses of tau in the Alzheimer's disease brain. *Journal of Biological Chemistry*, **267**, 17047–54.

Hornykiewicz, O. (1973). Parkinson's disease: from brain homogenate to treatment. *Federation Proceedings*, **32**, 183–190.

Hyman, B. T., Kromer, U., and Van Hoesen, G. W. (1988a). A direct demonstration of the perforant pathway terminal zone in Alzheimers disease using the monoclonal antibody Alz–50. *Brain Research*, **450**, 392–397.

Hyman, B. T., Van Hoesen, G. T., Wolozin, B. L., *et al.* (1988b). Alz-50 antibody recognizes Alzheimer-related neuronal changes. *Annals of Neurology*, **23**, 371–9.

Ihara, Y., Abraham, C., and Selkoe, DJ. (1983). Antibodies to paired helical filaments in Alzheimer's disease do not recognize normal brain proteins. *Nature*, **304**, 727–30.

Ikonomovic, M. D., Mizukami, K., Davies, P., *et a.l* (1997). The loss of GluR2(3) immunoreactivity precedes neurofibrillary tangles formation in the entorhinal cortex and hippocampus of Alzheimer's brains. *Journal of Neuropathology and Experimental Neurology*, **56**, 1018–27.

Jicha, G. A., Bowser, R., Kazam, I. G., and Davies, P. (1997*a*). Alz-50 and MC-1, a new monoclonal antibody raised to paired helical filaments, recognize conformational epitopes on recombinant tau. *Journal of Neuroscience Research*, **48**, 128–32.

Jicha, G. A., Lane, E.,Vincent, I. J., *et al.* (1997*b*). Conformation and phosphorylation dependent antibody recognizing the paired helical filaments of Alzheimer's Disease. *Journal of Neurochemistry*, **69**, 2087–95.

Johnston, M. V., McKinney, M., and J. T. Coyle. (1979). Evidence for a cholinergic projection to neocortex from neurons in basal forebrain. *Proceedings of National Academy of Science (USA)*, **76**, 5392–6.

Kalcheva, N., Albala, J., and O'Guin, K. *et al.* (1995). Genomic structure of human microtubule associated protein 2 (MAP-2) and charecterisation of additional MAP-2 isoforms. Proceedings of the National Academy of Sciences (USA), **92**, 10894–10898.

Ladner, C. J., and Lee, J. M. (1998). Pharmacological drug treatment of Alzheimer disease: the cholinergic hypothesis revisited. *Journal of Neuropathology and Experimental Neurology*, **57**, 719–31.

Lehmann, J. J. I., Nagy, S., Atmadja, and H. C. Fibiger. (1980). The nucleus basalis magnocellularis: the origin of a cholinergic projection to the neocortex of the rat. *Neuroscience*, **5**, 1161–74.

McKinney, M., Davies, P., and Coyle, J. T. (1982). Somatostatin is not co-localized in cholinergic neurons innervating the rat cerebral cortex — hippocampal formation. *Brain Research*, **243**, 169–72.

Mizukami, K., Ikonomovic, M. D., Grayson, D. R., *et al.* (1997). Immunohistochemical study of GABA(A) receptor beta2/3 subunits in the hippocampal formation of aged brains with Alzheimer-related neuropathologic changes. *Experimental Neurology,* 147, 333–45.

Nagy, Z., Vatter-Bittner, B., Braak, H., *et al.* (1997). Staging of Alzheimer-type pathology: an inter-rater-intrarater study *Dementia and Geriatric Cognitive Disorders,* 8, 248–51.

Perry, E. K., Perry, R. H., Blessed, G., and Tomlinson, B. E. (1977*a*) Necropsy evidence of central cholinergic deficits in senile dementia. *Lancet,* 1, 189.

Perry, E. K., Gibson, P. H., Blessed, G., *et al.* (1977*b*). Neurotransmitter enzyme abnormalities in senile dementia. Choline acetyltransferase and glutamic acid decarboxylase activities in necropsy brain tissue. *Journal of Neurological Science,* 34, 247–65.

Perry, R. H., Dockray, G. J., Dimaline, R., *et al.* (1981). Neuropeptides in Alzheimer's disease, depression and schizophrenia. A post mortem analysis of vasoactive intestinal peptide and cholecystokinin in cerebral cortex. *Journal of Neurological Science,* 51, 465–72.

Perry, R. H., Perry, E. K., Smith, C. J., *et al.* (1987). Cortical neuropathological and neurochemical substrates of Alzheimer's and Parkinson's Disease. *Journal of Neural Transmission,* 24, 131–6.

Perry, E. K., Smith, C. J., Perry, R.H. *et al.* (1989). Regional distribution of muscarinic and nicotinic cholinergic receptor binding activities in the human brain. *Journal of Chemical Neuroanatomy,* 2, 189–199.

Sassin, I., Schultz, C., Koppers, D., *et al* (1998). Evolution of Alzheimer-related neurofibrillary pathology in the nucleus basalis meynert-Ch4 complex. *Neurobiology of Aging,* 19, suppl4S abstract no. 1012

Shafit-Zagardo, B., and Kalcheva, N. (1998). Making sense of the multiple MAP-2 transcripts and their role in the neuron. *Molecular Neurobiology,* 16, 149–162.

Sims, N. R., Marek, K. L., Bowen, D. M., and Davison, A. N. (1982). Production of [14C]acetylcholine and [14C]carbon dioxide from [U-14C] glucose in tissue prisms from aging rat brain. *Journal of Neurochemistry,* 38, 488–92.

Smith, C. M. and Swash, M. (1978). Possible biochemical basis of memory disorder in Alzheimer disease. *Annals of Neurology,* 36, 471–3.

Struble, R. G., Lehmann, J., Mitchell, S. J., *et al.* (1986). Basal forebrain neurons provide major cholinergic innervation of primate neocortex. *Neuroscience Letters,* 66, 215–20.

Vincent, I. J., Rosado, M., and Davies, P. (1996). Mitotic mechanisms in Alzheimer's Disease? *Journal of Cell Biology,* 132, 413–25.

Vincent, I. J., Zheng, J-H, Dickson, D. W., *et al.* (1998). Mitotic phosphoepitopes precede paired helical filaments in Alzheimer's Disease. *Neurobiology of Aging,* 19, 287–96.

Wallace, W. C., Bragin, V., Robakis, N. K., *et al.* (1991). Increased biosynthesis of Alzheimer amyloid precursor protein in the cerebral cortex of rats with lesions of the nucleus basalis of Meynert. *Molecular Brain Research,* 10, 173–8.

Whitehouse, P. J., Price, D. L., Clark, A. W., *et al.* (1981). Alzheimer disease: evidence for selective loss of cholinergic neurons in the nucleus basalis. *Annals of Neurology,* 10,122–6.

Wolozin, B. L. and Davies, P. (1987). Alzheimer related neuronal protein A68: Specificity and distribution. *Annals of Neurology,* 22, 521–6.

Wolozin, B. L., Pruchnicki, A., Dickson, D. W., and Davies, P. (1986). A neuronal antigen in the brains of patients with Alzheimer's disease. *Science,* 232; 648–50.

Chapter 11

Clinical assessment of Alzheimer's disease

Suzanne Jeffries and Alistair Burns

11.1 Clinical assessment of dementia

The clinical diagnosis of Alzheimer's disease (AD) is a two-stage process. First, a diagnosis of dementia is made; the main conditions from which it should be differentiated being delirium, depression, concomitant physical illness, drug treatment, and normal ageing. Determining the aetiology of the syndrome is the second stage — AD, vascular dementia, Lewy body dementia, frontal lobe dementia, or the many and relatively rare secondary causes of dementia.

The manifestation of the clinical syndrome can be divided into three parts. First, a neuropsychological element consisting of *amnesia* (loss of memory); *aphasia* (either a receptive aphasia or expressive aphasia, the latter being more apparent in conversation and nominal aphasia tested by direct questioning of naming of objects); *apraxia* (the inability to carry out tasks despite intact sensory and motor nervous systems, manifest in dementia most usually by an inability to dress often described as putting on a shirt or coat back to front, or the inability to use a knife and fork correctly); and *agnosia* (the inability to recognize things such as ones own mirror reflection or a family member — this is different to forgetting the name of someone).

Second, a neuropsychiatric component with associated symptoms such as psychiatric disturbances and behavioural disorders which are present in a substantial proportion of patients. The commonest are (approximate frequencies in brackets): depression (up to 66% at some point during their dementia); paranoid ideation (30%); misidentifications (usually based on agnosia, 20%); hallucinations (most commonly auditory, suspect an intercurrent delirium or Lewy body dementia if persistent visual hallucinations are present, 15%); aggression (20%); and wandering (20%).

Third, deficits in activities of daily living. Towards the later stages of dementia these are manifest by obvious problems in dressing, eating, and going to the toilet. In the early stages they may be manifest by a failure to wash or dress to a person's usual standard and in people living alone, self neglect of the diet can lead to weight loss and neglect of household tasks lead to comments about cleanliness of the house.

This triad of presentation is common to all types of dementia, the differentiation being based on the clinical presentation, the presence of other features and other aspects of the history and examination.

11.2 **Clinical presentation of the dementias**

The main clinical manifestation of AD is short-term memory loss. This can be manifest by repeating questions (which can be particularly stressful and irritating for carers), forgetting a hitherto remembered birthday or anniversary (be careful to document whether forgetting such an event is unusual or not), needing to be reminded of the day or date and forgetting appointments to meet with friends or family. Occasionally the first signs can be more obvious such as forgetting the names of grandchildren or even children, getting lost (either while driving or when visiting a strange place), or failure to recognize a family member (misrecognition of a spouse to whom a patient has been married for 50 years is particularly distressing for all concerned). Emerging difficulties in activities of daily living can also be present — failure to work the controls on a washing machine, microwave, or video recorder are noticed by family members and this can sometimes be brought to attention when the purchase of a new gadget completely dumbfounds the patient. Commonly, changes in personality and general demeanour take place, (a coarsening of affect, mild irritability, mild disinhibition) but these are only usually apparent in retrospect, unless very marked as in the case of frontal lobe dementia

Personality changes which are seen include: increased rigidity; increased egocentricity; impairment of regard for the feelings of others; coarsening of affect; impairment of emotional control; hilarity in inappropriate situations; diminished emotional responsiveness; sexual misdemeanour; hobbies relinquished; diminished initiative, or growing apathy and purposeless hyperactivity (Blessed *et al.* 1968). Oppenheim (1994) found that in one third of patients, a psychiatric presentation was the primary difficulty. Memory impairment is a problem with short-term memory and the significance of such a change is sometimes not fully appreciated by families and others (including professionals) and is considered by many as a normal age related change. Changes in personality may, retrospectively, be regarded as one of the earliest signs of dementia and are well documented in the later stages. In the later stages, motor signs are evident with increased muscle tone, hyper- reflexia and extensor plantar responses. During these stages, emotional and neuropsychiatric manifestations may present, such as hallucinations, delusions and mood disturbances. Agitation, wandering, aggression, and incontinence very often accompany a diagnosis of AD and is often the most problematical.

In AD, these symptoms evolve over a relatively long period of time, posssibly two or more years before the patient comes for help. Characteristically, relatives are unable to date accurately when the first symptoms started. In vascular dementia, the presentation is usually more sudden and the time of onset can be timed more accurately than the onset of AD. The progression over time may follow a more stepwise decline, with periods of weeks, or even months, of no obvious decline followed by a sudden deterioration (presumably coinciding with a cerebrovascular event). Symptomatology is much the same as in AD although aphasia can be more prominent, personality changes less marked and depression more often apparent in vascular dementia as are catastrophic reactions (extreme tearfulness when faced with failure on cognitive tests) and emotional lability occurring. Features discriminating AD from vascular dementia are summarized in Table 11.1. Patients with frontal lobe dementia characteristically present with personality changes, repetitive behaviour, and depression. Patients with Lewy body dementia often present with acute or subacute confusional states, falls, florid visual hallucinations, and persecutory ideas with Parkinsonian features including sensitivity to neuroleptic medication. The reader should not take away the

Table 11.1 Some features which help distinguish Alzheimer's disease from vascular dementia.

Alzheimer's disease	Vascular dementia
Focal disease absent	Focal disease present
Fits and hypertension rare	Fits and hypertension common
Generalized atherosclerosis rare	Generalized atherosclerosis common
Personality disorganization	Personality preservation
Loss of insight	Insight remains, catastrophic reactions
Blunted affect	Affective symptoms common
Females > males	Males > females
Genetic factors important in some cases	No clear genetic causes
Insidious onset	Relatively sudden onset
Gradual and progressive course	Stepwise
Somatic complaints rare	Somatic complaints common

impression that these defined syndromes are always clearly clinically differentiated and commonly there is considerable clinical overlap, for example patients with AD who appear to have prominent aphasia, patients with vascular dementia who have frontal lobe symptoms etc.

11.3 **The diagnostic process**

The most important parts, in an assessment where AD is suspected, is a history from an informant, a physical examination with special relevance to the central nervous system (CNS), mental state examination to include a detailed assessment of cognitive function and investigations. It is important to establish the nature and timing of the initial problem and this in itself gives an important clue to the diagnosis. Gradual impairment suggests AD, sudden onset is in favour of vascular disease. The investigations which should be carried out have been well discussed in Corey Bloom *et al.* (1995) and Doraiswamy *et al.* (1998).

11.4 **Clinical diagnostic criteria for dementia**

Many regard the gold standard for the diagnosis of AD as neuropathological examination and the success of clinical criteria to predict pathological changes are generally taken as a marker of their validity. However, there is significant overlap in the histological changes seen in dementia (Holmes *et al.* 1999) and increasing understanding of molecular biology has probably diminished the importance of classical descriptive neuropathological examination in research terms, but it remains the gold standard in terms of pathological diagnosis.

The most commonly used clinical diagnostic criteria in practice are the North American based Diagnostic and Statistical Manual currently in its fourth edition (American Psychiatric Association 1994) and the European based International Classification of Disease, currently in the tenth revision (WHO). The main criteria are summarized in

Table 11.2 ICD-10 and DSM-IV criteria for dementia.

ICD-10[1,2]	DSM-IV[3,4]
A syndrome due to disease of the brain, usually of a chronic (at least six months) or progressive nature with disturbance of memory and one or more higher cortical functions including thinking, orientation, comprehension, calculation, learning capacity, language, and judgement.	The development of multiple cognitive deficits manifested by memory impairment and at least one of: aphasia, apraxia, agnosia, and disturbance in executive functioning (e.g. planning and sequencing).
Consciousness is not clouded.	These cognitive deficits cause significant impairment in social and occupational functioning.
The cognitive impairments are commonly accompanied by deterioration in emotional control, social behaviour, or motivation.	Deficits do not occur exclusively during delirium and are not accounted for by depression.
There is usually some interference with personal activities of daily living, the exact nature of which will depend on the social and cultural setting in which the patient lives.	

1 Adapted from: *The ICD-10 Classification of Mental and Behavioural Disorders*. World Health Organization, Geneva 1992.

2 Unlike DSM-IV, ICD-10 specifically defines general criteria for dementia, prior to further criteria specific to particular types such as Alzheimer's disease and vascular dementia.

3 Adapted from: *Diagnostic and statistical manual of mental disorders*. 4th edition. American Psychiatric Association, Washington DC. 1995

4 The above criteria are common to all categories classified under dementia in DSM-IV, viz dementia of the Alzheimer type; vascular dementia: dementia due to other general medical conditions; substance-induced persisting dementia and dementia due to multiple aetiologies.

Table 11.2. Both require the memory problems to be evident in the absence of delirium and the exclusion of other diseases which may cause memory problems. In DSM IV, a person has to have multiple cognitive deficits rather than simply a decline in memory and thinking. Both emphasize that the deficits should interfere with activities of daily living and social functioning but only ICD 10 puts a time estimate of six months on the duration of illness. Erkinjunti *et al.* (1997) compared the DSM criteria (version III, 1980, the revision of version III, 1987, and version IV, 1994) and ICD criteria (version 9, 1977 and version 10, 1992) with CAMDEX criteria (Roth *et al.* 1986). The percentage of people receiving a diagnosis of dementia decreased with successive revisions of the DSM — 29.1% with DSM III, 17.3% with DSM IIIR and 13.7% with DSMIV. The rates with ICD 9 and 10 were 5% and 3.1% respectively. Subtle changes in the criteria over time are apparent: in the earliest DSM criteria, either short or long term memory loss was required for the diagnosis but later, both were required. The comparative low rates for ICD reflect the fact that more factors are required for the diagnosis.

Only a minority of clinicians use diagnostic criteria, 25% and 11% respectively in the studies of Somerfield *et al.* (1991) and Smith *et al.* (1992). Garcia *et al.* (1981) noted that the use of diagnostic criteria improved diagnostic accuracy, the main reasons for incorrect diagnosis being related to the failure to recognize depression, equating cerebral atrophy as seen on computed tomography with clinical dementia (avoided with the NINCDS/ADRDA criteria as atrophy is supportive rather than diagnostic) and focal impairment being regarded as synonymous with global impairment.

Instruments have been developed to provide a structured diagnosis of dementia. The geriatric mental state schedule (GMSS, Copeland *et al.* 1976) relies on features of the mental state but with the computer assisted algorithm (AGECAT) can provide an accurate diagnosis. The Cambridge examination for mental disorders of the elderly (CAMDEX, Roth *et al.* 1986) is divided into a number of sections — a structured psychiatric interview, cognitive evaluation (often referred to separately as the CAMCOG), mental state examination, informant interview, physical examination, physical investigations, and a list of medication. The Canberra interview for the elderly (CIE, Henderson *et al.* 1992) was designed for lay interviewers, has computer algorithms and is based on DSM and ICD criteria. SIDAM (Zaudig *et al.* 1991) is the structured interview for the diagnosis of dementia of the Alzheimer type, multi-infarct dementia, and other dementias. It is a semi-structured diagnostic interview, which allows for a diagnosis in accordance with ICD10 and DSM IIIR (the third edition revised, the predecessor to DSM IV) and includes standardized cognitive testing, taking into account medical history and severity of dementia.

11.5 Alzheimer's disease

Alzheimer's disease was first described by Alois Alzheimer in 1907 (Alzheimer 1907), the most prominent symptoms being those of behavioural disturbance (screaming, dragging her bedding around her hospital ward) and psychiatric symptoms (delusional ideas directed against her husband and Alzheimer, her physician), along with rapid onset of memory loss (Berrios 1994). Alzheimer considered that he had described a novel combination of features in terms of clinical features and pathological changes (plaques and tangles), not because of their combination, but the fact that they had occurred in a young person (the illness had started aged 51, coincidentally the age at which Alzheimer died). Until the clinical studies of the late 1960s (Blessed *et al.* 1968) which showed that AD pathology was the commonest determinant of dementia in older people and that the severity of the clinical picture correlated with the extent of the pathological change, AD was considered a diagnosis of younger people, the dementia affecting the elderly population being cerebrovascular in origin and termed senile dementia. This influenced the diagnostic process and AD was regarded as a diagnosis of exclusion, one which was made after all other diagnoses had been ruled out. However, there is now an appreciation that AD can be diagnosed positively (Reisberg *et al.* 1997) following a straightforward and simple clinical approach based on history, examination, and investigations.

11.6 Clinical diagnostic criteria for Alzheimer's disease

The most widely used set of diagnostic criteria for AD are those of the National Institute of Neurological and Communicative Disorders and Stroke and the Alzheimer's disease and Related Disorders Association (NINCDS/ADRDA, McKhann *et al.* 1984). Describing the deliberations of a workgroup, they reflected current clinical practice and the criteria are summarized in Table 11.3. The criteria are divided into probable, possible, and definite (requiring a histological diagnosis alongside a clinical picture). They require documentation of dementia using a scale such as the mini-mental state examination (Folstein *et al.* 1975) or the Blessed scale (Blessed *et al.* 1968). Two or more cognitive deficits are required, a curious feature being the inclusion of an age range of 40–90 years (reflecting diagnostic uncertainty outside these ages). Physical investigations such as blood tests and a computed tomography (CT) scan to rule out secondary causes is recommended. Tierney *et al.* (1988) validated these criteria against neuropathological features of AD. Their overall accuracy was 81–88%, with sensitivity of 64–86% (those patients diagnosed as having the disease clinically who had the pathological features) and a specificity of 89–91% (those patients who did not have the disease clinically who did not have the pathological changes). They differed with plaques and tangles in the hippocampus. Rates of accuracy of 78–88% (using possible and probable categories) have been described (Burns *et al.* 1990) and 87% have been described. Gearing *et al.* (1995) and Morris *et al.* (1988) found 100% accuracy of clinical diagnosis compared to histological changes. In other words, the criteria are useful in defining a sample of patients who are highly likely to have AD.

11.7 Clinical diagnostic criteria for other dementias

The other major dementias for which there are diagnostic criteria are vascular dementia, Lewy body dementia, and dementia of frontal type. The two main criteria for vascular dementia are the ADDTC (Chui *et al.* 1992) and NINCDS/AIREN (Roman *et al.* 1993) schemes. Each is summarized in the Table 11.4, the main differences being the definition of dementia, the requirement for brain imaging or neurological signs to support the diagnosis. The criteria for the diagnosis of Lewy body dementia are in Table 11.5 (after McKeith *et al.* 1992). Features of dementia of frontal lobe type appear in Table 11.6 (Lund and Manchester group 1994).

11.8 Assessment instruments for dementia

There are a plethora of instruments available for the assessment of various aspects of dementia and only very few are mentioned below. A more extensive summary of over 150 scales appears in Burns *et al.* (1999).

11.8.1 Cognitive function

The Mini-Mental State Examination: (MMSE, Folstein *et al.* 1975) is the most widely used test of cognitive function. It is scored out of 30, and tests the domains of orientation, language, writing, memory and praxis. It is reproduced in Table 11.7.

The Standardized Mini Mental State Examination: (Molloy *et al.* 1991) is a standardized version of the mini mental state examination which comes with complete rating instructions leading to slightly improved validity.

The Abbreviated Mental Test Score (AMTS, Hodkinson 1972) is a much briefer screening tool, is scored out of 10 and tests only orientation and memory.

Alzheimer's disease assessment scale: (ADAS, Rosen *et al.* 1984). This is now a standard cognitive scale used in drug trials. It assesses a number of cognitive functions including

Table 11.3 NINCDS-ADRDA criteria for clinical diagnosis of Alzheimer's disease (from McKhann *et al.* 1984).

I	The criteria for the clinical diagnosis of probable Alzheimer's disease include:

- dementia established by clinical examination and documented by the mini mental test, Blessed dementia scale or some similar examination, and confirmed by neuropsychological tests.

- deficits in two or more areas of cognition;

- progressive worsening of memory and other cognitive functions;

- no disturbance of consciousness;

- onset between ages 40 and 90, most often after age 65; absence of systemic disorders or other brain diseases that in and of themselves could account for the progressive deficits in memory and cognition.

II	Other clinical features consistent with the diagnosis of probable Alzheimer's disease, after exclusion of causes of dementia other than Alzheimer's disease, include:

- progressive deterioration of specific cognitive functions such as language (aphasia), motor skills (apraxia), and perception (agnosia);

- impaired activities of daily living and altered patterns of behaviour;

- family history of similar disorders, particularly if confirmed neuropathologically;

- laboratory results of:

    normal lumbar puncture as evaluated by standard techniques

    normal pattern or non-specific changes in EEG such as increased slow-wave activity;

    evidence of cerebral atrophy on CT with progression documented by serial observation

III	Other clinical features consistent with the diagnosis of probable Alzheimer's disease after exclusion of causes of dementia rather than Alzheimer's disease, include

- plateaus in the course of progression of the illness;

- other neurological abnormalities in some patients especially with more advanced disease and including motor signs such as increased muscle tone, myoclonus, or gait disorder;

- seizures in advanced diseases;

- CT normal for age.

IV	Features that make the diagnosis of probable Alzheimer's disease uncertain or unlikely include:

- sudden apoplectic onset;

- focal neurological findings such as hemiparesis, sensory loss, visual field deficits, and uncoordination early in the course of the illness

- seizures or gait disturbance at the onset or very early in the course of the illness

V	Clinical diagnosis of possible Alzheimer's disease.

- may be made on the basis of the dementia syndrome, in the absence of other neurological, psychiatric or systemic disorders sufficient to cause dementia and in the presence of variations in the onset, in the presentation, or in the clinical course;

- may be made in the presence of a second systemic or brain disorder sufficient to produce dementia, which is not considered to be the cause of the dementia;

- should be used in research studies when a single gradually progressive severe cognitive deficit is identified in the absence of other identifiable cause.

Table 11.3 (*continued*) NINCDS-ADRDA criteria for clinical diagnosis of Alzheimer's disease (from McKhann et al. 1984).

VI Criteria for diagnosis of definite Alzheimer's disease are:
• the clinical criteria for probable Alzheimer's disease and histopathological evidence obtained from a biopsy or autopsy.
VII Classification of Alzheimer's disease for research purposes should specify features that may differentiate subtypes of the disorder, such as:
• familial occurrence;
• onset before the age of 65;
• presence of trisomy-21.

memory, language, and praxis and also has a section devoted to non-cognitive features.

Clock drawing test: (Brodaty and Moore 1997; Shulman *et al.* 1986; Sunderland *et al.* 1989) This is a relatively new development which is easy to administer and is popular in primary care because of its simplicity.

11.8.2 Global measures

Clinical Dementia Rating: (Hughes *et al.* 1983; Morris 1993). This is probably the most widely used global scale to give an overall severity rating in dementia, ranging from 0 (none), 0.5 (questionable dementia), through mild (1) and moderate, (2) to severe (3) dementia. Each is rated in 6 domains — memory, orientation, judgement and problem solving, community affairs, home and hobbies, and personal care.

Global Deterioration Scale: (Reisberg *et al.* 1982). This scale consists of the description of 7 stages of dementia from 1 being normal to 7 where all verbal ability is lost. The scale has been used extensively and validated with post-mortem findings.

11.8.3 Psychopathology

Cornell Scale for Depression and Dementia: (Alexopoulos *et al.* 1988). This is a 19 item scale which specifically assesses depression in people with dementia in 5 main domains — mood related signs, behavioural disturbance, physical signs, cyclic functions, and ideation disturbance. A mixture of informant rated and observational ratings makes it ideal for the assessment in patients with cognitive impairment where information from the patient might not always be available. A score of 8 or above suggests significant depressive symptoms.

BEHAVE-AD: (Reisberg *et al.* 1987). This is a 25 item scale which measures many of the psychiatric symptoms in behavioural disturbances associated with dementia. They are rated on a 3 point scale and a second part of the scale is a global rating of the severity of the symptoms. The BEHAVE-AD is particularly useful in the assessment of patients in drug trials.

NeuroPsychiatric Inventory: (NPI, Cummings *et al.* 1994). Twelve behavioural areas are assessed in the NPI (delusions, hallucinations, agitation, depression, anxiety, euphoria,

Table 11.4 From: Amar *et al.* (1986). Reproduced with kind permission.

	The ADDTC criteria	The NINCDS-AIREN criteria
Dementia definition	Deterioration from a known level of intellectual function sufficient to interfere with the patient's customary affairs of life and which is not isolated to a single category of intellectual performance.	Impairment of memory plus at least two other areas of cognitive domains which should be severe enough to interfere with activities of daily living and not due to physical effects of stroke alone.
Probable vascular dementia	Requires all the following: Dementia	Requires all the following: Dementia
	Evidence of two or more strokes by history, neurological signs and/ or neuroimaging, or a single stroke with a clear temporal relationship to the onset of dementia.	Cerebrovascular disease (CVD); focal signs on examination + evidence of relevant CVD by brain imaging (CT/MR)
	Evidence of at least one infarct outside the cerebellum by CT or TI-weighted MRI	Relationship between the above two disorders, manifested by one or more of the following:
		(a) dementia onset within 3 months of a stroke
		(b) abrupt deterioration in cognitive functions, or fluctuating stepwise course
Possible vascular dementia	Dementia and one or more of the following: a) History or evidence of a single stroke without a clear temporal relationship to dementia onset or (b) Binswanger's disease that includes all the following: (i) early onset of urinary incontinence or gait disturbance; (ii) vascular risk factors; (iii) extensive white matter changes on neuroimaging	May be made in the presence of dementia and focal neurological signs in patients with: No evidence of CVD on neuroimaging; or In the absence of clear temporal relationship between stroke and dementia; or In patients with subtle onset and variable course of cognitive deficit and evidence of CVD

apathy, disinhibition, irritability, aberrant motor behaviour, night time behaviours, and appetite/eating disorders), each of which is rated on a 4 point scale of frequency and a 3 point scale of severity. Distress in carers is also measured.

MOUSEPAD: (Allen *et al.* 1996). This is based on the longer 'present behavioural examination' and measures a number of behaviour and psychiatric symptoms, with particular reference to their development over the life of the dementia syndrome.

Table 11.5 Operational criteria for senile dementia of the Lewy body type. (after McKeith *et al.* 1992)

Fluctuating cognitive impairment affecting both memory and higher cortical functions (such as 1anguage, visuospatial ability, praxis, or reasoning skills). The fluctuation is pronounced with both episodic confusion and lucid intervals, as in delirium, and is evident either on repeated tests of cognitive function or by variable performance in daily living skills.

At least one of the following:

visual or auditory hallucinations or both, which are usually accompanied by secondary paranoid delusions;

mild spontaneous extrapyramidal features or neuroleptic sensitivity syndrome- that is exaggerated adverse responses to standard doses of neuroleptics;

repeated unexplained falls, or transient clouding, or loss of consciousness, or both.

Despite this fluctuating pattern, the clinical features persist over a long period of weeks or months, unlike delirium which rarely persists as long. The illness progresses, often rapidly, to an end stage of severe dementia.

Exclusion by appropriate examination and investigation of any underlying physical illness adequate to account for the fluctuating cognitive state.

Exclusion of past history of confirmed stroke or evidence of cerebral ischaemic damage or both, on physical examination or brain imaging.

Table 11.6 Clinical features of fronto-temporal dementia.

Insidious onset and slow progression

Early loss of personal and social awareness and insight

Early signs of disinhibition

Mental rigidity and inflexibility

Hyperorality

Stereotyped and perserverative behaviour

Unrestrained exploration of objects and the environment (hypermetormorphosis)

Distractibility and impulsivity

Depression and anxiety

Hypochondriasis

Emotional unconcern

Inertia

Disorders of speech

Preserved abilities of spatial orientation

(Lund and Manchester groups 1994).

Table 11.7 Mini-mental state examination (MMSE) (Folstein *et al.* 1975)

Max score	Score	
		ORIENTATION
5	[ ]	What is the (year) (season) (date) (month) (day)?
5	[ ]	Where are we: (state) (county) (town) (hospital) (floor)?
		REGISTRATION
3	[ ]	Name 3 objects: (1 second to say each). Then ask the patient all three after you have said them.Give 1 point for each correct answer. Then repeat them until the patient learns all 3. Count trials and record.
		Number of trials ....
		ATTENTION AND CALCULATION
5	[ ]	Serial 7s. 1 point for each correct. Stop after 6 answers. If the patient refuses, spell 'world' backwards.
		RECALL
3	[ ]	Ask for 3 objects repeated above. Give 1 point for each correct.
		LANGUAGE
9	[ ]	Name a pencil; name a watch. (2 points)
		Repeat the following: 'No ifs, ands or buts' (1 point)
		Follow a three stage command; 'Take this paper in your right hand, fold it in half, and put it on the floor.' (3 points)
		Read and obey the following: 'Close your eyes' (1 point)
		Write a sentence (1 point)
		Copy a design (1 point)

TOTAL SCORE ———— Assess level of consciousness along a continuum Alert...Drowsy...Stupor...Coma

11.8.4 **Functional ability**

Bristol Activities of Daily Living Scale: (Bucks *et al.* 1996). A 20-item scale rated on a 5 point severity looking at basic activities of daily living (such as feeding, eating, and toiletting) and instrumental activities of daily living (which refer to the performance of more complex tasks such as shopping, travelling, answering the telephone, and handling finances)

Interview for Deterioration in Daily Living Activities in Dementia: (IDDD, Tuenisse *et al.* 1991). This contains 33 self-care items rated on a 4 point scale and has been used extensively to assess the effects of drugs.

Disability Assessment for Dementia: (DAD, Galineas *et al.* 2000). A rating of activities of daily living in dementia separating them into the different areas of initiation, planning and organisation and affective performance. ADL and instrumental ADL are assessed.

Alzheimer's Disease Functional Assessment and Change Scale: (ADFACS, Galasko *et al.* 1997) An 18 item scale looking at a wide range of basic activities and instrumental activities of daily living.

11.9 Conclusion

Contrary to widespread belief, the diagnosis of AD is a relatively simple process involving a straightforward clinical approach without necessarily the need for complex and detailed investigations or examinations except where the presentation or clinical course is atypical. Validated diagnostic criteria are available for all the major dementias, adherence to which increases diagnostic accuracy. Standardized scales are also becoming increasingly used to assess all aspects of the dementia syndrome.

Acknowledgements

We are grateful to Barbara Dignan, Sue Whalley and Barbara Woodyatt for secretarial help.

References

Alexopolous, G., Abrams, R., Young, R., and Shamoian, C. (1998). Cornell scale for depression in dementia. *Biological Psychiatry*, **232**, 271–84.

Allen, N. H. P., Gordon, S., Hope, T., and Burns, A. (1996). Manchester and Oxford Universities scale for the psychopathological assessment of dementia (MOUSEPAD). *British Journal of Psychiatry*, **169**, 293–307.

Alzheimer, A. (1907). Uber eigenartige ertrankungder Hirnrinde. *Allgmeine Zeitschrift fur Psychiatrie*, **64**, 146–8.

Amar, K., Wilcock, G. K., and Scott, M. (1986). The diagnosis of vascular dementia in the light of the main criteria. *Age and Ageing*, **25**, 51–5.

American Psychiatric Association (1994). In *Diagnostic and statistical manuals of mental disorders*, 4th edn Washington DC.

Baldereschi, M., Amato, M. P., Nencini, P., *et al.* (1994). Cross-national inter-rater agreement on the clinical diagnostic criteria for dementia. *Neurology*, **44**, 239–42.

Berrios, G. (1994). *Dementia: historical overview in dementia.* (ed. A. Burns and R. Levy), pp. 5–20.

Blessed, G., Tomlinson, B., and Roth, M. (1968). The association between quantitative measures of dementia and of senile change in the cerebral grey matter of elderly subjects. *British Journal of Psychiatry*, **114**, 797–811.

Brodaty, H. and Moore, C. M. (1997). The clock drawing test for dementia of the Alzheimer's type: a comparison of three scoring methods in memory disorders clinic. *International Journal of Geriatric Psychiatry*, **12**, 619–27.

Bucks, R., Ashworth, D., Wilcock, G., and Siegfrid, K. (1996). Assessment of activities of daily living in dementia. *Age and Ageing*, **25**, 113–20.

Burns, A., Luthert, P., Levy, R., *et al.* (1990). Accuracy of clinical diagnosis of Alzheimer's disease. *British Medical Journal*, **301**, 1026.

Burns, A., Lawlor, B., and Craig, S. (1999). Assessment Scales in Old Age Psychiary. Dunitz.

Chui, H., Victoroff, J., and Margolin, D., *et al.* (1992). Criteria for the diagnosis of ischaemic vascular dementia proposed by the State of California Alzheimer's Disease Diagnostic and Treatment Centres. *Neurology*, **42**, 473–80.

Copeland, J., Kelleher, M., Kellett, J., *et al.* (1976). The Geriatric Mental State Schedule. *Psychological Medicine*, **6**, 439–49.

Corey-Bloom, J., Thal, L. J., Galasko, D., *et al.* (1995). Diagnosis and evaluation of dementia. *Neurology*, **45**, 211–18.

Cummings, J. L., Mega, M., Gray, K., *et al.* (1994). The Neuropsychiatric Inventory — comprehensive assessment of psychopathology in dementia. *Neurology*, **44**, 2308–14.

Doraiswamy, P. M., Steffens, D. C., Pitchumoni, S., and Tabrizi, S. (1998). Early recognition of Alzheimer's disease. *Journal of Clinical Psychiatry*, **59**, 6–18.

Erkinjuntti, T., Ostbye, T., Steenhuis, R., and Hachinski, V. (1997). The effect of different diagnostic criteria on the prevalence of dementia. *The New England Journal of Medicine*, **337**, 1667–74.

Folstein, M., Folstein, S., and McHugh, P. (1975). Mini-mental state. A practical method for grading the cognitive state of patients for the clinician. *Journal of Psychiatric Research*, **12**, 189–98.

Galasko, D., Bennett, D., Sanor, M., *et al.* (1997). An inventory to assess activities of daily living for clinical trials in Alzheimer's disease. *Alzheimer's Disease and Associated Disorders*, **11** S33–9.

Galineas, I., Cofia, L., Mackintyre, M., and Cofia, S. (2000). Development of a functional measure for persons with Alzheimer's disease. *American Journal of Occupational Therapy*, (in press).

Garcia, C. A., Reding, M. J., and Blass, J. P. (1981). Overdiagnosis of dementia. *Journal of the American Geriatrics Society*, **29**, 407–10.

Gearing, M., Mirra, S. S., Hedreeen, J. C., *et al.* (1995). The consortium to establish a registry for Alzheimer's disease (CERAD) — part X — Neuropathology confirmations of the clinical diagnosis of Alzheimer's disease. *Neurology*, **45**, 461–6.

Hachinski, V. C., Iliff, L. D., Zilkha, E., *et al.* (1975). Cerebral blood flow in dementia. *Archives of Neurology*, **32**, 632–7.

Henderson, A. S. *et al.* (1992). The Canberra Interview for the Elderly: a new field instrument for the diagnosis of dementia and depression by ICD-10 and DSM-III-R. *Acta Psychiatrica Scandinavica*, **85**, 105–13.

Hodkinson, H. M. (1972). Evaluation of a mental test score or assessment of mental impairment in the elderly. *Age and Ageing*, **1**, 233–8.

Holmes, C., Cairns, N., Lantos, P., and Mann, S. (1999). Validity of current clinical criteria for Alzheimer's disease vascular dementia and dementia with Lewy bodies. *British Journal of Psychiatry*, **174**, 45–50.

Hughes, C., Berg, L., Danziger, W. L., *et al.* (1982). A new clinical scale for the staging of dementia. *British Journal of Psychiatry*, **140**, 566–72.

Lund and Manchester Groups (1994). Clinical and neuropathological criteria for frontotemporal dementia. *Journal of Neurology, Neurosurgery and Psychiatry*, **57**, 416–18.

McKeith, I., Perry, R., Fairbairn, A., *et al.* (1992). Operational criteria for senile dementia of Lewy body type *Psychological Medicine*, **22**, 911–22.

McKeith, I. G., Galasko, D., Kosaka, K., *et al.* (1996). Consensus guidelines for the clinical and pathologic diagnosis of dementia with Lewy bodies (DLB): Report of the consortium on DLB international workshop *Neurology*, **47**, 1113–24.

McKhann, G., Drachman, D., Folstein, M., *et al.* (1984). Clinical diagnosis of Alzheimer's disease: Report of the NINCDS-ADRDA workgroup under the auspices of Department of Health and Human Services task force on Alzheimer's disease. *Neurology*, **34**, 939–44.

Molloy, D., Alemayehu, E., and Roberts, R. (1991). Reliability of a standardized Mini Mental State Examination. *American Journal of Psychiatry*, **148**, 102–5.

Morris, J. (1993). The CDR: current version and scoring rules. *Neurology*, 43, 2412–3.

Morris, J. C., McKeel, D. W., Fulling, K., *et al.* (1988). Validation of clinical diagnostic criteria for Alzheimer' s disease. *Annals of Neurology*, 24, 17–22.

Oppenheim, G. (1994). The earliest signs of Alzheimer's disease. *Journal of Geriatric Psychiatry and Neurology*, 7, 116–20.

Reisberg, B., Borenstein, J., Salob, S. P., *et al.* (1987). Behavioural symptoms in Alzheimer's disease: phenomenology and treatment. *Journal of Clinical Psychiatry*, 48, 9–15.

Reisberg, B., Ferris, S. H., DeLeon, M. J., and Crook, T. (1982). The global deterioration scale for assessment of primary degenerative dementia. *American Journal of Psychiatry*, 139, 1136–9.

Roman, G., Tatemichi, T., Erkinjuntti, T., *et al.* (1993). Vascular dementia: diagnostic criteria for research studies. *Neurology*, 43, 250–60.

Rosen, W. G., Mohs, R. C., and Davis, K. L. (1984). A new rating scale for Alzheimer's disease. *American Journal of Psychiatry*, 141, 1356–64.

Roth, M., Tym, E., Mountjoy, C. Q., *et al.* (1986). CAMDEX — A standardized instrument for the diagnosis of mental disorder in the elderly with special reference to the early detection of dementia. *British Journal of Psychiatry*, 149, 698–709.

Shulman, K., Shedletsky, R., and Silver, I. (1986). The challenge of time. Clock drawing and cognitive function in elderly. *International Journal of Geriatric Psychiatry*, 1, 135–40.

Smith, C. W., Byrne, E. J., Arie, T., and Lilley, J. M. (1992). Diagnosis of dementia II — Diagnostic Methods: a Survey of Current Consultant Practice and Review of the Literature *International Journal of Geriatric Psychiatry*, 7, 323–9.

Somerfield, M. R., Wiesman, C. S., Ury, W., *et al.* (1991). Physician practices in the diagnosis of dementing disorders. *Journal of the American Geriatrics Society*, 39, 172–5.

Sunderland, T., Hill, J., Mellow, A., *et al.* (1989). Clock drawing in Alzheimer's disease *Journal of the American Geriatrics Society*, 37, 725–9.

Teunisse, S., Derix, M. M. A., and Van Crevel, H. (1991). Assessing the severity of dementia — patient and caregiver. *Archives of Neurology*, 48, 274–7.

Tierney, M. C., Fisher, R. H., Lewis, A. J., *et al.* (1988). The NINCDS-ADRDA work group outcome for the clinical diagnosis of probable Alzheimer's disease: A clinicopathologic study of 57 cases. *Neurology*, 38, 359–64.

World Health Organization (1992). *International classification of mental and behavioural disorders*. 10th edn.WHO.

Zaudig, M., Mittelhammer, J., Hiller, W., *et al.* (1991). SIDAM — a structured interview for the diagnosis of dementia of the Alzheimer type, multi-infarct dementia and dementia of other aetiology according to ICD 10 and DSMIIIR. *Psychological Medicine*, 21, 225–36.

Chapter 12

Molecular and biological markers for diagnosing and monitoring the progression of Alzheimer's disease

Hiroyuki Arai, Makoto Higuchi, Nobuyuki Okamura, Yu-ichi Morikawa, Susumu Higuchi, Takeshi Iwatsubo, Eugeen Vanmechelen, Hugo Vanderstichele, John Q. Trojanowski, and Hidetada Sasaki

12.1 Introduction

Alzheimer's disease (AD) is a chronic neurodegenerative disease characterized by common clinical features (such as progressive memory loss and other cognitive impairments) and distinct neuropathological lesions (that is massive degeneration of selectively vulnerable neurons as well as abundant senile plaques, neurofibrillary tangles (NFT), and related neurofibrillary lesions) within the central nervous system (Trojanowski *et al.* 1996; Ginsberg *et al.* 1999). In typical cases, AD begins with insidious memory impairments followed by disturbances in other cognitive domains including language and visuospatial skills. These impairments gradually progress to the extent that patients are not able to live independently. Finally, patients are unable to feed themselves, and they may develop aspiration pneumonias or other infections which are the proximal cause of death. The criteria most commonly used for the clinical diagnosis of AD in living patients include the National Institute of Neurological and Communicative Disorders and Stroke and the Alzheimer's disease and Related Disorders Association (NINCDS-ADRDA) criteria (McKhann *et al.* 1984) or Diagnostic and Statistical Manual (DSM-IV) criteria (American Psychiatric Association 1994). However, a definite diagnosis of AD can only be made if post-mortem examination of the affected brain reveals abundant senile plaques and NFT in many cortical regions as proposed in an initial consensus document (Khachaturian 1985) which was updated and clarified recently in another consensus report (NIA Working Group 1997). Both the NINCDS-ADRDA criteria and the DSM-IV criteria require the presence of memory impairment and at least one of several other cognitive dysfunctions that are severe enough to disturb social and occupational activities.

Clinico-pathological studies have shown that the accuracy of criteria for the clinical diagnosis of AD is about 85% (Tierney *et al.* 1989). These diagnostic criteria have been well accepted by many researchers and they appear to minimize false-positive diagnoses of AD in living patients. None the less, it is still nearly impossible to detect AD accurately in its very mild or presymptomatic stages before extensive brain damage occurs, and improved strategies to accomplish this are desperately needed, especially for the conducting clinical trials of new therapeutics. Indeed, the most important clinical applications of a reliable biological marker of AD would be to use it to develop accurate tests for the early diagnosis of AD, to monitor the response of AD patients to new therapeutic interventions, to track the progression of AD, and rule out the presence of other dementing neurodegenerative disorders that resemble AD. As suggested in another recent consensus report (Reagan Institute 1998), the ideal biological marker should be reliable, reproducible, non-invasive, simple to perform, inexpensive, and with a sensitivity >80% and a specificity >80%. Unfortunately, no ideal biological markers have been reported and confirmed in follow-up studies.

However, among the proposed molecular and biological markers, mutations in presenilin-1 (*PS-1*), presenilin-2 (*PS-2*), and amyloid precursor protein (*APP*) genes for early-onset familial AD (FAD) have some diagnostic value, and cerebrospinal fluid (CSF) levels of tau and amyloid β-protein ending at amino acid 42 (Aβ1–42) appear to have the most promise for the diagnosis of sporadic and possibly FAD (Reagan Institute 1998). This review focuses on the potential uses and further development of CSF assays of CSF tau and Aβ, as well as genetic polymorphisms or allelic variants for the diagnosis of AD.

12.2 **Cerebrospinal fluid tau protein**

Tau proteins are a group of developmentally regulated microtubule-associated proteins that bind to microtubules to stabilize them and facilitate the polymerization of tubulin into microtubules. Tau consists of six alternatively spliced proteins encoded by the gene on chromosome 17. The paired helical filaments (PHF) that accumulate in AD NFT were isolated from the AD brain and shown to comprise hyperphosphorylated tau (Lee *et al.* 1991; Ginsberg *et al.* 1998). Since there is a correlation between the abundance of neurofibrillary lesions and severity of dementia in AD (Arriagata *et al.* 1992), it seemed plausible to measure CSF levels of tau (CSF-tau) in living patients for the diagnosis of AD. In 1993, Vandermeeren *et al.* established a new technology to detect CSF-tau by enzyme-linked immunosorbent assay (ELISA). The ELISA (Innotest™ hTAUAg, Innogenetics, Belgium) was constructed to detect both normal and PHF-tau using three different phosphorylation independent antibodies (AT120, HT7, and BT2) to tau (Vandermeeren *et al.* 1993). The ELISA is sensitive in detecting tau in a range from 10–160 pg/ml on a human brain tau basis, and in a range from 70–1120 pg/ml on a recombinant tau basis. Subsequently, several independent groups have reported that the CSF-tau is significantly increased in patients with AD compared to patients with other neurological diseases and normal control subjects (Arai *et al.* 1995; Jensen *et al.* 1995; Mori *et al.* 1995; Motter *et al.* 1995; Munroe *et al.* 1995; Rosler *et al.* 1996). We have extended our earlier studies and additional patients are included and re-analysed here.

In the present analysis, a total of 410 demented and non-demented patients were examined. As shown in Table 12.1, they included 143 patients with AD (73.9 ± 7.8 years), 45 patients with meningo-encephalitis (36.6 ± 15.9 years), 27 patients with Parkinson's disease (68.0 ± 7.6 years), 22 patients with alcohol-induced dementia (59.2± 6.5 years),

Table 12.1 Case material examined here

	Number of patients	Age(Years)
Alzheimer's disease	143	73.9 ± 7.8
Cortico-basal degeneration	3	64.0 ± 7.2
Dementia with Lewy bodies	9	65.3 ± 8.1
Frontotemporal dementia	11	64.2 ± 11.4
Multisystem atrophy	12	60.4 ± 7.6
Menigo-encephalitis	45	36.6 ± 15.9
Motor neuron disease	21	65.1 ± 9.2
Multiple sclerosis	11	39.3 ± 9.5
Alcoholic dementia	22	59.2 ± 6.5
Progressive supranuclear palsy	6	64.0 ± 4.6
Vascular dementia	21	72.0 ± 7.2
Parkinson's disease	27	68.0 ± 7.6
Myopathy	5	49.2 ± 22.1
Others	22	63.2 ± 13.7
Mild cognitive impairment	9	76.8 ± 5.9
Memory complainer	7	64.3 ± 16.0
Normal control	28	54.3 ± 20.7
Total	410	64.2 ± 16.1

21 patients with motor neuron disease (65.1 ± 9.2 years), 21 patients with vascular dementia (72.0 ± 7.2 years), 12 patients with multi-system atrophy (60.4 ± 7.6 years), 11 patients with frontotemporal dementia (FTD, 64.2 ± 11.4 years), 11 patients with multiple sclerosis (39.3 ± 9.5 years), 9 patients with dementia with Lewy bodies (DLB, 65.3 ± 8.1 years), 9 patients with mild cognitive impairments (76.8 ± 5.9 years), 8 non-demented patients with cerebrovascular disease (66.4 ± 10.5 years), 7 memory complainers without dementia (64.3 ± 16.0), 6 patients with progressive supranuclear palsy (PSP, 64.0±4.6 years), 5 patients with miscellaneous myopathy (49.2 ± 22.1 years), 3 patients with cortico-basal degeneration (64.0 ± 7.2 years), 22 patients with other neurological diseases (63.2 ± 13.6 years) and 28 normal control subjects without major medical and neuropsychiatric diseases (54.3 ± 20.7 years). Diagnostic criteria and/or guidelines used here included NINCDS-ADRDA criteria for AD, ADDTC criteria for vascular disease, Lund and Manchester criteria for FTD (Lund and Manchester Groups 1994), consensus guidelines by McKeith *et al.* for DLB (McKeith *et al.* 1996), and DSM-IV criteria for alcohol-induced dementia (American Psychiatric Association 1994). The diagnosis of PSP and cortico-basal degeneration were established based on the original descriptions by Steele *et al.* for PSP (Steele *et al.* 1964) and Gibb *et al.* for cortico-basal degeneration (Gibb *et al.* 1989), respectively. Each of the other neurological diseases were diagnosed by well-documented neurological signs and symptoms described in the literature. Other neurological disease groups included 4 patients with epilepsy, 4 patients with depression, 3 patients with Creutzfeldt-Jakob disease, 3 patients

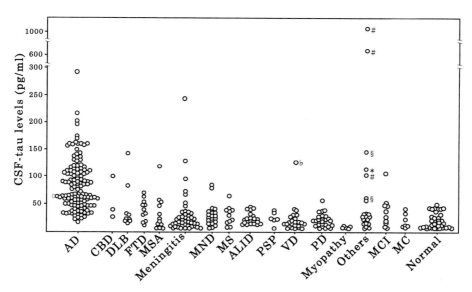

Fig. 12.1 Cerebrospinal fluid tau (CSF-tau) protein levels in diverse neurological diseases and controls. Values were expressed using bovine tau standards. One patient with vascular dementia showed a high CSF-tau level which may suggest the presence of combined dementia (indicated by b). #: Creutzfeldt-Jakob disease, §: dementia due to B_{12} deficiency, *: normal pressure hydrocephalus

with Neuro-Beçhet disease, 2 patients with vitamin B_{12} deficiency, 1 patient with cerebellitis, 1 patient with chronic inflammatory demyelinating polyneuropathy, 1 patient with neurosyphilis, and 3 patients who had an uncertain diagnosis of dementia. The AD patients were enrolled from 1991 until 1998 in The Tohoku University Outpatient clinic for dementia, and they were either sporadic or late-onset FAD cases. As shown in Fig. 12.1, CSF-tau levels (Mean ± standard deviation) were 86.1 ± 68.3 in AD, 54.4 ± 37.6 in cortico-basal degeneration, 43.2 ± 40.5 in DLB, 39.0 ± 18.8 in FTD, 40.0 ± 32.4 in MSA, 30.7 ± 39.1 in meningo-encephalitis, 30.3 ± 19.7 in motor neuron disease, 29.9 ± 17.2 in multiple sclerosis, 24.6 ± 10.0 in alcoholic dementia, 24.1 ± 13.7 in PSP, 30.0 ± 27.3 in vascular dementia, 20.4 ± 11.7 in Parkinson's disease, 8.1 ± 2.7 in myopathy, 118.3 ± 268.8 in Others, 41.5 ± 33.7 in mild cognitive impairments, 22.4 ± 12.6 in memory complainers, and 15.7 ± 12.9 in the normal control group.

The CSF-tau levels in AD were significantly elevated compared to those in vascular disease (p = 0.0016), alcohol-induced dementia (p = 0.0005), meningo-encephalitis (p<0.0001), Parkinson's disease (p<0.0001), motor neuron disease (p = 0.0021), non-demented cerebrovascular disease patients (p = 0.016), multisystem atrophy (p = 0.02), multiple sclerosis (p = 0.02), myopathy (p = 0.03), patients with memory complaints (p = 0.03) and normal controls (p<0.0001). There was a trend toward a lower CSF-tau level in so-called tauopathies including cortico-basal degeneration (p = 0.48), DLB (p = 0.11), FTD (p = 0.05), PSP (p = 0.05) as well as others (p = 0.07), and mild cognitive impairments (p = 0.09), but they did not reach a statistically significant level due to a small sample size. Using a 41.5 pg/ml (mean+2 standard deviations of normal control) as a cut-off, AD can be detected with a sensitivity of 81.5% and a specificity of 88%. The specificity of the CSF-tau assay for discriminating AD from other neurodegenerative conditions is not enhanced by combination of tau with two other neuron-specific proteins i.e. neuron-specific enolase and neuromodulin (Vanmechelen *et al.* 1997). Although the number of samples from non-AD groups including cortico-basal degeneration, myopathy, and PSP is limited and CSF-tau measurements may have less diagnostic value in the differential diagnosis between AD and some of the non-AD neurological diseases (including the group of neurodegenerative 'tauopathies' characterized by abundant tau pathology) several important observations from recent studies are worth emphasizing here.

First, a subset of patients with mild cognitive impairments showed a borderline or an AD range of their CSF-tau levels. If disturbances in memory and other cognitive functions are very mild and patients are still independent in their social and occupational life, these patients are referred to as having 'mild cognitive impairments', but not dementia. In such instances, we are uncertain if they represent patients with early and subtle signs of AD or if they reflect benign forgetfulness associated with age or other non-progressive mild memory disorders such as that due to anxiety. Despite an extensive evaluation by computerized tomography (CT) and/or magnetic resonance imaging (MRI), there is limited information in the diagnostic work-up in most cases. Therefore, patients are often asked for a re-evaluation in 6–12 months.

In order to examine whether an elevated CSF-tau level might be a potential predictor of progression to dementia in patients with questionable dementia (clinical dementia rating 0.5), we carefully followed up 15 patients for a mean period of three years after an initial assessment of CSF-tau was completed (Arai *et al.* 1997c). Ten of the patients progressed to manifest further cognitive deficits, meeting the DSM-IV or the NINCDS-ADRDA criteria for AD upon follow-up (Fig. 12.2). In the 'progressive group', the CSF-tau levels at entry

	Non-Progressive	Progressive	p<
Number	5	10	
Male/female ratio	2:3	3:7	
Entry MMSE score	25.4 ± 2.5	25.7 ± 2.4	0.83
Age at entry (years)	73.0 ± 13.9	68.2 ± 9.8	0.45
Follow-up period (months)	35.0 ± 21.0	33.0 ± 25.0	0.91
CSF-tau (pg/ml)	21.2 ± 12.4	88.2 ± 41.0	0.005

MMSE: Mini-mental state examination

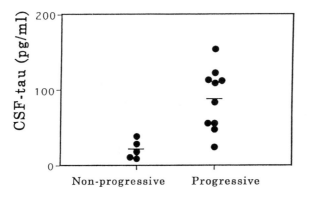

Fig. 12.2 Above: baseline patient profiles in the progressive (left) and non-progressive group (right) of patients that presented with questionable dementia. Below: the baseline CSF-tau levels were significantly higher in the progressive group compared to the non-progressive group. See Arai *et al.* (1997c). for further details.

were significantly increased (88.2 ± 41.0 pg/ml) and were in an AD range compared to the other 5 patients who remained non-demented or even better than the initial evaluation (21.2 ± 12.4 pg/ml). These 10 patients who progressed to AD are included in the AD group in Fig. 12.1. Three out of nine patients with mild cognitive impairments in Fig. 12.1 show CSF-tau levels above the upper range of the normal control group and we are attempting to follow-up such patients. Two of these have been described by Terajima et al. (Terajima et al. 1996). If effective therapies for AD are to be developed they must be administered in the early stages of the disease before a massive and extensive loss of neurons has taken place. As to cholinergic therapy using acetylcholine esterase inhibitors or cholinomimetic drugs, we demonstrated that pre-and/or post-synaptic acetylcholine receptors visualized by positron emission tomography (PET) started degenerating in the early stage of AD, and the receptor binding was progressively lost as the disease progressed (Higuchi et al. unpublished data). Since efforts to develop assays that enable an accurate diagnosis of AD in its earliest stages are considered an important future goal in the consensus recommendations of the working group of The Ronald and Nancy Reagan Institute of Alzheimer's Association on biological markers of AD (1998), especially for conducting clinical trials of emerging therapeutic interventions, it appears that measurement of CSF-tau levels may become an appropriate strategy for this purpose.

Second, CSF-tau measurements can be a useful diagnostic marker in combination with other clinical findings in the differential diagnosis between AD and vascular disease (Arai et al. 1998). There was only a small overlap in the CSF-tau levels between AD and vascular disease, and the CSF-tau levels were in a normal range in our vascular disease patients except for one who showed 83.5 pg/ml (Fig. 12.1b). This is particularly important in Japan, because vascular disease is still the most predominant type of dementia, and because vascular disease and AD collectively account for approximately 80–90% of all dementia cases in Japan. Further, our findings imply that ischaemia alone may not cause a massive and progressive death of neurons required for the increase in the CSF-tau levels in most AD patients. The CSF-tau levels were transiently elevated in patients with acute cerebral infarction when CSF samples were taken 2–3 weeks after the onset of stroke (Arai et al. unpublished observation), suggesting that CSF samples obtained on near occasions of acute stroke should be interpreted with caution. There was no significant difference in the CSF-tau levels between multiple lacunar infarctions and other types of vascular disease, whereas Andreasen et al. reported that vascular disease patients with progressive leukoaraiosis showed relatively lower CSF-tau levels compared to those without such progressive leukoaraiosis (Andreasen et al. 1998). Despite common features shared by AD and vascular disease, both underlying mechanisms leading to dementia and genetic or other risk factors should be considered separately in the aetiology of AD and vascular disease.

Thirdly, it remains unknown why there is a wide range in CSF-tau levels in AD. The CSF-tau levels in AD were increased irrespective of age at onset, gender, and apolipoprotein E (APOE)genotype (Fig. 12.3). Several independent groups demonstrated that the CSF-tau levels are elevated in such mild stages of AD (Arai et al. 1997c; Galasko et al. 1997; Riemenschneider et al. 1997) and they continued to be abnormally high during the progression of the disease (Arai et al. 1997a; Isoe et al. 1996). There was no correlation between the CSF-tau levels and dementia severity as assessed by mini-mental state examination (MMSE) as described in a small sample size (Munroe et al. 1995). Therefore, an interval between the onset of AD and spinal tap does not appear to influence diagnostic accuracy. Further, the CSF-tau levels alone did not correlate with global deterioration of cerebral glucose utilization, suggesting that the CSF-tau levels did not simply reflect the rate of

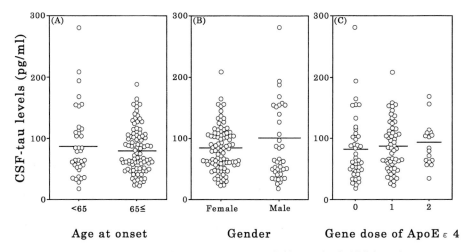

Fig. 12.3 The CSF-tau levels according to age at onset (left), gender (middle), and *APOE* genotype (right). Each bar represents the mean value.

neuron loss, but rather complicated mechanisms may exist in the regulation of the CSF-tau (Okamura N, unpublished data).

Finally, there is a potential limitation in the use of the ELISA to differentiate AD from certain neurological diseases, especially the tauopathies (Arai *et al.* 1997*b*). An accurate distinction between AD and other primary degenerative dementia including DLB, FTD, cortico-basal degeneration, and PSP may not be possible by monitoring CSF-tau levels alone. This is not surprising, because all of these disorders are characterized by a progressive degeneration of specific populations of neurons, and because the ELISA has been constructed to detect both normal and PHF-tau. In AD, it is as yet unclear whether the increase in the CSF-tau levels is related to a progressive accumulation of PHF-tau in neurons or if it simply reflects more generalized neuron damage. Therefore, it remains to be determined if the accumulation and release of PHF-tau can be distinguished from an increase in the release of normal tau from neurons by measuring CSF-tau levels by the ELISA. The diagnosis of DLB apart from AD is particularly important, because DLB patients have a greater sensitivity to neuroleptics than AD patients, and because the parkinsonian motor features of DLB patients often respond to L-dopa therapy. Recently, functional neuroimaging using positron emission tomography (PET) or single photon emission computed tomography (SPECT) have shown that occipital hypometabolism or hypoperfusion has a diagnostic value in the distinction between AD and DLB (Albin *et al.* 1996; Ishii *et al.* 1998). Abnormal CSF-tau levels have also seen in certain acute neurological conditions including vitamin B_{12} deficiency, Creutzfeldt-Jakob disease and hypoxic brain damage (Ohrui *et al.* 1997). However, the rate of cognitive decline and other neurological features as well as laboratory and neuroimaging findings should enable the distinction of these disorders. Therefore, it is necessary to refine an ELISA that is highly specific to AD-PHF/tau. Mutations in the α-synuclein gene in sporadic DLB cases are unlikely to be found (Higuchi *et al.* 1998), but in a small group of familial FTD cases, it is appropriate to search for mutations in the tau gene on chromosome 17 (Hutton *et al.* 1998).

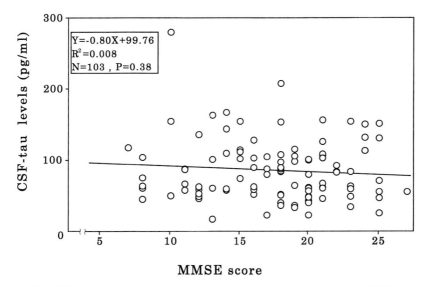

Fig. 12.4 The CSF-tau levels as a function of mini-mental state examination (MMSE) scores in 113 Alzheimer's disease patients. No significant correlation was noted between the MMSE scores and the CSF-tau levels.

12.3 **Cerebrospinal fluid amyloid-β protein (Aβ)1–42**

The deposition of amyloid β protein (Aβ) in abundant senile plaques that accumulate in selected brain regions is the second pathological hallmark brain lesion required for the definite diagnosis of AD brain (Selkoe 1994; NIA Consensus Report 1997). Aβ is a 40–43 amino acid long peptide that is proteolytically cleaved from APP by β and γ secretase enzymes. Aβ is secreted into extracellular space and the CSF by normal metabolic processes (Seubert *et al.* 1992; Shoji *et al.* 1992). Two main forms of Aβ have been identified, Aβ1–40 and Aβ1–42 (Suzuki *et al.* 1994). Immunohistochemical studies have shown that Aβ1–42 deposits initially and predominantly in senile plaques of AD, Down syndrome and normal aged brains (Iwatsubo *et al.* 1994). Furthermore, a recent study has shown that an elevation in the levels of soluble Aβ1–42 in brain tissue precedes the formation of senile plaques in Down syndrome brains (Teller *et al.* 1996). Several studies using cultured cells transfected with mutant *APP* genes have shown that the APP670/671 mutations increase Aβ secretion by 5–8 fold, whereas the APP717 mutation increases the percentage of Aβ1–42 in the total pool of Aβ. If Aβ1–40 or Aβ1–42 and their derivatives are produced by neurons affected by AD pathology, and this is reflected in the species of Aβ that are secreted into extracellular space, then measures of the relative abundance of different Aβ species in the CSF may enable the early diagnosis of AD and for monitoring the progression of the disease as well as the response of AD patients to treatment. Initial studies have reported that total CSF-Aβ levels did not differ significantly from those in normal control subjects (Nitsch *et al.* 1995; Van Gool *et al.* 1995). However, subsequent studies to quantify the levels of total Aβ and the pools of Aβ1–40 and Aβ1–42 in CSF by ELISA using well-characterized antibodies to each of these two Aβ species have concluded that CSF-Aβ1–42 levels are preferentially reduced in

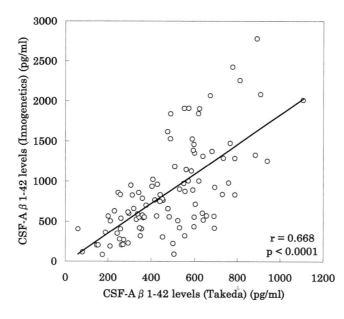

Fig. 12.5 A significant positive correlation was noted between values obtained by two independent ELISAs for CSF-Aβ1–42 provided by Takeda Chemical and Innogenetics. See Suzuki *et al.* 1994 and Vanderstichele *et al.* 1998 for original antibodies.

AD (Motter *et al.* 1995; Tamaoka *et al.* 1997; Galasko *et al.* 1998; Hock *et al.* 1998; Kanai *et al.* 1998; Andreasen *et al.* 1999). The ELISAs have been developed independently by Takeda Chemical, Japan (Suzuki *et al.* 1994) and Innogenetics, Belgium (Vanderstichele *et al.* 1998). Data from these two independent ELISAs correlated well with each other ($n = 99$, $r = 0.668$, $p < 0.0001$), although the absolute values obtained with each of these assays differed (Fig. 12.5)

The exact reason for the difference in the absolute values is not clear, but it could be due to several factors for example the use of different antibodies in the assays, or different assay protocols, or different methods for the preparation of Aβ peptides used as standards. In the assay of CSF-Aβ, care must be taken to use polypropylene tubes for handling and storage of CSF samples, and to avoid repeated freeze-thawing cycles. Treatment of CSF samples by heating for 3 min at 100°C before measurement did not affect absolute values. Using the Innognetics' ELISA, we investigated CSF-Aβ1–42 levels from a total of 135 patients, and we divided them into 7 groups for analysis: mild AD (mini mental score examination MMSE score>20 points, $n = 30$), moderate AD (MMSE score between 13–19 points, $n = 24$), advanced AD (MMSE score<12 points, $n = 26$), neurodegenerative dementia other than AD ($n = 24$) including FTD ($n = 8$), DLB ($n = 8$), PSP ($n = 5$) and cortico-basal degeneration ($n = 3$), vascular disease ($n = 8$), mild cognitive impairment ($n = 6$), and non-demented normal controls ($n = 17$). The CSF-Aβ1–42 levels were 374.2 ± 147.2 pg/ml (mean $\pm$ SD) in the mild AD group, 360.8 ± 105.9 pg/ml in the moderate AD group, 306.1 ± 117.1 pg/ml in the advanced AD group, 308.3 ± 193.9 pg/ml in the non-AD neurodegenerative dementia group, 451.5 ± 115.4 pg/ml in the vascular disease group, 542.3 ± 355.1 pg/ml in the mild cognitive impairment group and 562.8 ± 272.7 pg/ml in the non-demented normal group (Fig.12.6).

A significant reduction of CSF-Aβ1–42 levels was observed in all of the groups except for the vascular disease and the mild cognitive impairment groups when compared with

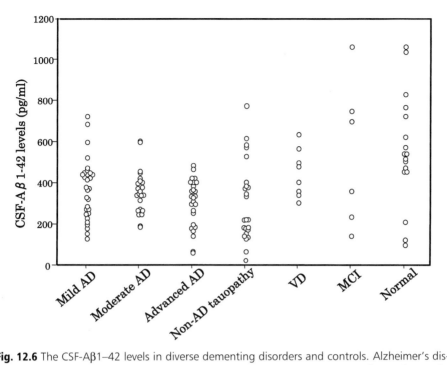

Fig. 12.6 The CSF-Aβ1–42 levels in diverse dementing disorders and controls. Alzheimer's disease (AD) was divided into mild, moderate, and advanced groups based on dementia severity. Dementia with Lewy bodies, frontotemporal dementia, progressive supranuclear palsy and corticobasal degeneration are collectively referred to as 'non-AD tauopathy' here. VD: vascular dementia, MCI: mild cognitive impairment.

non-demented normal patients. Among three AD subgroups with different clinical stages, the CSF-Aβ1–42 levels showed a non-significant trend towards declining values as the disease progressed. Furthermore, there was no correlation between the CSF-Aβ1–42 levels and the duration of dementia, and the CSF-Aβ1–42 levels obtained on two separate occasions were stable at the baseline and follow-up assays (Andreasen *et al.* 1999). The CSF-Aβ1–42 levels in AD patients were significantly lower than those of the aged normal (p<0.001) and the MCI (p<0.05) groups. In addition, CSF-Aβ1–42 levels in the severe AD group were significantly lower from those in the vascular disease group (p<0.05). Despite an overlap in these levels in some of the groups, our data demonstrated that measurement of CSF-Aβ1–42 levels could differentiate AD from normal patients. However the CSF-Aβ1–42 levels in the neurodegenerative dementia group also decreased to nearly a comparable degree as in the AD patients. It remains enigmatic whether these reductions in CSF-Aβ1–42 levels reflect a progressive deposition of Aβ within senile plaque or the alteration of Aβ clearance in the AD brain. The CSF-Aβ1–42 in the vascular disease group also showed a trend of slight reduction compared to normal controls. These results indicate that the reduction of CSF-Aβ1–42 levels is not necessarily specific for AD patients. Since the total CSF-Aβ levels including both CSF-Aβ1–40 and 1–42 are inversely correlated with dementia severity (Nitsch *et al.* 1995; Hock *et al.* 1998), the reduction of the CSF-Aβ1–42 might be better explained by the decreased production of Aβ1–42 from residual but diseased and progressively dysfunctional neurons. Combinatorial analysis of tau and Aβ1–42 in CSF may provide a strategy for a more accurate diagnosis of AD than using the individual markers alone (Motter *et al.* 1995; Galasko *et al.* 1998; Kanai *et al.* 1998).

12.4 Apolipoprotein E and α_1-antichymotrypsin polymorphisms

ApoE, a plasma protein which plays an important role in cholesterol transport, exists as three different isoforms encoded by ε *2*, ε *3*, and ε *4* alleles. The *APOE* ε *4* allele confers an increased risk of AD, and appears to lower the age at which patients with late-onset familial and sporadic AD show clinical signs of the disease in a dose-dependent fashion (Strittmatter *et al.* 1993). Further, the type A allele in the gene of α_1-antichymotrypsin (ACT), which belongs to the class of serine proteinase inhibitors, has recently been suggested to increase the risk of sporadic AD either independently of or in combination with the *APOE* genotype (Kamboh *et al.* 1995; Muramatsu *et al.* 1996; Talbot *et al.* 1996).

The apoE and ACT proteins have both been shown to co-localize with Aβ deposits in senile plaques (Abraham *et al.* 1988; Bao *et al.* 1996), and have been reported to promote the assembly of native Aβ into amyloid fibrils (Ma *et al.* 1994). These observations suggest that the two molecules play substantial roles in the pathogenesis of AD, and it is possible to formulate a hypothesis that the presence of the *APOE* ε *4* and ACT type A alleles may accelerate the neurodegenerative process in AD, and the presence of different combinations of these risk factor alleles in different groups of AD patients may account for the heterogeneity in the clinical and pathological manifestations of AD.

Our recent investigation has demonstrated that the *APOE* ε *4* allele exists in sporadic AD cases approximately four times as frequently as in age-matched controls (36.6% *vs.* 9.4%) (Higuchi *et al.* 1999). In the same study, however, sensitivity of the ε *4* allele for differentiating AD patients from normal subjects was estimated to be only 60%, since there was a considerable proportion of non- ε 4 carriers in the AD cases. Moreover, a recent multi-centre analysis of autopsy-confirmed AD cases showed that the sensitivity of the ε *4* allele as a test for the pathological diagnosis of AD is approximately 65% (Mayeux *et al.* 1998), and a recent consensus report suggests that *APOE* genotyping cannot be used alone as an antemortem diagnostic marker for AD (Reagan Institute 1998). However, the specificity of the *APOE* ε *4* allele for differentiating AD patients from normal cases was approximately 90% in our recent analysis (Higuchi *et al.* 1999), and the positive predictive value of the ε *4* allele has been reported to be more than 90% in other studies (Saunders *et al.* 1996; Welsh-Bohmer *et al.* 1997). None the less, approximately 10% of normal cases may be misdiagnosed as having AD if the ε *4* allele is applied as a predictor of AD among individuals who are cognitively normal. Thus, *APOE* genotyping may not be an appropriate screen for AD in individuals without cognitive impairments.

In contrast to the *APOE* genotyping, the diagnostic significance of determing the ACT genotype is more controversial. Several independent studies have failed to show a significant association between ACT polymorphisms and AD (Haines *et al.* 1996; Itabashi *et al.* 1998). However, further studies may demonstrate how ACT genotyping can be exploited in combination with other laboratory data to increase the accuracy of the antemortem diagnosis of AD.

With regard to predicting the rate of progression of AD among different cohorts of patients, there has been little evidence that the cognitive decline in AD patients carrying the *APOE* ε *4* allele is more rapid or aggressive than that in AD patients who carry no ε *4* allele. One study has demonstrated no difference in the rate of disease progression between AD patients with and without the ε *4* allele (Growdon *et al.* 1996). Other research groups have indicated an accelerated disease progression in ε *4*-negative AD patients compared to ε *4*-positive patients (Frisoni *et al.* 1995; Stern *et al.* 1997). Functional imaging techniques, including positron emission tomographic measurements, enable *in vivo* assessments of the extent and severity of neuronal metabolic dysfunction in the AD brain. A PET study using ¹⁸F-fluorodeoxyglucose (FDG) has indicated that the cerebral glucose metabolism in AD patients with the ε *4* allele does not differ from that in AD patients carrying no ε *4* (Corder *et al.* 1997). Our recent study with PET and FDG has demonstrated that the cerebral glucose metabolism in the frontal and temporal regions in AD patients with the ε *4* allele is better preserved than those without ε *4* allele (Higuchi *et al.* 1997). These findings suggest that the presence of the *APOE* ε *4* allele does not appear to influence deleteriously the progression of AD.

Although the risk for AD that might be conferred by the ACT genotype remains to be determined, the ACT polymorphism may contribute to the heterogeneity in the progression of AD among different patients. For example, Murphy and coworkers reported no relationship between the ACT type A allele and rate of cognitive decline in AD patients (Murphy *et al.* 1996), but cerebral glucose metabolism in the temporal and parietal regions was shown to be especially decreased in patients with the type A allele in a PET study (Higuchi *et al.* 1997). In addition, post-mortem brain analysis has revealed that cerebral amyloid angiopathy is more frequent in AD patients with the type A allele than in AD patients without this allele (Yamada *et al.* 1998). Therefore, the ACT type A allele may modify neuronal functions in several regions of the AD brain by accelerating specific pathological changes including cerebral amyloid angiopathy. The correlation between the cerebral metabolic rate for glucose and the gene dose of the *APOE* ε *4* or ACT type A allele among the AD patients examined in our earlier PET study has been re-analysed on a voxel-by-voxel basis, as depicted in Fig. 12.7, indicating that the *APOE* and ACT alleles play distinct roles in the progression of AD.

In addition to the effect of the *APOE* ε *4* allele on the brain glucose metabolism, we showed that the *APOE* ε *4* allele is not associated with the temporal progression of hippocampal atrophy in AD, suggesting that the *APOE* ε *4* allele is not a critical factor in mechanisms that contribute to the death of specific populations of hippocampal neurons (Yamaguchi *et al.* 1996). Since a deficit in cholinergic neurotransmission has been proposed to account for at least some of the cognitive impairments in AD (Perry, 1986; Bierer *et al.* 1995), this hypothesis has prompted the development of treatments for AD using cholinesterase inhibitors and agonists of muscarinic acetylcholine receptors. Several post-mortem brain studies have suggested that the choline acetyltransferase (ChAT) activity and the nicotinic acetylcholine receptor binding decline in the AD brain with an increasing dose of the *APOE* ε *4* allele, whereas the muscarinic acetylcholine receptor binding does not appear to be modulated by the ε *4* allele (Poirier *et al.* 1995). Our *in vivo* analysis for AD patients using PET and [¹¹C]benztropine (a selective radiotracer for muscarinic M_1/M_2 receptors) demonstrated that the muscarinic receptor binding is not associated with the ε *4* allele, but correlates strongly with the severity of dementia, as shown in Fig. 12.8. However, the

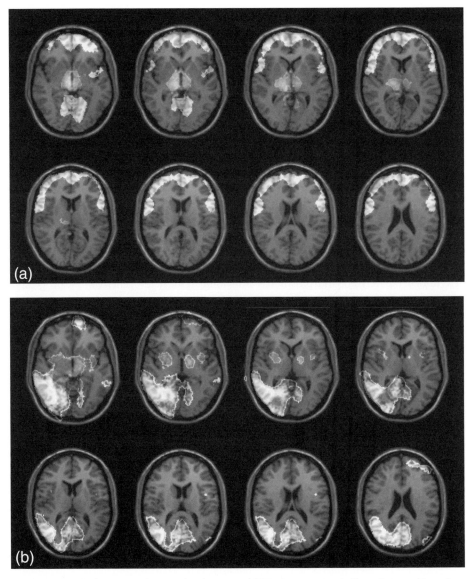

Fig. 12.7 Statistical parametric mapping images of PET glucose metabolism. Areas with a significant positive correlation between the glucose utilization (estimated as regional cerebral metabolic rate for glucose (rCMRglc)) and gene dose of the *APOE* ε4 allele (A), or a significant negative correlation between the rCMRglc and gene dose of the ACT type A allele (B) in 20 patients with AD (see Higuchi *et al.* for more detailed profiles of the patients). These brain maps are constructed by using Statistical Parametric Mapping (SPM96) software. The SPM{Z} maps are thresholded at p value of 0.01.

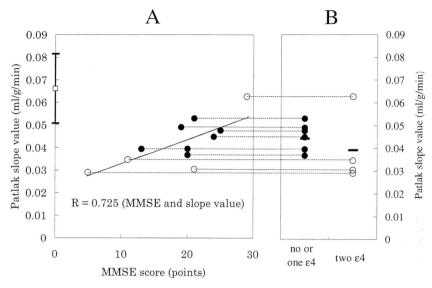

Fig. 12.8 Muscarinic (M1/M2) acetylcholine receptor binding estimated as a Patlak slope value in the whole brain of 11 patients with AD. The data were obtained from dynamic PET scans with [^{11}C]benztropine. (A) The receptor binding shows a significant correlation with the severity of dementia as measured by Mini-Mental State Examination (MMSE) score ($p < 0.05$ by t-test). Mean±SD values of the receptor binding are indicated on the y-axis. (B) No significant difference in the receptor binding is observed between the patients with no or one copy of ε4 (closed circles) and two copies of ε4 (open circles) ($p = 0.58$ by t-test). Horizontal bars represent the mean values. Correspondence of the patients in (A) and (B) is indicated by the broken lines.

practical utility of correlating the *APOE* genotype with these metabolic measures of brain function for improving the management of AD patients remains to be determined by future studies.

12.5 **Summary**

The CSF-tau measurement can be used alone or in combination with the CSF-Aβ1–42 measurement to detect AD accurately in its early stages and to rule out some of dementing disorders that resemble AD. The CSF-tau levels are increased throughout the progression of the disease. A future direction of CSF study would be to address the issue if the CSF-tau or the CSF-Aβ1–42 be used to monitor the response of AD patients to therapeutic interventions. Since CSF markers are not ideal biological markers for AD, we have to continue our efforts to develop a simpler and less invasive technology including functional neuroimaging for general screening of dementia in the elderly population.

References

Abraham, C. R., Selkoe, D. J., and Potter, H. (1988). Immunochemical identification of the serine protease inhibitor α1-antichymotrypsin in the brain amyloid deposits of Alzheimer's disease. *Cell*, 52, 487–501.

Albin, R. L., Minoshima, S., D'Amato, C. J., *et al.* (1996). Fluoro-deoxyglucose positron emission tomography in diffuse Lewy body disease. *Neurology*, **47**, 462–6.

American Psychiatric Association (1994). In *Diagnostic and statistical manuals of mental disorders*, 4th edn. Washington DC.

Andreasen, N., Vanmechelen, E., Van de Voorde, A., *et al.* (1998). Cerebrospinal fluid tau protein as a biochemical marker for Alzheimer disease, a community based follow up study. *Journal of Neurology, Neurosurgery and Psychiatry*, **64**, 298–305.

Andreasen, N., Hesse, C., Davidsson, P., *et al.* (1999). Cerebrospinal fluid β-amyloid 1–42 in Alzheimer's disease. Differences between early-onset and late-onset AD and stability during the course of disease. *Archives of Neurology*, **56**, 673–80.

Arai, H., Terajima, M., Miura, M., *et al.* (1995). Tau in cerebrospinal fluid. A potential diagnostic marker in Alzheimer's disease. *Annals of Neurology*, **38**, 649–52.

Arai, H., Terajima, M., Miura, M., *et al.* (1997*a*). Effect of genetic risk factors and disease progression on the cerebrospinal fluid tau levels in Alzheimer's disease. *Journal of the American Geriatric Society*, **45**, 1228–31.

Arai, H., Morikawa, Y., Higuchi, M., *et al.* (1997*b*). Cerebrospinal fluid tau levels in neurodegenerative diseases with distinct tau-related pathology. *Biochemical and Biophysical Research Communications*, **236**, 262–4.

Arai, H., Nakagawa, T., Kosaka, Y., *et al.* (1997*c*). Elevated cerebrospinal fluid tau protein level as a predictor of dementia in memory-impaired individuals. *Alzheimer's Research*, **3**, 211–13.

Arai, H., Satoh-Nakagawa, T., Higuchi, M., *et al.* (1998). No increase in cerebrospinal fluid tau protein levels in patients with vascular dementia. *Neurocience Letters*, **256**, 1–3.

Arriagata, P. V., Growdon, J. H., Hedley-Whyte, T., and Hyman, B. T. (1992). Neurofibrillary tangles but not senile plaques parallele duration and severity of Alzheimer's disease. *Neurology*, **42**, 631–9.

Bao, F., Arai H., Matsushita, S., *et al.* (1996). Expression of apolipoprotein E in normal and diverse neurodegenerative disease brain. *NeuroReport*, **7**, 1733–9.

Bierer, L. M., Haroutunian, V., Gabriel, S., *et al.* (1995). Neurochemical correlates of dementia severity in Alzheimer's disease, Relative importance of the cholinergic deficits. *Journal of Neurochemistry*, **64**, 749–60.

Chui, H. C., Victoroff, J. I., Margolin, D., *et al.* (1992) Criteria for the diagnosis of ischemic vascular dementia proposed by the State of California Alzheimer disease diagnostic and treatment centres. *Neurology*, **42**, 473–80.

Corder, E. H., Jelic, V., Basun, H., *et al.* (1997). No difference in cerebral glucose metabolism in patients with Alzheimer disease and differing apolipoprotein E genotypes. *Archives of Neurology*, **54**, 273–7.

Frisoni, G. B., Govoni, S., Geroldi, C., *et al.* (1995). Gene dose of the epsilon 4 allele of apolipoprotein E and disease progression in sporadic late-onset Alzheimer's disease. *Annals of Neurology*, **37**, 596–604.

Galasko, D., Clark, C. M., Chang, L., *et al.* (1997). Assessment of CSF levels of tau protein in mildly demented patients with Alzheimer's disease. *Neurology*, **48**, 632–5.

Galasko, D., Chang, L., Motter, R., *et al.* (1998). High cerebrospinal fluid tau and low amyloid β42 levels in the clinical diagnosis of Alzheimer disease and relation to apolipoprotein E genotype. *Archives of Neurology*, **55**, 937–45.

Gibb, W. R. G., Luthert, P. J., and Marsden, C. D. (1989). Corticobasal degeneration. *Brain*, **112**, 1171–92.

Ginsberg, S. D., Schmidt, M. L., Crino, P. B., *et al.* (1999). Molecular pathology of Alzheimer's disease and related disorders. In *Cerebral cortex: neurodegenerative and age-related changes in structure and function of cerebral cortex*, vol. 14 (ed. J. H. Morrison and A. Peters). pp 603–653 Plenum Press, New York, NY.

Growdon, J. H., Locascio, J. J., Corkin, S., *et al.* (1996). Apolipoprotein E genotype does not influence rates of cognitive decline in Alzheimer's disease. *Neurology*, 47, 444–8.

Haines, J. L., Pritchard, M. L., Saunders, A. M., *et al.* (1996). No genetic effect of alpha 1-antichymotrypsin in Alzheimer disease. *Genomics*, 33, 53–6.

Higuchi, M., Arai, H., Nakagawa, T., *et al.* (1997). Regional cerebral glucose utilization is modulated by the dosage of apolipoprotein E type 4 allele and α_1-antichymotrypsin type A allele in Alzheimer's disease. *NeuroReport*, 8, 2639–44.

Higuchi, M., Arai, H., Okamura, N., and Sasaki, H. (1999). Apolipoprotein E and Alzheimer's disease: therapeutic implications. *CNS Drugs*, 11, 411–20.

Higuchi, S., Arai, H., Matsushita, S., *et al.* (1998). Mutation in the α-synuclein gene and sporadic Parkinson's disease, Alzheimer's disease, and dementia with Lewy bodies in Japanese. *Experimental Neurology*, 153, 164–6.

Hock, C., Golombowski, S., Mullerspahn, F., *et al.* (1998). Cerebrospinal fluid levels of amyloid precursor protein and amyloid beta-peptide in Alzheimer's disease and major depression-Inverse correlation with dementia severity. *European Neurology*, 39, 111–18.

Hutton, M., Lendon, C. L., Rizzu, P., *et al.* (1998). Association of missense and 5'-splice- site-mutations in tau with the inherited dementia FTDP-17. *Nature*, 393, 702–5.

Isoe, K., Urakami, K., Shimomura, T., *et al.* (1996). Tau proteins in cerebrospinal fluid from patients with Alzheimer's disease, A longitudinal study. *Dementia*, 7, 175–6.

Ishii, K., Imamura, T., Sasaki, M., *et al.* (1998). Regional cerebral glucose metabolism in dementia with Lewy bodies and Alzheimer's disease. *Neurology*, 51, 125–30.

Itabashi, S., Arai, H., Matsui, T., *et al.* (1998). Absence of association of α_1-antichymotrypsin polymorphisms with Alzheimer's disease. A report on autopsy-confirmed cases. *Experimental Neurology*, 151, 237–40.

Iwatsubo, T., Odaka, A., Suzuki, N., *et al.* (1994). Visualization of Aβ42(43) and Aβ40 in senile plaques with end-specific Aβ nomoclonals, evidence that an initially deposited species is Aβ42(43). *Neuron*, 13, 45–53.

Jensen, M., Basun, H., and Lannfelt, L. (1995). Increased cerebrospinal fluid tau in patients with Alzheimer's disease. *Neuroscience Letters*, 186, 189–91.

Kamboh, M. I., Sanghera, D. K., Ferrell, R. E., and DeKosky, S. T. (1995). APOE4-associated Alzheimer's disease risk is modified by α_1-antichymotrypsin polymorphism. *Nature Genetics*, 10, 486–8.

Kanai, M., Matsubara, E., Isoe, K., *et al.* (1998). Longitudinal study of cerebrospinal fluid levels of tau, Aβ1–40, and Aβ1–42(43) in Alzheimer's disease. A study in Japan. *Annals of Neurology*, 44, 17–26.

Khachaturian, Z. S. (1985). Diagnosis of Alzheimer's disease. *Archives of Neurology*, 42, 1097–105.

Lee, V. M-Y., Balin, B. J., Otvos, L. Jr., and Trojanowski, J. Q. (1991). A68, a major subunit of paired helical filaments and derivatized forms of normal tau. *Science*, 251, 675–8.

Lund and Manchester Groups (1994). Clinical and neuropathological criteria for frontotemporal dementia. *Journal of Neurology, Neurosurgery and Psychiatry*, 57, 416–18.

Ma, J., Yee, A., Brewer, H. B. Jr., *et al.* (1994). Amyloid-associated proteins α1-antichymotrypsin and apolipoprotein E promote assembly of Alzheimer β-protein into filaments. *Nature*, 372, 92–4.

Mayeux, R., Saunders, A. M., Shea, S., *et al.* (1998). Utility of the apolipoprotein genotype in the diagnosis of Alzheimer's disease. *New England Journal of Medicine*, 338, 506–11.

McKeith, I. G. and anonymous (1996). Consensus guidelines for the clinical and pathological diagnosis of dementia with Lewy bodies (DLB). Report of the consortium on DLB international workshop. *Neurology*, 47, 1113–24.

McKhann, G., Drachman, D., Folstein, M., *et al.* (1984). Clinical diagnosis of Alzheimer's disease, Report of the NINCDS-ADRDA work group under auspices of the Department of Health and Human Services Task Force on Alzheimer's disease. *Neurology*, 34, 939–44.

Mori, H., Hosoda, K., and Matsubara, E. (1995). Tau in cerebrospinal fluid, Establishment of the sandwich ELISA with antibody specific to the repeat sequence in tau. *Neuroscience Letters*, **186**, 181–3.

Motter, R., Vigo-Pelfrey, C., Kholodenko, D. *et al.* (1995). Reduction of β-amyloid42 in the cerebrospinal fluid of patients with Alzheimer's disease. *Annals of Neurology*, **36**, 903–11.

Munroe, W. A., Southwick, P. C., Chang, L., *et al.* (1995). Tau protein in cerebrospinal fluid as an aid in the diagnosis of Alzheimer's disease. *Annals of Clinical Laboratory Science*, **25**, 207–17.

Muramatsu, T., Matsushita, S., Arai, H., *et al.* (1996). Alpha 1-antichymotrypsin gene polymorphism and risk for Alzheimer's disease. *Journal of Neural Transmission*, **103**, 1205–10.

Murphy, G. M. Jr., Yang, L., Yesavage, J., and Tinklenberg, Jr. (1996). Rate of cognitive decline in Alzheimer's disease is not affected by the alpha-1-antichymotrypsin A allele or the CYP2D6 B mutant. *Neuroscience Letters*, **217**, 200–2.

National Institute on Aging and Reagan Institute Working Group on Diagnostic Criteria for the Neuropathological Assessment of Alzheimer's Disease (Phelps, C., Khachaturian, Z., and Trojanowski, J. Q., Working Group Chairs). (1997). Consensus recommendations for the postmortem diagnosis of Alzheimer's disease. *Neurobiology of Aging*, **18** (4S), S1-S2.

Nitsch, R. M., Rebeck, W., Deng, M., *et al.* (1995). Cerebrospinal fluid levels of amyloid β-protein in Alzheimer's disease: Inverse correlation with severity of dementia and effect of apolipoprotein E genotype. *Annals of Neurology*, **37**, 512–18.

Ohrui, T., Yamaya, M., Arai, H., *et al.* (1997). Disturbed consciousness and asthma. *Lancet*, **349**, 652.

Perry, E. K. (1986). The cholinergic hypothesis — ten years on. *British Medical Bulletin*, **42**, 63–9.

Poirier, J., Delisle, M-C., Quirion, R., *et al.* (1995). Apolipoprotein E4 allele as a predictor of cholinergic deficits and treatment outcome in Alzheimer disease. *Proceedings of the National Academy of Science (USA)*, **92**, 12260–4.

Riemenschneider, N. M., Buch, K., Schmolke, M., *et al.* (1997). Cerebrospinal fluid tau is elevated in early Alzheimer's disease. *Neuroscience Letters*, **212**, 209–11.

The Ronald and Nancy Reagan Institute of the Alzheimer's Association and the National Institute on Aging working Group. (1998) Consensus report of the working group on, Molecular and biochemical markers of Alzheimer's disease. *Neurobiology of Aging*, **19**, 109–16.

Rosler, N., Wichart, I., and Jellinger, K. A. (1996). Total tau protein immunoreactivity in lumbar cerebrospinal fluid of patients with Alzheimer's disease. *Journal of Neurology, Neurosurgery and Psychiatry*, **60**, 237–8.

Saunders, A. M., Hulette, C., Welsh-Bohmer, K. A., *et al.* (1996). Specificity, sensitivity, and predictive value of apolipoprotein E genotyping for sporadic Alzheimer's disease. *Lancet*, **348**, 90–3.

Selkoe, D. J. (1994). Cell biology of the amyloid β-protein precursor and the mechanism of Alzheimer's disease. *Annual Reviews in Cell Biology*, **10**, 373–403.

Seubert, P., Vigo-Pelfrey, C., and Esch, F. (1992). Isolation and quantification of soluble Alzheimer's β-peptide from biological fluids. *Nature*, **359**, 325–7.

Shoji, M., Golde, T. E., and Ghiso, J., (1992). Production of the Alzheimer amyloid β-protein by normal proteolytic processing. *Science*, **258**, 126–9.

Steele, J. C., Richardson, L. C., and Olszewski, J. (1964). Progressive supranuclear palsy. A heterogenous degeneration involving the brain stem, basal ganglia and cerebellum, with vertical gaze and pseudobulbar palsy, nuchal dystonia and dementia. *Archives of Neurology*, **10**, 333–59.

Stern, Y., Brandt, J., Albert, M., *et al.* (1997). The absence of an apolipoprotein ε 4 allele is associated with a more aggressive form of Alzheimer's disease. *Annals of Neurology*, **41**, 615–20.

Strittmatter, W. J., Saunders, A. M., Schmechel, D., *et al.* (1993). Apolipoprotein E, high-avidity binding to β-amyloid and increased frequency of type 4 allele in late-onset familial Alzheimer disease. *Proceedings of the National Academy of Science (USA)*, **90**, 1977–81.

Suzuki, N., Cheung, T. T., Cai, X-D., *et al.* (1994). An increased percentage of long amyloid β-protein is secreted by familial amyloid β-protein precursor (β-App717) mutants. *Science*, 264, 1336–40.

Talbot, C., Houlden, H., Craddock, N., *et al.* (1996). Polymorphism in AACT gene may lower age of onset of Alzheimer's disease. *NeuroReport*, 7, 534–6.

Tamaoka, A., Sawamura, N., Fukushima, T., *et al.* (1997). Amyloid β-protein 42(43) in cerebrospinal fluid of patients with Alzheimer's disease. *Journal of Neurological Science*, 148, 41–7.

Teller, J. K., Russo, C., and DeBusk, L. M. (1996). Presence of soluble amyloid β-peptide precedes amyloid plaque formation in Down syndrome. *Nature Medicine*, 2, 93–5.

Terajima, M., Arai, H., Itabashi, S., *et al.* (1996). Elevated cerebrospinal fluid tau, Implications for early diagnosis of Alzheimer's disease. *Journal of the American Geriatric Society*, 44, 1012–23.

Tierney, M. C., Fisher, R. H., Lewin, A. J., *et al.* (1989). The NINCDS-ADRDA work group criteria for the clinical diagnosis of probable Alzheimer's disease. *Neurology*, 38, 359–64.

Trojanowski, J. Q., Clark, C. M., Arai, H., and Lee, V. M-Y. (1996). Elevated levels of tau in cerebrospinal fluid: implications for the antemortem diagnosis of Alzheimer's disease. *Alzheimer's Disease Reviews*, 1, 77–83.

Van Gool, W. A., Kuiper, M. A., Walstra, G. J. M., *et al.* (1995). Concentrations of amyloid β-protein in cerebrospinal fluid of patients with Alzheimer's disease. *Annals of Neurology*, 37, 277–9.

Vandermeeren, M., Mercken, M., Vanmechelen, E., *et al.* (1993). Detection of τ protein in normal and Alzheimer's disease cerebrospinal fluid with a sensitive sandwich enzyme-linked immunosorbent assay. *Journal of Neurochemistry*, 61, 1828–34.

Vanderstichele, H., Blennow, K., D'Heuvaert, N., *et al.* (1998). Development of a specific diagnostic test for measurement of β-amyloid (1–42) [βA$_4$(42)] in CSF. *Neurobiology of Aging*, 19, S163.

Vanmechelen, E., Blennow, K., Davidsson, P., *et al.* (1997). Combination of tau/phospho-tau with other intracellular proteins as diagnostic markers for neurodegeneration. In *Alzheimer's disease, Biology, Diagnosis and Therapeutics* (ed K. Iqbal, B. Winblad, T. Nishimura, M. Takeda, and H. M. Wisniewski), pp 197–203 John Wiley& Sons Ltd.

Welsh-Bohmer, K. A., Gearing, M., Saunders, A. M., *et al.* (1997). Apolipoprotein E genotype in a neuropathological series from the Consortium to Establish a Registry for Alzheimer's Disease. *Annals of Neurology*, 42, 319–25.

Yamada, M., Sodeyama, N., Itoh, Y., *et al.* (1998). Association of α1-antichymotrypsin polymorphism with cerebral amyloid angiopathy. *Annals of Neurology*, 44, 129–31.

Yamaguchi, S., Nakagawa, T., Arai, H., *et al.* (1996). Temporal progression of hippocampal atrophy and apolipoprotein E gene in Alzheimer's disease. *Journal of the American Geriatric Society*, 44, 1012–23.

Chapter 13

Alzheimer's disease and neuroimaging

Nick Fox, Rachael Scahill, Peter Høgh, and
Martin N Rossor.

13.1 Introduction

Neuroimaging already plays an important supporting role in the clinical diagnosis of Alzheimer's disease (AD). This role is likely to grow with imaging becoming a mandatory part of the diagnostic work-up in dementia and as a research tool it will increasingly be used to monitor disease progression and evaluate therapeutic responses to novel medication. Neuroimaging relevant to AD can conveniently be divided into structural and functional techniques. Structural imaging provides an image of the brain which allows differentiation of tissue types and the identification of different cerebral structures. In this way it may be used to exclude structural lesions, identify ischaemic changes and/or patterns of atrophy which point towards a particular cause of degenerative dementia. The two structural modalities are computed tomography (CT) and magnetic resonance imaging (MRI). By contrast, functional imaging can identify patterns of hypometabolism which indicate the presence of a degenerative process and implicate a particular disease. Functional imaging changes may exist in the absence of structural changes and may be complementary to them. Functional imaging is still largely a research tool or confined as a diagnostic aid to a small but growing number of centres. The functional imaging modalities discussed here are Positron Emission Tomography (PET), Single Photon Emission Computed Tomography (SPECT) and functional MRI (fMRI). This chapter will consider the relevance of structural and functional imaging to the understanding of AD.

13.2 Structural imaging

13.2.1 X - Ray computed tomography

CT involves the reconstruction of a cross-sectional image of the brain from X-ray attenuation data, reflecting tissue densities. A narrow (collimated) X-ray beam rotates around the head and attenuation is measured by an array of detectors. The attenuation of tissues is expressed in terms of a CT number, or Hounsfield Units, giving a numerical value for each picture element (pixel) within the image.

CT scans are widely available, cheap and relatively rapid. A disadvantage of CT is the radiation dose necessary for acquisition of images, but CT also has limitations in terms of image quality (DeCarli *et al.* 1990). Tissue contrast and resolution are inferior to MRI. Partial volume effects, that is the mixing of signal from neighbouring tissues (e.g. cerebrospinal fluid (CSF) and brain), produces practical problems for the delineation of structures. Beam hardening effects, due to the increased absorption of lower energy X-rays by the skull, mean that the medial temporal lobe is poorly visualised with conventional CT scanning. Temporal-lobe-oriented CT scanning improves visualisation and measurement of this region (Jobst *et al.* 1992). The recent development of spiral CT has reduced scan times and allows 3D reconstruction, but as yet image quality remains inferior to conventional CT (Bahner *et al.* 1998).

13.2.2 Magnetic resonance imaging

Structural MRI utilises the fact that hydrogen nuclei, in a magnetic field, emit a radio signal following excitation by a radiofrequency pulse at their resonant frequency. The MR dataset can give a display of the density of hydrogen nuclei (commonly referred to as proton density), slice by slice through the brain. In addition the MR signal is influenced by the mobility of the protons within a particular tissue. Each type of tissue thereby produces a relatively characteristic signal with different T1 and T2 values (longitudinal spin-lattice and transversal spin-spin relaxation times, respectively). Tissues with a large amount of freely mobile water appear dark in T1-weighted images but bright in proton density and T2-weighted images (Fig. 13.1 and 13.2).

These variations in MR signal allow sensitive differentiation of tissue types and the detection of inhomogeneities within tissues. High spatial resolution (better than 1 mm), the absence of artefact due to bone and improved tissue contrast allows better visualisation and more accurate quantification of smaller cerebral structures. There is an increasing range of different MRI procedures for acquiring images offering improved sensitivity to tissue characteristics (physical or chemical), thinner slices, or increased speed of imaging, in particular

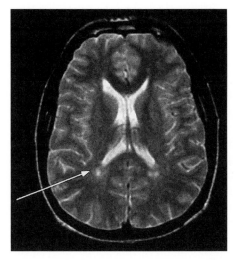

Fig. 13.1 Axial, T2-weighted MR scan of a patient who had just become symptomatic for early familial AD at the age of 42, showing bilateral, symmetrical signal change in the white matter adjacent to the posterior parts of the body of the lateral ventricles (arrow), and less conspicuous but similar changes adjacent to each anterior horn.

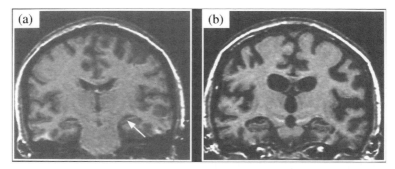

Fig. 13.2 (a) Coronal, T1-weighted MR scan of a normal control showing good differentiation between grey and white matter. The arrow points to the left hippocampus. (b) Coronal, T1-weighted MR scan of patient with moderately severe AD. Generalized cerebral atrophy is evident with ventricular enlargement and widening of the cortical sulci. The atrophy is greater than would be expected in a person of this age (mid-50s).

echo planar imaging (EPI) (Reiser and Faber, 1997). MRI avoids X-ray irradiation, but scanners are more expensive than CT and more likely to produce claustrophobia. Longer scanning times mean MR images are sensitive to patient movement artefact which is a particular problem in dementia where patients may forget instructions and have difficulty keeping still. Because of the powerful magnetic fields employed (20,000 times the earth's magnetic field), patients with pacemakers or certain metallic implants cannot be scanned.

13.2.3 Differential diagnosis of Alzheimer's disease using structural imaging

The contribution of neuroimaging to the differential diagnosis in AD has in practice three aspects to it, each complementary to the clinical assessment. The first is to exclude structural and potentially reversible conditions. The second is to distinguish normal individuals with age-related changes in memory, particularly when these are compounded by anxiety or depression, from patients with a degenerative dementia such as AD. The final aspect is to distinguish AD from other degenerative dementias; this has been referred to as the real differential diagnosis of AD.

13.2.4 Excluding structural lesions

Until recently the sole role of neuroimaging in dementia was to exclude potentially treatable structural lesions. The most important of these are cerebral tumours, hydrocephalus and subdural haematomata (Fig. 13.3a-d). These are all relatively rare, but are nevertheless the most common surgically treatable lesions that may present as dementia. Most of these pathologies will be detected by routine unenhanced CT or MR scanning. Both modalities will identify space-occupying lesions such as a frontal meningioma which may mimic frontotemporal degeneration. Subdural haematomata, which can cause problems in the elderly, may also occur in the setting of degenerative dementia. Normal pressure hydrocephalus may produce AD-like symptoms, but can be treated with ventriculo-peritoneal shunting. The typical imaging appearances of normal pressure hydrocephalus are enlarged ventricles with prominent periventricular white matter changes without corresponding sulcal widen-

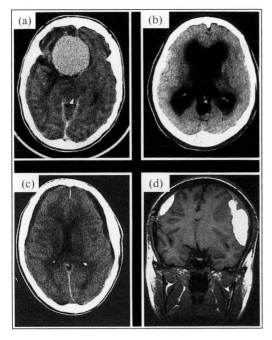

Fig. 13.3 (a) Axial, contrast-enhanced CT scan showing a large meningioma. The patient presented with confusion and behavioural (frontal) changes. (b) CT scan showing hydrocephalus. (c) CT scan of bilateral, low-density subdural haematomas with diffuse compression of the lateral ventricles. (d) MR, T1-weighted, coronal image showing large, bilateral, subacute, subdural haematomata.

ing. An unexpected scan result, for example extensive white matter changes, better seen on T2-weighted MRI, may also suggest the need for further investigation. On rare occasions this may include cerebral biopsy, to exclude a treatable condition such as cerebral vasculitis. Infectious causes of cognitive decline, particularly in the immunocompromised, may mimic a degenerative dementia and MRI and then CSF examination are essential to avoid over-looking a treatable condition in this setting.

13.2.5 Differentiating Alzheimer's disease from normal ageing: atrophy as a diagnostic marker

Neuroimaging has proved valuable in discriminating memory and other cognitive deficits due to, for example depression (pseudo-dementia), from true degenerative diseases. Cortical atrophy (greater than that expected for age) should not be a feature of depression (Zubenko *et al.* 1990). However, the distinction between normal ageing and AD is problem-atic as there is often overlap on imaging between these two groups. The use of CT and MRI for positive diagnostic (as opposed to purely exclusionary) purposes in established AD has been confirmed by numerous reports, but their utility must be judged by their ability to improve the diagnosis of AD in the early stages of the disease. In order to be clinically useful any method needs to distinguish mild AD from normal ageing and ideally from other causes of cognitive impairment. Validation of a diagnostic test for AD requires comparison of an AD group with age- and sex-matched controls, where histological confirmation is available for both. Ideally the subjects should be matched for pre-morbid intelligence as sig-nificant correlations between intelligence and intracranial, cerebral, temporal lobe, hip-pocampal and cerebellar volumes have been reported (Andreasen *et al.* 1993).

The histopathological hallmarks of AD include neurofibrillary tangles (NFT) and senile amyloid plaques, neuronal death, dendritic pruning and synaptic loss accompanied by axonal dropout in the white matter (Braak *et al.* 1993; Hyman and Gomez-Isla 1994; Swaab *et al.* 1994). Unfortunately, there are still no methods of directly imaging these microscopic changes *in vivo*. However, concomitant macroscopic changes, such as gross cerebral atrophy particularly involving the parietal, temporal and frontal cortices and enlargement of CSF spaces can be assessed with neuroimaging. Pathological studies have shown cortical atrophy, reduced brain weight and ventricular enlargement all to be more prominent in AD patients. However, considerable overlap is present when compared with age-matched controls. Normal ageing is also associated with a reduction in brain volume and increases in ventricular and sulcal volumes. These features are not linearly related to age, but become more important sometime after the fifth decade. The reported age at which atrophy accelerates remains controversial but tends to be put between the 5th and the 7th decades (Dekaban, 1978; Ho *et al.* 1980; Pfefferbaum *et al.* 1994; Blatter *et al.* 1995). Some studies suggest that age-related atrophy appears to be greater in men than in women (Kaye *et al.* 1992; Cowell *et al.* 1994), but this is contradicted by other work (Blatter *et al.* 1995; Jack *et al.* 1997; Mu *et al.* 1999). Several reports suggest that different regions of the brain are more susceptible to age-related loss than others, with the frontal lobes being more affected than temporal lobes (Coffey *et al.* 1992; DeCarli *et al.* 1994). Imaging studies of the cerebral volume changes in normal ageing have shown good correspondence with neuropathological findings, but longitudinal studies are relatively lacking.

The histopathological changes of AD can involve nearly all cerebral areas but particularly affect the medial temporal and limbic lobes. Large numbers of neuritic plaques and NFT are found in the grey matter of the temporal lobe, the entorhinal (parahippocampal) cortex, the hippocampus and the amygdala. The hippocampal formation is invariably involved in severe cases; so much so that AD has been called a 'hippocampal dementia' (Hyman *et al.* 1984; Ball *et al.* 1985). Memory impairment is one of the earliest manifestations of AD and temporal limbic lobe structures, in particular the entorhinal cortex and hippocampus, are closely involved in those aspects of memory function that fail in AD (Squire, 1986). Other areas, however, are severely affected too. The amygdala, particularly its magnocellular portion, contains large numbers of plaques and tangles and suffers disproportionate atrophy in advanced AD (Scott *et al.* 1991). The regions of earliest involvement and the degree of variability in the patterns of progression are still unclear. Postmortem attempts at staging disease progression suggest changes start in the entorhinal cortex and hippocampus before progressing to the association cortices (Braak *et al.* 1993). Although the causal links and time course of this process are not established these histopathological changes are clearly associated with atrophy. Furthermore, this atrophy can be quantified with imaging and has been taken to have a direct relationship to the underlying disease process. In addition to quantifying generalised cortical atrophy, imaging studies have focused on region specific atrophy and in particular, atrophy of the hippocampus and adjacent regions.

13.2.6 Measures of cerebral atrophy

Whether imaged using CT or MRI, atrophy may be assessed qualitatively by visual inspection or by linear, area or volumetric measurements. These assessments may either be applied directly to loss of brain tissue or indirectly through the measurement of increased CSF spaces (compare Fig. 13.2a with 13.2b).

13.2.7 Qualitative assessments of atrophy

Computed tomography

Visual inspection of scans is the only method of assessment used by radiologists and neurologists in a case of possible AD. Qualitative ratings of atrophy, when formalised, use a scoring system for the size of ventricles or degree of cortical atrophy. Higher scores of atrophy are more often found in patients with a clinical diagnosis of AD and the extent of atrophy increases with severity of dementia. However, there is considerable overlap with normal controls and a significant number of patients are rated as having no atrophy on CT or MRI. A review by DeCarli suggested the sensitivity of qualitative assessments of generalised cerebral atrophy on CT for differentiating AD and controls are no better than 60%, with a specificity of 90% (DeCarli et al. 1990). The separation of AD from other causes of dementia is much poorer. The criteria for clinical diagnosis of AD drawn up for the National Institute of Neurological and Communicative Disorders and Stroke (NINCDS) and the Alzheimer's Disease and Related Disorders Association (ADRDA) reflect the observed association between atrophy and AD and also the overlap with normal ageing (McKhann et al. 1984). These criteria state that 'the diagnosis of *probable* AD is supported by evidence of cerebral atrophy on CT with progression documented by serial observation'. However, the criteria do not require imaging evidence of atrophy and allow a scan 'normal for age' as being consistent with this diagnosis.

Qualitative assessments of temporal lobe atrophy (temporal horn enlargement, reductions in the size of the hippocampus, medial and lateral temporal cortex) result in improved sensitivity and specificity, although at least 20% of subjects are incorrectly classified (George et al. 1990). Longitudinal CT studies show that qualitative assessment of hippocampal atrophy is a marker for AD in the presence of memory or other cognitive impairment (de Leon et al. 1993). All qualitative ratings depend on the skill and experience of the raters and have variable inter-observer reliability.

Magnetic resonance imaging

The Consortium to Establish a Registry for Alzheimer's Disease (CERAD) assessed the reliability of standardised (axial T2-weighted and coronal T1-weighted sequences) qualitative MRI evaluation for AD, having concluded 'that the use of CT to differentiate AD from changes caused by normal ageing had not been successful'. Their multi-centre study found that inter-rater agreement of the MR scans was unsatisfactory and decided that 'eyeball' interpretation of MR scans was highly subjective and that more objective techniques were required (Davis et al. 1992).

Various qualitative rating scales used to assess temporal lobe atrophy on MRI give a specificity of 90%, whereas sensitivity of atrophy ratings vary from 40% to 95%, with the entorhinal cortex having arguably the highest sensitivity. Several authors have shown significant differences between patients with AD and controls using subjective ratings of medial temporal lobe atrophy on MRI suggesting this may be the most useful region to assess with a rating scale (Scheltens et al. 1992; Convit et al. 1993; Scheltens et al. 1997). Equally it has been shown that while the presence of atrophy on visual inspection makes the diagnosis of AD more likely, the absence of atrophy does not exclude the diagnosis (Erkinjuntti *et al.* 1993).

13.2.8 Quantitative measures of atrophy

Several quantitative measurements of atrophy have been developed in an attempt to produce greater objectivity. Whether these measurements are linear, of cross-sectional area or volumetric, they should be normalised to correct for the variation in brain size that is present before atrophy (Pfefferbaum *et al.* 1994; Free *et al.* 1995). The most commonly used denominators (for normalisation) are total intracranial width, area or volume. A few studies have not controlled at all for pre-morbid normal variation and their conclusions must therefore be treated more cautiously.

Linear measurements

Linear measurements have the advantage of speed and simplicity and require the identification of two recognisable anatomical landmarks and the measurement of the distance between them. Using this method the widths of the lateral ventricles and the third ventricle have been shown to differ significantly in AD from normal controls in several CT studies, although the sensitivity was no better than 70% (DeCarli *et al.* 1990). Jobst *et al.* used temporal-lobe-oriented CT to investigate the minimum width of the medial temporal lobe. A single linear measurement differentiated severe AD from normal controls but not from other causes of dementia (Jobst *et al.* 1992), and serial measurements showed a greater rate of reduction in this measure in AD patients compared to controls (Jobst *et al.* 1994). Other linear measures that have been advocated include the height of the hippocampus and parahippocampal gyrus (Pucci *et al.* 1998), the width of the temporal horn (Erkinjuntti *et al.* 1993; Frisoni *et al.* 1996) and the thickness of the corpus callosum (Vermersch *et al.* 1994). Claims that MRI measures of interuncal distance are useful for the detection of AD have not been substantiated (Dahlbeck *et al.* 1991; Early *et al.* 1993; Howieson *et al.* 1993). Generally, linear measurements produce considerable overlap between normal controls and patients with mild AD.

Cross-sectional area measurements

Area measurements may provide a better estimate of atrophy than linear measures and are generally less time-consuming to perform than volumetric analysis. However, because they involve the choice of a single slice for assessment they will not accurately estimate volume change if it is not uniform along the length of the measured structure (Cook *et al.* 1992). Furthermore, normal anatomical variation between subjects means it is difficult to determine the equivalent section of a structure. The ventricular-brain ratio has been estimated by measuring the area of the ventricles divided by total brain area at a single defined level on CT or MRI, and has been shown to increase with age in normal controls. Patients with AD have significantly increased areas of the third ventricle, lateral ventricles and inter-hemispheric fissure area when compared to normal controls. These measures have been used with CT to distinguish AD patients from controls, and are more sensitive (60-80%) than linear measures, but have not been shown to be clinically useful in early AD or in the differential diagnosis of dementia (DeCarli *et al.* 1990). The sagittal cross-sectional area of the corpus callosum (particularly posteriorly) has been shown to be reduced on MRI in AD patients (n=10) compared to controls (n=14) (Yamauchi *et al.* 1993). Seab *et al.* used coronal MR imaging to measure the cross-sectional area of the hippocampus at the level of the lateral geniculate body and found a 40% reduction in mean normalised hippocampal area in the AD patients compared to controls (Seab *et al.* 1988). Ikeda *et al.* showed significant differences between both probable and possible AD cases and controls using a single normalised area measurement of the hippocampal formation and parahippocampal gyrus although there was some overlap (Ikeda *et al.* 1994).

Volumetric measures

Estimating the volumes of cerebral structures usually involves defining a region of interest on a number of slices and then summing the area measurements and multiplying by the distance between the cross-sections measured (Cavalieri's principle). The methods used to define the structure seen on the slice vary from manual outlining using anatomical landmarks, to an automated segmentation based on Hounsfield units (CT), or grey scale level (MRI), whereby thresholds are chosen that distinguish CSF, grey and white matter on the basis of signal intensity. MR imaging produces greater distinction between tissue types, although structure boundaries and thus calculated volumes are influenced by the intensity level set for each image. Partial volume averaging limits accuracy but may be compensated for when two or more imaging sequences are combined (Rusinek *et al.* 1991).

Cerebrospinal fluid volumes

Mean CSF volume as measured by CT appears to increase with severity of AD resulting in significant differences in CSF spaces when AD patients were compared with normal controls (sensitivity and specificity almost 90%) (DeCarli *et al.* 1990). These age-adjusted differences are most marked with younger patients, and of the CSF spaces, measures of the Sylvian fissure and temporal horn are the most discriminating (Sandor *et al.* 1992; Sullivan *et al.* 1993). When comparable CSF regions in the same subjects are assessed, MRI is better than CT at separating AD from controls (Sandor *et al.* 1992), and in particular MRI gives better separation of extra-ventricular (sulcal) CSF. Validation studies suggest reasonably high accuracy and low inter-observer variability (Jack 1991).

Grey and white matter volumes

Concomitant with increasing ventricular and sulcal spaces, total MRI brain volume measurements are reduced in AD compared with controls, and this loss correlates with severity of cognitive impairment (Murphy *et al.* 1993). Rusinek *et al.* used two MR inversion recovery sequences to compensate for partial signal averaging and found that the percentage of brain tissue identified as grey matter in AD patients is significantly lower than in control subjects, 45% as opposed to 50% (Rusinek *et al.* 1991). Several studies have shown a strong association between the loss of grey matter in AD and the increase in CSF in each cortical lobe.

Volumes of the temporal lobe, hippocampus and the amygdala

Due to their prominent pathological involvement in AD, atrophy of the temporal lobes and the hippocampal formation have been extensively studied. Several studies have shown reduction in temporal lobe volumes to be disproportionately greater than reduction in whole brain volume in AD (Jernigan *et al.* 1991; Rusinek *et al.* 1991). Anatomical definitions of the structures measured tend to vary between studies making valid comparisons difficult. The amygdala is comparatively difficult to define, whereas the hippocampus can be separated more easily from surrounding tissue by manual outlining and consistently shows

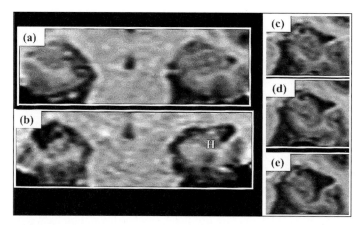

Fig. 13.4 (a) Magnified MR image of normal hippocampus. (b) In this case of AD, the hippocampi (H) are shrunken with a deep excavation on the medial aspect. 4c–e. Left hippocampus in an AD patient at (c) baseline scan (d) 19 months after baseline, and (e) 30 months after baseline.

volume loss in moderate to severe AD (Fig. 13.4a-e). Numerous studies have shown that in AD both the amygdala (Pearlson *et al.* 1992; Cuenod *et al.* 1993; Maunoury *et al.* 1996) and the hippocampus (Kesslak *et al.* 1991; Jack, Jr. *et al.* 1992; Pearlson *et al.* 1992) are reduced by 40% in advanced cases. Measurements of these structures have also shown differentiation of mildly affected individuals from normal controls (Convit *et al.* 1993; Killiany *et al.* 1993; Soininen *et al.* 1994; Jack *et al.* 1997). Lehericy *et al.* showed a 36% reduction in the amygdala and 25% reduction in the hippocampal formation in mildly affected patients (mean mini mental state examination (MMSE) of 24/30) compared to normal controls (Lehericy *et al.* 1994). Most studies found overlap between the two groups, but there was better differentiation when a combination of measures was used (Lehericy *et al.* 1994; Krasuski *et al.* 1998). Hippocampal losses have been detected in presymtomatic familial AD cases (Fox *et al.* 1996b; Convit *et al.* 1997). By contrast, Kaye *et al.* found in a longitudinal study of elderly subjects that volume losses in the temporal lobe, but not the hippocampus, distinguished those individuals who were developing cognitive impairment (Kaye *et al.* 1997).

White matter changes

White matter changes, on both CT and MRI, are commonly found in AD and have been subject to much speculation as to their significance. It has been suggested that white matter changes reflect 'incomplete infarction' and may be due to hypoperfusion (Brun and Englund, 1986), which in turn may be influenced by amyloid angiopathy (Haan *et al.* 1990). In addition, Wallerian degeneration, secondary to cortical neuronal loss, has been suggested as a cause of the white matter changes. On CT, focal or diffuse areas of low density in the white matter are termed leuko-araiosis, or periventricular lucencies when surrounding the ventricles. Neuropathologically, these areas show evidence of pallor, mild demyelination, astrocytosis and axonal loss but no evidence of frank infarction. On T2-weighted MR

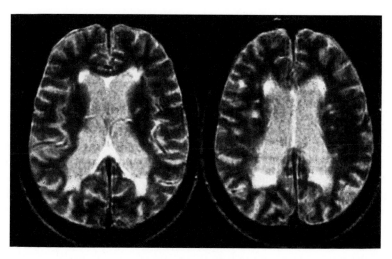

Fig. 13.5 Axial, T2-weighted MR images showing multiple discrete infarcts in the basal ganglia and corona radiata bilaterally, and confluent areas of signal change in the white matter adjacent to the lateral ventricles that probably represents chronic ischaemic damage.

images areas of high signal are usually referred to as white matter hyperintensities (WMH). WMHs are frequently seen both periventricularly and in the deep white matter, and pathological examination of these regions may have a variety of histological features from lacunar infarcts to vacuolated myelin around the perivascular spaces (Scarpelli *et al.* 1994). MRI demonstrates many more abnormalities in the white matter than are seen with CT.

White matter changes correlate with age and vascular disease and with the presence of vascular risk factors such as hypertension and diabetes. White matter changes on MRI are common in AD patients (Figure 13.5) even when those with evidence of cerebrovascular disease are excluded (Bennett *et al.* 1992). These white matter changes correlate with severity of disease (Stout *et al.* 1996) and longitudinal studies seem to suggest that periventricular WMHs become more prominent with disease progression (Fox *et al.* 1997a). Equally WMHs are frequent incidental findings in the elderly and studies comparing the prevalence of white matter lesions in AD with normal controls have reached conflicting conclusions. Thirty to 80% of elderly individuals have focal white matter abnormalities on MRI (Drayer, 1988). Excluding subjects with vascular risk factors seems to result in a lack of any significant difference between patients with mild AD and controls (Erkinjuntti *et al.* 1994). Hyperintensities in the basal ganglia are much more common in vascular dementia than in AD and together with the extent of deep WMHs are the best imaging markers of vascular dementia (Barber *et al.* 1999). Qualitative assessments of white matter changes may point to a diagnosis of vascular dementia but appear to be neither specific nor sensitive in distinguishing AD from controls, particularly in the early stages of the disease.

Measurement of progression

The majority of neuroimaging studies in AD have been cross-sectional, which has the disadvantage that small changes in brain structure tend to be masked by the large variation within normal individuals, and in many cases scans of affected patients are reported as normal. Longitudinal studies use serial scans to measure changes in cerebral structure over time in a single individual either for diagnostic purposes or to measure rates and patterns of disease progression. Rate of ventricular enlargement and hippocampal and medial temporal lobe atrophy have all been shown to be significantly greater in AD than in normal controls when subjects are rescanned after an interval of a year or more (Luxenberg *et al.* 1987; de Leon *et al.* 1989; Jobst *et al.* 1994; Fox *et al.* 1996b; Jack *et al.* 1998). Even with longitudinal studies, detection of small, diffuse changes remains difficult. Manual volumetric measurement involves outlining particular regions of interest and there is a critical dependence on the reproducibility of identifying anatomical structures and on prior decisions about which areas to measure. The development of automated image registration and subtraction algorithms allows even small amounts of atrophy to be shown. Such atrophy can also be quantified to give regional or global measures of disease progression. Subjects with AD have been found to have rates of global cerebral volume loss that are very significantly greater than in age-matched controls, with individual rates of atrophy in mild to moderate AD being 20 times the mean for the controls (Fox *et al.* 1996a; Fox and Freeborough, 1997). Rates of global atrophy measured with this technique have been shown to correlate closely with cognitive decline (Fox *et al.* 1999). The ability to visualise atrophy even in the early stages of the degenerative process may also allow distinctive patterns of atrophy to be identified to help in the differential diagnosis. Additionally sensitive measures of disease progression are likely to be of importance in the assessment of new and potentially disease-modifying therapies for these diseases (Leber 1997).

Differentiating Alzheimer's disease from other dementias

Neuroimaging studies in AD have tended to concentrate on comparing AD patients with normal subjects. What is lacking is detailed comparison of the imaging features of the different degenerative dementias with each other. Kitagaki *et al.* used MRI to show that frontotemporal dementia can be distinguished from AD by the presence of asymmetrical degeneration of the frontal and anterior temporal lobes (Kitagaki *et al.* 1998). Left temporal lobe atrophy is commonly found in the neuropsychological syndrome of semantic dementia which usually has Pick's disease as the underlying pathology (Hodges *et al.* 1992) (Figure 13.6). In

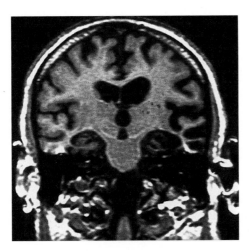

Fig. 13.6 Coronal T1-weighted MR image: Pick's disease with marked asymmetrical atrophy of the whole left temporal lobe and almost complete loss of the left hippocampus. On the right there is definite but less severe atrophy confined mainly to the hippocampus and parahippocampal gyrus.

corticobasal degeneration the asymmetrical para-central (frontoparietal) pattern of atrophy found at autopsy is best seen with MRI but may not be prominent in the early stages (Caselli and Jack, 1992; Tokumaru *et al.* 1996). The contribution of neuroimaging to the diagnosis of Huntington's disease has largely been overtaken by the discovery of genetic markers for this disease.

In Creutzfeldt-Jakob disease (CJD) scans may show non-specific atrophy, signal abnormalities or appear normal. Early CT studies reported scans to be normal in up to 80% of cases and MRI is normal in almost 50% (Galvez and Cartier, 1984; Zeidler *et al.* 1996). Overall, CT is insensitive to changes in CJD, even in relatively late stages. With any imaging movement artefact, as may be expected, is a major problem. Very rapidly progressive atrophy may be seen with serial scans (Uchino *et al.* 1991; Fox *et al.* 1997b). Increased signal intensity on T2-weighted MR images has been reported in the peripheral cortex (Falcone *et al.* 1992) and in the basal ganglia in CJD patients (Milton *et al.* 1991; Barboriak *et al.* 1994; Bahn *et al.* 1997; Hutzelmann and Biederer, 1998). However, Zeidler *et al.* found that such signal abnormalities were detected in routine clinical reporting in only 4 out of 96 autopsy-confirmed CJD cases (Zeidler *et al.* 1996). However when specifically looked for with appropriate MR sequences signal changes may be more common. Finkenstaedt *et al.* showed symmetrical increases in signal intensities in the caudate head and putamen on long TR sequences in 80% of cases in a series of 29 patients (Finkenstaedt *et al.* 1996). Less frequent changes were found in the globus pallidus (24%) and thalamus (14%). In new variant CJD, Collie *et al.* found over 85% of proven cases showed high signal intensities in the pulvinar of the thalamus on T2-weighted and proton density images (Collie *et al.* 1998).

Structural imaging now has an established position in the diagnosis of vascular dementia, since clinical differentiation from AD or dementia with Lewy bodies (DLB) is difficult without imaging due to the considerable overlap of features. These pathologies are the most common causes of dementia and share an increasing prevalence with age; they therefore frequently coexist - giving rise to the catch-all description of 'mixed dementia'. A diagnosis of vascular dementia is supported by the presence of relevant vascular changes on CT or MRI (Roman *et al.* 1993). Both the extent and location of changes are important (Amar and Wilcock 1996). Multiple infarcts and/or high signal foci in the basal ganglia and thalamus are very suggestive of vascular lesions (Schmidt 1992). In vascular or mixed dementia white matter changes are extensive, confluent and irregular (Schmidt 1992), compared to the small foci (<5 mm) seen in AD and elderly controls (Bennett *et al.* 1992; Erkinjuntti *et al.* 1994). The absence of vascular change on imaging, particular if proton density and T2-weighted MRI are employed, essentially excludes a diagnosis of vascular dementia. Structural imaging may provide strong supporting evidence for a diagnosis of vascular dementia when extensive white matter changes are seen. Clearly focal atrophy of the frontal or temporal lobe suggests frontotemporal degeneration.

13.3 **Functional imaging**

Scans that assess brain morphology are central to the differential diagnosis of dementia. In many instances of dementia, however, brain anatomy appears normal even though clinical examinations indicate that function is impaired. In these situations, functional neuroimaging has the potential to complement morphologic brain imaging and provide a biological measure of the behavioural abnormalities observed in dementia. Functional neuroimaging measures neural activity indirectly using glucose metabolism (CMR-glu) or cerebral blood flow (CBF) as surrogate markers. Regional or global measures may be used either to assess resting brain activity or response to a cognitive task.

13.3.1 Positron emission tomography

PET is used to determine CMR-glu and CBF by radioactive tracers which emit positrons. An emitted positron collides with an electron to produce gamma rays. The PET scanner converts these gamma rays into visible photons which can be used to construct a 3D image showing the location and concentration of the tracer. Two different techniques have been developed to measure cerebral metabolism or blood flow with PET. The use of ^{18}F fluorodeoxyglucose (^{18}F-FDG) enables cerebral glucose metabolism to be estimated after intravenous injection of radio-labelled glucose. Alternatively, $^{15}O_2$ oxygen can be used to measure both cerebral oxygen metabolism and CBF following inhalation of ^{15}O-labelled oxygen or following infusion of ^{15}O-labelled water. Complex kinetic models allow both methods to quantify absolute values for metabolism and CBF from the reconstructed images. PET scan analysis may use visual assessment of colour-coded images, although this may be insufficiently sensitive for diagnostic purposes. For inter-subject comparison it is necessary to normalise data, to take into account the wide variations in global cerebral metabolism. This may be done by comparison of the regional with the global cerebral metabolic rate for glucose. Alternatively, data may be normalised to a cerebellar or pons internal reference standard since these areas are thought to be unaffected by the majority of degenerative diseases (Minoshima *et al.* 1995; Kushner *et al.* 1987). The variation in normalisation methods may account for some of the discrepancies between studies. Statistical parametric mapping (SPM) (Friston *et al.* 1995), which involves analysis of scans on a voxel-by-voxel basis, is increasingly being applied to PET data (Kennedy *et al.* 1995; Desgranges *et al.* 1998; Signorini *et al.* 1999).

The main advantage of PET is the ability to provide high resolution images, with modern PET cameras having resolutions approaching 4mm full-width-half-maximum (FWHM)(Levin and Hoffman, 1999). It also allows sensitive quantitative measures of brain function and the assessment of physiological parameters such as receptor binding. However, its clinical application is limited, mainly because a cyclotron is required to produce the radioactive isotopes on which the techniques are based. It is expensive and scanning is time-consuming. For these reasons it is primarily a research tool.

Single photon emission computed tomography

SPECT is similar to PET in that it involves the detection of gamma rays produced by radioactive tracers. Absolute quantification of regional CBF (rCBF) may be obtained using the ^{133}Xenon inhalation technique. High resolution SPECT uses lipophilic tracers of CBF such as technetium ^{99m}Tc hexamethyl propyleneamine oxamine (^{99m}Tc-HMPAO), which cross the blood-brain barrier where they are metabolised to less lipid-soluble products. The distribution of the breakdown products are thought to reflect CBF at the time of injection, as the tracer is metabolised within a few minutes after injection. Some of the methods used to analyse PET data have been employed for SPECT and include visual assessments of images by blinded observers (Waldemar *et al.* 1994) and the use of regions of interest and normalisation of CBF to reference values (Krausz *et al.* 1998; Asenbaum *et al.* 1998; Fleming *et al.* 1999). SPM has not been applied widely to SPECT due to its poor spatial resolution.

In contrast to PET, the radioactive tracers used in SPECT are relatively inexpensive and easy to prepare and administer. The use of a standard gamma ray detection camera means SPECT brain scans are widely available, and modern SPECT cameras have image resolutions approaching that of PET. Overall, the technical limitations of SPECT have to be compared with the expense and restricted availability of PET. It remains to be determined whether the tracers used in SPECT, which in general have poorer resolution, will limit its ability to distinguish the CBF changes associated with early AD.

13.3.2 Functional magnetic resonance imaging

Unlike PET and SPECT, fMRI does not require a tracer. It utilises the magnetic properties of oxygenated and deoxygenated blood to estimate CBF, with a high signal intensity indicating a high level of blood oxygenation. It can be used to assess abnormalities in resting blood flow as well as during activation by cognitive tasks. The difference in signal intensities between oxygenated and deoxygenated haemoglobin is slight, necessitating the summation of several scans for analysis. Generally SPM is used for this analysis using a series of scans in the activated and resting state to determine regions of significant activation associated with a specific cognitive task. This functional image is superimposed onto a conventional morphological MR image. The information provided by fMRI is comparable to PET. Gonzalez *et al* (Gonzalez *et al*. 1995) conducted a study to determine the correlation between perfusion abnormalities in patients with dementia detected by functional magnetic resonance imaging and PET, and found an overall concordance of 78%.

In addition, Magnetic Resonance Spectroscopy (MRS) is a research technique for measuring specific metabolites in the brain. N-acetyl aspartate, a marker of neuronal integrity, has been shown to be reduced in AD. Some studies have used this technique to differentiate AD patients and controls (Lazeyras *et al*. 1998; Parnetti *et al*. 1997; Pettegrew *et al*. 1997), but as yet MRS has had little clinical application. The technique may assume greater importance in the future.

Functional MRI is multi-modal, giving perfusion and diffusion images. Functional MRI provides high resolution images, but is less expensive and invasive than PET. No radioactive tracers are required, reducing radiation risks. Moseley and colleagues (Moseley *et al*. 1996) reviewed its clinical use and predicted that its application would grow exponentially in the near future.

13.3.3 Diagnosis of Alzheimer's disease using functional imaging

Functional imaging can complement structural information in the diagnosis of AD by showing regions with metabolic deficits. The prevailing hypothesis is that metabolic deficits in some way reflect neuronal dysfunction because they parallel the distribution of AD histopathology, showing predilection for the association neocortices. Rapoport *et al* .reported five out of six subjects who showed a clear relationship between the antemortem pattern of regional hypometabolism and the density of NFT found at postmortem (Rapoport *et al*. 1991). There is considerable heterogeneity in the distribution of functional deficits within AD groups (Waldemar *et al*. 1997). Deficits in the temporoparietal (TP) region, common in AD, may reflect 'disconnection' possibly as a result of lesions at distant locations. For example, even the earliest metabolic changes in AD may not be in the brain region that shows the earliest or most severe pathologic changes, such as the entorhinal cortex and hippocampus. Minoshima *et al*, using ^{18}F-FDG PET, found functional deficits in the posterior cingulate cortex prior to those in the parahippocampal region in early AD cases (Minoshima *et al.* 1997).

13.3.4 Excluding structural lesions

Functional imaging has a less important role in the exclusion of treatable causes of dementia, as it is generally inferior to results provided by structural imaging. Patients suspected of normal pressure hydrocephalus will often have increased extension of sub-cortical low perfusion areas, which do not correspond to a similar degree of central atrophy registered by CT or MRI. Functional imaging (in particular SPECT) may add evidence for the diagnosis of normal pressure hydrocephalus and may help patients most likely to benefit from ventriculo-peritoneal shunting.

13.3.5 Differentiating Alzheimer's disease from normal ageing

Functional imaging studies investigating normal ageing have been inconclusive in establishing typical patterns of hypometabolism. Waldemar *et al.* (Waldemar *et al.* 1991) found no age-associated decline in global CBF, also using ^{99m}Tc-HMPAO SPECT, but a reduction in rCBF in the frontal cortex. Martin *et al.* (Martin *et al.* 1991) used PET to show there was a decrease in rCBF in the association cortices in normal ageing. PET studies have shown an age-related reduction in CMR-glu in the frontal cortex (Moeller *et al.* 1996), whilst Petit *et al* showed there was a significant decline in CMR-glu in all brain areas except for most of the occipital lobes and part of the cerebellum (Petit *et al.* 1998). Most severely affected were the anterior temporal and frontal regions.

AD is characterised by hypometabolism of the temporal and parietal cortices. This pattern was first shown by Frackowiak *et al.* (Frackowiak *et al.* 1981) using [15]O PET in 20 patients with degenerative dementia. There was a global reduction in CBF and oxygen metabolism, most marked in the temporal and parietal cortices, with additional frontal hypometabolism in those more severely demented. Similar results have since been obtained using ^{18}F-FDG PET (Friedland *et al.* 1984), SPECT (van Gool *et al.* 1995; Banyu *et al.* 1997) plate 2 and fMRI studies (Sandson *et al.* 1996). The deficits are usually bilateral (Haxby *et al.* 1986), although unilateral temporal-parietal (TP) hypometabolism has been noted (Duara *et al.* 1986; Holman *et al.* 1992). Hypometabolism in frontal association cortices is usually less severe and is most apparent in patients with advanced disease (Frackowiak *et al.* 1981; Duara *et al.* 1986; Haxby *et al.* 1988). The sensorimotor, visual cortices, basal ganglia, and cerebellum usually have metabolic values that are not significantly different from those found in controls (Frackowiak *et al.* 1981). In addition, Ishii *et al* found no significant differences in rCBF and cerebral blood volume in the hippocampus between mild-to-moderate AD patients and controls (Ishii *et al.* 1998c).

The sensitivity and specificity of diagnosis achieved by functional imaging is generally inferior to that of stuctural imaging. SPECT has obtained a wide range of sensitivities and specificities: 82% and 89% (Hanyu *et al.* 1993), 89% and 80% (Jobst *et al.* 1998), 91% and 86% (Johnson *et al.* 1993), 86% and 91% (Banyu *et al.* 1997) respectively. Greene *et al.* (Greene *et al.* 1996) reported that approximately one-third of the AD patients had normal perfusion patterns. Van Gool *et al* found a specificity of 89% gave a sensitivity of only 43% when discriminating AD from controls using SPECT (van Gool *et al.* 1995). Comparing the value of SPECT to that of neuropsychological assessment in the diagnosis of AD, Villa *et al.* noted that they showed similar degrees of sensitivity (91%), but a SPECT hippocampal CBF deficit was considerably less specific (71% versus 81%) than cognitive testing (Villa *et al.* 1995). The sensitivity and specificity of SPECT may be inferior to that found in PET, although few studies have directly compared the two modalities with similar resolution cameras using patients with early disease. Visual analysis of PET data is widely used but may not be sufficiently sensitive. Consequently, the use of metabolic patterns in the diagnosis of AD will remain a subject of controversy until large, randomly chosen samples can be studied and followed to a definitive pathologic diagnosis.

13.4 Correlations between neuropsychological markers and metabolic patterns in Alzheimer's disease

Correlation between regional hypometabolism and neuropsychological measures of disease severity has been shown in PET (Frackowiak *et al.* 1981; Haxby *et al.* 1988; Ishii *et al.* 1998c; Mielke and Heiss, 1998), SPECT (Jagust *et al.* 1997) and fMRI (Sandson *et al.* 1996); however, a significant association is not always found (Sachdev *et al.* 1997). Individuals who have greater language deficits have been shown to have more pronounced left frontotemporal asymmetry, whilst those who have impairment in visuospatial function show right parietal asymmetry. Although most investigators have not reported overall asymmetries in metabolism, Lowenstein and colleagues did note predominant left hemisphere hypometabolism in 33 AD subjects that was unrelated to severity or duration of dementia (Lowenstein *et al.* 1989). This striking observation supports *a priori* speculation that in AD the left hemisphere is more vulnerable than the right (Rossor *et al.* 1982).

An association between the pattern of regional blood flow pattern and more specific cognitive tests, such as explicit memory (Greene *et al.* 1996), visuospatial function, and frontal lobe function have been reported (Eberling *et al.* 1993). Some studies have correlated CBF with scores from structured neuropsychological batteries (O'Brien *et al.* 1992). The idea that AD may have a focal onset has been supported by a study that showed that six probable AD patients with circumscribed neuropsychological impairments had focal cerebral perfusion deficits (Celsis *et al.* 1987). Pietrini *et al* showed that PET measurements of glucose metabolism during activation gave a more sensitive indication of neuronal dysfunction in AD patients than that measured during rest (Pietrini *et al.* 1999). The scarcity of such studies in AD reflects the practical difficulties associated with asking cognitively impaired patients to perform intricate behavioural tasks during functional imaging.

13.5 Imaging of neurotransmitter systems

PET and SPECT radioligand studies have been used to try and quantify the loss of cholinergic receptors in AD. Data interpretation from these studies has been complicated because apparent reductions in receptor binding may be secondary to tissue loss or alterations in receptor regulation and not merely due to the loss of receptors themselves. The uptake of a radioligand by a muscarinic acetylcholinergic receptor (mAch-R) was investigated by Yoshida *et al.* (Yoshida *et al.* 1998). They found a significant reduction in mAch-Rs in AD subjects when compared to controls. Nordberg *et al* showed that binding of ^{11}C-nicotine was reduced in AD patients compared to controls, but that treatment with tacrine increased uptake after 3 months (Nordberg 1993). Some investigators have tried to develop ligands specific for amyloid (Friedland *et al.* 1997) which would provide a direct window on the molecular pathology but so far this has remained elusive.

13.6 **Differentiating Alzheimer's disease from other dementias**

A bilateral TP deficit is common but by no means universal in AD patients. Furthermore, other dementias may exhibit similar deficits. TP deficits have also been shown in multi-infarct dementia (Weinstein *et al.* 1991), Parkinson's disease (PD) without dementia (Eberling *et al.* 1994), PD with dementia (Goto *et al.* 1993), DLB (Donnemiller *et al.* 1997), and CJD (Goto *et al.* 1993). Masterman *et al* found that a TP deficit was not specific to AD and obtained a sensitivity of 75% and specificity of 52% for differentiating AD from other dementias with ^{99m}Tc-HMPAO SPECT (Masterman *et al.* 1997). However, the combination of medial temporal lobe atrophy and TP deficit is relatively more specific for AD (Jobst *et al.* 1998).

Pseudo-dementia caused by depression may be differentiated from AD by involvement of the frontal and cingulate regions as well as the amygdala (Kennedy *et al.* 1997). Ishii *et al.* used ^{18}F-FDG PET to differentiate between AD and FTD (Ishii *et al.* 1998b). They found FTD cases had a significant reduction in CMR-glu in the frontal and anterior temporal lobes, basal ganglia and thalamus when compared to AD. Pickut used ^{99m}Tc-HMPAO SPECT to show frontal rather than parietal deficits in FTD compared to AD (Pickut *et al.* 1997) (Plate 11).^{18}F-FDG PET has also been used for the differential diagnosis of AD from DLB (Imamura *et al.* 1997; Ishii *et al.* 1998a) with AD patients having lower CMR-glu in the medial temporal and cingulate areas. Mielke and Heiss used PET to show that rCBF was reduced in both AD and vascular dementia cases, but that the pattern in vascular dementia was more scattered, occurring in cortical and subcortical regions (Mielke and Heiss, 1998).

Based on our current knowledge, it is reasonable to conclude that bilateral TP deficits are frequently, but not exclusively, found in AD and this pattern has some utility in distinguishing AD patients from those with FLD and from depression.

13.7 **Conclusion**

Functional imaging is not yet established in the diagnostic process for AD. A TP deficit may add weight to a clinical diagnosis of AD, but cannot in itself differentiate between AD and other types of dementia. The pattern of hypometabolism involved in the normal ageing process is uncertain, making differentiation between AD and healthy elderly groups problematic. Activation studies may increase our understanding of the disease process in the early stages, but has limited use when patients are more severely affected. PET and SPECT have limitations in terms of resolution and practicality, but fMRI is likely to assume a more prominent role in the future.

Structural imaging already has an established role in excluding potentially treatable causes such as tumours, hydrocephalus or haematomata. However, despite improvements in imaging, there remains considerable overlap between early AD and normal ageing. Disproportionate atrophy of medial temporal lobe structures (hippocampus, parahippocampus or amygdala) appear to provide the earliest marker of AD, and improving methods for the identification of these regions of interest could prove valuable in the future.

However, distinguishing AD and dementia with Lewy bodies remains difficult. Vascular dementia is suggested by 'extensive' white matter changes and frontotemporal dementia patients usually exhibit relatively focal frontal and/or temporal atrophy. Nevertheless, in some cases structural imaging may be inconclusive in the differential diagnosis of AD.

As specific drug therapies for AD are developed there will be increasing pressure to make an early diagnosis. Furthermore, objective imaging measures of disease progression will be important in assessing new treatments. Longitudinal studies will also be needed to develop and validate objective measures of disease progression. In the future, structural imaging may be combined with functional imaging to establish early diagnoses in the degenerative dementias and to monitor responses to therapy.

References

Amar, K., and Wilcock, G. (1996). Vascular dementia. *British Medical Journal*, **312**, 227–231.

Andreasen, N. C., Flaum, M., Swayze, V., Swayze V. O'Leary, D. S., Cohen, G. *et al.* (1993). Intelligence and brain structure in normal individuals. *American Journal of Psychiatry*, **150**, 130–134.

Asenbaum, S., Brucke, T., Pirker, W., Pietrzyk U., and Podreka, I. (1998). Imaging of cerebral blood flow with technetium-99m-HMPAO and technetium-99m-ECD: a comparison. *Journal of Nuclear Medicine*, **39**, 613–618.

Bahn, M. M., Kido, D. K., Lin, W., and Pearlman, A. L. (1997). Brain magnetic resonance diffusion abnormalities in Creutzfeldt-Jakob disease. *Archives of Neurology*, **54**, 1411–1415.

Bahner, M. L., Reith, W., Zuna, I., *et al.* (1998). Spiral CT vs incremental CT: Is spiral CT superior in imaging of the brain? *European Journal of Radiology*, **8**, 416–420.

Ball, M. J., Fisman, M., Hachinski, V., *et al.* (1985). A new definition of Alzheimer's disease: a hippocampal dementia. *Lancet*, **325**, 14–16.

Banyu, H., Asano, T., Abe, S., Arai, H., Takasaki, M., Shindo, H. *et al.* (1997). Single photon emission computed tomography in the diagnosis of Alzheimer's disease. *Japanese Journal of Geriatrics*, **34**, 468–473.

Barber, R., Scheltens, F., Gholkar, A., Ballard, C., McKeith, I., Ince, P. *et al.* (1999). White matter lesions on magnetic resonance imaging in dementia with Lewy bodies, Alzheimer's disease, vascular dementia, and normal aging. *Journal of Neurology, Neurosurgery, and Psychiatry*, **67**, 66–72.

Barboriak, D. P., Provenzale, J. M., and Boyko, O. B. (1994). MR diagnosis of Creutzfeldt-Jakob disease: significance of high signal intensity of the basal ganglia. *American Journal of Roentgenology*, **162**, 137–140.

Bennett, D. A., Gilley, D. W., Wilson, R. S., Huckman, M. S., and Fox, J. H. (1992). Clinical correlates of high signal lesions on magnetic resonance imaging in Alzheimer's disease. *Journal of Neurology*, **239**, 186–190.

Blatter, D. D., Bigler, E. D., Gale, S. D., Johnson, S. C., Anderson, C. V., Burnett, B. M. *et al.* (1995). Quantitative volumetric analysis of brain MR: Normative database spanning 5 decades of life. *American Journal of Neuroradiology*, **16**, 241–251.

Braak, H., Braak, E. and Bohl, J. (1993). Staging of Alzheimer-related cortical destruction. [Review]. *European Neurology*, **33**, 403–408.

Brun, A., and Englund, E. (1986). A white matter disorder in dementia of the Alzheimer type: a pathoanatomical study. *Annals of Neurology*, **19**, 253–262.

Caselli, R. J., and Jack, C. R. (1992). Asymmetric cortical degeneration syndromes - a proposed clinical classification. *Archives of Neurology*, **49**, 770–780.

Celsis, P., Agniel, A., Rascol, A., Rascol, A., and Marc-Vergnes, J. P. (1987). Focal cerebral hypoperfusion and selective cognitive deficit in dementia of the Alzheimer type. *Journal of Neurology, Neurosurgery, and Psychiatry*, **50**, 1602–1612.

Coffey, C. E., Wilkinson, W. E., and Parashos, I. A. (1992). Quantitative cerebral anatomy of the aging human brain: a cross-sectional study using Magnetic Resonance Imaging. *Neurology*, 42, 527–536.

Collie, D. A., Sellar, R. J., and Ironside, J. (1998). New variant Creutzfeldt-Jakob disease: Diagnostic features on MR Imaging with histopathologic correlation. *Proceedings of American Society of Neuroradiology*, 139

Convit, A., de Leon, M. J., Golomb, J., De Santi, S., Tsui, W., Rusinek, H. *et al.* (1993). Hippocampal atrophy in early Alzheimer's disease: anatomic specificity and validation. *Psychiatric Quarterly*, 64, 371–387.

Convit, A., De Leon, M. J., Tarshish, C., De Santi, S., Tsui, W., Rusinek, H. *et al.* (1997). Specific hippocampal volume reductions in individuals at risk for Alzheimer's disease. *Neurobiology of Aging*, 18, 131–138.

Cook, M. J., Fish, D. R., Shorvon, S. D., Straughan, K., and Stevens, J. M. (1992). Hippocampal volumetric and morphometric studies in frontal and temporal lobe epilepsy. *Brain*, 115, 1001–1015.

Cowell, P. E., Turetsky, B. I., Gur, R. C., Grossman, R. I., Shtasel, D. L., and Gur, R. E. (1994). Sex differences in aging of the human frontal and temporal lobes. *Journal of Neuroscience*, 14, 4748–4755.

Cuenod, C. A., Denys, A., Michot, J. L., *et al.* (1993). Amygdala atrophy in Alzheimer's disease. An in vivo magnetic resonance imaging study. *Archives of Neurology*, 50, 941–945.

Dahlbeck, J. W., McCluney, K. W., Yeakley, J. W., *et al.* (1991). The interuncal distance: a new MR measurement for the hippocampal atrophy of Alzheimer disease. *American Journal of Neuroradiology*, 12, 931–932.

Davis, P. C., Gray, L., Albert, M., Wilkinson, W., Hughes, J., Heyman, A. *et al.* (1992). The Consortium to Establish a Registry for Alzheimer's Disease (CERAD). Part III. Reliability of a standardized MRI evaluation of Alzheimer's disease. *Neurology*, 42, 1676–1680.

De Leon, M. J., George, A. E., Reisberg, B., Ferris, S. H., Kluger, A., Stylopoulos, L. A. *et al.* (1989). Alzheimer's disease: longitudinal CT studies of ventricular change. *American Journal of Roentgenology*, 152, 1257–1262.

De Leon, M. J., Golomb, J., George, A. E., Convit, A., Tarshish, C. Y., McRae, T. *et al.* (1993). The radiologic prediction of Alzheimer disease: the atrophic hippocampal formation. *American Journal of Neuroradiology*, 14 , 897–906.

DeCarli, C., Kaye, J. A., Horwitz, B., and Rapoport, S. I. (1990). Critical analysis of the use of computer-assisted transverse axial tomography to study human brain in aging and dementia of the Alzheimer type. [Review]. *Neurology*, 40, 872–883.

DeCarli, C., Murphy, D. G., Gillette, J. A., Haxby, J. V., Teichberg, D., Schapiro, M. B. *et al.* (1994). Lack of age-related differences in temporal lobe volume of very healthy adults. *American Journal of Neuroradiology*, 15, 689–696.

Dekaban, A. S. (1978). Changes in brain weights during the span of human life: relation of brain weights to body heights and body weights. *Annals of Neurology*, 4, 345–356.

Desgranges, B., Baron, J. C., De-La, S. V., Petit-Taboue, M. C., Benali, K., Landeau, B. *et al.* (1998). The neural substrates of memory systems impairment in Alzheimer's disease. A PET study of resting brain glucose utilization. *Brain*, 121, 611–631.

Donnemiller, E., Heilmann, J., Wenning, G. K., Bergera, W., Decristoforo, C., Moncayo, R. *et al.* (1997). Brain perfusion scintigraphy with 99mTc-HMPAO or 99mTc-ECD and 123I-beta-CIT single-photon emission tomography in dementia of the Alzheimer-type and diffuse Lewy body disease. *European Journal of Nuclear Medicine*, 24, 320–325.

Drayer, B. P. (1988). Imaging of the aging brain. Part I. Normal findings. [Review]. *Radiology*, 166, 785–796.

Duara, R., Grady, C., Haxby, J., *et al.* (1986). Positron emission tomography in Alzheimer's disease. *Neurology*, 36, 879–887.

Early, B., Escalona, P. R., Boyko, O. B., Doraiswamy, P. M., Axelson, D. A., Patterson, L. *et al.* (1993). Interuncal distance measurements in healthy volunteers and in patients with Alzheimer's disease. *American Journal of Neuroradiology*, **14**, 907–910.

Eberling, J .L., Reed, B. R., Baker, M. G., and Jagust, W. J. (1993). Cognitive correlates of regional cerebral blood flow in Alzheimer's disease. *Archives of Neurology*, **50**, 761–766.

Eberling, J. L., Richardson, B. C., Reed, B. R., Wolfe, N., and Jagust, W. J. (1994) Cortical glucose metabolism in Parkinson's disease without dementia. *Neurobiology of Aging*, **15**, 329–335.

Erkinjuntti, T., Gao, F., Lee, D. H., Eliasziw, M., Mershey, H., and Hachinski, V. C. (1994). Lack of difference in brain hyperintensities between patients with early Alzheimer's disease and control subjects. *Archives of Neurology*, **51**, 260–268.

Erkinjuntti, T., Lee, D. H., Gao, F., Steenhuis, R., Eliasziw, M., Fry, R. *et al.* (1993). Temporal lobe atrophy on magnetic resonance imaging in the diagnosis of early Alzheimer's disease. *Archives of Neurology*, **50**, 305–310.

Falcone, S., Quencer, R. M., Bowen, B., Bruce, J. H., and Naidich, T. P. (1992). Creutzfeldt-Jakob disease: focal symmetrical cortical involvement demonstrated by MR imaging. *American Journal of Neuroradiology*, **13**, 403–406.

Finkenstaedt, M., Szudra, A., Zerr, I., Poser, S., Hise, J. H., Stoebner, J. M. *et al.* (1996). MR imaging of Creutzfeldt-Jakob disease. *Radiology*, **199**, 793–798.

Fleming, J. S., Kemp, P. M. and Bolt, L. (1999). A technique for manual definition of an irregular volume of interest in single photon emission computed tomography. *Physical and Medical Biology*, **44**, N15–N20

Fox, N. C. and Freeborough, P. A. (1997). Brain atrophy progression measured from registered serial MRI: validation and application to Alzheimer's disease. *Journal of Magnetic resonance Imaging*, 7, 1069–1075.

Fox, N. C., Freeborough, P. A. and Rossor, M. N. (1996). Visualisation and quantification of atrophy in Alzheimer's disease. *The Lancet*, **348**, 94–97.

Fox, N. C., Warrington, E. K., Freeborough, P. A., Hartikainen, P., Kennedy, A. M., Stevens, J. M. *et al.* (1996). Presymptomatic hippocampal atrophy in Alzheimer's disease: a longitudinal MRI study. *Brain*, **119**, 2001–2007.

Fox, N.C., Kennedy, A. M., Harvey, R. J., Lantos, P. L., Roques, P. K., Collinge, J. *et al.* (1997a). Clinicopathological features of familial Alzheimer's disease associated with the M139V mutation in the presenilin 1 gene. Pedigree but not mutation specific age at onset provides evidence for a further genetic factor. *Brain*, **120**, 491–501.

Fox, N. C., Freeborough, P. A., Mekkaoui, K. F., Stevens, J. M., and Rossor, M. N. (1997b). Cerebral and cerebellar atrophy on serial magnetic resonance imaging in an initially symptom free subject at risk of familial prion disease. *British Medical Journal*, **315**, 856–857.

Fox, N. C., Scahill, R. I., Crum, W. R., and Rossor, M. N. (1999). Correlation between rates of brain atrophy and cognitive decline in Alzheimer's disease. *Neurology*, **52**, 1687.

Frackowiak, R. J., Pozzilli, C., Legg, N. J., *et al.* (1981). Regional cerebral oxygen supply and utilization in dementia. A clinical and physiological study with oxygen-15 and positron tomography. *Brain*, **104**, 753–778.

Free, S. L., Bergin, P. S., Fish, D. R., Cook, M. J., Shorvon, S. D., and Stevens, J. M. (1995). Methods for normalization of hippocampal volumes measured with MR. *American Journal of Neuroradiology*, **16**, 637–643.

Friedland, R. P., Budinger, T., Brant-Zawadzki, M., and Jagust, W. J. (1984). The diagnosis of Alzheimer Type dementia. A preliminary comparison of Positron Emission Tomography and proton Magnetic resonance. *Journal of the American Medical Association*, **252**, 2750–2752.

Friedland, R. P., Kalaria, R., Berridge, M., Miraldi. F., Hedera, P., Reno, J. *et al.* (1997). Neuroimaging of vessel amyloid in Alzheimer's disease. *Annals of the NewYork Academy of Science*, **826**, 242–247.

Frisoni, G. B., Beltramello, A., Weiss, C., Geroldi, C., Bianchetti, A., and Trabucchi, M. (1996). Usefulness of simple measures of temporal lobe atrophy in probable Alzheimer's disease. *Dementia,*. 7, 15–22.

Friston, K. J., Holmes A. P., Worsley K. J. *et al.* (1995). Statistical parametric maps in functional imaging: A general linear approach. *Human Brain Mapping*, 2, 189–210.

Galvez, S., and Cartier, L. (1984). Computed Tomography findings in 15 cases of Creutzfeld-Jacob Disease with histological verification. *Journal of Neurology, Neurosurgery, and Psychiatry*, 47, 1244–1246.

George, A. E., de Leon, M. J., Stylopoulos, L. A., Geroldi, C., Bianchetti, A., Trabucchi, M. *et al.* (1990). CT diagnostic features of Alzheimer disease: importance of the Choroidal/Hippocampal fissure complex. *American Journal of Neuroradiology*, 11, 101–107.

Gonzalez, R. G., Fischman, A. J., Guimaraes, A. R., Carr, C. A., Stern, C. E., Halpern, E. F. *et al.* (1995). Functional MR in the evaluation of dementia: correlation of abnormal dynamic cerebral blood volume measurements with changes in cerebral metabolism on positron emission tomography with fludeoxyglucose F 18. *American Journal of Neuroradiology*, 16, 1763–1770.

Goto, I., Taniwaki, T., Hosokawa, S., Otsuka, M., Ichiya, Y., and Ichimiya, A. (1993). Positron emission tomographic (PET) studies in dementia. *Journal of Neurological Science*, 114, 1–6.

Greene, J. D., Miles, K., and Hodges, J. R. (1996). Neuropsychology of memory and SPECT in the diagnosis and staging of dementia of Alzheimer type. *Journal of Neurology*, 243, 175–190.

Haan, J., Lanser, J., Zijderveld, I., Van der Does, I. G. F., and Roos, A.C. (1990). Dementia in heredi-tary Cerebral Haemorrhage with Amyloidosis dutch type. *Archives of Neurology*, 47, 965–967.

Hanyu, H., Abe, S., Arai, H., Asano, T., Iwamoto, T., and Takasaki, M. (1993). Diagnostic accuracy of single photon emission computed tomography in Alzheimer's disease. *Gerontology*, 39, 260–266.

Haxby, J. V., Grady, C., Durara, R., *et al.* (1986). Neocortical metabolic deficit precede non memory cognitive defects in early Alzheimer's type dementia. *Archives of Neurology*, 43, 882–885.

Haxby, J. V., Grady, C., Koss, E., Horwitz, B., Schapiro, M., Friedland, R. P. *et al.* (1988). Heterogeneous anterior-posterior metabolic patterns in Dementia of the Alzheimer type. *Neurology*, 38, 1853–1863.

Ho, K., Roessmann, U., Straumfjord, J. V., and Monroe, G. (1980) Analysis of brain weight. I. Adult brain weight in relation to sex, race, and age. *Archives of Pathology and Laboratory Medicine*, 104, 635–639.

Hodges, J. R., Patterson, K., Oxbury, S., and Funnell, E. (1992). Semantic dementia. Progressive fluent aphasia with temporal lobe atrophy. *Brain*, 115, 1783–1806.

Holman, B. L., Johnson, K. A., Gerada, B., Carvalho, P. A., and Satlin, A. (1992). The scintigraphic appearance of Alzheimer's disease: A prospective study using technetium-99m-HMPAO SPECT. *Journal of Nuclear Medicine*, 33, 181–185.

Howieson, J., Kaye, J. A., Holm, L., and Howieson, D. (1993). Interuncal distance: marker of aging and Alzheimer disease. *American Journal of Neuroradiology*, 14, 647–650.

Hutzelmann, A. and Biederer, J. (1998) MRI follow-up in a case of clinically diagnosed Creutzfeld-Jakob disease. *European Journal ofRadiology*, 8, 421–423.

Hyman, B .T., Damasio, A. R., VanHoesen, G. W., and Barnes, C. L. (1984). Alzheimer's disease: cell-specific pathology isolates the hippocampal formation. *Science*, 298, 83–95.

Hyman, B. T. and Gomez-Isla, T. (1994). Alzheimer's disease is a laminar, regional, and neural system specific disease, not a global brain disease. *Neurobiology of Aging*, 15, 353–354.

Ikeda, M., Tanabe, H., Nakagawa, Y., Kazui, H., Oi, H., Yamazaki, H. *et al.* (1994). MRI-based quanti-tative assessment of the hippocampal region in very mild to moderate Alzheimer's disease. *Neuroradiology*, 36, 7–10.

Imamura, T., Ishii, K., Sasaki, M., Kitagaki, H., Yamaji, S., Hirono, N. *et al.* (1997) Regional cerebral glucose metabolism in dementia with Lewy bodies and Alzheimer's disease: a comparative study using positron emission tomography. *Neuroscience Letters*, **235**, 49–52.

Ishii, K., Imamura, T., Sasaki, M., Yamaji, S., Sakamoto, S., Kitagaki, H. *et al.* (1998a) Regional cerebral glucose metabolism in dementia with lewy bodies and Alzheimer's disease. *Neurology*, **51**, 125–130.

Ishii, K., Sakamoto, S., Sasaki, M., Kitagaki, H., Yamaji, S., Hashimoto, M. *et al.* (1998b) Cerebral glucose metabolism in patients with frontotemporal dementia. *Journal of Nuclear Medicine*, **39**, 1875–1878.

Ishii, K., Sasaki, M., Yamaji, S., Sakamoto, S., Kitagaki, H., and Mori, E. (1998c) Paradoxical hippocampus perfusion in mild-to-moderate Alzheimer's disease. *Journal of Nuclear Medicine*, **39**, 293–298.

Jack, C. R. (1991) Brain and cerebrospinal fluid volume: measurement with MR imaging [editorial; comment]. *Radiology*, **178**, 22–24.

Jack, C. R., Petersen, R. C., Xu, Y., O'Brien, P. C., Smith, G. E., Ivnik, R. J. *et al.* (1998) Rate of medial temporal lobe atrophy in typical aging and Alzheimer's disease. *Neurology*, **51**, 993–999.

Jack, C. R., Petersen, R. C., Xu, Y. C., Waring, S. C., O'Brien, P. C., Tangalos, E. G. *et al.* (1997) Medial temporal atrophy on MRI in normal aging and very mild Alzheimer's disease. *Neurology*, **49**, 786–794.

Jack, C. R., Jr., Petersen, R. C., O'Brien, P. C., and Tangalos, E. G. (1992) MR-based hippocampal volumetry in the diagnosis of Alzheimer's disease. *Neurology*, **42**, 183–188.

Jagust, W. J., Eberling, J. L., Reed, B. R., Mathis, C. A., and Budinger, T. F. (1997). Clinical studies of cerebral blood flow in Alzheimer's disease. *Annals of New York Academy of Science*, **826**, 254–262.

Jernigan, T. L., Salmon, D. P., Butters, N., *et al.* (1991). Cerebral structure on MRI, Part II: Specific changes in Alzheimer's and Huntington's diseases. *Biological Psychiatry*, **29**, 68–81.

Jobst, K. A., Barnetson, L. D. and Shepstone, B. J. (1998). Accurate prediction of histologically confirmed Alzheimer's disease and the differential diagnosis of dementia: The use of NINCDS-ADRDA and DSM-III-R criteria, SPECT, X-ray CT, and Apo E4 in medial temporal lobe dementias. *International Psychogeriatrics*, **10**, 271–302.

Jobst, K. A., Smith, A. D., Szatmari, M., Esiri, M. M., Jaskowski, A., Hindley, N. *et al.* (1994). Rapidly progressing atrophy of medial temporal lobe in Alzheimer's disease. *Lancet*, **343**, 829–830.

Jobst, K. A., Smith, A. D., Szatmari, M., Molyneux, A., Esiri, M. E., King, E. *et al.* (1992). Detection in life of confirmed Alzheimer's disease using a simple measurement of medial temporal lobe atrophy by computed tomography. *Lancet*, **340**, 1179–1183.

Johnson, K. A., Kijewski, M. F., Becker, J. A., Garada, B., Satlin, A., Holman, B. L. *et al.* (1993). Quantitative brain SPECT in Alzheimer's disease and normal aging. *Journal of Nuclear Medicine*, **34**, 2044–2048.

Kaye, J. A., DeCarli, C., Luxenberg, J. S., and Rapoport, S. I. (1992). The significance of age-related enlargement of the cerebral ventricles in healthy men and women measured by quantitative computed X-ray tomography. *Journal of the American Geriatrics Society*, **40**, 225–231.

Kaye, J. A., Swihart, T., Howieson, D., *et al.* (1997). Volume loss of the hippocampus and temporal lobe in healthy elderly persons destined to develop dementia. *Neurology*, **48**, 1297–1304.

Kennedy, A. M., Newman, S. K., Frackowiak, R. S. J., Cunningham, V. J., Roques, P., Stevens, J. *et al.* (1995). Chromosome 14 linked familial Alzheimer's disease: A clinico-pathological study of a single pedigree. *Brain*, **118**, 185–205.

Kennedy, S. H., Javanmard, M. and Vaccarino, F. J. (1997). A review of functional neuroimaging in mood disorders: positron emission tomography and depression. *Canadian Journal of Psychiatry*, **42**, 467–475.

Kesslak, J. P., Nalcioglu, O. and Cotman, C. W. (1991). Quantification of magnetic resonance scans for hippocampal and parahippocampal atrophy in Alzheimer's disease [see comments]. *Neurology*, **41**, 51–54.

Killiany, R. J., Moss, M. B., Albert, M. S., Sandor, T., Tieman, J., and Jolesz, F. (1993). Temporal lobe regions on magnetic resonance imaging identify patients with early Alzheimer's disease. *Archives of Neurology*, **50**, 949–954.

Kitagaki, H., Mori, E., Yamaji, S., Ishii, K., Hirono, N., Kobashi, S. *et al.* (1998). Frontotemporal dementia and Alzheimer disease: evaluation of cortical atrophy with automated hemispheric surface display generated with MR images. *Radiology*, **208**, 431–439.

Krasuski, J. S., Alexander, G. E., Horwitz, B., Daly, E. M., Murphy, D. G. M., Rapoport, S. I. *et al.* (1998). Volumes of medial temporal lobe structures in patients with Alzheimer's disease and mild cognitive impairment (and in healthy controls). *Biological Psychiatry*, **43**, 60–68.

Krausz, Y., Bonne, O., Gorfine, M., Karger, H., Lerer, B., and Chisin R. (1998). Age-related changes in brain perfusion of normal subjects detected by 99mTc-HMPAO SPECT. *Neuroradiology*, **40**, 428–434.

Kushner, M., Tobin, M., Alavi, A. *et al.* (1987). Cerebellar glucose consumption in normal and pathologic states using fluorine-FDG and PET. *Journal of Nuclear Medicine*, **28**, 1667–1670.

Lazeyras, F., Charles, H. C., Tupler, L. A., Erickson, R., Boyko, O. B., and Krishnan KRR. (1998). Metabolic brain mapping in Alzheimer's disease using proton magnetic resonance spectroscopy. *Psychiatry Research*, **82**, 95–106.

Leber, P. (1997). Slowing the progression of Alzheimer disease: methodologic issues. *Alzheimer Disease Assococian Disorders*, 11 Suppl 5, S10–S21.

Lehericy, S., Baulac, M., Chiras, J., *et al.* (1994). Amygdalohippocampal MR volume measurements in the early stages of Alzheimer disease. *American Journal of Neuroradiology*, **15**, 929–937.

Levin, C. S. and Hoffman, E. J. (1999). Calculation of positron range and its effect on the fundamental limit of positron emission tomography system spatial resolution. *Physical and Medical Biology*, **44**, 781–799.

Lowenstein, D., Barker, Chang, J., *et al.* (1989). Predominant Left hemishere metabolic dysfunction in dementia. *Archives of Neurology*, **46**, 146–152.

Luxenberg, J. S., Haxby, J. V., Creasey, H., *et al.* (1987). Rate of ventricular enlargement in dementia of the Alzheimer type correlates with rate of neuropsychological deterioration. *Neurology*, **37**, 1135–1140.

Martin, A., Friston, K., Colebatch, J., *et al.* (1991). Decreases in regional cerebral blood flow with normal aging. *Journal of Cerebral Blood Flow and Metabolism*, **11**, 684–689.

Masterman, D. L., Mendez, M. F., Fairbanks, L. A., and Cummings, J. L. (1997). Sensitivity, specificity, and positive predictive value of technetium 99–HMPAO SPECT in discriminating Alzheimer's disease from other dementias. *Journal of Geriatric Psychiatry and Neurology*, **10**, 15–21.

Maunoury, C., Michot, J. L., Caillet, H., Parlato, V., Leroy-Willig, A., Jehenson, P. H. *et al.* (1996). Specificity of temporal amygdala atrophy in Alzheimer's disease: quantitative assessment with magnetic resonance imaging. *Dementia*, **7**, 10–14.

McKhann, G., Drachman, D., Folstein, M., *et al.* (1984). Clinical diagnosis of Alzheimer's Disease: Report of the NINCDS- ADRDA work group under the auspices of Department of Health and Human Services Task Force on Alzheimer's Disease. *Neurology*, **34**, 939–944.

Mielke, R. and Heiss, W. D. (1998). Positron emission tomography for diagnosis of Alzheimer's disease and vascular dementia. *Journal of Neural Transmission*, Suppl. 53, 237–250.

Milton, W. J., Atlas, S. W., Lavi, E., and Mollman, J. E. (1991). Magnetic resonance imaging of Creutzfeldt-Jacob disease [see comments]. *Annals of Neurology*, **29**, 438–440.

Minoshima, S., Frey, K. A., Foster, N. L., and Kuhl, D. E. (1995). Preserved pontine glucose metabolism in Alzheimer disease: a reference region for functional brain image (PET) analysis. *Journal of Computer Assisted Tomography*, **19**, 541–547.

Minoshima, S., Giordani, B., Berent, S., Frey, K. A., Foster, N. L., and Kuhl, D. E. (1997). Metabolic reduction in the posterior cingulate cortex in very early Alzheimer's disease. *Annals of Neurology*, **42**, 85–94.

Moeller, J. R., Ishikawa, T., Dhawan, V., Spetsieris, P., Mandel, F., Alexander, G. E. *et al.* (1996). The metabolic topography of normal aging. *Journal of Cerebral Blood Flow Metabolism*, **16**, 385–398.

Moseley, M. E., deCrespigny, A., Spielman, D. M., Dobben, G., Alperin, N., Mafee, M. F. (1996). Magnetic resonance imaging of human brain function. *Surgical Neurology*, **45**, 385–391.

Mu, Q., Xie, J., Wen, Z., *et al.* (1999). A quantitative MR study of the hippocampal formation, the amygdala, and the temporal horn of the lateral ventricle in healthy subjects 40 to 90 years of age. *American Journal of Neuroradiology*, **20**, 207–211.

Murphy, D. G., DeCarli, C. D., Daly, E., Gillette, J. A., McIntosh, A. R., Haxby, J. V. *et al.* (1993). Volumetric magnetic resonance imaging in men with dementia of the Alzheimer type: correlations with disease severity. *Biological Psychiatry*, **34**, 612–621.

Nordberg, A. (1993). In-vivo detection of neurotransmitter changes in Alzheimers- disease. *Annals of New York Academy of Science*, **695**, 27–33.

O'Brien, J. T., Eagger, S. A., Syed, G. M. S., Sahakian, B. J., and Levy R. A. (1992). A study of regional cerebral blood flow and cognitive performance in Alzheimer's disease. *Journal of Neurology, Neurosurgery, and Psychiatry*, **55**, 1182–1187.

Parnetti, L., Tarducci, R., Presciutti, O., Lowenthal, D. T., Pippi, M., Palumbo, B. *et al.* (1997). Proton magnetic resonance spectroscopy can differentiate Alzheimer's disease from normal aging. *Mechanisms of Ageing and Development*, **97**, 9–14.

Pearlson, G. D., Harris, G. J., Powers, R. E., Barta, P. E., Camargo, E. E., Chase, G. A. *et al.* (1992). Quantitative changes in medial temporal volume, regional cerebral blood flow, and cognition in Alzheimer's disease. *Archives of General Psychiatry*, **49**, 402–408.

Petit, T. M., Landeau, B., Desson, J. F., Desgranges B., and Baron, J. C. (1998). Effects of healthy aging on the regional cerebral metabolic rate of glucose assessed with statistical parametric mapping. *Neuroimage*, **7**, 176–184.

Pettegrew, J. W., Klunk, W. E., Panchalingam, K., McClure, R. J., and Stanley, J. A. (1997). Magnetic resonance spectroscopic changes in Alzheimer's disease. *Annals of New York Academy of Science*, **826**, 282–306.

Pfefferbaum, A., Mathalon, D. H., Sullivan, E. V., Rawles, J. M., Zipursky, R. B., and Lim, K. O. (1994). A quantitative Magnetic Resonance Imaging study of changes in brain morphology from infancy to late adulthood. *Archives of Neurology*, **51**, 874–887.

Pickut, B. A., Saerens, J., Marien, P., Borggreve, F., Goeman, J., Vandevivere, J. *et al.* (1997). Discriminative use of SPECT in frontal lobe-type dementia versus (senile) dementia of the Alzheimer's type. *J Nucl.Med* **38**, 929–934.

Pietrini, P., Furey, M. L., Alexander, G. E., Mentis, M. J., Dani, A., Guazzelli, M. *et al.* (1999). Association between brain functional failure and dementia severity in Alzheimer's disease: resting versus stimulation PET study. *American Journal of Psychiatry*, **156**, 470–473.

Pucci, E., Belardinelli, N., Regnicolo, L., Nolfe, G., Signorino, M., Salvolini, U. *et al.* (1998). Hippocampus and parahippocampal gyrus linear measurements based on magnetic resonance in Alzheimer's disease. *Journal of European Neurology*, **39**, 16–25.

Rapoport, S. I., Horwitz, B., Grady, C. L., Haxby, J. V., DeCarli, C., and Schapiro, M. B. (1991). Abnormal brain glucose metabolism in Alzheimer's disease, as measured by position emission tomography. [Review]. *Advances in Experimental Medicine & Biology*, **291**, 231–248.

Reiser, M. and Faber, S. C. (1997). Recent and future advances in high-speed imaging. *European Radiology*, **7**, Suppl 5, 166–173.

Roman, G. C., Tatemichi, T. K., Erkinjuntti, T., Cummings, J. L., Masdeu, J. C., Garcia, J. H. *et al.* (1993). Vascular Dementia: Diagnostic criteria for research studies. Report of the NINDS-AIREN International Workshop. *Neurology*, **43**, 250–260.

Rossor, M. N., Garrett, N. J., Johnson, A. L., *et al.* (1982). A post-mortem study of the cholinergic and GABA systems in senile dementia. *Brain*, **105**, 313–330.

Rusinek, H., de Leon, M. J., George, A. E., Stylopoulos, L. A., Chandra, R., Smith, G.*et al.* (1991). Alzheimer disease: measuring loss of cerebral gray matter with MR imaging. *Radiology*, **178**, 109–114.

Sachdev, P., Gaur, R., Brodaty, H., Walker, A., Meares, S., Koder, D. *et al.* (1997). Longitudinal study of cerebral blood flow in Alzheimer's disease using single photon emission tomography. *Psychiatry Research*, **68**, 133–141.

Sandor, T., Jolesz, F., Tieman, J., Kikinis, R., Jones, K., and Albert, M. (1992). Comparative analysis of computed tomographic and magnetic resonance imaging scans in Alzheimer patients and controls. *Archives of Neurology*, **49**, 381–384.

Sandson, T. A., O'Connor, M., Sperling, R. A., Edelman, R. R., and Warach, S. (1996). Noninvasive perfusion MRI in Alzheimer's disease: a preliminary report. *Neurology*, **47**, 1339–1342.

Scarpelli, M., Salvolini, V., Diamanti, L., Montironi, R., Chiaromoni, L., and Maricotti, M. (1994). MRI and pathological examination of post-mortem brains: the problem of white matter high signal areas. *Neuroradiology*, **36**, 393–398.

Scheltens, P., Leys, D., Barkhof, F., Huglo, D., Weinstein, H. C., Vermersch, P. *et al.* (1992). Atrophy of medial temporal lobes on MRI in 'probable' Alzheimer's disease and normal ageing: diagnostic value and neuropsychological correlates. *Journal of Neurology, Neurosurgery, and Psychiatry*, **55**, 967–972.

Scheltens, P., Pasquier, F., Weerts, J. E., Barkhof, F., and Leys, D. (1997). Qualitative assessment of cerebral atrophy on MRI: Inter- and intra-observer reproducibility in dementia and normal aging. *Journal of European Neurology*, **37**, 95–99.

Schmidt, R. (1992). Comparison of magnetic resonance imaging in Alzheimer's disease, vascular dementia and normal aging. *European Neurology*, **32**, 164–169.

Scott, S., Dekosky, S. and Scheff, S. (1991). Volumetric atrophy of the amygdala in Alzheimer's disease: Quantitative serial reconstructions. *Neurology*, **41**, 351–356.

Seab, J. B., Jagust, W. J., Wong, S. T. S., Roos, M. S., Reed, B. R., and Budinger, T. F. (1988). Quantitative NMR Measurements of hippocampal atrophy in Alzheimer's disease. *Magnetic Resonance in Medicine*, **8**, 200–208.

Signorini, M., Paulesu, E., Friston, K., Perani, D., Colleluori, A., Lucignani, G. *et al.* (1999). Rapid assessment of regional cerebral metabolic abnormalities in single subjects with quantitative and nonquantitative [18F]FDG PET: A clinical validation of statistical parametric mapping. *Neuroimage*, **9**, 63–80.

Soininen, H. S., Partanen, K., Pitkanen, A., Vainio, P., Hanninen, T., Hallikainen, M. *et al.* (1994). Volumetric MRI analysis of the amygdala and the hippocampus in subjects with age-associated memory impairment: Correlation to visual and verbal memory. *Neurology*, **44**, 1660–1668.

Squire, L.R. (1986). Mechanisms of memory. *Science*, **232**, 1612–1619.

Stout, J. C., Jernigan, T. L., Archibald, S. L., and Salmon, D. P. (1996). Association of dementia severity with cortical gray matter and abnormal white matter volumes in dementia of the Alzheimer type. *Archives of Neurology*, **53**, 742–749.

Sullivan, E. V., Shear, P. ., Mathalon, D. H., Lim, K. O., Yesavage, J. A., Tinklenberg, J. R. *et al.* (1993). Greater abnormalities of brain cerebrospinal-fluid volumes in younger than in older patients with Alzheimers-disease. *Archives of Neurology*, **50**, 359–373.

Swaab, D. F., Hofman, M. A., Lucassen, P. J., Salehi, A., and Uylings, H. B. M. (1994). Neuronal atrophy, not cell death, is the main hallmark of Alzheimer's disease. *Neurobiology of Aging*, 15, 369–371.

Tokumaru, A. M., O'uchi, T., Kuru, Y., Maki, T., Murayama, S., and Horichi, Y. (1996). Corticobasal degeneration: MR with histopathologic comparison. *American Journal of Neuroradiology*, 17, 1849–1852.

Uchino, A., Yoshinaga, M., Shiokawa, O., Hata, H., and Ohno, M. (1991). Serial MR imaging in Creutzfeldt-Jakob disease. *Neuroradiology*, 33, 364–367.

Van Gool, W. A., Walstra, G. M., Teunisse, S., Van der Zant, F. M., Weinstein, H. C., and Van Royen, E. A. (1995). Diagnosing Alzheimer's disease in elderly, mildly demented patients: The impact of routine single photon emission computed tomography. *Journal of Neurology*, 242, 401–405.

Vermersch, P., Scheltens, P., Barkhof, F., Steinling, M., and Leys, D. (1994). Evidence for atrophy of the Corpus callosum in Alzheimer's disease. *Journal of European Neurology*, 34, 83–86.

Villa, G., Cappa, A., Tavolozza, M., Gainotti, G., Giordano, A., Calcagni, M. L. *et al.* (1995). Neuropsychological tests and [(99m)Tc]-HM PAO SPECT in the diagnosis of Alzheimer's dementia. *Journal of Neurology*, 242, 359–366.

Waldemar, G., Hasselbalch, S. G., Andersen, A. R., Delecluse, F., Petersen, P., Johnsen, A. *et al.* (1991). (99m)Tc-d,l-HMPAO and SPECT of the brain in normal aging. *Journal of Cerebral Blood Flow Metabolism*, 11, 508–521.

Waldemar, G., Hogh, P. and Paulson, O. B. (1997). Functional brain imaging with single-photon emission computed tomography in the diagnosis of Alzheimer's disease. *International Psychogeriatrics*, 9, Suppl 1, 223–227.

Waldemar, G., Walovitch, R. C., Andersen, A. R., Hasselbalch, S. G., Bigelow, R., Joseph, J. L. *et al.* (1994). ^{99m}Tc-Bicisate (Neurolite) SPECT brain imaging and cognitive impairment in dementia of Alzheimer type: a blinded read of image sets from a multicenter SPECT trial. *Journal of cerebral blood flow*, 14, S99–S105

Weinstein, H. C., Haan, J., van Royen, E. A., Derix, M. M. A., Lanser, J. B. K., Van der Zant, F. *et al.* (1991). SPECT in the diagnosis of Alzheimer's disease and multi-infarct dementia. *Clinical Neurology and Neurosurgery*, 93, 39–43.

Yamauchi, H., Fukuyama, H., Harada, K., Nabatame, H., Ogawa, M., Ouchi, Y. *et al.* (1993). Callosal atrophy parallels decreased cortical oxygen metabolism and neuropsychological impairment in Alzheimer's disease. *Archives of Neurology*, 50, 1070–1074.

Yoshida, T., Kuwabara, Y., Ichiya, Y., Sasaki, M., Fukumura, T., Ichimiya, A. *et al.* (1998). Cerebral muscarinic acetylcholinergic receptor measurement in Alzheimer's disease patients on 11C-N-methyl-4–piperidyl benzilate—comparison with cerebral blood flow and cerebral glucose metabolism. *Annals of Nuclear Medicine*, 12, 35–42.

Zeidler, M., Will, R. G., Ironside, J. W., *et al.* (1996). Creutzfeldt-Jakob disease and bovine spongiform encephalopathy. Magnetic resonance imaging is not a sensitive test for Creutzfeldt-Jakob disease [letter; comment]. *British Medical Journal*, 312, 844

Zubenko, G. S., Sullivan, P., Nelson, J. P., Belle, S. H., Huff, F. J., and Wolf, G. L. (1990). Brain imaging abnormalities in mental disorders of late life. *Archives of Neurology*, 47, 1107–1111.

Chapter 14

Current pharmacological approaches to treating Alzheimer's disease

Rebecca Eastley, Gordon Wilcock, and
David Dawbarn

14.1 Introduction

Pharmacological approaches to the treatment of Alzheimer's disease (AD) can be grouped broadly into those that aim for symptomatic treatment, those that attempt to modify the disease process, and those that may lower the risk or delay the onset of AD. The distinction between these approaches is not clear-cut as will become apparent.

Symptomatic treatments have mainly centred on neurotransmitter systems. The well established deficits in the cholinergic system in AD provided an obvious focus for pharmacological research, and led to the development of the first drugs to be licensed for the treatment of AD. However, numerous other neurotransmitter systems are affected in AD, including the noradrenergic, serotonergic, glutaminergic, and dopaminergic systems. These systems have physiological roles in normal cognitive functioning, and multiple neurotransmitter deficits probably contribute to the cognitive decline in AD.

The behavioural and psychiatric complications of AD are common, and may be related to monoamine dysfunction. Although they can have an important impact on both patients and carers, they have received considerably less attention than the cognitive symptoms. A small number of studies have investigated various medications for specific behavioural or psychiatric disorders, and measures of behavioural and psychiatric disturbance are beginning to be included in clinical trials of general treatments for AD.

The mechanisms which lead to neuronal death are complex, and undoubtedly multifactorial. Many different agents show promise as disease modifying treatments although their actions may not be specific for AD. Combination therapy with cognitive enhancers may be an avenue for future research. Some neuroprotective approaches may lower the risk for developing AD although the evidence for this remains inconclusive.

14.2 Issues in clinical drug research

There are several issues which need to be considered when interpreting the results of clinical trials in patients with AD. A definite diagnosis of AD can only be made with histopathological evidence. Antemortem diagnosis of probable AD relies on the use of standardized diagnostic criteria. Even using the most stringent diagnostic criteria, the error rate is still of the order of 10–15%. Additionally, AD is probably a syndrome rather than a single disease entity. This may account for some of the inter-individual variation in treatment responses in many drug trials. Group treatment effects can appear modest because the marked response of a subgroup of patients is masked by the non-response of others. No distinguishing characteristics have been identified to help predict which patients will benefit, and in clinical practice a trial of treatment is often required.

Outcome measures in drug trials have to be clinically meaningful. Changes in cognitive test scores may be statistically significant but meaningless in terms of the day to day life of patients and carers. Most drug trials now include instruments which at least attempt to measure 'global function'. Scales which measure the ability to perform activities of daily living (ADL) and neuropsychiatric function arguably provide the most relevant clinical information.

Ideally assessment schedules should include standard instruments. Common measures of cognitive function include the cognitive component of the Alzheimer's disease assessment scale (ADAS-cog) and the mini mental state examination (MMSE). Scales measuring non-cognitive items have been more varied making it harder to compare results.

A common criticism levelled at drug treatments for AD, is the lack of evidence for improvement in the quality of life for sufferers or their carers. Quality of life (QOL) is neither easy to define nor to quantify. Some studies have included QOL scales for patients, although these mainly reflect functional ability. Investigating well-being in carers is equally complex but probably more amenable to future evaluation.

14.3 Cholinergic strategies

One of the earliest neurochemical changes to be seen in AD is the loss of choline acetyl-transferase (ChAT) activity in the cerebral cortex and hippocampus seen post-mortem (Bowen *et al.* 1976; Davies *et al.* 1976) and in biopsy specimens (Bowen *et al.* 1982; Sims *et al.* 1983). Most of the ChAT in these regions is located in nerve terminals; the cell bodies of these fibres are found in the medial septal nucleus, the diagonal band of Broca (DBB) and the nucleus basalis of Meynert (NBM) (Mesulam *et al.* 1983, 1986; Mesulam and Geula 1988). Many lines of evidence indicate that this cholinergic system is involved in cognitive processes in rats, monkeys, and humans. Lesions of the NBM and DBB in rats result in a range of behavioural impairments including retention of passive avoidance (Dunnett *et al.* 1987), acquisition of delayed no matching to position (Dunnett *et al.* 1989), maze performance (Wenk *et al.* 1989; Connor *et al.* 1991; Turner *et al.* 1992) and attention to brief stimuli (Robbins *et al.* 1989). Similarly, cognitive impairment has been observed following lesions to the NBM and DBB in primates (Ridley *et al.* 1985, 1986).

In addition to lesion studies impairment of the central cholinergic system with drugs (scopolamine, hemicholinium-3) has also been shown to result in impaired acquisition of new information in primates (Ridley *et al.* 1984a, b). Furthermore, the cholinergic antagonist scopolamine has been shown to cause learning impairments in human volunteers (Crow and Grove-White 1973). Since cognitive deficits appear early in AD patients and because cholinergic deficits also appear early it has been assumed that these events are linked and that it is the loss of cholinergic function in the cerebral cortex and hippocampus that is responsible for the observed memory deficits. In addition the available drug treatments nearly all work by augmenting cholinergic synaptic transmission. If ways could be found to stop the degeneration of the basal forebrain cholinergic neurons disease progression might be slowed.

14.3.1 Acetylcholine precursors

Choline is a precursor for acetylcholine (ACh). Animal studies reported that choline and lecithin (phosphatidyl choline) increased the production the brain ACh. It was therefore logical to attempt to treat the cholinergic deficit in AD with ACh precursors. This strategy proved unsuccessful (Higgins and Flicker 1998), possibly because once the disease process in AD had become symptomatic, there were too few presynaptic cholinergic neurons for precursor loading to have any clinical effect.

14.3.2 Cholinesterase inhibitors

Cholinesterase inhibitors (CEIs) have been the most widely investigated and so far the most successful therapeutic agents for the symptomatic treatment of AD. ACh is hydrolysed by acetylcholinesterase (AChE) and butyrylcholinesterase. Cholinesterase inhibition increases the availability of ACh for synaptic transmission. Cholinesterases are widely distributed throughout the central and peripheral nervous systems, plasma, and liver. AChE is the predominant enzyme in the central nervous system (CNS).

Physostigmine

Physostigmine is a non-selective, reversible CEI in the carbamate class. It is reasonably well absorbed after oral administration and crosses the blood–brain barrier satisfactorily. However, physostigmine has a plasma half-life of approximately 30 minutes, necessitating the use of parenteral administration, high frequency oral dosing schedules, or sustained release preparations.

Early double-blind trials reported a significant improvement in memory function (Davis *et al.* 1979; Christie *et al.* 1981) but these findings were not universal. More recent studies have also yielded conflicting results, possibly reflecting differences in study design. Asthan *et al.* (1995) found that continuous intravenous infusion of physostigmine improved memory in five of nine AD patients. Marin *et al.* (1995) reported no significant improvement in cognitive functioning in AD patients receiving intermittent physostigmine infusions when compared to controls receiving placebo. Supporting evidence for the beneficial effects of physostigmine is provided by studies which have reported increased cerebral blood flow particularly in those areas of the brain most affected in AD (Geaney *et al.* 1990; Wilson *et al.* 1991; Gustafson 1993).

The short half-life of physostigmine has limited its clinical applications but attempts have been made to overcome this. Fairly stable plasma concentrations were achieved by a continuous transdermal delivery system (Levy *et al.* 1994) in a single-blind study of 12 AD patients. Four of these patients improved on all four cognitive tests employed, and two patients on two tests. No major adverse effects were reported. A controlled-release preparation of physostigmine was evaluated in a double-blind, placebo controlled trial in 1111 patients with mild or moderate AD by Thal *et al.* (1996). A modest improvement in cognitive and global function was observed in a subset of patients after six weeks active treatment. Common adverse effects included nausea and vomiting, diarrhoea, and anorexia.

Tacrine

Tacrine or tetrahydroaminoacridine (THA) is a centrally active, reversible CEI in the acridine class. It is licensed for the treatment of AD in countries including the USA and UK (although it is not available in the UK). Acridines are not specific for AChE but also inhibit butyrylcholinesterase. Tacrine is reasonably well absorbed after oral administration but has a relatively short half life of approximately three and a half hours in the elderly. Its main metabolite is 1-hydroxytacrine (velnacrine). Steady state plasma concentrations are reached within 24 hours with four times daily dosing (Davis and Powchik 1995).

Interest in cholinergic therapies had flagged in the 1980s but was rekindled by promising results for tacrine treatment in 17 AD patients (Summers *et al.* 1986). Early optimism was lost when a series of studies failed to replicate Summers and colleagues' findings (Chatellier and Lacomblez 1990; Fritten *et al.* 1990). The first convincing study after Summers' paper was that by Eagger and colleagues (1991). In their study, 65 of 89 patients completed a 7-month trial of treatment with tacrine and lecithin. They were able to demonstrate an improvement in cognitive functioning equivalent to the decline which would be expected with disease progression over 6 to 12 months.

Nearly all the early studies were subjected to fierce criticism, but subsequently larger multicentre studies were published suggesting that tacrine treatment had modest beneficial effects on cognitive function (Davis *et al.* 1992; Farlow *et al.* 1992). Both of these studies were relatively short in duration and the maximum dosage of tacrine was limited to 80 mg daily. The next major study enrolled 663 patients and evaluated the effects of tacrine in doses up to 160 mg daily over 30 weeks (Knapp 1994). Only 263 patients completed the study, 133 being withdrawn due to transaminase elevation which suggested liver damage. Intention-to-treat (ITT) analysis revealed significant dose dependent improvements on measures of cognitive and global function. Arrieata and Artalejo (1998) analysed the results of 49 trials published between 1981 and 1997 and concluded that just over 20% of patients showed significant improvements in cognitive and functional ability after 3–6 months with tacrine.

Current research is attempting to identify factors which can be used to predict response. The influence of genotyping was an obvious avenue for exploration but findings have not been consistent. The possession of the apolipoprotein (*APOE*) ε 4 allele has been reported to be associated with a positive response to tacrine (Lucotte *et al.* 1996; Oddoze *et al.* 1998) and a predictor of poor response to tacrine (Poirier *et al.* 1995). MacGowan *et al.* (1998) found that gender was a more powerful determinant CEI response than *APOE* status in the short term. Men were more likely to respond than women in the first three months of CEI treatment but thereafter genotype may have had an effect. An analysis of the treatment outcome of tacrine in 528 patients indicated that both gender and genotype may influence response (Farlow *et al.* 1998). This study found that the treatment effect in women was larger among those with ε2 or ε3 allele rather than the ε4 allele. This interaction was not found in men. The situation is further complicated by the wide inter-individual variation in the penetration of tacrine into the cerebrospinal fluid (CSF) (Grothe *et al.* 1998).

The most significant problem of tacrine is its side-effect profile and potential for hepatotoxicity. Analysis of multicentre clinical trial data revealed that transaminase elevation occurred in approximately 50% participants, and was more than three times the upper limit of normal in 25% patients (Watkins *et al.* 1994). Transaminase levels usually return to normal after tacrine is discontinued and many patients can successfully resume treatment on careful re-challenge (O'Brien *et al.* 1991; Watkins *et al.* 1994). However a case of fatal hepatotoxicity possibly secondary to long-term treatment with tacrine has been reported (Blackart *et al.* 1998).

Cholinergic adverse effects are dose dependent and probably related to tacrine's lack of central specificity. Those affecting the gastrointestinal system may be particularly troublesome and include nausea, vomiting, diarrhoea, anorexia, dyspepsia, abdominal pain, and weight loss. Dose reduction or discontinuation brings rapid relief and patients are often able to tolerate lower maintenance doses.

Tacrine was the first drug to be approved for the symptomatic treatment of AD and as such represented a landmark development. However second generation CEIs with better side-effect profiles have now been licensed and undoubtedly the clinical use of tacrine will be limited.

Donepezil

Donepezil (Aricept), a second generation CEI, is a piperidine-based agent which was developed specifically for the treatment of AD and is now licensed for clinical use in several countries. It is a non-competitive, reversible antagonist of AChE and is highly selective for AChE as opposed to butyrylcholinesterase. It is well absorbed after oral administration and peak plasma concentration is reached in 3 to 4 hours. Donepezil is metabolized by the hepatic isoenzymes CYP2D6 and CYP3A4 and undergoes glucuronidation. The plasma half-life is approximately 70 hours thus allowing once daily dosing.

The first phase II clinical trial to be published indicated that donepezil improved cognitive and global function in patients with mild to moderate AD (Rogers *et al.* 1996). These promising findings have now been replicated in three large, multicentre studies. The shortest of these was a 12 week, double-blind, placebo-controlled, parallel-group trial (Rogers *et al.* 1998*a*). 468 patients with mild to moderate AD were randomized to receive placebo, 5 mg/day or 10 mg/day (5 mg/day during the first week) donepezil. ITT analysis, which included 97% of the patients who were enrolled, revealed a statistically significant improvement in cognitive and global function. Clinically significant improvements in cognitive function were found for between 48% and 57% patients who received donepezil, and 30% patients who received placebo. A trend towards a dose related effect was apparent but did not reach statistical significance. Plasma concentrations of donepezil were significantly correlated with red cell membrane AChE inhibition (thought to be indicative of cerebral AChE inhibition), and red cell AChE inhibition was correlated with change in the cognitive and global function test scores. In general donepezil was well tolerated and the only adverse effects which occurred more commonly than in the placebo group were nausea, insomnia, and diarrhoea. Many of these events were mild and resolved within one to two days with continued treatment. A decrease in group mean heart rate was observed (2.7/minute in the 5 mg/day group, and 2.3/minute in the 10 mg/day group) but this was not clinically significant. No evidence of hepatotoxicity was found.

The results of a 24-week phase III trial (Rogers *et al.* 1998*b*) provided further evidence of donepezil's clinical efficacy and good tolerability. 473 patients with mild to moderate AD were randomly assigned to treatment with placebo, 5 mg/day donepezil or 10 mg/day donepezil. Clinically significant improvements in cognitive test scores were achieved in 38% of the patients receiving 5 mg/day donepezil and 54% patients receiving 10 mg/day donepezil, compared to 27% patients in the placebo group. Lack of deterioration in cognitive function was observed in over 80% of the donepezil treated patients, and 58% of those who received placebo. Measures of global function also improved in the donepezil treatment groups. At the end of the 6-week placebo washout which followed the treatment phase, there were no significant differences on cognitive or global function measures between any of the three groups. The only adverse effects which occurred significantly more frequently in the active treatment groups were fatigue, diarrhoea, nausea, vomiting, and muscle cramps.

The first analysis (at 98 weeks) of the effects of long-term treatment with donepezil in an open-label study of 133 patients has now been published (Rogers and Friedhoff 1998). Improvements from baseline levels in cognitive and global function were still evident after 38 and 26 weeks respectively. Thereafter the deterioration was slower than would be expected in untreated AD patients. There was no evidence of hepatotoxicity.

The evidence to date indicates that donepezil is generally well tolerated and can improve cognitive symptoms and functional ability in a subgroup of AD patients. Long-term use may slow the rate of cognitive deterioration.

Rivastigmine

Rivastigmine (ENA 713, Exelon), also a second generation CEI, is a centrally selective carbamate CEI that is already licensed as a symptomatic treatment for mild to moderate AD. It binds to the esteratic site of the AChE enzyme but dissociates more slowly than ACh and so has pseudo-irreversible activity. Cholinesterase inhibition thereby lasts approximately 10 hours although the plasma half-life is only about two hours (Anand and Gharabawi 1996). Rivastigmine is inactivated mainly by the interaction with AChE, and its cleavage product is excreted by the kidneys. This reduces the potential for interaction with drugs which are metabolized by the hepatic cytochrome P450 system. Rivastigmine is well absorbed and peak plasma levels are reached in one to two hours after ingestion.

The first large multicentre clinical trial recruited 699 patients with mild to moderate AD (Corey-Bloom 1998). Patients with concomitant illnesses were eligible for inclusion unless the illness was severe or unstable. Concurrent medication was allowed with the exception of anticholinergic drugs, any potential memory enhancers, and all psychotropics apart from chloral hydrate. Patients were randomly allocated to receive either placebo, low dose rivastigmine (1–4 mg daily) or high dose rivastigmine (6–12 mg daily). The study consisted of an initial seven week fixed dose-titration phase, followed by a flexible dose phase up to week 26. Overall 78% of patients completed the study. At 26 weeks 56% of the patients who had received high dose rivastigmine had either improved or not deteriorated on tests of cognitive function, compared to 27% of those who received placebo. The improvement in cognitive function relative to the patients receiving placebo represented a delay in cognitive deterioration of about 6 months. As a group the patients who received active treatment deteriorated less on global function measures than those on placebo. One quarter of the patients in the high dose rivastigmine group had shown clinically significant improvements in their ability to perform activities of daily living compared to 15% patients in the placebo group. The commonest adverse effects were dose related, and cholinergic in origin, mainly nausea, vomiting, diarrhoea, and anorexia. Most were mild or moderate in severity, transient, and occurred on initiation or dose escalation. Weight loss too appeared to be dose related and equalled or exceeded 7% body weight in 21% of the high-dose treatment group, 6% of the low dose treatment group, and 2% of the placebo group. There was no evidence of any organ toxicity.

Rivastigmine is currently undergoing extensive investigation as part of the phase III clinical trial programme. Because there have been few exclusion criteria the patients who have participated in studies are much more representative of 'typical' AD patients. The findings so far demonstrate that rivastigmine has beneficial effects on cognitive and global function, and may delay the worsening in ability to perform activities of daily living.

Metrifonate

Metrifonate is an organophosphate and has been available as a treatment for schistosomiasis since 1962. Metrifonate itself is a prodrug and has no intrinsic CEI activity. It is not metabolized by the cytochrome P450 system but hydrolysed nonenzymatically to 2,2-dimethyl dichlorovinyl phosphate (DDVP). DDVP binds irreversibly to the catalytic site of AChE and competitively inhibits its activity. Although metrifonate has a short plasma half life of about 2 hours it can be given once a day because of the long action of DDVP. Butyrylcholinesterase is also inhibited by DDVP.

A small placebo-controlled study over three months indicated that metrifonate had beneficial effects on cognition in AD (Becker et al. 1996). Two larger clinical trails have provided further evidence of its efficacy. Cummings et al. (1998) reported the findings of a prospective, double-blind, parallel-group, dose-finding study. 480 patients with mild to moderate AD were randomly allocated to receive either placebo or metrifonate once a day. Active treatment patients received loading doses of 0.5 mg/kg (25–45 mg), 0.9 mg/kg (45–80 mg), or 2.0 mg/kg (100–180 mg) for two weeks, followed by maintenance doses of 0.2 mg/kg (10–20 mg), 0.3 mg/kg (15–25 mg), or 0.65 mg/kg (30–60 mg) for ten weeks. Metrifonate was well tolerated even at high doses and 94%, 90%, and 89% of the active treatment patients completed the study. Significant treatment effects for cognition and global function were demonstrated for high and mid dose metrifonate. The relative improvement in cognitive function for the patients receiving high dose metrifonate equated to a five month delay in the progression of cognitive deterioration. Both cognitive and global function treatment effects were positively correlated with red blood cell AChE inhibition, which in turn was dose related. Most adverse events were mild and transient, and occurred early on in the study. Adverse events exceeding the rate in the placebo group by 5% were abdominal pain, diarrhoea, flatulence, nausea, and leg cramps. A dose-related reduction in mean heart rate was observed and necessitated the withdrawal of three patients.

The second clinical trial to be published was a randomized, double blind, parallel group placebo-controlled study (Morris et al. 1998). This multicentre trial enrolled 408 patients with mild to moderate AD. The metrifonate treatment group received a loading dose of 2.0 mg/kg/day (100–180 mg/day) for two weeks followed by maintenance 0.65 mg/kg/day (30–60 mg/day) for 24 weeks. Only 12% of the treatment group were withdrawn because of adverse events and 79% completed the study. Significant treatment effects were achieved on measures of cognitive and global function and sustained over the 26 week treatment period. This study also included a test item measuring behavioural disturbance. The patients who received metrifonate showed less behavioural disturbance than those receiving placebo, particularly as evidenced by hallucinatory experiences. The only adverse events occurring at a rate greater than 5% that of the placebo group were diarrhoea, leg cramps, and rhinitis. A lowering in the mean heart rate of about 7 beats per minute was observed for the metrifonate patients but this was not thought to be clinically significant.

Although metrifonate has not been tested concurrently with other CEIs, its efficacy for the cognitive and global symptoms of AD appear to be comparable to tacrine, donepezil, and rivastigmine (Knopman 1998). It has also been shown to have some beneficial effect on the behavioural manifestations of AD. Recent suggestions that adverse effects may be problematic are under investigation.

Galanthamine

Galanthamine (Reminyl) is a tertiary alkaloid derived from the bulbs of snowdrop and narcissi. Apart from its action as a specific, reversible inhibitor of brain AChE it appears to allosterically modulate nicotinic receptors. Early open studies (Wilcock and Wilkinson 1993) indicated that galanthamine showed promise as a symptomatic treatment for AD. Phase II trials confirmed the efficacy and good tolerability of galanthamine (Wilcock *et al.* 1997). Over 1100 patients have now been treated with galanthamine 24 mg or 32 mg daily, for six months, in double-blind trials. Patients who received galanthamine showed a significant improvement on measures of cognition, global function, and behavioural disturbance compared to those who received placebo. The patients who received treatment with galanthamine 24 mg daily over 12 months showed no deterioration from their baseline level of functioning. Cholinergic side-effects mainly affected the gastrointestinal system and their incidence was influenced by the titration rate and dose.

Galanthamine may actually modify the disease process in AD, and the dual mode of action may contribute to this. The publication of further clinical trials is awaited.

14.3.3 **Muscarinic agonists**

The degeneration of cholinergic neuronal systems in AD primarily affects the projections from the basal forebrain to the hippocampus and cerebral cortex. Presynaptic muscarinic ACh receptors are reduced in number but neocortical post-synaptic muscarinic receptors are relatively spared. Direct action on muscarinic receptors by-passes the dysfunctional presynaptic terminals and theoretically agonists could offer therapeutic advantages over CEIs (Avery *et al.* 1997).

The results of early studies with muscarinic agonists such as arecoline, oxotremorine, bethanechol and RS86 were disappointing (Spiegel 1991). Compounds had a narrow therapeutic window and activity on peripheral muscarinic receptors led to high rates of side-effects. These included cardiovascular problems and hyperidrosis (increased sweating).

The discovery of subtypes of muscarinic receptor which were differently distributed, was an important development. M1 receptors (mainly post-synaptic) were found to predominate in the frontal cortex and hippocampus, and M2 (mainly pre-synaptic) and M3 subtypes peripherally.

Xanomeline, an M1/M4 agonist has been evaluated in a multicentre trial of 343 patients with AD (Bodick *et al.* 1997). This study used a randomized, parallel-group, double-blind, placebo controlled design. Patients received placebo or xanomeline in doses of 25, 50, or 75 mg three times a day for six months. Significant treatment effects on cognitive and global function were demonstrated for high dose xanomeline, and there were significant dose-dependent reductions in behavioural disturbance and psychotic symptomatology. However adverse effects, particularly gastrointestinal, were troublesome, and led to the withdrawal of 52% patients in the high dose group. Syncope occurred in 12.6%, 13.3%, and 3.5% of patients receiving high, medium or low dose xanomeline, and 4.6% of patients on placebo. Mild to moderate elevations in transaminase levels occurred in 13% of patients who received xanomeline. In view of the poor tolerability and side-effect profile of the oral preparation, a transdermal formulation was developed and is undergoing further evaluation.

Other muscarinic compounds have similar profiles and our present level of knowledge about them does not allow us to predict whether they will prove to be effective and safe treatments for AD.

14.3.4 Nicotinic agonists

Some cognitive processes involve nicotinic receptors, and the density of these receptors is reduced in AD. Initial case-control studies found a negative association between smoking and AD and this helped to increase research interest in the possible therapeutic role of nicotinic agonists . However the negative association between smoking and AD was not confirmed in later studies, and a population based, cohort study of 6870 elderly people, found that smoking actually doubled the risk of dementia and AD (Ott *et al.* 1998). Despite the lack of convincing evidence that smoking protects against the development of AD, nicotine may have neuroprotective properties (Shimohama *et al.* 1996). *In vitro* studies suggest that nicotine may exert an effect on amyloid processing. Nicotine is able to inhibit formation of the amyloid beta-peptide (Aβ) (Salomon *et al.* 1996), and stimulates the release of amyloid precursor protein (APP) (Kim *et al.* 1997). Additional support for this hypothesis comes from a post-mortem study of brain tissue from 301 people over the age of 65 (Ulrich *et al.* 1997). Smoking appeared to protect against senile plaque formation but correlated with neurofibrillary changes.

There are numerous subtypes of nicotinic receptors which probably have differing effects on neurotransmitter systems. Stimulation of the presynaptic nicotinic receptors increases ACh release. Nicotine is an unselective agonist for nicotinic receptors. In addition to increasing the release of ACh, it may also increase the release of noradrenaline, serotonin, and dopamine. A small, pilot study in patients with AD found that nicotine patches improved learning (Wilson *et al.* 1995), but a placebo-controlled, double-blind, cross-over study in 18 patients with AD failed to demonstrate any benefits on cognitive function (Snaedal *et al.* 1996).

As our knowledge about the function of different nicotinic receptors and their relationship to AD increases, it may be possible to target particular receptor subtypes selectively. At present we can not judge what the clinical applications will be.

14.3.5 Acetylcholine releasers

Linopirdine is a phenylindolinone which enhances the depolarization-induced release of ACh, dopamine, serotonin, and glutamate, possibly via potassium channel blockade. Basal neurotransmitter release is not increased so theoretically it should enhance normal brain activity. The results of clinical trials however, have been disappointing. In a double-blind parallel group study, 375 patients with mild to moderate AD were randomized to receive either placebo or linopirdine 30 mg three times a day (Rockwood *et al.* 1997). A small difference in cognitive function in favour of linopirdine was observed but this was not clinically significant. More potent anthracenone analogues of linopirdine have now been identified and are under further investigation.

14.3.6 **Neurotrophins and acetylcholine**

Structure and function

The development and maintenance of the nervous system is controlled by a series of neu-rotrophic factors which control cell targeting, proliferation, differentiation, and phenotypic expression of cell markers (Purves 1989). Particularly pertinent here are the neurotrophins which include nerve growth factor (NGF) (Thoenen and Barde 1980; Scott *et al.* 1983; Ullrich *et al.* 1983; Thoenen *et al.* 1987; Thoenen 1991), brain derived neurotrophic factor (BDNF) (Barde *et al.* 1982; 1987; Leibrock *et al.* 1989), neurotrophin-3 (NT-3) (Hohn *et al.* 1990; Maisonpierre *et al.* 1990*a*) and neurotrophin-4 (NT-4) (Birkmeier *et al.* 1991; Hallbook *et al.* 1991; Ip *et al.* 1992). These proteins are structurally similar and share approximately 50% sequence homology at the amino acid level. They are all basic proteins with pIs above 9.0 and are processed from preprohormones to give monomers of approxi-mately 120 amino acids (Maisonpierre *et al.* 1990*b*). All of the neurotrophins exist as homodimers and the crystal structures of all of them have been determined (McDonald *et al.* 1991; Holland *et al.* 1994; Robinson *et al.* 1995, 1996; Butte *et al.* 1998). They are all part of the cystine knot superfamily which includes transforming growth factor-β (TGF-β), platelet-derived growth factor (PDGF), and human choriogonadotrophin (McDonald and Hendrickson 1993). Each neurotrophin monomer consists of four antiparallel β-strands, with the fourth β-strand twisted around the third, a feature conserved across all the cystine knot growth factors. The cystines are arranged such that Cys(III-VI) penetrates the ring formed by Cys(I–IV) and Cys(II–V).

Neurotrophin receptors

All of the neurotrophins bind to the p75^{NGFR} receptor with a Kd of about 10^{-9} M (Rodrigues-Tebar *et al.* 1992). Specificity is defined through their interaction with tyrosine receptor kinases (Trk) where the Kd is approximately 10^{-10}–10^{-11} M. NGF binds to Trk A (Kaplan *et al.* 1991), BDNF and NT-4 bind to TrkB (Klein *et al.* 1992; Ip *et al.* 1993) and NT-3 binds to TrkC (Lamballe *et al.* 1991) and an alternatively spliced version of TrkA (Clary and Reichardt 1994). Following ligand binding the Trk receptors dimerize (Jing *et al.* 1992) and intracellular tyrosines are phosphorylated which leads to signal transduction through a complex cascade involving Cγ1, PI-3 kinase, ERK, Raf1, Ras, and SHC (Loeb *et al.* 1994; Stephens *et al.* 1994). The extracellular region of the Trk receptors can be subdivided into different domains using protein structure prediction programmes (Schneider and Schweiger 1991). Thus at the N-terminus there are three leucine rich motifs which are flanked by two cysteine rich regions. These are then followed by two immunoglobulin like domains and a proline rich region adjacent to the membrane. It has been shown using mutagenesis studies that if the immunoglobulin like domains of TrkA are swapped with those from TrkB then ligand specificity is altered indicating that these domains represent the binding domain (Perez *et al.* 1995). If all of the extracellular domains except for the second Ig domain of TrkA are deleted, addition of NGF leads to phosphorylation and cell signalling (Urfer *et al.* 1995). Furthermore, recombinant Ig domains made in *E. coli* are able to bind NGF with a similar affinity to the wild type membrane bound receptor (Holden *et al.* 1997) and that all of the binding activity resides in the Ig domain nearest to the membrane (Robertson *et al.* 1999). Subsequent crystallization and structure determination of this domain shows it to be of the I-set of Ig-like domains with an unusual exposed disul-phide bridge linking two neighbouring strands in the same β-sheet (Ultsch *et al.* 1999).

Distribution of NGF

In the brain the levels of NGF mRNA have been shown to correlate with the degree of basal forebrain cholinergic innervation (Korsching *et al.* 1985). Thus the highest levels of NGF and NGF mRNA in the brain are found within the cerebral cortex and hippocampus. Injection of [^{125}I]NGF into the hippocampus or cerebral cortex reveals that it is taken up by the terminals of basal forebrain cholinergic cells and retrogradely transported back to the cell bodies (Seiler and Schwab 1984). Immunohistochemical and *in situ* analysis of the distribution of p75[NGFR] in rat brain and human brain show that it is almost exclusively located on basal forebrain neurones (Riopelle *et al.* 1987; Dawbarn *et al.* 1988a; Kordower *et al.* 1988; Schatteman *et al.* 1988; Allen *et al.* 1989). Co-localisation studies with antibodies to ChAT and p75[NGFR] demonstrates that nearly all of the basal forebrain cholinergic neurons express p75[NGFR] (Dawbarn *et al.* 1988b; Kordower *et al.* 1988). Examination of the distribution of TrkA protein and mRNA in rat and human brain shows that TrkA is also expressed on basal forebrain cholinergic neurons (Steininger *et al.* 1993; Sobreviela *et al.* 1994). Administration of NGF to basal forebrain cholinergic neurons *in vitro* results in increased survival and up regulation of ChAT (Gnahn *et al.* 1983; Hefti *et al.* 1985; Martinez *et al.* 1987; Hartikka and Hefti, 1988a; b; Hatanaka *et al.* 1988).

Knockout mice have been generated to investigate the function of both NGF and TrkA in the brain (Crowley *et al.* 1994; Smeyne *et al.* 1994). The phenotypes show dramatic cell loss, similar to that seen after administration of neutralizing antibodies to NGF *in utero*. Both phenotypes survive but show weight loss compared to unaffected littermates and usually die by the end of the third month. In the peripheral nervous system there is cell loss in the superior cervical, dorsal root, and trigeminal ganglia. Surprisingly, in the CNS there is no cell loss in the cholinergic basal forebrain cells in either the NGF or TrkA knockout mice. There are however marked reductions in basal forebrain ChAT staining and axonal cholinesterase activity in both the hippocampal and cortical target fields. These results suggest that NGF may not be necessary for the development of basal forebrain cholinergic cells. Mice which are heterozygous for the NGF deletion exhibit aberrations in spatial memory function in the Morris water maze (Chen *et al.* 1993, 1994). These behavioural deficits correlated with losses in both the size and number of basal forebrain cholinergic neurons.

Rescue of cholinergic function by NGF

Since the memory loss seen in AD patients is thought to be a reflection of basal forebrain cholinergic cell loss, several attempts have been made to produce such lesions in rodents and primates. Lesion of the fimbria-fornix in rats severs the septal cholinergic fibres such that the terminals are not able retrogradely to transport NGF back to the cell bodies resulting in cell loss. Intracerebroventricular administration of NGF has been shown to stop this degeneration completely(Haroutunian *et al.* 1986; Hefti, 1986; Kromer 1987; Williams *et al.* 1987; Gage *et al.* 1988) and the cognitive deficits arising from such lesions (Will and Hefti 1985; Williams *et al.* 1987; Mandel *et al.* 1989). A subpopulation of aged rats has been shown to perform poorly in the Morris water maze. Infusion of NGF increases the performance of these animals to within the normal range (Fischer *et al.* 1987, 1991, 1994). It appears that NGF can protect cells from degenerating after lesions and have direct effects on cognition by acting specifically on basal forebrain cholinergic neurons via its receptors.

Because of this early loss of cholinergic function in AD, infusion of NGF into the brains of patients might increase ChAT levels, prevent further degeneration of cholinergic cells, and thereby prevent further decline in memory function. However for NGF to be efficacious it will be necessary for the basal forebrain cells still to be present to some extent and also to possess NGF receptors. Some considerable effort has been made to address these issues.

NGF receptors in AD

Immunohistochemical staining for p75[NGFR] in basal forebrain cholinergic neurons has revealed a range of results. A large decrease in neuronal number has been reported (Hefti and Mash 1989; Mufson *et al.* 1989) although we (Allen *et al.* 1990) have also shown that even severely demented patients may have very little cell loss, most of which occurs in the posterior region of the NBM. The main differences in these studies is the age of onset of the disease and it may be that an earlier onset of AD gives rise to much greater basal forebrain cell loss. Analysis of the mRNA for p75[NGFR] in normal basal forebrain and AD basal forebrain by Northern blotting showed no loss of p75[NGFR] mRNA in AD (Goedert *et al.* 1989). In support of this, our determination of p75[NGFR] receptors by ligand binding showed there to be no difference between normal and AD brain (Treanor *et al.* 1991). Although studies examining the number of TrkA positively staining cells in AD basal forebrain have generally shown a reduction in AD (Mufson *et al.* 1997a; b; Boissiere *et al.* 1997; Mufson *et al.* 1997a; b), in all cases there are still a significant number of viable cells remaining. The observed degeneration of these cholinergic cells in AD may be due to reduced trophic support, that is a lack of production of NGF in the cerebral cortex and hippocampus. Measurements of the content of NGF protein in AD brain have shown non-significant or significant increases in cerebral cortex in AD (Allen *et al.* 1991; Crutcher *et al.* 1993) and no change in hippocampus (Allen *et al.* 1991). Similarly no change in NGF mRNA level was found in AD cerebral cortex and hippocampus compared with normal brains (Goedert *et al.* 1986). One possibility for the degeneration of basal forebrain cholinergic neurons in AD is disruption of the ability to transport NGF retrogradely from the target tissues to the cell bodies. Support for this hypothesis comes from a study which shows that NGF content, although normal in the cerebral cortex and hippocampus, is reduced in the basal forebrain (Mufson *et al.* 1995).

Phase I clinical trials with NGF

Thus if recombinant hNGF were to be administered to AD patients intracerebroventricularly it is likely that basal forebrain cholinergic function would be increased via the interaction of NGF with its receptors since although there is a reduction in the number of cholinergic cells in the basal forebrain those that are left express both p75[NGFR] and TrkA.

Regime To date, three AD patients have been given mouse NGF intracerebroventricularly (Olsen *et al.* 1992; Jonhagen *et al.* 1998). All of the patients were diagnosed using diagnostic and statistical manual (DSM-III-R) and National Institute of Neurological and Communicative Disorders and Stroke and Alzheimer's disease and Related Disorders Association, (NINCDS-ADRDA) criteria and all were evaluated using a cognitive test battery, electroencephalography (EEG), magnetic resonance imaging (MRI), and positron emission tomography (PET). In patient I the NGF infusion was started immediately after the operation, but was delayed 2 and 4 weeks postoperatively in patients II and III respectively. A total of 6.6 mg of NGF was infused continuously for three months in the first 2 patients. In patient III 0.21 mg of NGF was infused for 2 weeks, then the infusion was stopped and after 5 weeks NGF was restarted with a total of 0.24 mg NGF for a period of 10 weeks. A third treatment period was started 8 months later with a total NGF dose of 0.11 mg over 10 weeks.

Patient assessment All of the patients were tested for cognitive function before NGF administration using MMSE and had scores of 18, 23, and 23. These scores did not stabilize over the time of treatment but declined with time. However patient I showed a slight improvement in the selective reminding test and delayed recognition of word list. Patient II showed a slight improvement in delayed recognition of faces and word list. Patient III did not show any improvement in any sub-test. Patient I was again tested ten weeks after the NGF infusion had been stopped, and the improved results in selective reminding and delayed recall of word list found during treatment were no longer seen.

In patient I a marked increase in the cerebral blood flow in the frontal and temporal cortices that outlasted the NGF treatment by several months was observed. The other two patients did not show such improved cerebral blood flow. A general improvement of glucose metabolism was observed in patient II after the end of the NGF treatment. No marked effect on glucose metabolism was observed in patient III. However, the glucose metabolism in cortical brain regions remained constant during the whole period of NGF treatments compared to the decrease in glucose metabolism that had been observed during the year prior to the initiation of the NGF treatment.

Examination of ^{11}C nicotine binding in the brain (a measure of cholinergic synapses) showed an increase in frontal and temporal cortices of patient I after three months of NGF treatment and also at three months after infusion compared to the pre-infusion value. Similarly increased binding was observed in the frontal, temporal, and parietal cortices as well as in the hippocampus in patient II after three months of NGF treatment and also three months after the end of treatment. In patient III nicotine binding was generally decreased in the frontal, temporal, and parietal cortices during and after the end of the different periods of NGF treatments. Increased binding was however observed in the hippocampus of patient III seven months after the end of the second period of NGF treatment.

Neurophysiological evaluation showed reduction in slow-wave activity expressed as an increased alpha/theta ratio in patients I and II. In patient III there were no significant changes in EEG activity before, during or after the three treatment periods.

Side effects Two types of side-effects occurred during NGF treatment. All three patients reported the development of pain. The first patient complained of muscle pain in the lower back that appeared 11–14 days after the start of NGF infusion. Similar symptoms were also reported by patient II 11 days after the start of NGF infusion. When the NGF infusion was stopped the pain disappeared within two days. In the third patient receiving a lower dose of NGF (16 µg/24 hours) a constant muscle pain in the lumbar region was reported. The NGF infusion was stopped after two weeks and the pain disappeared in two days. When the NGF dose was lowered to 3.4 µg/24 hours and restarted 5 weeks later the pain returned after four days but was reported to be less in intensity and could be alleviated with Dextropropoxyphene. When the NGF infusion was stopped 2 months later the pain disappeared. Eight months later the patient received a lower dose of NGF (1.6 µg/24 hours) for ten weeks. Again the pain returned but was reported to be of low intensity and also stopped completely following cessation of NGF treatment.

In the first two patients NGF infusion was also associated with a loss of weight and appetite: 6.7 kg in 3 months (12% patient I) and 6.5 kg in 3 months (15% patient II). In the third patient there was a clear reduction in weight over time but no correlation with the treatment periods and no marked weight gain after the treatment periods.

Toxicological side-effects in animals It is uncertain how these side-effects are brought about although weight loss has been reported following infusion of NGF into the cerebral ventricles of rats (Day-Lollini *et al.* 1997) and primates (Fernandez *et al.* 1998). However, in the rodent study it was only observed at the higher dose (300 ng/24 hour). It is difficult to project from rodent to man in terms of dosage but it is likely that the CSF concentration obtained here would be higher than those achieved above. In the primate study the dose used was 2.5 μg/kg/24 hours which is substantially higher than used in AD patients. Other studies where lower doses of NGF have been infused into primates have not resulted in weight loss. Furthermore the weight loss reported in primates was reversible following cessation of NGF infusion similar to that seen in patients.

Two studies have shown that NGF infusion into rats and primates also results in Schwann cell hyperplasia. In one study (Day-Lollini *et al.* 1997) recombinant human NGF (5 μg/24 hours) was administered intracerebroventricularly (icv) to rats for 12 weeks and then the rats were histologically examined immediately, 2, 8, 12, and 52 weeks after termination of the NGF infusion. Examination of tissue sections showed that from the caudal part of the medulla, at the hypoglossal nerve to the C3 level of the cervical cord was surrounded by atypical hyperplastic tissue. The hyperplastic tissue was predominately attached to the dorsal and lateral surface of the medulla and the spinal cord underneath the pia arachnoid. The tissue was primarily composed of densely packed spindle shaped cells, up to 30 layers thick. No mitotic figures or malignant transformed cells were observed.

Immunohistochemical analysis of the cells showed that they stained for p75[NGFR] but not TrkA. In addition a strong cellular S-100 immunoreactivity was observed together with vimentin and GFAP positive fibres, suggesting that the hyperplasia consisted of proliferating Schwann cells. Associated neuronal fibres were also observed which were immunopositive for either tyrosine hydroxlase or calcitionin gene related protein indicating the presence of sympathetic and sensory fibres. Following stopping the NGF infusion the hyperplasia, measured as mean thickness of the pia-arachnoid at the most affected place, was shown to be completely reversible. Thus it was significantly reduced after 8 weeks and completely abolished after 52 weeks.

In the second study (Winkler *et al.* 1997) recombinant human NGF was infused into both rat and primate cerebral ventricles. The doses used were 0, 6, 60 or 300 ng per day for rats and 0, 0.6, 6 or 60 μg per day for primates; both groups were infused for 6 months. Similar hyperplasia was reported except that the effects were shown to be dose related such that at the lowest dose used for rodents the hyperplasia was completely absent.

Conclusions

If we compare the doses of NGF used in the clinical trials to the CSF concentrations measured we can see that a 75 μg dose over 24 hours results in a CSF concentration of 200 ng/ml. A 16μg dosing schedule results in a CSF concentration of 50 ng/ml. The concentration of NGF in human brain is 459 pg/g wet weight in Brodman area 22 (Allen *et al.* 1991) which is ~100 fold lower than that achieved in CSF using a dose of 16 μg/24 hours. Although it is difficult to estimate the concentration of NGF which enters into the brain parenchyma it has been shown that injection of [125I]NGF icv in rats (Lapchack *et al.* 1993) and primates (Emmett *et al.* 1996) leads to specific labelling of basal forebrain cholinergic neurons indicating that brain penetration occurs readily. Since the hyperplasia observed in animals is dose related and is possibly the cause of the observed side-effects in humans it may be possible to maintain a therapeutic effect of NGF without the side-effects by using alternative dosing, starting with lower doses and delivering the NGF intermittently.

An alternative strategy might be to give NGF via an intranasal route. Recent reports have shown that following injection of [^{125}I]NGF into the olfactory bulb of rats radiolabelled NGF was found to be specifically retrogradely transported to basal forebrain cholinergic nuclei (Altar and Bakhit 1991). Similarly it has been shown that radiolabelled NGF can be transported into the brain following administration as nose drops (Frey *et al.* 1997; Chen *et al.* 1998)

14.4 **Other neurotransmitter approaches**

14.4.1 **Monoamines**

Although the cholinergic system has been investigated the most extensively, other neuro-transmitter systems are involved in both cognitive processing and AD. Dopaminergic activity influences working memory, and the noradrenergic systems are involved in maintaining attention and concentration. Monoamine oxidases (MAO) occur in two forms, MAO-A and MAO-B. Noradrenaline and serotonin (5-HT) are deaminated by MAO-A, and dopamine by MAO-B. MAO-B accounts for about 80% of human brain MAO, and the highest concentrations are found in the hippocampus. Patients with AD have higher MAO-B activity than healthy elderly people (Alexopolous *et al.* 1984) and so strategies aimed at increasing monoamine availability have a logical rationale.

Selegiline

Selegiline (L-deprenyl) is a MAO inhibitor. At low doses (10 mg/day) it acts as an irreversible inhibitor of MAO-B. At higher doses (40 mg/day) it loses its selectivity for MAO-B and also inhibits MAO-A. The possible beneficial effects of selegiline may not rely solely on its ability to enhance monoamine activity (Tolbert and Fuller 1996). Selegiline is metabolized in the liver to desmethylselegiline and metamphetamine, which are subsequently metabolized to amphetamine. The stimulant effects of these metabolites may exert some effect on mood and arousal. Additionally selegiline may have neuro-protective attributes as MAO-B inhibition helps to decrease the production of oxidative free radicals (Cohen and Spina 1989).

Birks and Flicker (1998) reviewed 14 randomized, double-blind, placebo-controlled studies of the effects of selegiline in dementia. Eleven of the trials examined behavioural and mood symptoms in addition to cognitive function. Nine studies found beneficial effects for cognitive function and four demonstrated improvements in behaviour and mood. The meta-analysis revealed significant improvements in memory function for selegiline treated patients compared with those who received placebo.

The findings so far are promising but larger trials using standardized rating scales are needed before selegiline can be considered for routine clinical use in AD.

Moclobemide

The antidepressant moclobemide is a reversible MAO-A inhibitor. Its efficacy as an antidepressant in patients with dementia or cognitive impairment has been demonstrated in a double-blind, placebo-controlled trial which enrolled 694 elderly people (Roth *et al.* 1996). In this study the moclobemide treated patients improved significantly on tests of cognitive function compared to those who received placebo. The improvement in cognitive function may have been secondary to treatment of the depressive symptoms, but a mood-independent effect was a possibility.

Selective serotonin reuptake inhibitors

Most pharmacological research has focused on the cognitive symptoms of AD, but depression, psychosis, and behavioural changes are common features. Many of the non-cognitive symptoms may be caused by neurobiological changes.

The selective serotonin reuptake inhibitors (SSRIs) are effective treatments for depression, anxiety, and obsessive-compulsive disorder. They have minimal anti-cholinergic activity which makes them a good choice for AD patients. Citalopram, a highly selective serotonin reuptake inhibitor, has been shown to produce modest improvements in cognitive function when used as an antidepressant in elderly people (Nyth *et al.* 1992). SSRIs have also been used to treat psychotic symptoms in demented patients (Burke *et al.* 1997).

14.4.2 **Glutamate**

L-glutamate is the major excitatory neurotransmitter in the central nervous system.

The ionotropic glutamate receptors can be distinguished by the binding of three agonists: N-methyl-D-aspartate (NMDA), alpha-amino-3-hydroxy-5-methyl-4-isoxazole propionic acid (AMPA), and kainate. The metabotropic glutamate receptors, of which there are several subtypes, act via a G protein on secondary messenger systems.

Glutamate is involved in both learning and memory, but is also a powerful neurotoxin and has been implicated in the pathogenesis of AD. *In vitro* studies have demonstrated that NMDA antagonists such as amantadine and memantine have neuroprotective properties, and the results of clinical trials are awaited. Cycloserine, an indirect glutamate agonist, modulates the NMDA receptor-associated glycine site. Animal studies indicated that cycloserine had beneficial effects on learning and memory functions, and one study in AD patients found that it improved implicit memory (Schwartz *et al.* 1996). However the results of clinical trials have been disappointing (Fakouhi *et al.* 1995; Mohr *et al.* 1995).

14.5 **Neuroprotective strategies**

14.5.1 **Oestrogen replacement therapy**

Oestrogen replacement therapy (ERT) may have a role in the treatment or prophylaxis of AD. Indirect evidence supporting the potential benefits of ERT comes from a number of observational studies and can be inferred from the physiological actions of oestrogen and the results of animal experiments.

Animal studies indicate that oestrogens have a direct effect on neuronal development and neurotransmitter systems. Oestrogen receptors are found in the equivalent areas of rat brain to those that are preferentially damaged in humans suffering from AD. The poor performance on tests of memory and learning of ovariectomized rats is associated with reduced cholinergic activity, but can be prevented by oestrogen replacement (Singh *et al.* 1994). In rats 17β oestradiol modulates CA1 hippocampal dendritic spine density (Woolley and McEwen 1994). Oestrogen may exert some of its effects through its actions on nerve growth factor (NGF). Rodent mRNA for NGF declines after ovariectomy but is restored by replacement therapy (Singh *et al.* 1995).

The effects of oestrogen on processes thought to be relevant in the pathogenesis of AD gives further credence to the oestrogen hypothesis (Henderson 1997). Regional vascular insufficiency may contribute to the disease process in AD (Birge 1997b), and oestrogen improves cerebral blood flow in post menopausal women. In cell cultures with oestrogen receptors, 17β oestradiol promotes the metabolism of amyloid precursor protein to the soluble fragments, thus reducing the accumulation as the neurotoxic Aβ amyloid fragment (Jaffe et al. 1994). In addition, oestrogens have potent anti-oxidant properties.

Clinic based case control studies on the effects of ERT on the development of AD have yielded inconsistent results. Some of these studies were open to criticism because different methods were used to determine ERT usage in patients and controls. Moreover prescribing practices may have been different for female AD patients compared to their controls. The population-based studies have been more consistent in their findings that ERT has beneficial effects on the development of AD, but not universally so. Brenner and colleagues (1994) compared ERT usage as determined by computerized pharmacy data in 107 female AD sufferers and 120 age-matched controls, and found no significant differences between the two groups. Paganini-Hill and Henderson (1996) conducted a case-control study nested within a prospective cohort study of 8877 women. The participants were sent a health questionnaire at the beginning of the study period. 3760 of the female cohort died in the following 14 years. AD or other terms likely to indicate AD were recorded on the death certificates of 248 women. Each case was matched with five women for year of birth and death. The risk of AD was reduced in those who had received ERT (odds ratio 0.65, 95% C.I. 0.49–0.88). Increased doses and duration of therapy with oral conjugated equine oestrogen were associated with increased risk reduction. The main limitation of this study was the use of death certificates to define the cases.

In the study by Tang and colleagues (1996), ERT use in 1124 non-demented elderly women was ascertained by personal interview at the beginning of the study. The women were then followed up annually for between one and five years. The diagnosis of AD was made by an independent group of clinicians based on information from the assessments, medical records, and imaging studies. The relative risk (RR) of developing AD was reduced in ERT users (RR 0.40, 95% CI 0.22–0.85). The RR was reduced most for women who had taken ERT for more than one year. ERT use was also documented prospectively in the Baltimore Longitudinal Study of Aging (Kawas et al. 1997). 472 post- or perimenopausal women were assessed every two years for up to 16 years. The RR for AD among women who had ever used ERT (oral or transdermal oestrogen) was 0.46 (95% CI 0.209–0.997). The authors did not find any correlation with duration of ERT use but this had been recorded in broad time-period categories.

There have been so few treatment trials of ERT that no firm conclusions can be drawn about its effects on the symptoms of AD. Observational studies in non-demented, post-menopausal women suggest that ERT may help to preserve cognitive function (Resnick et al. 1997; Jacobs et al. 1998).

The earliest treatment study in AD patients was an open-label, uncontrolled trial of unopposed conjugated oestrogens (Fillit et al. 1986). Three of seven women improved on cognitive test scores. Ohkura et al. (1995) reported on the effects of long-term (5 to 45 months), low dose, ERT given to seven women with mild -to moderate AD. Four women improved in areas of cognition and ability to perform activities of daily living.

ERT may also act synergistically with other cholinergic treatments. Schneider *et al.* (1996) retrospectively analysed the effects of ERT usage in a 30 week, randomized, double-blind, placebo-controlled, parallel-group, clinical trial of tacrine. Of 318 women with mild to moderate AD, 14.5% were receiving ERT prior to randomization. The women who were taking ERT and received tacrine improved significantly more on cognitive tests than women not on ERT who received tacrine or placebo.

Undoubtedly ERT holds promise as a treatment and may even have a role in the prevention of AD. Clinical trials are under way, and a randomized, prospective study to determine the effects of ERT on the development of AD has been included in the Women's Health Initiative (Birge 1997*a*). The results of these investigations will determine the future of ERT in the management of this illness.

14.5.2 **Anti-inflammatory drugs**

Inflammatory and immune mechanisms are implicated in the pathological processes which lead to nerve cell death in AD (Aisen and Davis 1994). Early reports of a decreased incidence of AD among rheumatoid arthritis sufferers led to the hypothesis that anti-inflammatory drugs might be protective for AD. A number of studies examining arthritis, non-steroidal anti-inflammatory drugs (NSAIDs) and steroid use as risk factors for AD followed. A meta-analysis of case-control studies (McGeer *et al.* 1996) found that the chance of developing AD was lower than in the general population for individuals who had suffered from arthritis (odds ratio 0.56), or who had taken NSAIDs (odds ratio 0.5) or steroids (odds ratio 0.66).

The findings of population based studies have been harder to interpret due to differences in methodologies. Anderson *et al.* (1995) examined the cross-sectional relation between NSAID use and the risk for AD in a large population based study of elderly people. The relative risk for AD in NSAID users (n = 365) compared to non-users (n = 5893) was 0.38. The Baltimore Longitudinal Study of Aging also found an inverse association between aspirin and NSAID use and the onset of AD (Stewart *et al.* 1997). Among NSAID users, the relative risk of AD was influenced by the duration of drug use. Treatment with NSAIDs for more than two years was associated with a lower relative risk for AD than treatment of less than two years duration.

Prince *et al.* (1998) examined the relationship between NSAID use and cognitive function in 2651 people aged 65 to 74, who were enrolled in the UK MRC treatment trial of hypertension. NSAID use was ascertained at three monthly intervals for up to 8 years, by a nurse interviewer. NSAID users showed less decline on the paired associate learning test than non-users, with younger patients benefiting most. Other longitudinal, observational studies have found no evidence that NSAIDs protect against the development of dementia, or cognitive decline (Fourrier *et al.* 1996; Henderson *et al.* 1997).

Pilot studies of prednisone and indomethacin have been published, but only randomized, controlled trials can confirm whether anti-inflammatory drugs can protect against the development of AD or alter the course of cognitive decline.

14.5.3 **Antioxidants**

Brain tissue has low levels of endogenous antioxidants and is therefore particularly vulnerable to free-radical damage (Lethem and Orrell 1997). Oxidative stress has been implicated in the pathogenesis of AD (Smith *et al.* 1996) and this has inevitably aroused interest in the possible therapeutic benefits of antioxidants. A number of medications with actions which include antioxidant activity have been investigated.

Ginkgo biloba

Ginkgo biloba (Egb 761) is a plant extract that has been approved as a treatment for dementia in Germany. Several studies have reported on the beneficial effects of ginkgo biloba but few have used standard assessments of cognitive function or behaviour.

Maurer *et al.* (1997) conducted a randomized, double-blind, placebo-controlled trial in 20 patients with AD over three months. The active treatment group received 240 mg/day of ginkgo biloba extract. A significant treatment effect was found on tests of attention and memory, but the sample size was too small to demonstrate any other treatment effects. A recent placebo-controlled, double-blind, randomized trial of ginkgo biloba, which used standard measures of cognition and behaviour, included patients with AD and multi-infarct dementia (Le Bars *et al.* 1997). 327 patients with mild to moderate dementia were enrolled in the 52 week study (251 with AD). 166 patients were allocated to receive Egb 120 mg/day, and 161 patients to the placebo group. In the ITT analysis, the active treatment group deteriorated less than the placebo group on measures of cognitive function, activities of daily living, and social behaviour. Similar results were demonstrated for the subgroup of AD patients. A clinically significant improvement in cognitive function was achieved in 27% of patients treated with Egb compared with 14% of patients who received placebo. Adverse events were generally mild to moderate and, with the exception of gastrointestinal symptoms, equally distributed between the two groups.

The availability of ginkgo biloba extract in over-the-counter herbal supplements has raised concern due to the potential risk of adverse events (Vale 1998). The bioavailability of the active compound varies in different preparations, and in addition to its anti-oxidant properties, ginkgo biloba inhibits platelet-activating factor. Long-term use has been associated with an increased bleeding time, and spontaneous haemorrhage (Rowin and Lewis 1996). The efficacy of ginkgo biloba appears to be comparable to that of tacrine but it should not be used without clinical supervision.

Idebenone

Idebenone is a benzoquinone derivative with several possible modes of action. It probably acts as a free radical scavenger, protecting cell membranes against lipid peroxidation, and appears to improve cerebral metabolism and correct neurotransmitter defects (Adkins and Nobel 1998). It may also exert some beneficial effects secondary to its ability to stimulate nerve growth factor synthesis. A randomized, double-blind, placebo-controlled trial in 300 patients with mild to moderate AD evaluated the effects of two doses of idebenone over six months (Weyer *et al.* 1997). Active treatment was with idebenone 30 mg three times per day or 90 mg three times per day. Patients receiving the higher dose of idebenone improved significantly on cognitive function testing. In a second double-blind study, 450 patients with mild to moderate AD were randomized to receive placebo three times per day or active treatment with idebenone 90 mg three times per day or 120 mg three times per day for up to 12 months (Gutzmann *et al.* 1997). 379 patients participated for 12 months. Significant dose-dependent effects on cognitive and global function, were apparent after six months of active treatment. In both studies six months of active treatment was required to achieve maximum effect, and the most severely impaired patients benefited most. The treatment effect was maintained in the 12 month study and showed a trend towards further improvement. The results of a two year study are awaited.

Alpha-tocopherol

Alpha-tocopherol (vitamin E) is a lipid-soluble vitamin with potent anti-oxidant activity.

Animal and *in vitro* studies have suggested that alpha-tocopherol has neuro-protective properties. It has been evaluated in a double-blind, placebo-controlled trial in patients with moderate AD (Sano *et al.* 1997). 341 patients were randomly assigned to receive selegiline 5 mg twice a day, alpha-tocopherol 1000 IU twice a day, selegiline and alpha-tocopherol, or placebo. The primary outcome measure was the time to the occurrence of one end point: death; institutionalization; loss of ability to perform two of three activities of daily living (i.e. eating, grooming, using the toilet). Adjusting for base-line functioning, all three active treatments significantly delayed the primary outcome (risk ratio for alpha-tocopherol 0.47; risk ratio for selegiline 0.57; risk ratio for combination treatment 0.69). Only alpha-tocopherol delayed institutionalization (risk ratio 0.42) when individual end-points were examined. Falls and syncope were commoner in the treatment groups but did not lead to discontinuation of therapy.

Antioxidants may have a potential role as neuroprotective agents but further investigation is required to clarify their method of action, efficacy, and long-term safety.

14.5.4 Glial cell modulation

Immune mechanisms contribute to neuronal death in both AD and ischaemia, and ischaemia can enhance the beta-amyloidogenic reaction. Propentofylline, a xanthine derivative, is an adenosine re-uptake/phosphodiesterase inhibitor, with a broad range of effects. It appears to inhibit the cytotoxic functions of activated microglia and reinforce the neuro-protective properties of astrocytes by stimulating NGF secretion. It may have additional beneficial activity as an anti-oxidant.

Animal studies indicate that propentofylline may have benefits on some aspects of cognitive functioning. Randomized, double-blind, placebo-controlled, studies including 901 patients with mild to moderate AD, have shown significant treatment effects for propentofylline in tests of global and cognitive function, and activities of daily living (Kittner *et al.* 1997). Treatment effects were comparable in patients with vascular dementia. Adverse effects, most commonly gastrointestinal disturbance, headaches and dizziness, were mainly mild.

14.5.5 Calcium channel blockers

Calcium dysregulation may play a role in neuronal cell degeneration. High intracellular calcium concentrations are neurotoxic, and the enhancement of glutamate toxicity by $A\beta$ may be calcium-dependent. Two randomized trials in 1648 patients with AD failed to demonstrate any significant benefits for nimodipine, a calcium channel blocker, over placebo on primary outcome measures (Morich *et al.* 1996).

14.6 Summary and conclusions

Of the symptomatic treatments for AD, CEIs have been the most successful so far. However most clinical trials have been confined to patients with mild or moderately severe dementia.

The most severely impaired patients, and those with minor degrees of cognitive impairment possibly representing subclinical AD have been largely excluded. The efficacy of individual CEIs appears broadly similar although direct comparative studies have not been conducted.

Drugs which target other neurotransmitter systems, particularly those using monoamines, may prove helpful, especially for the behavioural and psychiatric manifestations of the illness.

Advances in our understanding of the neuropathological processes involved in AD have paved the way for new and exciting opportunities to alter the disease progression, or even delay the onset of AD. The people who may benefit most from neuroprotective treatments, are those who are asymptomatic but at risk of developing the illness. The next challenge will be to find a sensitive and specific marker for the prediction of AD.

References

Adkins, J. C. and Noble, S. (1998). Idebenone: A review of its use in mild to moderate Alzheimer's disease. *CNS Drugs*, 9, 5, 403–19.

Aisen, P. S. and Davis, K. L. (1994). Inflammatory mechanisms in Alzheimer's disease: Implications for therapy. *American Journal of Psychiatry*, 151, 8, 1105–13.

Alexopoulos, G. S., Lieberman, K. W., and Young, R. C. (1984). Platelet MAO activity in primary degenerative dementia. *American Journal of Psychiatry*, 141, 97–9.

Allen, S. J., Dawbarn, D., Spillantini, M. G., *et al.* (1989). The distribution of β-nerve growth factor receptors in the human basal forebrain. *Journal of Comparative Neurology*, 289, 626–40.

Allen, S. J., Dawbarn, D., MacGowan, S. H., *et al.* (1990). A Quantitative morphometric analysis of basal forebrain neurons expressing β-NGF receptors in normal and Alzheimer's disease brains. *Dementia*, 1, 125–37.

Allen, S. J., MacGowan, S. H., Treanor, J. J. S., *et al.* (1991). Normal NGF content in Alzheimer's disease cerebral cortex and hippocampus. *Neuroscience Letters*, 131, 135–9.

Altar, C. and Bakhit, C. (1991). Receptor mediated transport of human recombinant nerve growth factor from olfactory bulb to basal forebrain cholinergic nuclei. *Brain Research*, 541, 82–8.

Anand, R., and Gharabawi, G. (1996). Clinical development of Exelon (ENA–713): The ADENA programme. *Journal of Drug Development and Clinical Practice*, 8, 117–122.

Anderson, K., Launer, L. J., Ott, A., *et al.* (1995). Do nonsteroidal anti-inflammatory drugs decrease the risk for Alzheimer's disease? The Rotterdam Study. *Neurology*, 45, 1441–5.

Arrieata, J. L. and Artalejo, F. R. (1998). Methodology, results, and quality of clinical trials of tacrine in the treatment of Alzheimer's disease: a systematic review of the literature. *Age and Ageing*, 27, 161–79.

Asthana, S., Raffaele, K. C., Berardi, A., *et al.* (1995) Treatment of Alzheimer disease by continuous intravenous infusion of physostigmine. *Alzheimer disease and Associated Disorders*, 9, (4), 223–32

Avery, E. E., Baker, L. D., and Asthana, S. (1997). Potential role of muscarinic agonists in Alzheimer's disease. *Drugs and Aging*, 11, (6), 450–9.

Barde, Y.-A., Davies, A. M., Johnson, J. E., *et al.* (1982). Brain derived neurotrophic factor. *Progress in Brain Research*, 71, 185–9.

Barde, Y.-A., Edgar, D., and Thoenen, H. (1987). Purification of a new neurotrophic factor from mammalian brain. *European Molecular Biology Organisation Journal*, 1, 549–53.

Becker, R. E., Colliver, J. A., Markwell, S. J., *et al.* (1996). Double-blind, placebo-controlled study of metrifonate, an acetylcholinesterase inhibitor, for Alzheimer's disease. *Alzheimer's Disease and Associated Disorders*, 10, 124–31.

Berkemeier, L. R., Winslow, J. M., Kaplan, D. R., *et al.* (1991). Neurotrophin-5: a novel neurotrophic factor that activates trk and trkB. *Neuron*, 7, 857–66.

Birge, S. J. (1997*a*). The role of ovarian hormones in cognition and dementia. *Neurology*, **48**, suppl. 7, 1.

Birge, S. J. (1997*b*). The role of estrogen in the treatment of Alzheimer's disease. *Neurology*, **48**, suppl. 7, 36–41.

Birks, J. and Flicker, L. (1998). The efficacy and safety of selegiline for the symptomatic treatment of Alzheimer's disease: a systematic review of the evidence. Cochrane Review, In: *The Cochrane Library*, Issue 3. Oxford: Update Software.

Blackart, W. G., Sood, G. K., Crowe, D. R., and Fallon, M. B. (1998). Tacrine a cause of fatal hepato-toxicity? *Journal of Clinical Gastroenterology*, **26**, 1, 57–9.

Bodick, N. C., Offen, W. W., Shannon, H. E., *et al.* (1997). The selective muscarinic agonists xanome-line improves both the cognitive deficits and behavioural symptoms of Alzheimer's disease. *Alzheimer Disease and Associated Disorders*, 11, Suppl. 4, S16–22.

Boissiere, F., Faucheux, B., Ruberg, M., *et al.* (1997). Decreased TrkA gene expression in cholinergic neurons of the striatum and basal forebrain of patients with Alzheimer's disease. *Experimental Neurology*, **145**, 245–52.

Bowen, D. M., Smith, C. B., White, P., and Davison, A. N. (1976). Neurotransmitter related enzymes and indices of hypoxia in senile dementia and other abiotrophies. *Brain*, **99**, 459–96.

Bowen, D. M., Benton, J. S., Spillane, J. A., *et al.* (1982). Choline acetyltransferase activity and histopathology of frontal neocortex from biopsies of demented patients. *Journal of Neurological Science*, 57, 191–202.

Brenner, D. E., Kukull, W. A., Stergachis, A., *et al.* (1994). Postmenopausal estrogen replacement therapy and the risk of Alzheimer's disease: a population-based case-control study. *American Journal of Epidemiology*, **140**,262–7.

Burke, W. J., Dewan, V., Wengel, S. P., *et al.* (1997). The use of selective serotonin reuptake inhibitors for depression and psychosis complicating dementia. *International Journal of Geriatric Psychiatry*, 12, 5, 519–25.

Butte, M. J., Hwang, P. K., Mobley, W. C., and Fletterick, R. J. (1998). Crystal structure of Neurotrophin-3 homodimer shows distinct regions are used to bind its receptors. *Biochemistry, 37,* 16846–52.

Chatellier, G. and Lacomblez, L. (1990). Tacrine (tetrahydroaminoacridine; THA) and lecithin in senile dementia of the Alzheimer type: a multicentre trial. Groupe Francais d'Etude de la Tetrahydroaminoacridine. *British Medical Journal*, 300, 495–9.

Chen, K. S., Nishimura, M. C., Broz, S., *et al.* (1993). Assessment of learning and memory perfor-mance in mice heterozygous for nerve growth factor deletion. *Society for Neuroscience Abstracts*, 19, 1963.

Chen, K. S.,Nishimura, M. C., Spencer, S., *et al.* (1994). Learning memory and the basal cholinergic system in aged mice heterozygous for nerve growth factor deletion. *Society for Neuroscience Abstracts*, 28, 856.

Chen, X. Q., Fawcett, J. R., Ala, T. A., *et al.* (1998). Olfactoey route: a new pathway to deliver nerve growth factor to the brain. 6th International Conference on Alzheimer's disease, Amsterdam, Abstact 1086.

Christie, J. E., Shering, A., Ferguson, J., and Glen, AI. (1981). Physostigmine and arecoline: effects of intravenous infusions in Alzheimer presenile dementia. *British Journal of Psychiatry*, 138, 46–50.

Clary, D. O. and Reichardt, L. F. (1994). An alternatively spliced form of the nerve growth factor receptor trkA confers an enhanced response to neurotrophin-3. *Proceedings of the National Academy of Sciences (USA)*, **91**, 11133–7.

Cohen, G. and Spina, M. B. (1989). Deprenyl suppresses the oxidant stress associated with increased dopamine turnover. *Annals of Neurology*, **26**, 689–90.

Connor, D. J., Langlais, P. L., and Thal, L. J. (1991). Behavioural impairments after lesions of the nucleus basalis by ibotenic acid and quisqualic acid. *Brain Research*, **555**, 84–90.

Corey-Bloom, J., Anand, R., and Veach, J. for the ENA 713 B352 Study Group. (1998). A randomized trial evaluating the efficacy and safety of ENA 713 (rivastigmine tartrate), a new acetyl-cholinesterase inhibitor, in patients with mild to moderately severe Alzheimer's disease. *International Journal of Geriatric Psychopharmacology*, **1**, 55–65.

Crow, T. J. and Grove-White, I. G. (1973). An analysis of the learning deficit following hyoscine administration to man. *British Journal of Pharmacology*, **49**, 322–7.

Crowley, C., Spencer, S. D., Nishimura, M. C., *et al.* (1994). Mice lacking nerve growth factor display perinatal loss of sensory and sympathetic neurons yet develop basal forebrain cholinergic neurons. *Cell*, **76**, 1001–11.

Crutcher, K. A., Scott, S. A., Liang, S., *et al.* (1993). Detection of NGF-like activity in human brain tissue: Increased levels in Alzheimer's disease. *Journal of Neuroscience*, **13**, 2540–50.

Cummings, J. L., Cyrus, P. A., Bieber, F., *et al.* and the Metrifonate Study Group. (1998). Metrifonate treatment of the cognitive deficits of Alzheimer's disease. *Neurology*, **50**, 1214–21.

Davies, P. and Malony, A. J. F. (1976). Selective loss of central cholinergic neurons in Alzheimer's disease. *Lancet,* ii, 1403.

Davis, K. L. and Powchik, P. (1995). Tacrine. *The Lancet*, **345**, 625–30.

Davis, K. L., Mohs, R. C., and Tinlenberg, J. R. (1979). Enhancement of memory by physostigmine. *New England Journal of Medicine*, **301**, 946.

Davis, K. L., Thal, L. J., Gamzu, E. R., *et al.* (1992). A double-blind, placebo-controlled multicentre study of tacrine for Alzheimer's disease. *New England Journal of Medicine*, **327**, 1253–9.

Dawbarn, D., Allen, S. J., and Semenenko, F. M. (1988*a*). Immunohistochemical localisation of β-nerve growth factor receptors in the forebrain of the rat. *Brain Research*, **440**, 185–189.

Dawbarn, D., Allen, S. J., and Semenenko, F. M. (1988*b*). Coexistence of choline acetyltransferase and β-nerve growth factor receptors in the forebrain of the rat. *Neuroscience Letters*, **94**, 138–44.

Day-Lollini, P. A., Stewart, G. R., Taylor, M. J., *et al.* (1997). Hyperplastic changes within the lep-tomeninges of the rat and monkey in response to chronic intracerebroventricular infusion of nerve growth factor. *Experimental Neurology*, **145**, 24–37.

Dunnett, S. B., Whishaw, I. Q., Jones, G. H., and Bunch, S. T. (1987). Behavioural, biochemical and histochemical effects of different neurotoxic amino acids injected into nucleus basalis magnocellu-laris of rats. *Neuroscience*, **20**, 653–69.

Dunnett, S. B., Rogers, D. C. and Jones, G. H. (1989). Effects of nucleus basalis magnocellularis lesions in rats on delayed matching and non-matching to position tasks. *European Journal of Neuroscience*, **1**, 395–406.

Eagger, S. A., Levy, R., and Sahakian, B. J. (1991). Tacrine in Alzheimer's disease. *The Lancet*, **337**, 989–92.

Emmett, C. J., Stewart, G. R., Johnson, R. M., *et al.* (1996). Distribution of radioiodinated recombi-nant human nerve growth factor in primate brain following intracerebroventricular infusion. *Experimental Neurology*, **40**, 151–60.

Fakouhi, T. D., Jhee, S. S., Sramek, J. J., *et al.* (1995). Evaluation of cycloserine in the treatment of Alzheimer's disease. *Journal of Geriatric Psychiatry and Neurology*, **8**, 226–30.

Farlow, M., Gracon, S. T., Hershey, L. A., *et al.* (1992). A controlled trial of tacrine in Alzheimer's disease. *Journal of the American Medical Association*, **268**, 2523–9.

Farlow, M. R., Lahiri, D. K., Poirier, J., *et al.* (1998). Treatment outcome of tacrine therapy depends on apolipoprotein genotype and gender of the subjects with Alzheimer's disease. *Neurology*, **50**, 669–77.

Fernandez, C. I., Gonzalez, O., Diaz, E., *et al.* (1998). Systemic and side-effects of intracerebroventricular infusion of nerve growth factor in aged rodents and monkeys: Cautionary evidence for its therapeutic use. *Alzheimer's Disease Review*, **3**, 95–9.

Fillit, H., Weinreb, H., Cholst, I., *et al.* (1986). Observations in a preliminary open trial of estradiol therapy for senile dementia (Alzheimer's type). *Psychoneuroendocrinology*, **11**, 337–45.

Fischer, W., Wictorin, K., Bjorklund, A., *et al.* (1987). Amelioration of cholinergic neuron atrophy and spatial memory impairment in aged rats by nerve growth factor. *Nature*, **328**, 65–8.

Fischer, W., Bjorklund, A., Chen, K., and Gage, F. H. (1991). NGF improves spatial memory in aged rodents as a function of age. *Journal of Neuroscience*, **11**, 1889–906.

Fischer, W., Sirevaag, A., Wiegand, S. J., *et al.* (1994). Reversal of spatial memory impairments in aged rats by nerve growth factor and neurotrophins 3 and 4/5 but not by brain-derived neurotrophic factor. *Proceedings of the National Academy of Sciences (USA)*, **91**, 8607–11.

Fourrier, A., Letenneur, L., Begaud, B., and Dartigues, J. F. (1996). Nonsteroidal antiinflammatory drug use and cogntive function in the elderly: Inconclusive results from a population-based cohort study. *Journal of Clinical Epidemiology*, **49**, 1201.

Frey II, W. H., Liu, J., Chen, X., *et al.* (1997). Delivery of 125I-NGF to the brain via the olfactory route. *Drug Delivery: Journal of Delivery & Targeting of Therapeutic Agents*, **4**, 87–92.

Fritten, L. J., Perryman, K. M., Gross, P. M., *et al.* (1990). Treatment of Alzheimer's disease with short- and long-term oral THA and lecithin: a double-blind study. *American Journal of Psychiatry*, **2**, 239–42.

Gage, F. H., Armstrong, D. M., Williams, L. R., and Varon, S. (1988). Morphological response of axotomized septal neurons to nerve growth factor. *Journal of Comparative Neurology*, **269**, 147–55.

Geaney, D. P., Soper, N., Shepstone, B. J., Cowan, P. J. (1990). Effect of cholinergic stimulation on regional cerebral blood flow in Alzheimer's disease. *The Lancet*, **335**, 1484–7.

Gnahn, H., Hefti, F., Heumann, R., *et al.* (1983). NGF-mediated increase of choline acetyltransferase (ChAT) in the neonatal rat forebrain: evidence for a physiological role of NGF in the brain. *Brain Research*, **285**, 45–52.

Goedert, M., Fine, A., and Ullrich, A. (1986). Nerve growth factor RNA in peripheral and central rat tissues and in the human central nervous system: lesion effects in the rat brain and levels in Alzheimer's disease. *Molecular Brain Research*, **1**, 85–92.

Goedert, M., Fine, A., Dawbarn, D., *et al.* (1989). Nerve growth factor receptor mRNA distribution in human brain: normal levels in basal forebrain in Alzheimer's disease. *Molecular Brain Research*, **5**, 1–7.

Grothe, D. R., Piscitelli, S. C., Dukoff, R., *et al.* (1998). Penetration of tacrine into cerebrospinal fluid in patients with Alzheimer's disease. *Journal of Clinical Psychopharmacology*, **18**, (1), 78–81.

Gustafson, L. (1993). Physostigmine and tetrahydroaminoacridine treatment of Alzheimer's disease. *Acta Neurologica Scandinavica*, Supplementum. 149 (Rand):39–41.

Gutzman, H., Hadler, D., and Erzigkeit, H. (1997. Long-term treatment of Alzheimer's disease with idebenone. In *Alzheimer's disease: Biology, diagnosis and therapeutics*, (ed. K. Iqbal, B. Winblad, T. Nishimura, M. Takeda, and H. M. Wisniewski), pp. 687–705. Wiley, Chichester.

Hallbook, F., Ibanez, C. F., and Persson, H. (1991). Evolutionary studies of the nerve growth factor family reveal a novel member abundantly expressed in *Xenopus* ovary. *Neuron*, **6**, 845–58.

Hartikka, J. and Hefti, F. (1988*a*). Development of septal cholinergic neurons in culture: plating density and glial cells modulate effects of NGF on survival, fiber growth and expression of transmitter specific enzymes. *Journal of Neuroscience*, **8**, 2967–2985.

Hartikka, J. and Hefti, F. (1988*b*). Comparison of nerve growth factor effects on development of septum, striatum, and nucleus basalis cholinergic neurons *in vitro*. *Journal of Neuroscience Research*, 21, 352–64.

Haroutunian, V., Kanof, P. D., and Davis, K. L. (1986). Partial reversal of lesion-induced deficits in cortical cholinergic markers by nerve growth factor. *Brain Research*, 386, 397–9.

Hatanaka, H., Tsukui, H., and Nihonmatsu, I. (1988). Developmental change in nerve growth factor action from induction of choline acetyltransferase to promotion of cell survival in cultured basal forebrain cholinergic neurons from postnatal rats. *Brain Research*, 467, 85–95.

Hefti, F. (1986). Nerve growth factor promotes survival of septal cholinergic neurons after fimbrial transections. *Journal of Neuroscience*, 6, 2155–62.

Hefti, F. and Mash, D. C. (1989). Localisation of nerve growth factor receptors in the normal human brain and in Alzheimer's disease. *Neurobiology of Ageing*, 10, 75–87.

Hefti, F., Hartikka, J., Eckenstein, F., *et al.* (1985). Nerve growth factor increases choline acetyltransferase but not survival or fiber outgrowth of cultured fetal septal cholinergic neurons. *Neuroscience*, 14, 55–68.

Henderson, V. W. (1997). The epidemiology of estrogen replacement therapy and Alzheimer's disease. *Neurology*, 48, suppl 7, s27–35.

Henderson, A. S., Jorm, A. F., Christensen, H., *et al.* (1997). Aspirin, anti-inflammatory drugs and risk of dementia. *International Journal of Geriatric Psychiatry*, 12, 926–30.

Higgins, J. P. T. and Flicker, L. (1998). The efficacy of lecithin in the treatment of dementia and cognitive impairment. Cochrane Review, In: *The Cochrane Library*, Issue 3. Oxford: Update Software.

Hohn, A., Leibrock, J., Bailey, K., and Barde, Y-A. (1990). Identification and characterisation of a novel member of the nerve growth factor/brain derived-neurotrophic factor family. *Nature*, 344, 339–41.

Holden, P. H., Asopa, V., Robertson, A. G. S., *et al.* (1997). Immunoglobulin-like domains define the nerve growth factor binding site of the TrkA receptor. *Nature Biotechnology*, 15, 668–72.

Holland, D. R., Cousens, L. S., Meng, W., and Matthews, B. (1994). Nerve growth factor in different crystal forms displays structural flexibility and reveals zinc binding sites. *Journal of Molecular Biology*, 239, 385–400.

Ip, N. Y., Ibanez, C. F., Nye, S. H., *et al.* (1992). Mammalian neurotrophin-4: Structure, chromosomal localisation, tissue distribution, and receptor specificity. *Proceedings of the National Academy of Sciences (USA)*, 89, 3060–4.

Ip, N. Y., Stitt, T. N., Tapley, P., *et al.* (1993). Similarities and differences in the way neurotrophins interact with trk receptors in neuronal and non-neuronal cells. *Neuron*, 10, 137–49.

Jacobs, D. M., Tang, M-X., Stern, Y., *et al.* (1998). Cognitive function in nondemented older women who took estrogen after menopause. *Neurology*, 50, 368–73.

Jaffe, A. B., Toran-Allerand, C. D., Greengard, P., and Gandy, S. E. (1994). Estrogen regulates metabolism of Alzheimer amyloid beta-precursor protein. *Journal of Biological Chemistry*, 269, 13065–8.

Jing, S., Tapley, P., and Barbacid, M. (1992) Nerve growth factor mediates signal transduction through trk homodimer receptors. *Neuron*, 9, 1067–79.

Jonhagen, M. E., Nordberg, A., Amberla, K., *et al.* (1998). Intracerbroventricular infusion of nerve growth factor in three patients with Alzheimer's disease. *Dementia and Geriatric Cognitive Disorders*, 9, 246–57.

Kaplan, D. R., Hempstead, B. L., Martinzanca, D., *et al.* (1991). The *trk* protooncogene product-a signal transducing receptor for nerve growth factor. *Science*, 252, 554–8.

Kawas, C., Resnick, S., Morrison, A., *et al.* (1997). A prospective study of estrogen replacement therpy and the risk of developing Alzheimer's disease: The Baltimore Longitudinal Study of Aging. *Neurology*, 48, 1517–21.

Kim. S. H., Kim, Y. K., Jeong, S. J., *et al.* (1997). Enhanced release of secreted form of Alzheimer's amyloid precursor protein from PC12 cells by nicotine. *Molecular Pharmacology*, 52, 3, 430–6.

Kittner, B., Rossner, M., and Rother, M. (1997). Clinical trials in dementia with propentofylline. *Annals of the New York Academy of Sciences*, 826, 307–16.

Klein, R., Lamballe, F., Bryant, S., and Baebacid, M. (1992). The trkB tyrosine protein kinase is a receptor for neurotrophin-4. *Neuron*, 8, 947–56.

Knapp, M. J., Knopman, D. S., Solomon, P. R., *et al.* for the Tacrine Study Group. (1994). A 30-week randomized controlled trial of high-dose tacrine in patients with Alzheimer's Disease. *Journal of the American Medical Association*, 271, 985–91

Knopman, D. S. (1998). Metrofinate for Alzheimer's disease. Is the next cholinesterase inhibitor better? *Neurology*, 50, 1203–5.

Kordower, J. H., Bartus, R. T., Bothwell, m., *et al.* (1988). Nerve growth factor receptor immunoreactivity in the non-human primate *Cebus appella*: distribution, morphology and colocalisation with cholinergic enzymes. *Journal of Comparative Neurology*, 277, 465–86.

Korsching, S., Auburger, G., Heumann, R., *et al.* (1985). Levels of nerve growth factor and its mRNA in the central nervous system of the rat correlate with cholinergic innervation. *European Molecular Biology Organisation Journal*, 4, 1389–93.

Kromer, L. F. (1987). Nerve growth factor treatment after brain injury prevents neuronal death. *Science*, 235, 214–16.

Lamballe, F., Klein, R., and Barbacid, M. (1991). TrkC a new mender of the trk family of tyrosine protein-kinases is a receptor for neurotrophin-3. *Cell*, 66, 947–56.

Lapchak, P. A., Araujo, D. M., Carswell, S., and Hefti, F. (1993). Distribution of [125I]nerve growth factor in the rat brain following a single intraventricular injection: Correlation with the topographical distribution of trkA messenger RNA-expressing cells. *Neuroscience*, 54, 445–60.

Leibrock, J., Lottspeich, F., Hohn, A., *et al.* (1989). Molecular cloning and expression of brain –derived neurotrophic factor. *Nature*, 341, 149–52.

Le Bars, P. L., Katz, M. M., Berman, N., *et al.* for the North American Egb Study Group. (1997). A placebo-controlled, double-blind, randomized trial of an extract of an extract of ginkgo biloba for dementia. *Journal of the American Medical Association*, 278, 1327–32.

Lerner, A., Koss, E., Debanne, S., *et al.* (1997). Smoking and oestrogen-replacement therapy as protective factors for Alzheimer's disease. *The Lancet*, 349, 403–4.

Lethem, R. and Orrell, M. (1997). Antioxidants and dementia. *The Lancet*, 349, 1189.

Levy, A., Brandeis, R., Treves T. A., *et al.* (1994) Transdermal physostigmine in the treatment of Alzheimer's disease. *Alzheimer Disease and Associated Disorders*, 8, (1),15–21.

Loeb, D. M., Stephens, R. M., Copeland, T, *et al.* (1994). A trk nerve growth factor (NGF) receptor point mutation affecting interaction with phosphlipase C-gamma I abolishes NGF- promoted peripherin induction and not neurite outgrowth. *Journal of Biological Chemistry*, 269, 8901–10.

Lucotte, G., Oddoze, C., and Michel, B. F. (1996). Apolipoprotein E genotype allele E4 and response to tacrine in Alzheimer's disease. *Alzheimer Research*, 2, 101–2.

McDonald, N. Q. and Hendrickson, W. A. (1993). A structural superfamily of growth factors containing a cysteine knot motif. *Cell*, 73, 421–4.

McDonald, N. Q., Lapatto, R., Murray-Rust, J., *et al.* (1991) New protein fold revealed by a 2,3-A resolution crystal structure of nerve growth factor. *Nature*, 354, 411–14.

McGeer, P. L., Schulzer, M., and McGeer, E. G. (1996). Arthritis and anti-inflammatory agents as possible protective factors for Alzheimer's disease: a review of 17 epidemiological studies. *Neurology*, 47, 2, 425–32.

MacGowan, S. H., Wilcock, G. K., and Scott, M. (1998). Effect of gender and apolipoprotein E geno-type on response to anticholinesterase therapy in Alzheimer's disease. *International Journal of Geriatric Psychiatry*, 13, 585–90.

Maisonpierre, P. C., Belluscio, L., Squinto, S., *et al.* (1990*a*). Neurotrophin-3: a neurotrophic factor related to NGF and BDNF. *Science*, 247, 1446–51.

Maisonpierre, P. C., Le Beau, M. M., Espinosa, R., *et al.* (1990*b*). Human and rat brain-derived neu-rotrophic factor and neurotrophin-3: gene structures, distributions and chromosomal localisations. *Genomics*, 10, 558–68.

Mandel, R. J., Gage, F. H., and Thal, L. J. (1989) Spatial learning in rats: correlation with cortical choline acetyltransferase and improvement with NGF following NBM damage. *Experimental Neurology*, 104, 208–17.

Marin, D. B., Bierer, L. P., Lawlor, B. A., *et al.* (1995). L-deprenyl and physostigmine for the treatment of Alzheimer's disease. *Psychiatry Research*, 58, (3), 181–9.

Martinez, H. J., Dreyfus, C. F., Jonkait, G. M., and Black, I. B. (1987). Nerve growth factor selectively increase cholinergic markers but not neuropeptides in rat basal forebrain culture. *Brain Research*, 412, 295–301.

Maurer, K., Ihl, R., Dierks, T., and Frolich, L. (1997). Clinical efficacy of Ginkgo biloba special extract Egb 761 in dementia of the Alzheimer type. *Journal of Psychiatric Research*, 31, 6, 645–55.

Mesulam, M. M. and Geula, C. (1988). Nucleus basalis (CH4) and cortical cholinergic innervation in the human brain: Observations based on the distribution of acetylcholinesterase and choline acetyltransferase. *Journal of Comparative Neurology*, 275, 216–40.

Mesulam, M. M., Mufson, E. J., Levey, A. I., and Wainer, B. H. (1983). Cytochemistry and cortical con-nections of the septal area, diagonal band , nucleus basalis (substantia innominata), and hypothala-mus in the rheusus monkey. *Journal of Comparative Neurology*, 214, 170–97.

Mesulam, M. M., Mufson, E. J., and Wainer, B. H. (1986). Three-dimensional representation and cor-tical projection topography of the nucleus basalis (Ch4) in the macaque: Concurrent demonstra-tion of choline acetyltransferase and retrograde transport with a stabilised tetramethybenzidine method for horseradish peroxidase. *Brain Research*, 367, 301–8.

Mohr, E., Knott, V., Sampon, M., *et al.* (1995). Cognitive and quantified electroencephalographic correlates of cycloserine treatment in Alzheimer's disease. *Clinical Neuropharmacology*, 18, 1, 28–38.

Morich, F. J., Bieber, F., Lewis, J. M., *et al.* (1996). Nimodipine in the treatment of probable Alzheimer's disease. Results of two multicentre trials. *Clinical Drug Investigation*, 11, 4, 185–95.

Morris, J. C., Cyrus, P. A., Orazem, J., *et al.* (1998). Metrofinate benefits cognitive, behavioural, and global function in patients with Alzheimer's disease. *Neurology*, 50, 1222–30.

Mufson, E. J., Bothwell, M., and Kordower, J. H. (1989). Loss of nerve growth factor receptor-contain-ing neurons in Alzheimer's disease: A quantitative analysis across sub-regions of the basal forebrain. *Experimental Neurology*, 105, 221–32.

Mufson, E. J., Conner, J. M., and Kordower, J. H. (1995). Nerve growth factor in Alzheimer's disease — defective retrograde transport to nucleus basalis. *Neuroreport*, 6, 1063–6.

Mufson, E. J., Lavine, N., Jaffar, S., *et al.* (1997a). Reduction in p140-trkA receptor protein within the nucleus basalis and cortex in Alzheimer's disease. *Experimental Neurology*, 146, 91–103.

Mufson, E. J., Li, J-M., Sobreviela, T., and Kordower, J. H. (1997b). Decreased TrkA gene expression within basal forebrain neurons in Alzheimer's disease. *Neuroreport*, 8, 25–29.

Nyth, A. L., Gottfries, C. G., Lyby, K., *et al.* (1992). A controlled multicentre clinical study of citalo-pram and placebo in elderly depressed patients with and without concomitant dementia. *Acta Psychiatrica Scandinavia*, 86, 2, 138–45.

O'Brien, J. T., Eagger, S., and Levy, R. (1991). Effects of tetrahydroaminoacridine on liver function in patients with Alzheimer's disease. *Age and Ageing*, 20, 129–31.

Oddoze, C., Michel, B. F., Berthezene, P., *et al.* (1998). Apolipoprotein E ε4 allele predicts a positive response to tacrine in Alzheimer's disease. *Alzheimer's Reports*, 1, 13–6.

Ohkura, T., Isse, K., Akazawa, K., *et al.* (1995). Long-term estrogen replacement therapy in female patients with dementia of the Alzheimer-type: 7 case reports. *Dementia*, 6, 2, 99–107.

Olsen, L., Nordberg, A., Von Holst, H., *et al.* (1992). Nerve growth factor effects[11]C-nicotine binding, blood flow, EEG, and verbal episodic memory in an Alzheimer patient. (Case report). *Journal of Neural Transmission — Parkinson's Disease & Dementia Section*, 4, 79–95.

Ott, A., Slooter, A. J. C., Hofman, A., *et al.* (1998). Smoking and risk of dementia and Alzheimer's disease in a population-based cohort study: the Rotterdam Study. *The Lancet*, 351, 1840–3.

Paganini-Hill, A. and Henderson, V. W. (1996). Estrogen replacement therapy and risk of Alzheimer's disease. *Archives of Internal Medicine*, 156, 19, 2213–7.

Perez, P., Coll, P. M., Hempstead, B. L., *et al.* (1995). NGF binding to the trk tyrosine kinase receptor requires the extracellular immunoglobulin-like domains. *Molecular and Cellular Neuroscience*, 6, 97–105.

Poirier, J., Delisle, M. C., Quirion, R., *et al.* (1995). Apolipoprotein E4 allele as a predictor of cholinergic deficits and treatment outcome in Alzheimer disease. *Proceedings of the National Academy of Sciences (USA)*, 92, (26), 12260–4.

Prince, M., Rabe-Hesketh, S., and Brennan, P. (1998). Do antiarthritic drugs decrease the risk for cognitive decline? An analysis based on data from the MRC treatment trial of hypertension in older adults. *Neurology*, 50, 374–379.

Purves, D. (1989). *Body and Brain: a Theory of Neural Connectivity*. Oxford University press, Oxford.

Resnick, S. M., Metter, E. J., and Zonderman, A. B. (1997). Estrogen replacement therapy and longitudinal decline in visual memory. A possible protective effect? *Neurology*, 49, 1491–7.

Ridley, R. M., Barratt, N. G., and Baker, H. F. (1984*a*). Cholinergic learning deficits in the marmoset produced by scopolamine and ICV hemicholinium. P*sychopharmacology*, 83, 340–45.

Ridley, R. M., Bowes, P. M., Baker, H. F., and Crow, T. J. (1984*b*). An involvement of acetylcholine in object discrimination learning and memory in the marmoset. *Neuropsychologia*, 22, 253–63.

Ridley, R. M., Baker, H. F., Drewett, B., and Johnson, J. A. (1985). Effects of ibotenic acid lesions of the basal forebrain on serial reversal learning in marmosets. *Psychpharmacology*, 86, 438–43.

Ridley, R. M., Murray, T. K., Johnson, J. A., and Baker, H. F. (1986). Learning impairment following lesion of the basal nucleus of Meynert in the marmoset: modification by cholinergic drugs. *Brain Research*, 376, 108–16.

Riopelle, J. M., Richardson, P. M., and Verge, V. M. (1987). Distribution and characteristics of nerve growth factor binding on cholinergic neurons of rat and monkey forebrain. *Neurochemical Research*, 12, 923–8.

Robbins, T. W., Everitt, B. J., Marston, H. M., *et al.* (1989). Comparative effects of ibotenic acid and quisqualate acid induced lesions of the substantia innominata on attentional function in the rat: further implications for the role of the cholinergic neurons of the nucleus basalis in cognitive processes. *Behavioural Brain Research*, 35, 221–4.

Robertson, A. G. S., Banfield, M., Allen, S. J., Tyler, S., Bennet, G. S., Brain, S. D., Mason, G. G. F., Clarke, A. R., Naylor, R., Wilcock, G. K., Brady, L., and Dawbarn, D. (2000) Identification of the Nerve Growth Factor Binding Site on TrkA. *Proteins, Structure, Function and Genetics*. submitted

Robinson, R. C., Radziejewski, C., Stuart, D. I., and Jones, E. Y. (1995). Structure of the brain-derived neurotrophic factor/neurotrophin 3 heterodimer. *Biochemistry*, 34, 4139–46.

Robinson, R. C., Radziejewski, C., Stuart, D. I., and Jones, E. Y. (1996). Crystals of the neurotrophins. *Protein Science*, l5, 973–7.

Rodrigues-Tebar, A., Dechant, G., Gotz, R., and Barde, Y-A. (1992). Binding of neurotrophin-3 to its neuronal receptors and interactions with nerve growth factor and brain-derived growth factor. *European Molecular Biology Organisation Journal*, 11, 917–22.

Rockwood, K., Beattie, B. L., Eastwood, M. R., *et al.* (1997). A randomized, controlled trial of linopirdine in the treatment of Alzheimer's disease. *Canadian Journal of Neurological Sciences*, 24, 2, 140–5.

Rogers, S. L. and Friedhoff, L. T. (1998). Long-term efficacy and safety of donepezil in the treatment of A;zheimer's disease: an interim analysis of the results of a US multicentre open label extension study. *European Neuropsychopharmacology*, 8, 67–75.

Rogers, S. L., Friedhoff, L. T., the Donepezil Study Group. (1996). The efficacy and safety of donepezil in patients with Alzheimer's disease: results of a US multicenter, randomized, double-blind, placebo-controlled trial. *Dementia*, 7, 293–303.

Rogers, S. L., Doody, R. S., Mohs, R. C., *et al.* and the Donepezil Study Group. (1998*a*). Donepezil improves cognition and global function in Alzheimer's disease. A 15-week, double-blind, placebo-controlled study. *Archives of Internal Medicine*, 158, 1021–31.

Rogers, S. L., Farlow, M. R., Doody, R. S., *et al.* and the Donepezil Study Group. (1998*b*). A 24-week, double-blind, placebo-controlled trial of donepezil in patients with Alzheimer's disease. *Neurology*, 50, 136–45.

Roth, M., Mountjoy, C. Q., Amrein, R., and the international collaborative study group. (1996). Moclobemide in elderly patients with cognitive decline and depression. An international double-blind, placebo-controlled trial. *British Journal of Psychiatry*, 168, 149–57.

Rowin, J. and Lewis S. L. (1996). Spontaneous bilateral subdural haematomas associated with chronic ginkgo biloba ingestion. *Neurology*, 46, 1775–6.

Saloman, A. R., Marcinowski, K. J., Friedland, R. P., and Zagorski, M. G. (1996). Nicotine inhibits amyloid formation by the beta-peptide. *Biochemistry*, 35, 42, 13568–78.

Sano, M., Ernesto, C., Thomas, R. G., *et al.* (1997). A controlled trial of selegiline, alpha-tocopherol, or both as treatment for Alzheimer's disease. *The New England Journal of Medicine*, 336, 17, 1216–22.

Schatteman, G. C., Gibbs, L., Lanahan, A. A., *et al.* (1988). Expression of NGF receptors in the developing and adult primate central nervous system. *Journal of Neuroscience*, 8, 860–73.

Schneider, L. S., Farlow, M. R., Henderson, V. W., and Pogoda, J. M. (1996). Effects of estrogen replacement therapy on response to tacrine in patients with Alzheimer's disease. *Neurology*, 46, 6, 1580–4.

Schneider, R. and Schweiger, M. (1991). A novel modular mosaic of cell adhesion motifs in the extra-cellular domains of the neurogenic trk and trkB tyrosine kinase receptors. *Oncogene*, 6, 1807–11.

Schwartz, B. L., Hashtroudi, S., Herting, R. L., *et al.* (1996). D-cycloserine enhances implicit memory in Alzheimer's patients. *Neurology*, 42, 2, 420–4.

Scott, J., Selby, M., Urdea, M., *et al.* (1983). Isolation and nucleotide sequence of a cDNA encoding the sequence of mouse nerve growth factor. *Nature*, 302, 538–40.

Seiler. M. and Schwab, M. E. (1984). Specific retrograde transport of nerve growth factor (NGF) from neocortex to nucleus basalis in the rat. *Brain Research*, 300, 33–9.

Shimohama, S., Akaike, A., and Kimura, J. (1996). Nicotine-induced protection against glutamate cytotoxicity. Nicotinic cholinergic receptor-mediated inhibition of nitric oxide formation. *Annals of the New York Academy of Sciences*, 777, 356–61.

Sims, N. R., Bowen, D. M. Allen, S. J., *et al.* (1983). Presynaptic cholinergic dysfunction in patients with dementia. *Journal of Neurochemistry*, 40, 503–9.

Singh, M., Meyer, E. M., Millard, W. J., Simpkins, J. W. (1994). Ovarian steroid deprovation results in a reversible learning impairment and compromised cholinergic function in female Sprague-Dawley rats. *Brain Research*, **644**, 305–12.

Singh, M., Meyer, E. M., and Simpkins, J. W. (1995). The effect of ovariectomy and estradiol replacement on brain-derived neurotrophic factor messenger ribonucleic acid expression in cortical and hippocampal brain regions of female Sprague-Dawley rats. *Endocrinology*, **136**, 2320–4.

Smeyne, R. J., Klein, R., Schnapp, A., *et al.* (1994). Severe sensory and sympathetic neuropathies in mice carrying a disrupted Trk/NGF receptor gene. *Nature*, **368**, 246–9.

Smith, M. A., Perry, G., Richey, P. L., *et al.* (1996). Oxidative damage in Alzheimer's. *Nature*, **382**, 120–1.

Snaedal, J., Johannesson, T., Jonsson, J. E., and Gylfadottir, G. (1996). The effects of nicotine in dermal plaster on cogntive functions in patients with Alzheimer's disease. *Dementia*, **7**, 47–52.

Sobreviela, T., Clary, D. O., Reichardt, L. F., *et al.* (1994). TrkA-immunoreactive profiles in the central nervous system: Colocalisation with neurons containing p75 nerve growth factor receptor, choline acetyltransferase, and serotonin. *Journal of Comparative Neurology*, **350**, 587–611.

Spiegel, R. (1991). Cholinergic drugs, affective disorders and dementia: problems of clinical research. *Acta Psychiatrica Scandinavica*, Suppl **366**, 47–51.

Steininger, T'L., Wainer, B. H., Klein, R., *et al.* (1993). High affinity nerve growth factor receptor (trk) is localised in cholinergic neurons of the basal forebrain and striatum in the adult rat brain. *Brain Research*, **612**, 330–5.

Stephens, R. M., Loeb, D. M., Copeland, T. D., *et al.* (1994). Trk receptors use redundant signal transduction pathways involving SHC and PLC-gamma 1 to mediate NGF responses. *Neuron*, **12**, 691–705.

Stewart, W. F., Kawas, C., Corrada, M., and Metter, E. J. (1997). Risk of Alzheimer's disease and duration of NSAID use. *Neurology*, **48**, 626–32.

Summers, W. K., Majovski, L. V., Marsh, G. M., *et al.* (1986). Oral tetrahydroaminoacridine in long-term treatment of senile dementia, Alzheimer type. *New England Journal of Medicine*, **315**, 1241–45.

Tang, M. -X., Jacobs, D., Stern, Y., *et al.* (1996). Effect of oestrogen during menopause on risk and age at onset of Alzheimer's disease. *The Lancet*, **348**, 429–32.

Thal, L. J., Schwartz, G., Sano, M., *et al.* (1996). A multicenter double-blind study of controlled-release physostigmine for the treatment of symptoms secondary to Alzheimer's disease. *Neurology*, **47**, 6, 1389–95.

Thoenen, H. (1991). The changing scene of neurotrophic factors. *Trends in Neuroscience*, **14**, 165–70.

Thoenen, H. and Barde, Y-A. (1980). Physiology of nerve growth factor. *Physiological Reviews*, **60**, 1284–335.

Thoenen, H., Bandtlow, C., and Heumann, R. (1987). The physiological function of nerve growth factor in the central nervous system: comparison with the periphery. *Reviews in Physiology, Biochemistry and Pharmacology*, **109**, 145–78.

Tolbert, S. R. and Fuller, M. A. (1996). Selegiline in treatment of behavioural and cognitive symptoms of Alzheimer's disease. *The Annals of Pharmacotherapy*, **30**, 10, 1122–9.

Treanor, J. J. S., Dawbarn, D., Allen, S. J., *et al.* (1991). Nerve growth factor receptor binding in normal and Alzheimer's disease basal forebrain. *Neuroscience Letters*, **121**, 73–6.

Turner, J. J., Hodges, H., Sinden, J. G., and Grey, J. J. (1992). Comparison of radial maze performance of rats after ibotenate and quisqualate lesions of the forebrain cholinergic projection system: effects of pharmacological challenge and changes in training regime. *Behavioural Pharmacology*, **3**, 765–9.

Ulrich, A., Grey, A., Berman, C., and Dull, T. J. (1983). Human β-nerve growth factor sequence highly homologous to that of mouse. *Nature*, **303**, 821–5.

Ulrich, J., Johannson-Locher, G., Seiler, W. O., and Stahelin, H. B. (1997). Does smoking protect from Alzheimer's disease? Alzheimer-type changes in 301 unselected brains from patients with known smoking history. *Acta Neuropathologica*, **94**, 5, 450–4.

Ultsch, M. H., Wiesmann, C., Simmons, L. C., *et al.* (1999). Crystal structure of the neurotrophin-binding domain of TrkA, TrkB and TrkC. *Journal of Molecular Biology*, 290, 149–59.

Urfer, R., Tsoulfas, P., Occonnel, L., *et al.* (1995). An immunoglobulin-like domain determines the specificity of neurotrophin receptors. *European Molecular biology Organisation Journal*, 14, 2795–805.

Vale, S. (1998). Subarachnoid haemorrhage associated with ginkgo biloba. *The Lancet*, 352, 36.

Watkins, P. B., Zimmerman, H. J., Knapp, M. J., *et al.* (1994). Hepatotoxic effects of tacrine administration in patients with Alzheimer's disease. *Journal of the American Medical Association*, 271, 992–8.

Wenk, G. L., Markowska, A. L., and Olton, D. S. (1989). Basal forebrain lesions and memory: alteration in neurotensin not acetylcholine may cause amnesia. *Behavioural Neuroscience*, 103, 765–9.

Weyer, G., Babej-Dolle, R. M., Hadler, D., *et al.* (1997). A controlled study of 2 doses of idebenone in the treatment of Alzheimer's disease. *Neuropsychobiology*, 36, 2, 73–82.

Wilcock, G. K., Scott, M., Pearsall, T., *et al.* (1993). Galanthamine and the treatment of Alzheimer's disease. *International Journal of Geriatric Psychiatry*, 8, 781–2.

Wilcock, G. K. and Wilkinson, D. (1997). Galanthamine hydrobromide: Interim results of a group comparative, placebo-controlled study of efficacy and safety in patients with a diagnosis of senile dementia of the Alzheimer type. In *Alzheimer's disease: Biology, diagnosis and therapeutics*, (ed. K. Iqbal, B. Winblad, T. Nishimura, M. Takeda, and H. M. Wisniewski), pp. 661–4. Wiley, Chichester.

Will, B. and Hefti, F. (1985). Behavioural and neurochemical effects of chronic intraventricular injections of nerve growth factor in adult rats with fimbria lesions. *Behavioural Brain Research*, 17, 17–24.

Williams, L. R., Varon, S., Peterson, G. M., *et al.* (1987). Continuous infusion of nerve growth factor prevents basal forebrain neuronal death after fimbria fornix transection. *Proceedings of the National Academy of Sciences (USA)*, 83, 9231–5.

Wilson, A. L., Langley, L. K., Monley, J., *et al.* (1995). Nicotine patches in Alzheimer's disease: Pilot study on learning, memory, and safety. *Pharmacology, Biochemistry and Behavior*, 51, 509–14.

Wilson, K., Bowen, D., Francis, P., and Tyrell, P. (1991). Effect of central cholinergic stimulation on regional cerebral blood flow in Alzheimer's disease. *British Journal of Psychiatry*, 158, 558–62.

Winkler, J., Ramirez, G. A., Kuhn, H. G., *et al.* (1997). Reversible schwann cell hyperplasia and sprouting of sensory and sympathetic neurites after intraventricular administration of nerve growth factor. *Annals of Neurology*, 41, 82–93.

Woolley, C. S. and McEwen. B. S. (1994). Estradiol regulates hippocampal dendritic spine density via an N-methyl-D-aspartate receptor-dependent mechanism. *Journal of Neuroscience*, 14, 7680–7.

Chapter 15

Current perspectives and future directions

Stephen I. Gracon and Mark R. Emmerling

15.1 Introduction

This chapter provides an overview of near-term opportunities and long-term strategies for the discovery and development of drugs to treat, to delay, and to prevent the expression of symptoms of Alzheimer's disease (AD).

AD is a chronic, progressive degenerative disease of the ageing brain with an insidious onset and prolonged course. It afflicts an estimated 1 in 10 individuals over the age of 65 and approximately 1 in every 2 over 85. There is no reliable predictor of who is at risk for AD and when they will develop symptoms. Similarly there is no reliable predictor of who is not at risk; therefore, everyone is at risk. AD reduces life expectancy and dramatically reduces quality of life for patients and their families. It consumes an inordinate amount of a family's finances in addition to health care resources. AD is the fourth leading cause of death in the United States and kills more than 100 000 people per year. Today there are an estimated 4 million Americans with AD. The direct and indirect costs of care exceed US$100 billion annually. The single largest expense is nursing home care that averages US$42 000 per patient per year.

The prevalence and incidence of AD doubles every five years after age 60 through to 90 and beyond. Today the age group at risk (those over 65 years) is the fastest growing segment of the world population and by the year 2050 there will be more than 14 million Americans with AD, and in excess of 30 million patients world-wide. Most of the individuals who will have AD in the year 2050 are alive today and for many the underlying biological, if not the pathological, cascade has already begun.

Treatment of AD must be a 'therapeutic imperative' for the first decade of the new millennium. It is unrealistic to expect a cure, but a treatment that could reliably delay the onset of AD by five years would be an extraordinary achievement. Such a treatment would reduce the incidence and prevalence of AD by half; yet there would still remain an enormous unmet medical need (www.alz.org).

15.2 Current perspectives

Table 15.1 lists a number of cholinergic treatments evaluated in AD. Most of the cholinesterase inhibitors 'work' and quite consistently produce statistically significant, if

Table 15.1 Cholinergics in AD

Sponsor	Generic	Marketed	Status
Acetylcholinesterase inhibitors			
Parke-Davis	tacrine	Cognex	Approved US & International
Esai/Pfizer	donepezil	Aricept	Approved US & International
Novartis International	rivastigmine	Exelon	Approvable US; Approved
Forest	physostigmine	(Synapton)	Not approved
Bayer	metrifonate	(Bilarcil)	Under review
Shire/Jansen	galanthamine	(Nivalin) (Reminyl)	Under review US & International
Hoechst	velnacrine	–	d/c
Mediolanum	eptastigmine	–	d/c
AstraZeneca	quilostigmine	–	d/c
Layton Bioscience	methanesulfonyl fluoride	–	in development
Muscarinic agonists			
HMR/Parke-Davis	milameline	–	d/c
Parke-Davis	CI-1017	–	Phase 1
Lilly	xanomeline	–	d/c
Lundbeck	LU 25–109	–	d/c
Boehringer Ingelheim	talsaclidine	–	d/c
SKB	sabcomeline	–	d/c
Forest	AF-102B	–	d/c
Yamanouchi	YM-796	–	unknown
Nicotinic agonists			
Abbott	AB-418	–	d/c
Reynolds/Rhone Poulenc	RJR-2403 metanicotine		in development
Sibia	SIB 1553A	–	unknown
Taiho			
	GTS-21	–	unknown

not clinically significant, results versus placebo in patients with AD. The effect of the cholinesterase inhibitors is symptomatic and it remains speculative whether this class of drugs can alter the underlying progression of disease. Regardless, Aricept and Exelon are being evaluated for their potential to delay the onset of symptoms of AD in 'at risk' populations.

In contrast to the anticholinesterases, none of the muscarinic agonists or nicotinic agonists tested to date have shown clinical efficacy. This suggests that either the agonist approach is futile, an agonist with the 'right' profile has yet to be tested, or the agonists tested have not been administered 'in a physiologically relevant manner' to receptors.

Beyond cholinergic treatments a number of studies are evaluating the potential of anti-inflammatories and oestrogen to treat and/or prevent AD. This includes the Alzheimer's disease cooperative studies of prednisone and oestrogen, Searle/Monsanto evaluations of celecoxib, a cyclooxygenase-2 (COX-2) inhibitor, and Conpharm evaluations of Reumacon (an anti-inflammatory) in patients with disease. Merck is investigating Vioxx, a cox-2 inhibitor, and Wyeth-Ayerst, premarin in individuals at risk for disease.

Roche's lazabemide, an inhibitor of monoamine oxidase B with antioxidant properties, was recently discontinued for development for AD. However, the antioxidant gingko biloba (Schwabe), the glutamate-antagonist memantine (Merz), and the adenosine reuptake inhibitor propentofylline (HMR) continue in development. It is difficult to survey the literature and popular press and come up with a realistic and accurate perspective on all the drugs which may be in development for AD. In general, Phase 1 of clinical development, consisting of single and multiple dose studies to determine oral bioavailability and pharmacokinetics and the maximum well-tolerated dose for study in Phase 2, takes one year. Phase 2 of clinical development usually involves dose response studies in the target patient population to determine whether or not the drug is 'effective and safe' and whether it merits continued development. This phase can last 1–3 years. Phase 3 studies are carried out in substantially larger patient samples designed to confirm efficacy and safety of the drug in populations of patients similar to those who may be treated after approval. Phase 3 can add an additional 1–3 years of development time and more when findings in Phase 3 are anything less than anticipated from Phase 2. There can be extended periods of time where no new information is reaching the public and development status becomes uncertain.

Newer and different agents include neotrofin, a 'neurotrophic' agent which restores function in animal models of ageing, brain and spinal cord injury, and is reported in press releases as effective in cognitive and behavioural domains in short term (1 month) studies in patients with AD (www.neotherapeutics.com). CX516 (Cortex), an ampakine, which 'enhances' glutamate neurotransmission also shows promise in memory enhancement along with cerebrolysin (Ebewe). Although early results are tantalizing we have learned that clinical validity only comes from studies replicated over longer treatment periods in larger patient samples, which takes time. Producing a statistically significant effect is no longer adequate, since the magnitude and the duration of the treatment effect and their impact on major disease milestones are important for approval and reimbursement.

Researchers, health care providers, patients, and families are understandably frustrated by the limited progress made in the treatment of AD. There is a sense of uneasiness that treatment advances for AD might mirror those for Parkinson's disease in that decades may pass between introduction of the first generation of symptomatic treatments and the new generation of disease modifying agents. This concern is justified for AD since it has taken more than a quarter century just to explore the cholinergic hypothesis of AD. Although of modest therapeutic benefit, systematic dissection of the cholinergic system did lead to the first effective symptomatic treatments for AD.

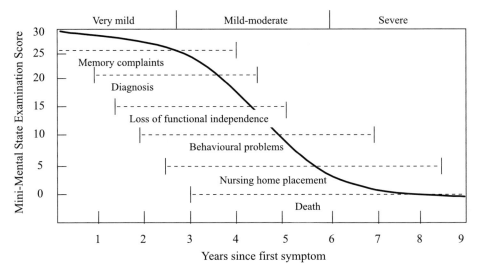

Fig. 15.1 The natural history of the clinical phases of AD, as measured by mini mental state examination score, from initial symptoms until death.

The core symptoms of AD are cognitive, while psychiatric, behavioural, and functional deficits, encompassing basic and complex activities of daily living (ADL), accompany the cognitive decline. Figure 15.1 illustrates a composite of the natural history of the clinical phases of AD from initial symptoms until death. Mini mental state examination score (MMSE; Folstein *et al.* 1975) is displayed on the vertical axis and time in years from first symptom is shown horizontally. The time from initial symptoms of short term memory impairment to diagnosis averages more than 3 years. Eventually, cognitive decline becomes obvious and leads to loss of concentration and confusion with disorientation to time and place and eventually loss of functional independence and ability to carry out complex and then even basic activities of self-care (Heyman *et al.* 1987; Drachman *et al.* 1990; Severson *et al.* 1994; Jost and Grossberg 1995; Piccini *et al.* 1995; Levy *et al.* 1996). There is evidence that the degree of specific regional pathology correlates with neuropsychologic function profile (Kanne *et al.* 1998).

Depression and anxiety are common early in the clinical course in more mildly impaired patients who may have insight into their cognitive loss (Levy *et al.* 1996). More troublesome neuropsychiatric symptoms such as delusions, hallucinations, paranoia, agitation, hostility, and aggression generally occur later and in more severely impaired patients (Heyman *et al.* 1987; Levy *et al.* 1996) reflecting more extensive pathology and involvement and imbalance of numerous neurotransmitter systems. These behavioural symptoms affect more than 70% of AD patients, are unpredictable and can wax and wane throughout the disease course (Levy *et al.* 1996).

These symptoms are not specific to AD and are reminiscent of symptoms in schizophrenia. Typical antipsychotic neuroleptics, such as haloperidol have been only modestly effective when used in AD patients and may result in moderate to severe extrapyramidal symptoms in a subgroup of patients (Devanand *et al.* 1998). The newer antipsychotics, Lilly's Zyprexa (olanzapine; American College of Neuropsychopharmacology (ACNP) Dec 1998), Janssen's Risperdal (risperidone; PINK SHEET Jan 1999) and Zeneca's Seroquel (quetiapine; ACNP Dec 1998) show promise in treating these behavioural symptoms in AD. Their ability to improve cognitive function must still be evaluated. In the United States three out of four patients will eventually enter a nursing home and remain there for an average of three years until death (Welch *et al.* 1992; Brodaty *et al.* 1993). The major predictors of nursing home placement are severe disability, incontinence, and behavioural problems (Knopman *et al.* 1988; Drachman *et al.* 1990). Until the time of nursing home placement the caregiver must bear the enormous task of 24 hour supervision and care.

15.3 **Challenges in Alzheimer's disease drug discovery**

Although the clinical course can last a decade or longer the underlying neurochemical, biochemical, and neuropathological changes begin years, if not decades, before symptoms appear (Fig. 15.2). The onset of symptoms may correspond with failure of compensatory processes. The pathology at the time the disease is clinically recognizable represents a cascade of pathologies that are much broader than were present when the disease process was first initiated (Mann *et al.* 1988). A much more detailed natural history of the biochemical, biological and structural changes from the pre-symptomatic stage through symptom development will be needed in the future to select patients for clinical trials and monitor the effectiveness of a new generation of treatments aimed at the pathological process.

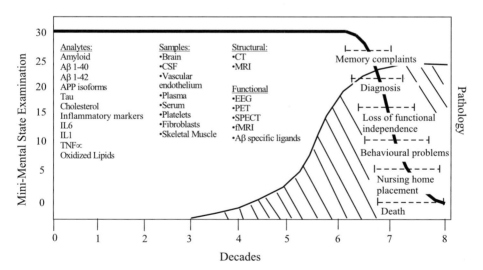

Fig. 15.2 Neurochemical, biochemical, and neuropathological markers of AD. Mini mental state examination score is shown as a line. Neuropathology, as measured by presence of neurofibrillary tangles (tau) and senile and diffuse plaques (Aβ1–42) is represented by the blocked curve. Appearance of symptoms begins with decline of mini mental score, but pathology has appeared perhaps decades before.

Optimism for new drug discovery in AD comes from advances in the understanding and treatment of cardiovascular disease that have taken place over the last quarter century. These advances in treatment occurred because of the identification, characterization, and validation of highly relevant and accessible biological markers, like serum cholesterol levels, against clinical endpoints. These markers signal risk in advance of disease and have provided an expanded array of potential drug targets for highly effective new preventive therapies.

A unifying hypothesis for the pathophysiology of AD in the ageing brain is emerging (Emmerling *et al.* 1999) that has the potential to change the treatment paradigm from symptomatic to disease modifying. The amyloidocentric model (Fig. 15.3) is the template for discussion of drug discovery strategies. The goal is early identification of those individuals at risk, early intervention, and disease prevention. Recent efforts to identify those individuals at immediate risk for AD has focused on mild cognitive impairment (MCI). MCI patients show modest cognitive problems but fail to qualify clinically as AD (Petersen *et al.* 1999). Once identified, MCI individuals typically reach the clinical criteria for AD sometime in the next 5 years and are therefore at immediate risk. Neuroimaging methods and measurements of relevant biomarkers of AD (e.g. Aβ, tau, and markers of oxidant stress) indicate that patients with MCI begin to exhibit some of the pathological hallmarks of AD. In general, imaging methods show a reduction in hippocampal volume and a shortening of entorhinal cortex in MCI patients compared to non-demented controls (Jack *et al.* 1999; Bobinski *et al.* 1999). On average, the CSF levels of tau are somewhat elevated (Imaging and biological markers for diagnosis and progression of Alzheimer's disease meeting, NIA

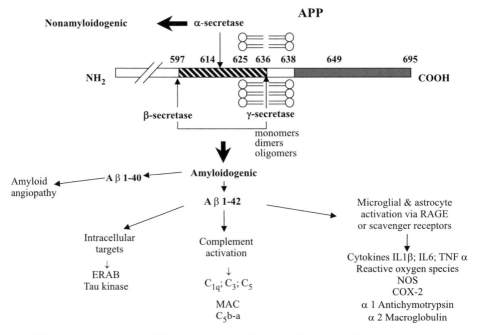

Fig. 15.3 Amyloidocentric model suggests areas of intervention in the disease process.

Workshop, Sept. 27–28, 1999, Bethesda, MD) and Aβ1–42 decreased (Andreasen *et al.* 1999; Jensen *et al.* 1999) in these individuals relative to controls, but not to the same extent as in AD. Serum levels of Aβ1–42 are also increased with MCI and the greater the level the increased likelihood of AD (Mayeux *et al.* 1999). Although preliminary, these results suggest that prodromal stages of AD can be detected, allowing for earlier implementation of therapies. Ultimately, these biomarkers may help to make an accurate identification of 'at-risk' patients, to provide predictable rates for conversion to disease and to act as surrogate markers of drug efficacy.

Ultimately, understanding AD will come from a systematic dissection of the mechanisms which cause the disease; discovering the multiple factors, genetic and environmental, which confer risk or protection by delaying the manifestation of the disease or modifying pathological processes of AD. Focusing on understanding the natural history of the ageing brain and AD at the level of its underlying pathology is key. New treatments will be evaluated in amyloid precursor protein (APP) transgenic animals in order to determine concentration–response relationships at the level of the centrally targeted event(s) (Games *et al.* 1995; Hsiao *et al.* 1996; Johnson-Wood *et al.* 1997; Schenk *et al.* 1999). Aβ1–42, or events associated with the accumulation of Aβ1–42, are critical for the development of AD. The questions are why does Aβ accumulate in the ageing brain and if accumulation were prevented, or if deposited amyloid were removed, would this result in prevention of disease in the first case and symptomatic improvement in the second?

In the near term, epidemiological studies have suggested new therapeutic opportunities employing non-steroidal anti-inflammatory drugs (McGeer and Rogers 1992; Rogers *et al.* 1993; Aisen and Davis 1994; Breitner 1996; McGeer *et al.* 1996), and oestrogen replacement (Birge 1997). If these agents prove effective, then, more important for future drug discovery, is an understanding of the precise mechanisms by which the pathological process is changed by drug treatment. Clinical studies must attempt to identify the relevant biological markers being altered by therapeutic intervention and their contribution to the specific pathology of AD.

Finding a treatment with the potential to prevent AD is the first step, proving it to be effective will be difficult. There is no diagnostic test for AD. Brain imaging, electroencephalogram (EEG), and genotyping may be useful adjuncts in diagnosis in cases with unusual presentation but are not definitive. Confirmation of the diagnosis comes from brain biopsy or histopathological examination after death that may be years if not decades removed in time from clinical diagnosis. Even the pathological diagnosis relies upon an increased expression of pathology beyond that which may occur in cognitively normal age-matched controls. In fact, normal controls may simply be on the same track but slightly behind those individuals expressing symptoms.

What are the biochemical processes that one could target within this pathological cascade? When during the pathogenesis of the disease must the intervention take place? To what degree must one alter the biochemical process to effect the desired clinical outcome? Who is at risk? When will they express clinical disease? When must treatment start? What are the treatable symptoms? What are the treatable pathologies? What are the biological markers for disease progression and treatment response? What are the risks of targeting these processes?

Developing cholinesterase inhibitors will appear to have been easy compared to the difficulties posed in developing compounds that alter pathological events.

15.4 **Pathology of Alzheimer's disease**

Gross pathological findings include reduced brain weight, brain atrophy, cortical atrophy, hippocampal atrophy, and selective loss of the medial temporal lobe. The histopathological correlates are synaptic loss, neuronal cell death, granulovacuolar degeneration, amyloid plaques and amyloid angiopathy, activated microglia and astrocytes, and neurofibrillary tangles consisting of paired helical filaments (PHF) of hyperphosphorylated tau protein and glycolipids (Feany and Dickson 1996; Goux *et al.* 1996; Wisniewski *et al.* 1997; Mann *et al.* 1988).

The most consistent change in AD brains is cholinergic loss in the CA1 region of the hippocampus, however the timing of this event and its relation to onset of symptoms has yet to be resolved. Cholinergic cells project from the basal forebrain to the cortex and hippocampus, and their loss is thought to contribute to memory and cognitive changes. Cholinergic neurons appear to be especially sensitive to Aβ compared to other cell types. This suggests neurochemical phenotype may play a central role in the early evolution of AD pathology (Olesen *et al.* 1998). As the pathology extends other neurodegenerative processes come into play and other neurotransmitter pathways are then affected.

15.5 **Genetic causes of AD**

The pathological lesions among patients with Down syndrome as well as patients with autosomal dominant mutations leading to AD appear indistinguishable from those in patients with early onset familial or late onset sporadic AD. Many non-demented elderly patients come to autopsy with significant pathology resembling AD (Lue *et al.* 1996; Mackenzie *et al.* 1996; Morris *et al.* 1996; Leverenz and Raskind 1998). These findings support the hypothesis that there is in fact a final common pathway between genetically determined AD, familial AD (FAD), sporadic AD, Down dementia, and ageing. It may be that the genetic background against which the pathology is expressed determines whether dementia occurs.

Genetic mutations account for less than 5% of all cases of AD. The APP gene is located on chromosome 21 and there are eight reported mutations of this gene that cause AD or amyloidosis. However, all known genetic causes of AD result in an increase in expression of Aβ peptide, Aβ1–42. Presenilin-1 (*PS1*) mutations on chromosome 14 account for up to 50% of early onset cases of FAD while *PS2* mutations on chromosome 1 are rare, having been identified in only a small number of families world-wide (Mann *et al.* 1996; Hardy 1997). These are autosomal dominant mutations. The exact mechanism by which PS mutations increase Aβ1–42 remains unclear but PS mutations most likely affect APP metabolism. PS may be a γ secretase and cleaves proteins other than APP like Notch protein. It is suggested that mutations in PS1 increase γ secretase activity and increase amyloidogenic fragments. In some mice models expressing these mutations it is reported that loss of neuronal or synaptic function precedes plaque formation (Hsaio *et al.* 1996; Borchelt 1998). This suggests that it is not only fully aggregated forms of Aβ that are toxic. A pathogenic role of soluble Aβ in AD brains is further indicated by recent work of Rogers and colleagues showing that the level of soluble Aβ correlates strongly with synaptophysin loss in AD brains (Lue *et al.* 1999).

However, Aβ alone can not explain AD pathology. Years or even decades before the diagnosis of AD, increases in Aβ1–42 are seen in brain, cerebrospinal fluid (CSF), and plasma. Diffuse plaques may be present for years or decades and not cause a cascade of pathological changes (Iwatsubo *et al.* 1995).The process of fibrilization/aggregation of Aβ is a nidus for generating the classic pathology of AD.

15.6 **Down syndrome**

Down syndrome occurs in approximately 1 in 1000 live births. It is the result of trisomy 21, there are three copies of chromosome 21, which includes the *APP* region. By age 12 Down patients have deposition of diffuse plaques which represent Aβ1–42 in a non-aggregated state (Iwatsubo *et al.* 1995). By the 3rd or 4th decade virtually all Down patients develop widespread AD pathology including neuritic plaques and neurofibrillary tangles (NFT). Clinical expression of dementia occurs about a decade later. Lesions are present before age 30 in about 15% of Down patients and half of these individuals are demented.

The importance of APP in disease expression is highlighted by a single case report in which a 78-year old woman with Down syndrome died with no evidence of dementia based upon thorough neuropsychologic testing (Prasher *et al.* 1998). There was no evidence of hippocampal atrophy on magnetic resonance imaging (MRI) and no evidence of AD pathology at autopsy or on histopathological examination. Further genetic analysis revealed that the gene sequence for the *APP* region was only present on two of the three copies of chromosome 21. These rare genetic events have the potential to provide insight to disease in a wider population of patients.

15.7 **Amyloid in Alzheimer's disease**

Amyloidosis in the brain is a central pathological event. Genetic mutations in APP or in PS protein lead to increased Aβ1–42 production and almost guarantee the development of AD in carriers. Once deposited, amyloid plaques of three progressive types are described (Gomez-Isla *et al.* 1997; Terry 1997). The earliest are diffuse plaques that are not associated with synaptic loss, neuronal injury, or reactive cell types. Second and most important pathologically are the neuritic plaques that have an aggregated amyloid core and evoke synaptic loss, reactive astrocytes, and microglia. These plaques also contain the remnants of degenerating neurons. The final stage is a mature or burnt out plaque which consists of an isolated dense amyloid core which now evokes little response from surrounding tissue. The underlying assumption is that the three plaque forms represent an evolution of plaque pathology determined by the local environment.

Neuritic plaques are made up of a central core of Aβ peptide, mainly Aβ1–42, heparan sulphate proteoglycan, alpha 1 antichymotrypsin, alpha 2 macroglobulin (α2M), apolipoprotein E (apoE), complement factors C1q, C3d, and C4d and components of cells dying directly or indirectly as a result of Aβ fibrillization and amyloid plaque formation (Cummings *et al.* 1998).

Amyloid peptides are derived from cleavage (proteolysis) of the larger APP parent molecule (Fig. 15.3). There are three putative enzymes (secretases) involved. The α secretase cleavage takes place at or near the plasma membrane and the product of this cleavage is non amyloidogenic. Products of α-cleavage have even been suggested to be neurotrophic or neuroprotective.

The β and γ secretase cleavage takes place at the level of endosomal/lysosomal structures, golgi derived vesicles, and ER and generates peptides either 40 or 42 amino acids in length. The levels of Aβ1–42 in patients with AD are estimated to be between 2 and 6 times that of controls but with considerable overlap, therefore implying interactions with other factors important to disease expression (Roher unpublished; Leverenz and Raskind 1998). Aβ alone is not sufficient for the expression of the pathology and clinical symptoms of AD. The amount of Aβ1–40 is *APOE* genotype dependent and if the patient does not carry an ε4 allele, the levels of Aβ1–40 in AD patients are indistinguishable from controls (Roher unpublished; Ishii *et al.* 1997).

Soluble Aβ monomers are consumed during formation of so called protofibrils, an intermediate in the formation of fibrillar β-amyloid. These protofibrils provide a nidus that accelerates conversion to fibrils and thence to plaques. The nature of the environment in which this occurs can delay, prevent, or accelerate fibril formation (Mantyh *et al.* 1993; Gearing *et al.* 1995; Webster *et al.* 1995; Alvarez *et al.* 1997; Castillo *et al.* 1997; Choo-Smith *et al.* 1997; Pirttila *et al.* 1997; Wilson and Binder 1997).

Establishing the natural history of formation of fibrils in the brain will be critical to the study of newer treatment approaches. Amyloid must not only be quantified but its nature be determined. The goal is to define the pharmacokinetics, metabolism, and pharmacodynamics of APP and its cleavage products in the brain and to develop strategies to modify this process to advantage.

15.8 **Consequences of amyloidogenesis**

Aβ can generate an inflammatory cascade causing complement activation resulting in increases in C1q, C3, C5, and membrane attack complex (MAC) (Bradt *et al.* 1996; Breitner 1996; Emmerling *et al.* 1997; Forloni *et al.* 1997; Watson *et al.* 1997; Webster *et al.* 1997*a, b*; Hu *et al.* 1998). Aβ can also cause microglial and astrocyte activation possibly through RAGE (receptor for advanced glycation endproducts) or Scavenger receptors, leading to generation of cytokines (IL-1β, IL-6, TNFα), reactive oxygen species (ROS), and cox-2 expression, alpha 1 antichymotrypsin, and α2M (El Khoury *et al.* 1996; Yan *et al.* 1996).

At the level of blood vessels Aβ1–40 leads to amyloid angiopathy while Aβ1–42 can interact with endothelial cells. Aβ can cause changes in vascular endothelium and changes in vasoactivity locally (Perry *et al.* 1997; Selwyn *et al.* 1997).

Aβ alone can suppress acetylcholine synthesis and may be responsible for some of the memory complaints observed in early AD (Hoshi *et al.* 1997). *In vitro* studies suggest that virtually any cellular insult is rendered worse by the presence of increasing concentrations of Aβ peptide (Mucke *et al.* 1995, 1996; Zhang *et al.* 1997). In stroke and head injury there may be massive over expression of Aβ1–42, and even minor insults to vascular endothelial cells can result in localized increased expression of Aβ1–42 (Zhang *et al.* 1997). It is the nature of the local environment in which the Aβ is produced that may be determining whether or not there is a pathological cascade.

15.9 **Genetic-modifiers**

Approximately 50% of patients recruited for Phase 2 and 3 clinical trials have a family history of AD or dementia in first degree relatives. The risk for AD is 2–4 fold higher among individuals with a first degree relative with AD and without known genetic risk factors (Mohs *et al.* 1987). Clinical trials of patients with AD and those at risk for AD provide an ideal setting in which to collect DNA from patients and spouses and other family members and collect longitudinal samples for proteomic determinations which could provide early markers of disease expression and targets for intervention.

Among 180 first-degree relatives of patients with late onset AD there was a highly significant increase in both Aβ1–40 and 1–42. An Aβ level greater than 190 pmol occurred in 34% of first degree relatives but only 7% of controls. Families with high Aβ had high values in three generations. Spouses of these patients did not show increases to help rule out an environmental effect (Graff-Radford *et al.* 1998). This type of data is critical for future drug development strategies.

Other chromosomes have been reported to alter the risk of developing AD. Chromosome 6 human leukocyte antigen (HLA), known to play a role in immune response, has been associated with earlier onset of AD. Chromosome 12 α2M may be involved in Aβ clearance and if inhibited reduces clearance. Polymorphisms in α, β, and γ secretases or in the α2M low density lipoprotein (LDL) receptor-related protein (LRP) may all be important in determining expression of AD. These genetic modulators will be examined as more DNA samples are collected and analytical approaches to identifying risk-modifying genes are resolved.

The single most important modifier of disease expression identified to date in sporadic and FAD is the *APOE* ε4 allele on chromosome 19. It was identified as candidate gene because of the increase in apoE levels observed in the CSF of AD patients and genotype dependent differential binding to Aβ (Pericak-Vance *et al.* 1991; Corder *et al.* 1993). The presence of the ε4 allele is a risk factor for both early and late onset AD as well as in Down syndrome but not apparently in other non-AD dementias, such as Parkinson's disease. The risk of AD is 3 fold higher for those with 1 copy and 15 fold higher for those who are homozygous for the ε4 allele. The age of onset differs by more that a decade. In addition to increased levels of Aβ1–42 there is a genotype dose dependent increase in Aβ1–40.

ApoE can serve as an antioxidant with a relative potency of E2 > E3 > E4. A similar profile is present for ability to transport lipids. E3 increases neurite outgrowth and supports microtubule formation whereas E4 has the opposite effect. E3 enters cells and neurites readily, but E4 does not. AD patients and Down syndrome patients, with ε4, deposit more amyloid. Amyloid accumulation may be a signal of defective repair or failure of repair (Strittmatter *et al.* 1993; Arendt *et al.* 1997).

15.10 Risk factors for AD

The single most important risk factor for AD is advancing age. Ischaemic events, hypoxic events, oxidative stress, free radical generation, inflammation, and repair are ongoing throughout life. These events lead to loss of neurons, loss of synapses, decreased cortical acetylcholine, and a never-ending demand for repair. The presence of Aβ in any of these situations makes a bad situation worse and 'like an oily rag may fuel the fires of AD'.

Small head size, small brain size, low IQ, lack of any education have all been shown to increase the risk for AD. These findings may be explained in the context of the threshold theory of neuronal reserve, in which individuals with more 'neurons' or more 'synaptic connections and greater neuronal plasticity' are able to establish alternate circuitry and therefore display symptoms later despite the presence of AD pathology (Fig. 15.4; Cummings *et al.* 1998). This seems reasonable given the finding of medial temporal lobe atrophy

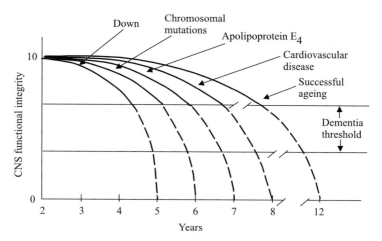

Fig. 15.4 Threshold theory of neuronal reserve, in which individuals with greater neuronal plasticity are able to establish alternate circuitry and therefore display symptoms later despite the presence of AD pathology.

predicting onset of clinical symptoms and lends support to the theory of a critical threshold for clinical expression of disease (Jobst *et al.* 1992).

The increased risk for women to develop AD is somewhat confounded by their longer life expectancy. However evidence of increasing risk associated with menopause and decreased risk for the 12% or so of women who take hormone replacement therapy may explain the apparent increased risk for AD. There are a number of studies ongoing that will investigate the use of oestrogen replacement in delaying the onset of cognitive decline and dementia.

Head trauma, especially associated with loss of consciousness, and particularly in later decades of life, confers a three to four fold increased risk for development of AD. The level of risk for AD is dramatically increased (ten fold) in subjects who carry one or two copies of the APOE ε4 allele. Severe head injury results acutely in significant elevations of Aβ1–42 which do not return to baseline levels. This increase is also associated with transforming growth factor β (TGF-β) and interleukin-6 (IL-6) expression. Milder forms of 'brain injury' resulting from coronary artery disease, heart attack, and strokes promote Aβ deposition in brain and also result in increased expression of Aβ1–42 (see Emmerling *et al.* 1999).

Transgenic mice overexpressing APP show increased susceptibility to brain damage as a result of stroke and head injury which may be mediated by Aβ effects on endothelium dependent vascular activity.

15.11 **Modulators**

Vascular lesions are present to some degree in up to 70% of AD cases (Kalaria and Hedera 1995; Scheibel 1987; Soneira and Scott 1996; de al Torre 1997; Sparks 1997; Perry *et al.* 1998). Epidemiological studies report increased risk for AD and dementia in both hypertension (Skoog *et al.* 1996) and hypotension (Guo *et al.* 1996), hypercholesterolemia (Kalmijn *et al.* 1997; Notkola *et al.* 1998), coronary artery disease (Sparks 1997), atherosclerosis (Hofman *et al.* 1997), cerebrovascular disease (Snowdon *et al.* 1997), atrial fibrillation (Ott *et al.* 1997), endoethelial cell (Kalaria and Hedera 1995), and blood–brain barrier damage (Claudio

1996), stroke and bypass surgery (Moody *et al.* 1997;Tardiff *et al.* 1997). Increases in cholesterol and LDL cholesterol, in particular, result in increased amyloid deposition.

Nutritional factors, which appear to increase risk, include low folate, resulting in increased serum homocysteine, and thiamine deficiency (Joosten *et al.* 1997). Thiamine deficiency causes vascular endothelial cell changes which result in local leakage and local expression of Aβ. Diets high in fats and cholesterol increase risk while low fat diets reduce risk. Antioxidants like vitamin E may confer a margin of benefit (Sano *et al.* 1997).

A multicentre study of antihypertensive therapy versus placebo on the risk of stroke was stopped early because of highly significant result in favour of antihypertensive therapy (Forette *et al.* 1998*a*, *b*). Although the sample size was small and the study was short there were also significantly reduced risks for dementia of any cause and specifically for AD.

Epidemiological studies provide evidence of increased risk for those with high cholesterol (Grant 1997). These findings are supported by *in vitro* studies which demonstrate high cholesterol levels interfere with α secretase cleavage of APP and may shift metabolism of APP to more amyloidogenic products (Racchi *et al.* 1997). Increased levels of LDL have been correlated to increased amyloid deposition (Kuo *et al.* 1998). Coronary artery disease patients, patients with atherosclerosis, and those with even subclinical disease, appear at increased risk for AD. Individuals showing midlife hyperglycaemia and presence of an *APOE ε4* allele experienced cognitive decline significantly greater than either alone (Poirier 1996; Roses 1997). ApoE4 exacerbates effects of cardiovascular risk factors on cognitive performance. By reducing the levels of cholesterol in living hippocampal neurons by 70% the formation of amyloidogenic fragments is completely inhibited (Simons 1998; Frears *et al.* 1999). This effect is reversible by adding back cholesterol. ApoE4 is associated with increased cholesterol and LDL, survivors from the Finnish seven countries study show previously high cholesterol results in a three-fold increased risk for AD (Notkola *et al.* 1998).

Non steroidal anti-inflammatory drugs such as ibuprofen, indomethacin, and dapsone have been reported to reduce the risk of AD by delaying the onset of symptoms (McGeer *et al.* 1996). This effect is presumably mediated by reducing the level of microglia cell activation by Aβ (Thomas *et al.* 1997; Mackenzie and Munoz 1998). The result of ongoing studies with prednisone and Cox-2 inhibitors should provide greater insight as to the potential of these treatment approaches.

The mechanism by which oestrogens are protective could relate directly to interactions through oestrogen receptors or indirectly through reduced risk for cardiovascular pathology (Birge 1996). Even modest differences in circulating oestradiol levels have significant effects on bone deposition and risk for fractures (Ettinger 1998). The question is not whether women should be placed on oestrogen replacement but what doses and regimens of replacement are most effective in providing optimal benefit in terms of bone, cardiovascular, and cognitive endpoints.

15.12 **The role of biological markers**

In order for a biological marker to be of value it must measure a fundamental contributor to AD neuropathology. The natural history of the marker must be validated against the natural history of the disease preclinically and clinically and it should be accessible and known to be relevant to clinical outcome. The marker must be validated in cross-section and longitudinally. It may seem trite to say but what is needed is the 'cholesterol' of AD.

Potential sources of biological markers include the brain itself, the CSF, plasma, serum, platelets, lymphocytes, and other cellular components of blood and other tissues. The technologies required to monitor these markers in the brain are likely to include a combination of structural and more importantly functional imaging and the development of specific imaging ligands and antibodies.

The list of possible markers may include APP itself, total Aβ, Aβ1–40, and Aβ1–42 or some combination of these necessary to quantify and describe the kinetics of amyloid production and clearance. Other targets include the putative secretases involved in APP cleavage, tau protein, apoE, cholesterol, inflammatory markers, antioxidant capacity, or an as yet to be identified substance. The techniques will have to encompass *in vitro* cellular assays and *in vivo* and *ex vivo* measures in small rodents, monkeys, and in man to expedite drug discovery.

The current emphasis on amyloid in drug discovery makes it a priority target as a biological marker. The techniques must be adequate to define quantitatively the kinetics for generation and clearance of both non-pathogenic and pathogenic pathways resolving the kinetics of monomers, dimers, and polymers. Altering this fundamental biological process carries theoretical benefits and unknown risks. Determining dose and degree to which one wants or needs to interfere with the process is an essential question that can only be addressed with certainty following trial and error.

Developing a cholinesterase inhibitor or other neurotransmitter based therapy today seems straightforward in comparison to the challenges provided by an amyloid modifier. Phase 1 and Phase 2 clinical development will be significantly more difficult and demanding, carry higher risks, and require new and innovative strategies and technologies.

15.13 **Outside the box**

Schenk and colleagues (Schenk *et al.* 1999) reported in July the successful immunization of *APP* transgenic mice against the development of AD-like pathology. Recently, the same group showed that passive immunization of *APP* transgenic mice with existing mouse monoclonal antibodies to Aβ, or antibodies isolated from mice immunized with Aβ, also showed a reduction in amyloid plaques (Bard *et al.* 2000). Expedited confirmation of the patential for immunization of patients with AD, and then at-risk populations, seems an absolute priority for the AD research community. Phase I clinical trials of the Aβ vaccine have been initiated.

Identification of possible secretases occurred in the past year. Evidence that PS1 and PS2 act as the γ-secretase gained additional support from reports showing that inhibitors of γ-secretase activity bind to and label the presenilin protein (De Strooper, 2000). In addition, four laboratories independently identified a protease thought to be responsible for the β-secretase cleavage of APP. BACE-1, also referred to as memapsin-2 and ASP-2, appears to be a likely candidate for the β-secretase (Potter and Dressler, 2000). It has been reported that some γ-secretase inhibitors are already in Phase I clinical trials.

15.14 **Conclusion**

Using epidemiological data to identify near-term opportunities and embracing the unified hypothesis provides drug discovery with numerous targets (Table 15.2). Focusing systematically on the underlying pathological process and biological markers appears to provide an avenue to guarantee future success in treating, delaying, and preventing AD.

A note of caution is important. The enthusiasm for investing in the discovery and development of drugs to treat AD has been dampened by the unimpressive success of the approved symptomatic therapies. The rewards of other disease targets are substantially larger than for AD and the level of risk less than for AD. In AD the magnitude of treatment effect that can be

Table 15.2 Therapeutic targets within the unifying hypothesis

1	Prevent access of β and γ secretases to APP cleavage sites
2	Inhibit β and/or γ secretases
3	Upregulate α secretase cleavage
4	Increase clearance of Aβ
5	Prevent fibrilization/aggregation of Aβ
6	Develop brain specific anti-inflammatories
7	Block Aβ microglial activation
8	Inhibit acute phase response
9	Antioxidants
10	Reduce serum cholesterol
11	Oestrogen replacement therapy
12	Target neuroprotection and nerve growth factors
13	Enhance cholinergic function
14	Stage and symptom specific treatments
15	Combination therapies

achieved is limited by the underlying pathology and loss of plasticity. Disease prevention is the goal, the reward, and a difficult task given our current level of understanding of the ageing brain and AD. Although there are short-term opportunities to explore potentially meaningful interventions in AD, only systematic investigation into the longitudinal development of the clinical symptoms, and biological and biochemical changes associated with this dementia will ultimately reveal the cause(s) and best treatments. It remains to be determined how to achieve this goal. However, an undertaking of this scope may best be achieved by a well-focused alliance of government, academia, and the private sector.

References

Aisen, P. S. and Davis, K. L. (1994). Inflammatory mechanisms in Alzheimer's disease: Implications for therapy. *American Journal of Psychiatry*, 151, 1105–13.

Alvarez, A., Opazo, C., Alarcon, R., *et al.* (1997). Acetylcholinesterase promotes the aggregation of amyloid-β-peptide fragments by forming a complex with the growing fibrils. *Journal of Molecular Biology*, 272, 348–61.

Andreasen, N., Hesse, C., Davidsson, P., *et al.* (1999). Cerebrospinal fluid beta-amyloid (1–42) in Alzheimer's disease: differences between early- and late-onset Alzheimer's disease and stability during the course of disease. *Archives of Neurology*, 56, 673–80.

Arendt, T., Schindler, C., Bruckner, M. K., *et al.* (1997). Plastic Neuronal Remodelling is Impaired in Patients with Alzheimer's Disease Carrying Apolipoprotein ε4 Allelle. *Journal of Neuroscience*, 17, 516–29.

Bard, F., cannon, C., Barbour, R. *et al.* (2000). Peripherally administered antibodies against amyloid β-peptide enter the central nervous system and reduce pathology in a mouse model of Alzheimer disease. *Nature Medicine*, 6, 916–919

Birge, S. J. (1996). Is there a role for oestrogen replacement therapy in the prevention and treatment of dementia? *Journal of American Geriatric Society*, 44, 865–70.

Birge, S. J. (1997). The role of oestrogen in the treatment of Alzheimer's disease. *Neurology*, **48**, S36–S41.

Bobinski, M., deLeon, M. J., Convit, A., *et al.* (1999). MRI of entorhinal cortex in mild Alzheimer's disease. *Lancet*, **353**, 38–40.

Borchelt, D. R. (1998). Accelerated amyloid deposition in the brains of transgenic mice co-expressing mutant presenilin 1 and amyloid precursor protein. In: *Alzheimer's Disease: New Drug Discovery Strategies*. Boston, MA: NMHCC Bio/Technology Conference Division.

Bradt, B. M., Bixby, T. S., and Cooper, N. R. (1996). The Alzheimer's disease Aβ peptide generates C5a and sC5b-9 via direct activation of both complement pathways. *Molecular Immunology*, **33**, 27.

Breitner J. C. S. (1996). Inflammatory Processes and antiinflammatory drugs in Alzheimer's disease: A current appraisal. *Neurobiology of Ageing.* **17**, 789–94.

Brodaty, H., McGilchrist, C., Harris, L., and Peters, K. E. (1993). Time until institutionalization and death in patients with dementia. Role of caregiver training and risk factors. *Archives of Neurology*, **50**, 643–50.

Castillo, G. M., Ngo, C., Cummings, J., *et al.* (1997). Perlecan binds to the β-amyloid protein (Aβ) of Alzheimer's disease, accelerates Aβ fibril formation, and maintains Aβ fibril stability. *Journal of Neurochemistry*, **69**, 2452–65.

Choo-Smith, L. P., Garzon-Rodriguez, W., Glabe, C. G., and Surewicz, W. K. (1997). Acceleration of amyloid fibril formation by specific binding of Aβ (1–40) peptide to ganglioside-containing membrane vesicles. *Journal of Biological Chemistry*, **272**, 22987–90.

Claudio, L. (1996). Ultrastructural features of the blood-brain barrier in biopsy tissue from Alzheimer's disease patients. *Acta Neuropathologicala*, **91**, 6–14.

Corder, E. H., Saunders, A. M., Strittmatter, W. J., *et al.* (1993). Gene dose of apolipoprotein E Type 4 allele and the risk of Alzheimer's disease in late onset families. *Science*, **261**, 921–3.

Cummings, J. L., Vinters, H. V., Cole, G. M., and Khachaturian, Z. S. (1998). Alzheimer's disease. Etiologies, pathophysiology, cognitive reserve, and treatment opportunities. *Neurology*, **51**, S2–S17.

de la Torre, J. C. (1997). Cerebromicrovascular pathology in Alzheimer's disease compared to normal ageing. *Gerontology*, **43**, 26–43.

DeStrooper, B. (2000). Alzheimer's disease. Closing in on gamma secretase. *Nature*, **405**, 627–629.

Devanand, D. P., Marder, K., Michaels K. S., *et al.* (1998). A randomized, Placebo-Controlled Dose-Comparison Trial of Haloperidol for Psychosis and Disruptive Behaviours in Alzheimer's Disease. *American Journal of Psychiatry*, **155**, 1512–20.

Drachman, D. A., O'Donnell, B. F., Lew, R. A., and Swearer, J. M. (1990). The prognosis in Alzheimer's disease. 'How far' rather than 'how fast' best predicts the course, *Archives of Neurology*, **47**, 851–6.

El Khoury, J., Hickman, S. E., Thomas, C. A., *et al.* (1996). Scavenger receptor-mediated adhesion of microglia to β-amyloid fibrils. *Nature*, **382**, 716–19.

Emmerling, M. R., Spiegel, K., and Watson, M. D. (1997). Inhibiting the formation of classical C3-convertase on the Alzheimer's β-amyloid peptide. *Immunopharmacology*, **38**, 101–9.

Emmerling, M. R., Gracon, S., and Roher A. E., (1999). Towards a Unifying Hypothesis of Alzheimer's Disease Pathogenesis and Pathophysiology. In Clinical Diagnosis and Management of Alzheimer's Disease edited by Serge Gauthier Martin Dunitz Publishers.

Ettinger, B., Pressman, A., Sklarin, P., *et al.* (1998). Associations between low levels of Serum Estradiol, Bone Density and Fractures among Elderly women: The Study of Osteoporotic Fractures. *Journal of Clinical Endocrinology and Metabolism*, **83**, 2239–43.

Feany, M. B., and Dickson, D. W., (1996). Neurodegenerative disorders with extensive tau pathology: a comparative study and review. *Annals of Neurology*, **40**, 139–48.

Folstein, M. F., Folstein, S. E., and McHugh, P. R. (1975). Mini-mental state, *Journal of Psychiatric Research*, **12**, 189–98.

Forette, F., Seux, M. L., Staessen, J. A., *et al.* (1998). Prevention of dementia in randomised double-blind placebo-controlled systolic hypertension in Europe (Syst-Eur) trial. *Lancet*, **352**, 1347–51.

Forette, F., Seux, M. L., Thijs, L., *et al.* (1998). Detection of cerebral ageing, an absolute need: predictive value of cognitive status. *European Neurology*, 39, 2–6.

Forloni, G., Mangiarotti, F., Angeretti, N., *et al.* (1997). β-Amyloid fragment potentiates IL-6 and TNF-α secretion by LPS in astrocytes but not in microglia. *Cytokine*, 9, 759–62.

Frears, E., Stephens, D., Walters, C., *et al.* (1999). The role of cholesterol in the biosynthesis of β-amyloid. *NeuroReport*, 10, 1699–05.

Games, D., Adams, D., Alessandrini, R., *et al.* (1995). Alzheimer-type neuropathology in transgenic mice overexpressing V717F β-amyloid precursor protein. *Nature*, 373, 523–7.

Gearing, M., Schneider, J. A., Robbins, R. S., *et al.* (1995). Regional variation in the distribution of apolipoprotein E and Aβ in Alzheimer's disease. *Journal of Neuropathology and Experimental Neurology*, 54, 833–41.

Gomez-Isla, T., Hollister, R., West, H., *et al.* (1997). Neuronal loss correlates with but exceeds neurofibrillary tangles in Alzheimer's disease. *Annals of Neurology*, 41, 17–24.

Goux, W. J., Rodriquez, S., and Sparkman, D. R. (1996). Characterization of the glycolipid associated with Alzheimer paired helical filaments. *Journal of Neurochemistry*, 67, 723–33.

Graff-Radford, N. R., Eckman, C., Hutton, M. L., *et al.* (1998). Plasma amyloid (A beta) levels in relatives of Alzheimer's disease patients. *Neurology*, 50, S4, 33005.

Grant, W. B. (1997). Dietary links to Alzheimer's disease. *Alzheimer Disease Reviews*, 2, 42–55.

Guo, Z., Viitanen, M., Fratiglioni, L., and Winblad, B. (1996). Low blood pressure and dementia in elderly people: the Kungsholmen project. *British Medical Journal*, 312, 805–8.

Hardy, J. (1997). Amyloid, the presenilins and Alzheimer's disease. *Trends in Neuroscience*, 20, 154–9.

Heyman A., Wilkinson, W. E., Hurwitz, B. J., *et al.* (1987). Early-onset Alzheimer's disease: clinical predictors of institutionalization and death, *Neurology*, 37, 980–4.

Hofman, A., Ott, A., Breteler, M. M., *et al.* (1997). Atherosclerosis, apolipoprotein E, and prevalence of dementia and Alzheimer's disease in the Rotterdam Study. *Lancet*, 349, 151–4.

Hoshi, M., Takashima, A., Murayama, M., *et al.* (1997). Nontoxic amyloid β peptide 1–42 suppresses acetylcholine synthesis. Possible role in cholinergic dysfunction in Alzheimer's disease. *Journal of Biological Chemistry*, 272, 2038–41.

Hsiao, K., Chapman, P., Nilsen, S., *et al.* (1996). Correlative memory deficits, Aβ elevation, and amyloid plaques in transgenic mice. *Science*, 274, 99–102.

Hu, J., Akama, K. T., Krafft, G. A., *et al.* (1998). Amyloid-β peptide activates cultured astrocytes: morphological alterations, cytokine induction and nitric oxide release. *Brain Research*, 785, 195–206.

Ishii, K., Tamaoka, A., Mizusawa, H., *et al.* (1997). Aβ1–40 but not Aβ1–42 levels in cortex correlate with apolipoprotein E ε4 allele dosage in sporadic Alzheimer's disease. *Brain Research*, 748, 250–2.

Iwatsubo, T, Mann, D. M., Odaka, A., *et al.* (1995). Amyloid beta protein (A beta) deposition: A beta 42(43) precedes A beta 40 in Down syndrome. *Annals of Neurology*, 37, 294–9.

Jack, C. R., Petersen, R. C., Xu, Y. C., *et al.* (1999). Prediction of AD with MRI-based hippocampal volume in mild cognitive impairment. *Neurology*, 52, 1397–403.

Jensen, M., Schroder, J., Blomberg, M., *et al.* (1999). Cerebrospinal fluid A beta 42 is increased early in sporadic Alzheimer's disease and declines with disease progression. *Annals of Neurology*, 4, 504–11.

Jobst, K. A., Smith, A. D., Szatmari, M., *et al.* (1992). Detection of Confirmed Alzheimer's Disease Using a Simple Measurement of Medial Temporal Lobe Atrophy by Computed Tomography. *Lancet*, 340, 1179–83.

Johnson-Wood, K., Lee, M., Motter, R., *et al.* (1997). Amyloid precursor protein processing and Aβ42 deposition in transgenic mouse model of Alzheimer's disease. *Proceedings of the National Academy of Science (USA)*, 94, 1550–55.

Joosten, E., Lesaffre, E., Riezler, R., *et al.* (1997). Is metabolic evidence for vitamin B-12 and folate deficiency more frequent in elderly patients with Alzheimer's disease? *Journal of Gerontological and Biological Science and Medical Science*, 52, M76-M79.

Jost, B. C. and Grossberg, G. T. (1995). The natural history of Alzheimer's disease: a brain bank study. *Journal of American Geriatric Society*, 43, 1248–55.

Kalaria, R. N. (1992). The blood-brain barrier and cerebral microcirculation in Alzheimer's disease. *Cerebrovascular Brain Metabolism Reviews*, 4, 226–260.

Kalaria, R. N. and Hedera, P. (1995). Differential degeneration of the cerebral microvasculature in Alzheimer's disease. *Neuroreport*, 6, 477–80.

Kalmijn, S., Launer, L. J., Ott, A., *et al.* (1997). Dietary fat intake and the risk of incident dementia in the Rotterdam Study. *Annals of Neurology*, 42, 776–82.

Kanne, S. M., Balota, D. A., Storandt, M., *et al.* (1998). Relating anatomy to function in Alzheimer's disease. Neuropsychological profiles predict regional neuropathology 5 years later. *American Academy of Neurology*, 50, 979–85.

Knopman, D. S., Kitto, J., Deinard, S., and Heiring, J. (1988). Longitudinal Study of Death and Institutionalization in Patients with Primary Degenerative Dementia. *Journal American Geriatric Society*, 36, 108–12.

Kuo, Y. M., Emmerling, M. R., Bisgaier, C. L., *et al.* (1998). Elevated low-density lipoprotein in Alzheimer's disease correlates with brain abeta 1–42 levels. *Biochemical and Biophysical Research Communications*, 252, 711–5.

Leverenz, J. B. and Raskind, M. A. (1998) Early amyloid deposition in the medial temporal lobe of young Down syndrome patients: a regional quantitative analysis. *Experimental Neurology*, 150, 296–304.

Levy, M. L., Cummings, J. L., Fairbanks, L. A., *et al.* (1996). Longitudinal assessment of symptoms of depression, agitation and psychosis in 181 patients with Alzheimer's disease. *American Journal of Psychiatry*, 153, 1438–43.

Lue, L. F., Brachova, L., Civin, W. H., and Rogers, J. (1996) Inflammation, Aβ deposition, and neurofibrillary tangle formation as correlates of Alzheimer's disease neurodegeneration. *Journal of Neuropathology and Experimental Neurology*, 55, 1083–8.

Lue, L. F., Kuo, Y. M., Roher, A. E., *et al.* (1999). Soluble amyloid β peptide concentration as a predictor of synaptic change in Alzheimer's disease. *American Journal of Pathology*, 155, 853–62.

McGeer, P. L. and Rogers, J. (1992). Anti-inflammatory agents as a therapeutic approach to Alzheimer's disease. *Neurology*, 42, 447–9.

McGeer, P. L., Schulzer, M., and McGeer, E. G. (1996). Arthritis and anti-inflammatory agents as possible protective factors for Alzheimer's disease: a review of 17 Epidemiological studies. *Neurology*, 47, 425–32.

Mackenzie, I. R., McLachlan, R. S., Kubu, C. S., and Miller, L. A. (1996). Prospective neuropsychological assessment of nondemented patients with biopsy proven senile plaques. *Neurology*, 46, 425–9.

Mackenzie, I. R. and Munoz, D. G. (1998). Nonsteroidal anti-inflammatory drug use and Alzheimer-type pathology in ageing. *Neurology*, 50, 986–90.

Mann, D.M., Marcyniuk, B., Yates, P.O., *et al.* (1988). The progression of the pathological changes of Alzheimer's disease in frontal and temporal neocortex examined both at biopsy and at autopsy. *Neuropathology and Applied Neurobiology*, 4, 177–95.

Mann, D. M. A., Iwatsubo, T., Cairns, N. J., *et al.* (1996). Amyloid beta protein (A beta) deposition in chromosome 14-linked Alzheimer's disease: Predominance of A beta(42(43). *Annals of Neurology*, 40, 149–56.

Mantyh, P. W., Ghilardi, J. R., Rogers, S., *et al.* (1993). Aluminium, iron, and zinc ions promote aggregation of physiological concentrations of β-amyloid peptide. *Journal of Neurochemistry*, 61, 1171–4.

Mayeux, R., Tang, M. X., Jacobs, D. M. *et al.* (1999). Plasma amyloid beta-peptide 1-42 and incipient Alzheimer's disease. *Annals of Neurology*, 46, 412–6.

Mohs, R. C., Breitner, J. C. S., Silverman, J. M., and Davis, K. L. (1987). Alzheimer's disease: morbid risk among first-degree relative approximates 50% by 90 years of age. *Archives of General Psychiatry*, 44, 405–8.

Moody, D. M., Brown, W. R., Challa, V. R., *et al.* (1997). Cerebral microvascular alterations in ageing, leukoaraiosis, and Alzheimer's disease. *Annals of NewYork Academy of Sciences*, 826, 103–16.

Morris, J. C., Storandt, M., McKeel, D. W. *et al.* (1996) Cerebral amyloid deposition and diffuse plaques in 'normal' ageing: evidence for presymptomatic and very mild Alzheimer's disease. *Neurology*, 46, 707–19.

Mucke, L., Abraham, C. R., Ruppe, M. D., *et al.* (1995). Protection against HIV-1 gp120-induced brain damage by neuronal expression of human amyloid precursor protein. *Journal of Experimental Medicine*, 181, 1551–6.

Mucke, L., Abraham, C. R., and Masliah, E. (1996). Neurotrophic and neuroprotective effects of hAPP in transgenic mice. *Annals of the New York Academy of Science*, 777, 82–8.

Notkola, I., Sulkava, R., Pekkanen, J., *et al.* (1998). Serum Total Cholesterol, Apolipoprotein E ε4 Allele, and Alzheimer's Disease. *Neuroepidemiology*, 17, 14–20.

Olesen, O. F., Lone D., and Mikkelsen, J. D. (1998). Amyloid β neurotoxicity in the cholinergic but not in the serotonergic phenotype of RN46A cells. *Molecular Brain Research*, 57, 266–74.

Ott, A., Breteler, M. M., de Bruyne, M. C., *et al.* (1997). Atrial fibrillation and dementia in a population-based study. The Rotterdam Study. *Stroke*, 28, 316–21.

Pericak-Vance M. A., Bebout J. L., Gaskell P. C. Jr, *et al.* (1991). Linkage studies in familial Alzheimer disease: evidence for chromosome 19 linkage. *American Journal of Human Genetics*, 48, 1034–50.

Perry, G., Smith, M. A., McCann, C. E., *et al.* (1998). Cerebrovascular muscle atrophy is a feature of Alzheimer's disease. *Brain Research*, 791, 63–6.

Perry, V. H., Anthony, D. C., Bolton, S. J., and Brown, H. C. (1997). The blood-brain barrier and the inflammatory response. *Molecular Medicine Today*, 3, 335–41.

Petersen, R. C., Smith, G. E., Waring, S. C., *et al.* (1999). Mild cognitive impairment: clinical characterization and outcome. *Archives of Neurology*, 56, 303–8.

Piccini, C., Bracco, L., Falcini, M., *et al.* (1995). Natural history of Alzheimer's disease: prognostic value of plateau. *Journal of the Neurological Sciences*, 131, 177–82.

Pirttila, T., Soininen, H., Mehta, P. D., *et al.* (1997). Apolipoprotein E genotype and amyloid load in Alzheimer's disease and control brains. *Neurobiology of Ageing*, 18, 121–7.

Poirier, J. (1996). Apolipoprotein E in the brain and its role in Alzheimer's disease. *Journal of Psychiatry and Neuroscience*, 21, 128–34.

Potter, H., and Dressler, D. (2000). The potential of BACE inhibitors for Alzheimer's therapy. *Nature Biotechnology*, 18, 125–6.

Prasher, V. P., Farrer, M. J., Kessling, A. M., *et al.* (1998). Molecular Mapping of Alzheimer's-type Dementia in Down Syndrome. *Annals of Neurology*, 43, 380–3.

Racchi, M., Baetta, R., Salvietti, N., *et al.* (1997). Secretory processing of amyloid precursor protein is inhibited by increase in cellular cholesterol content. *Biochemical Journal*, 322, 893–8

Rogers, J., Kirby, L. C., Hempelman, S. R., *et al.* (1993). Clinical trial of indomethacin in Alzheimer's disease. *Neurology*, 43, 1609–11.

Roses, A. D. (1997). Apolipoprotein E, a gene with complex biological interactions in the ageing brain. *Neurobiology of Disease*, 4, 170–85.

Sano, M., Ernesto, C., Thomas, R. G., *et al.* (1997). A controlled trial of selegiline, alpha-tocopherol, or both as treatment for Alzheimer's disease. *The New England Journal of Medicine*, 336, 1216–22.

Scheibel, A. B. (1987). Alterations of the cerebral capillary bed in the senile dementia of Alzheimer. *Italian Journal of Neurological Science*, 8, 457–63.

Schenk, D., Barbour, R., Dunn, W., *et al.* (1999). Immunization with amyloid-β attenuates Alzheimer-disease-like pathology in the PDAPP mouse. *Nature*, 400, 173–7.

Selwyn, A. P., Kinlay, S., Creager, M., *et al.* (1997). Cell dysfunction in atherosclerosis and the Ischaemic manifestations of coronary artery disease. *American Journal of Cardiology*, 79, 17–23.

Severson, M. A., Smith, G. E., Tangalos, E. G., *et al.* (1994). Patterns and predictors of institutionalization in community-based dementia patents. *Journal of the American Geriatric Society*, **42**, 181–5.

Simons, M., Keller, P., De Strooper, B., *et al.* (1998). Cholesterol depletion inhibits the generation of β-amyloid in Hippocampal neurons. *Proceedings of the National Academy of Science (USA)*, **95**, 6460–4.

Skoog, I., Lernfelt, B., Landahl, S., *et al.* (1996). 15-year longitudinal study of blood pressure and dementia. *Lancet*, **347**, 1141–5.

Snowdon, D. A., Greiner, L. H., Mortimer, J. A., *et al.* (1997). Brain infarction and the clinical expression of Alzheimer's disease. The Nun Study. *Journal of the American Medical Association*, **277**, 813–17.

Soneira, C. F. and Scott, T. M. (1996). Severe cardiovascular disease and Alzheimer's disease: senile plaque formation in cortical areas. (1996). *Clinical Anatomy*, **9**, 118–27.

Sparks, D. L. (1997). Coronary artery disease, hypertension, ApoE, and cholesterol: a link to Alzheimer's disease? *Annals of New York Academy of Science*, **826**, 128–46.

Strittmatter, W.J., Saunders, A.M., Schmechel, D., *et al.* (1993). Apolipoprotein E: high-avidity binding to beta-amyloid and increased frequency of type 4 allele in late-onset familial Alzheimer disease. *Proceedings of the National Academy of Science (USA)*, **90**, 1977–81.

Tardiff, B. E., Newman, M. F., Saunders, A. M., *et al.* (1997). Preliminary report of a genetic basis for cognitive decline after cardiac operations. The Neurologic Outcome Research Group of the Duke Heart Center. *Annals of Thoracic Surgery*, **64**, 715–20.

Terry R. D. (1997). The pathology of Alzheimer's disease: numbers count [letters]. *Annals of Neurology*, **41**, 7.

Thomas, T., Sutton, E. T., Bryant, M. W., and Rhodin, J. A. (1997). *In vivo* vascular damage, leukocyte activation and inflammatory response induced by β-amyloid. *Journal of Submicroscopic Cytology and Pathology*, **29**, 293–304.

Watson, M. D., Roher, A. E, Kim, K. S., *et al.* (1997). Complement interactions with amyloid-β1–42: a nidus for inflammation in AD brains. *Amyloid-International Journal of Experimental and Clinical Investigation*, **4**, 147–56.

Webster, S., Glabe, C., and Rogers, J. (1995). Multivalent binding of complement protein Clq to the amyloid β-peptide (Aβ) promotes the nucleation phase of Aβ aggregation. *Biochemical and Biophysical Research Communications*, **217**, 869–75.

Webster, S., Bradt, B., Rogers, J., and Cooper, N. (1997a). Aggregation state-dependent activation of the classical complement pathway by the amyloid β peptide. *Journal of Neurochemistry*, **69**, 388–98.

Webster, S., Lue, L. F., Brachova, L., *et al.* (1997b). Molecular and cellular characterization of the membrane attack complex, C5b-9, in Alzheimer's disease. *Neurobiology of Ageing*, **18**, 415–21.

Welch, H. G., Walsh, J. S., and Larson, E. B. (1992). The cost of institutional care in Alzheimer's disease: nursing home and hospital use in a prospective cohort. *Journal of the American Geriatric Society*, **40**, 221–4.

Wilson, D. M., and Binder, L. I. (1997). Free fatty acids stimulate the polymerization of tau and amyloid β peptides. In vitro evidence for a common effector of pathogenesis in Alzheimer's disease. *American Journal of Pathology*, **150**, 2181–95.

Wisniewski, T., Ghiso, J., and Frangione, B. (1997) Biology of Aβ amyloid in Alzheimer's disease. *Neurobiology of Disease*, **4**, 313–28.

Yan, S. D., Chen, X., Fu, J., *et al.* (1996). RAGE and amyloid-β peptide neurotoxicity in Alzheimer's disease. *Nature*, **382**, 685–91.

Zhang, F., Eckman, C., Younkin, S., *et al.* (1997). Increased susceptibility to Ischaemic brain damage in transgenic mice overexpressing the amyloid precursor protein. *Journal of Neuroscience*, **17**, 7655–61

AI Amyloid precursor protein (APP)

Protein name: Alzheimer's disease amyloid precursor protein or protease nexin-II
Gene name: *APP* or *A4* or *CVAP* or *AD1*
Swiss-Prot primary accession number: P05067

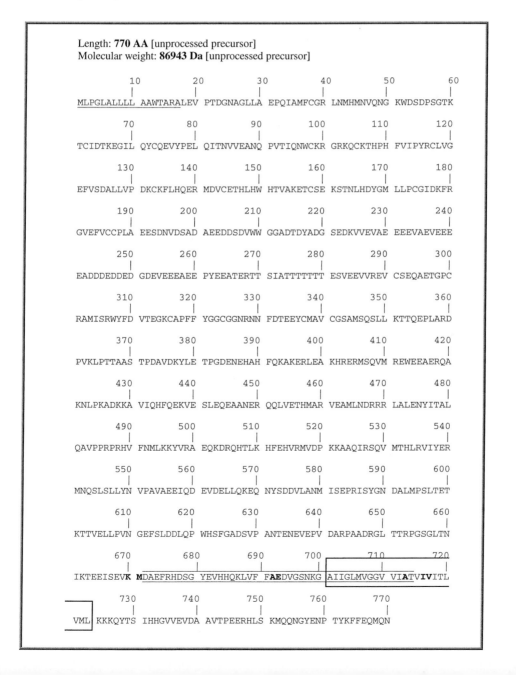

Length: **770 AA** [unprocessed precursor]
Molecular weight: **86943 Da** [unprocessed precursor]

```
            10         20         30         40         50         60
             |          |          |          |          |          |
      MLPGLALLLL AAWTARALEV PTDGNAGLLA EPQIAMFCGR LNMHMNVQNG KWDSDPSGTK

            70         80         90        100        110        120
             |          |          |          |          |          |
      TCIDTKEGIL QYCQEVYPEL QITNVVEANQ PVTIQNWCKR GRKQCKTHPH FVIPYRCLVG

           130        140        150        160        170        180
             |          |          |          |          |          |
      EFVSDALLVP DKCKFLHQER MDVCETHLHW HTVAKETCSE KSTNLHDYGM LLPCGIDKFR

           190        200        210        220        230        240
             |          |          |          |          |          |
      GVEFVCCPLA EESDNVDSAD AEEDDSDVWW GGADTDYADG SEDKVVEVAE EEEVAEVEEE

           250        260        270        280        290        300
             |          |          |          |          |          |
      EADDDEDDED GDEVEEEAEE PYEEATERTT SIATTTTTTT ESVEEVVREV CSEQAETGPC

           310        320        330        340        350        360
             |          |          |          |          |          |
      RAMISRWYFD VTEGKCAPFF YGGCGGNRNN FDTEEYCMAV CGSAMSQSLL KTTQEPLARD

           370        380        390        400        410        420
             |          |          |          |          |          |
      PVKLPTTAAS TPDAVDKYLE TPGDENEHAH FQKAKERLEA KHRERMSQVM REWEEAERQA

           430        440        450        460        470        480
             |          |          |          |          |          |
      KNLPKADKKA VIQHFQEKVE SLEQEAANER QQLVETHMAR VEAMLNDRRR LALENYITAL

           490        500        510        520        530        540
             |          |          |          |          |          |
      QAVPPRPRHV FNMLKKYVRA EQKDRQHTLK HFEHVRMVDP KKAAQIRSQV MTHLRVIYER

           550        560        570        580        590        600
             |          |          |          |          |          |
      MNQSLSLLYN VPAVAEEIQD EVDELLQKEQ NYSDDVLANM ISEPRISYGN DALMPSLTET

           610        620        630        640        650        660
             |          |          |          |          |          |
      KTTVELLPVN GEFSLDDLQP WHSFGADSVP ANTENEVEPV DARPAADRGL TTRPGSGLTN

           670        680        690        700        710        720
             |          |          |          |          |          |
      IKTEEISEVK MDAEFRHDSG YEVHHQKLVF FAEDVGSNKG AIIGLMVGGV VIATVIVITL

           730        740        750        760        770
             |          |          |          |          |
      VML KKKQYTS IHHGVVEVDA AVTPEERHLS KMQQNGYENP TYKFFEQMQN
```

Signal peptide is underlined
Putative transmembrane domain is boxed
43 amino acid beta-amyloid sequence is underlined and overlined
Mutations are shown in bold

Alternative splice products: Six alternative spliced variants including: APP(395), APP(563), APP(695), APP(751) and APP(770). APP (751) and APP(770) contain a protease inhibitor domain belonging to the kunitz family of inhibitors.

Mutations in the *APP* gene resulting in AD or HCHWA-D

Mutation	Common name	Age of onset
670K, 671M → 670N, 671L	Swedish double	44–59
692A → 692G	Flemish	40–60
693E → 693Q	Dutch (HCHWA-D)	~50
715V → 715M	French	40–60
716I → 716V	Florida	55
717V → 717I	London	50–60
717V → 717G	-	45–62
717V → 717F	-	42–52

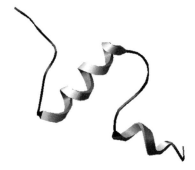

Fig. AI.1 Structure of amyloid peptide residues 1–40. Cartoon structure from NMR resolution of Aβ (1–40) showing mainly α-helix formation. [NCBI code 1AML]

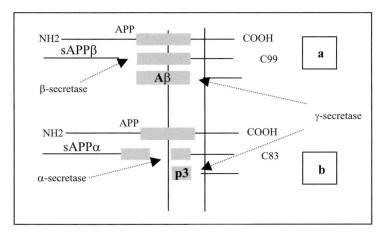

Fig. AI.2 Processing of APP may occur by cleaving with α-secretase as in (b) or β-secretase as in (a). This results in either an N-terminus of 83 (b) or 99 (a) amino acids. γ-secretase then cleaves within the transmembrane region to form p3 (b) or Aβ (a). α-secretase cleavage site is between M671 and D672. γ-secretase site is between V711 and I712 for Aβ1–40.

All Presenilin 1 (PS1)

Protein name: human presenilin 1 or PS-1 or S182
Gene name: *PSEN1* or *PSNL1* or *AD3* or *PS1*
Swiss-Prot primary accession number: P49768

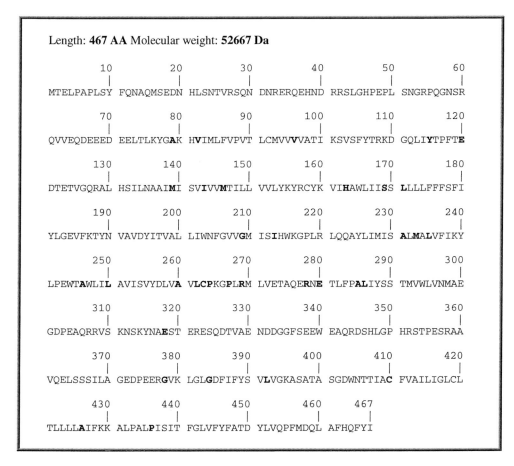

Length: **467 AA** Molecular weight: **52667 Da**

```
            10          20          30          40          50          60
             |           |           |           |           |           |
     MTELPAPLSY FQNAQMSEDN HLSNTVRSQN DNRERQEHND RRSLGHPEPL SNGRPQGNSR

            70          80          90         100         110         120
             |           |           |           |           |           |
     QVVEQDEEED EELTLKYGAK HVIMLFVPVT LCMVVVVATI KSVSFYTRKD GQLIYTPFTE

           130         140         150         160         170         180
             |           |           |           |           |           |
     DTETVGQRAL HSILNAAIMI SVIVVMTILL VVLYKYRCYK VIHAWLIISS LLLLFFFSFI

           190         200         210         220         230         240
             |           |           |           |           |           |
     YLGEVFKTYN VAVDYITVAL LIWNFGVVGM ISIHWKGPLR LQQAYLIMIS ALMALVFIKY

           250         260         270         280         290         300
             |           |           |           |           |           |
     LPEWTAWLIL AVISVYDLVA VLCPKGPLRM LVETAQERNE TLFPALIYSS TMVWLVNMAE

           310         320         330         340         350         360
             |           |           |           |           |           |
     GDPEAQRRVS KNSKYNAEST ERESQDTVAE NDDGGFSEEW EAQRDSHLGP HRSTPESRAA

           370         380         390         400         410         420
             |           |           |           |           |           |
     VQELSSSILA GEDPEERGVK LGLGDFIFYS VLVGKASATA SGDWNTTIAC FVAILIGLCL

           430         440         450         460         467
             |           |           |           |           |
     TLLLLAIFKK ALPALPISIT FGLVFYFATD YLVQPFMDQL AFHQFYI
```

No signal peptide
Positions of mutations are denoted in bold.

Mutations in PS-1 and age of onset (in years) when known

79A → V	64	260A → V	40
82V → L	55	262L → F	50
96V →F	-	263C → R	47
115Y → C/H	-/37	264P → L	45
120E → D/K	48/-	267P → S/T	35/-
139M→ K/T/V	-/49/40	269R → G/H	-/-
143I → F/T	-/35	278R → T	-
146M→ I/L/V	40/45/38	280E → A/G	47/42
163H → R/Y	50/47	285A → V	50
169S → L/P	-/-	286L → V	50
171L → P	40	318E → G	-
209G → V	-	378G → E	-
213I → T	-	384G → A	35
231A → T/V	52/-	392L → V	25–40
233M→ T	35	410C → Y	48
235L → P	32	426A → P	-
246A → E	55	436P → Q	-
250L → S	-		

AIII Presenilin 2 (PS2)

Protein name: human presenilin-2 or PS-2 or STM-2
Gene name: *PSEN2* or *PSNL2* or *AD4* or *PS2* or *STM2*
Swiss-Prot primary accession number: P49810

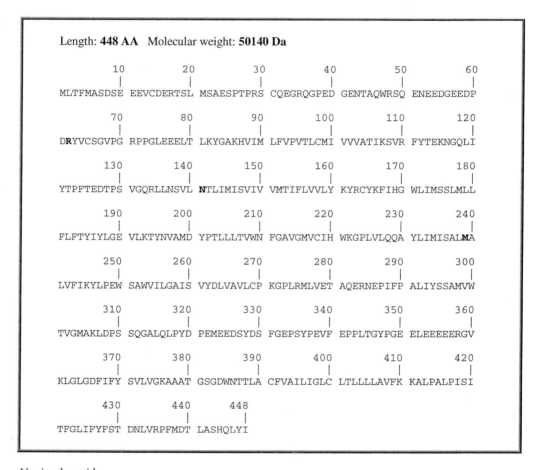

Length: **448 AA** Molecular weight: **50140 Da**

```
           10         20         30         40         50         60
            |          |          |          |          |          |
      MLTFMASDSE EEVCDERTSL MSAESPTPRS CQEGRQGPED GENTAQWRSQ ENEEDGEEDP

           70         80         90        100        110        120
            |          |          |          |          |          |
      DRYVCSGVPG RPPGLEEELT LKYGAKHVIM LFVPVTLCMI VVVATIKSVR FYTEKNGQLI

          130        140        150        160        170        180
            |          |          |          |          |          |
      YTPFTEDTPS VGQRLLNSVL NTLIMISVIV VMTIFLVVLY KYRCYKFIHG WLIMSSLMLL

          190        200        210        220        230        240
            |          |          |          |          |          |
      FLFTYIYLGE VLKTYNVAMD YPTLLLTVWN FGAVGMVCIH WKGPLVLQQA YLIMISALMA

          250        260        270        280        290        300
            |          |          |          |          |          |
      LVFIKYLPEW SAWVILGAIS VYDLVAVLCP KGPLRMLVET AQERNEPIFP ALIYSSAMVW

          310        320        330        340        350        360
            |          |          |          |          |          |
      TVGMAKLDPS SQGALQLPYD PEMEEDSYDS FGEPSYPEVF EPPLTGYPGE ELEEEEERGV

          370        380        390        400        410        420
            |          |          |          |          |          |
      KLGLGDFIFY SVLVGKAAAT GSGDWNTTLA CFVAILIGLC LTLLLLAVFK KALPALPISI

          430        440        448
            |          |          |
      TFGLIFYFST DNLVRPFMDT LASHQLYI
```

No signal peptide
Positions of mutations are denoted in bold.

Mutations in PS2

R62   →   H62

N141 →   I141

M239 →   V239

AIV Apolipoprotein E (apoE)

Protein name: human apolipoprotein E or Apo-E
Gene name: *APOE*
Swiss-Prot primary accession number: P02649

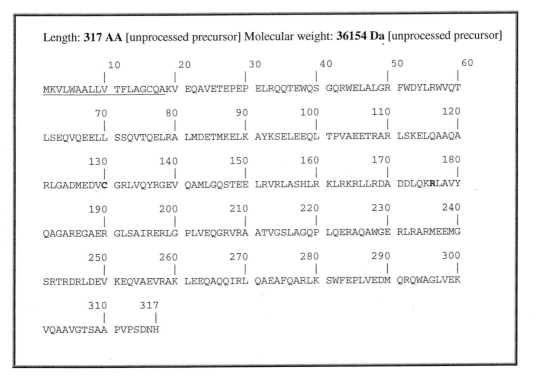

Length: **317 AA** [unprocessed precursor] Molecular weight: **36154 Da** [unprocessed precursor]

```
              10          20          30          40          50          60
               |           |           |           |           |           |
  MKVLWAALLV TFLAGCQAKV EQAVETEPEP ELRQQTEWQS GQRWELALGR FWDYLRWVQT

              70          80          90         100         110         120
               |           |           |           |           |           |
  LSEQVQEELL SSQVTQELRA LMDETMKELK AYKSELEEQL TPVAEETRAR LSKELQAAQA

             130         140         150         160         170         180
               |           |           |           |           |           |
  RLGADMEDVC GRLVQYRGEV QAMLGQSTEE LRVRLASHLR KLRKRLLRDA DDLQKRLAVY

             190         200         210         220         230         240
               |           |           |           |           |           |
  QAGAREGAER GLSAIRERLG PLVEQGRVRA ATVGSLAGQP LQERAQAWGE RLRARMEEMG

             250         260         270         280         290         300
               |           |           |           |           |           |
  SRTRDRLDEV KEQVAEVRAK LEEQAQQIRL QAEAFQARLK SWFEPLVEDM QRQWAGLVEK

             310         317
               |           |
  VQAAVGTSAA PVPSDNH
```

Signal peptide is underlined
Two amino acids in polymorphisms shown in bold
ε^3: C112, R158 (as shown here, including 18 aa signal peptide is C130 and R176)
ε^2: C112, C158
ε^4: R112, R158

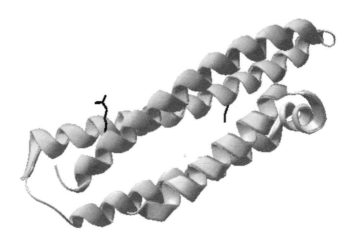

Fig. AIV.1 Structure of apoE3 showing side chains of C112 and R158. Cartoon of NMR resolved structure of apoE3 showing mainly α-helix formation (Brookhaven code 1LPE).

AV Tau

Protein name: microtubule associated protein tau
Gene name: *MAPT* or *MTBT1*

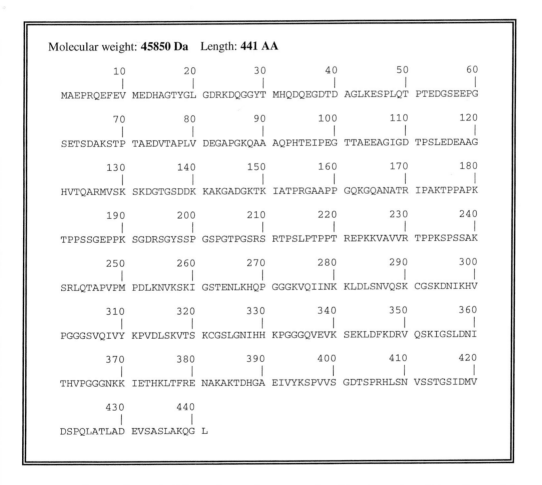

Molecular weight: **45850 Da**   Length: **441 AA**

```
            10           20           30           40           50           60
             |            |            |            |            |            |
   MAEPRQEFEV  MEDHAGTYGL  GDRKDQGGYT  MHQDQEGDTD  AGLKESPLQT  PTEDGSEEPG

            70           80           90          100          110          120
             |            |            |            |            |            |
   SETSDAKSTP  TAEDVTAPLV  DEGAPGKQAA  AQPHTEIPEG  TTAEEAGIGD  TPSLEDEAAG

           130          140          150          160          170          180
             |            |            |            |            |            |
   HVTQARMVSK  SKDGTGSDDK  KAKGADGKTK  IATPRGAAPP  GQKGQANATR  IPAKTPPAPK

           190          200          210          220          230          240
             |            |            |            |            |            |
   TPPSSGEPPK  SGDRSGYSSP  GSPGTPGSRS  RTPSLPTPPT  REPKKVAVVR  TPPKSPSSAK

           250          260          270          280          290          300
             |            |            |            |            |            |
   SRLQTAPVPM  PDLKNVKSKI  GSTENLKHQP  GGGKVQIINK  KLDLSNVQSK  CGSKDNIKHV

           310          320          330          340          350          360
             |            |            |            |            |            |
   PGGGSVQIVY  KPVDLSKVTS  KCGSLGNIHH  KPGGGQVEVK  SEKLDFKDRV  QSKIGSLDNI

           370          380          390          400          410          420
             |            |            |            |            |            |
   THVPGGGNKK  IETHKLTFRE  NAKAKTDHGA  EIVYKSPVVS  GDTSPRHLSN  VSSTGSIDMV

           430          440
             |            |
   DSPQLATLAD  EVSASLAKQG  L
```

Alternate splice products: Six different forms of tau are produced by alternative splicing of exons 2, 3 and 10.

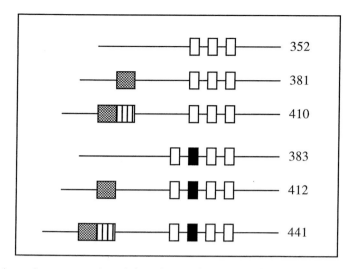

Fig. AV.1 Schematic representation of the 6 human brain tau isoforms. Protein inserts from exons 2 (shaded) 3 (vertical lines) and 10 (solid black) shown.

AVI α-, β- and γ-secretases

The identification and cloning of the enzymes (named α- and β- and γ-secretase) which cleave APP to produce Aβ or other products have been long sought after and recently these have been tentatively identified.

1 β-secretase

Four independent groups report that a novel transmembrane aspartyl protease is β-secretase. The first report from Amgen (Vassar *et al.* 1999) describes the construction of a directional cDNA library from HEK 293 cells (a cell line known to have β- and γ-secretase activity) in a cytomegalovirus promotor based expression vector. Pools of clones were then transiently transfected into a 293 cell line which overexpressed APP containing the Swedish double mutation. Conditioned media from the cells were then assayed for changes in Aβ levels, positives identified and subsequently subdivided into single cDNA clones. One positive clone showed significant sequence homology with the pepsin subfamily of aspartyl proteases and was termed BACE (β-site APP cleaving enzyme).

The sequence of the cDNA (Genbank accession number AF 190725) revealed an open reading frame of 501 amino acids. The protein has an amino terminal signal peptide of 21 amino acids followed by a preprotein domain, spanning amino acids 22–45. The luminal domain of the mature protein extends from residues 46 to 460 and is followed by one putative transmembrane domain of 17 residues and a short cytosolic tail of 24 amino acids.

BACE mRNA was shown to be highly expressed in brain and pancreas with much lower levels in other tissues. *In situ* hybridization studies showed that BACE mRNA was expressed throughout the brain and was predominately confined to neurons. BACE protein was also shown to be present in brain by immunoblotting. Double labelling immunocytochemical studies showed that BACE was mainly located within the Golgi and endosomes.

When BACE was overexpressed in HEK cells the amount of Aβ was increased two-fold. The amount of α-secretase cleavage was reduced suggesting that both enzymes compete for APP. Examination of the cleavage site of APP by BACE was checked by radiosequencing of both Aβ and C99 (the membrane bound fragment of APP left after β-secretase cleavage, before γ-secretase clipping) and in both cases was shown to be identical to that of β-secretase.

Finally expression and purification of the luminal domain of BACE fused to the Fc portion of human IgG allowed the demonstration of direct protease activity of BACE on synthetic peptides covering the β- secretase site. The results showed highly specific cleavage of APP peptides by BACE with the amount of cleavage of the Swedish double mutant peptide increased by 100-fold and no cleavage of peptides showing an M→V mutation at the β-secretase site. These results are identical to those expected of β-secretase and indicate that BACE is almost certainly this enzyme

The second report (Hussain *et al.* 1999) from SmithKline Beecham describes the identification of a novel transmembrane aspartyl proteinase in an EST database and the subsequent cloning of the full length cDNA and identification of this protein (called Asp 2) as β-secretase.

Transient transfection of SH-SY5Y APP-695 cells with Asp 2 cDNA resulted in an increase in sAPPβ. Mutation of either of the proposed catalytic Asp residues was shown to abolish this effect. Immunohistochemical analysis of the distribution of Asp 2 in human brain showed it to be localized to neurons. Using a myc tagged Asp2 cDNA it was possible to perform double labelling studies with APP in COS-7 cells to show that the two proteins co-localize to the Golgi/endoplasmic reticulum region of the cells.

The third report by Yan et al. (1999) examined the complete genome sequence of C. elegans for aspartyl protease motifs. By comparison of sequences on the database they identified human equivalents, two novel putative membrane- bound aspartyl proteases were named Asp1 and Asp2. Using a cell line engineered to secrete Aβ it was shown that antisense oligonucleotides to Asp2 but not Asp1 decreased the secretion of Aβ. Subsequent solubilization and purification of recombinant Asp2 from CHO cells showed that it was able to cleave synthetic peptides at the β-secretase site. Additionally the Asp2 gene was localized to chromosome 11q23–24.

Finally, using a more traditional approach, Sinha et al. (1999) identified β-secretase activity in triton solubilized membranes from a variety of tissues using an assay for sAPPβ. Interestingly, brain showed high activity whereas other tissue extracts showed little, including the pancreas where the corresponding mRNA levels are high. A 14 amino acid synthetic peptide was then made with the amino acid statine substiting for leucine at the P1 position, and a valine residue substituting for aspartic acid at the β-secretase site (P1' position). This was shown to inhibit the β-secretase activity and was subsequently used as an affinity matrix to purify the enzymatic activity from solubilized human brain extracts. An N-terminal sequence of the purified protein allowed the cloning of the cDNA. Overexpression, purification, and cleavage analysis of recombinant protein identified it to be β-secretase.

2 Putative identification of γ-secretase

Four recent reports, all presented in the same issue of Nature (DeStrooper et al. 1999; Struhl and Greenwald 1999; Wolfe et al. 1999b; Ye et al. 1999), provide strong evidence that PS1 is directly involved in γ-secretase activity and may even be γ-secretase itself. One of these papers (Wolfe et al. 1999b) shows that mutation of either of two transmembrane aspartate residues (Asp257 or Asp385) in PS1 results in a loss of γ-secretase activity. The other three investigate receptors of the Notch family and their processing, and centre on the role of PS1 in the processing of Notch.

The Notch receptor is synthesized as a 300-kDa precursor protein. It is a ligand-activated Type I transmembrane receptor, and is involved in cell fate decisions in invertebrates and vertebrates. The receptor exists at the plasma membrane as a heterodimer formed by the reassembly of the two parts of the receptor after cleavage by a furin-like convertase in the extracellular domain (Fig. AVI.1). Ligands, such as Delta, interact with epidermal growth factor (EGF) repeats in the extracellular domain resulting in the proteolytic release of the Notch intracellular domain (NICD) (Fig. AVI.1) and its translocation to the nucleus where it preferentially interacts with the CSL (CBF1, Su[H], Lag-1) family of DNA-binding proteins.

PS1 knockout (-/-) mice die shortly after birth with defects in somite segmentation and differentiation as PS1 is required for proper formation of the axial skeleton, normal neurogenesis, and neuronal survival (Shen et al. 1997; Wong et al. 1997). Expression of mRNA encoding Notch1 and Dll1 (delta-like gene 1), a vertebrate Notch ligand, is markedly reduced in the presomitic mesoderm of PS1(-/-) embryos. Hence, PS1 is required for the spatiotemporal expression of Notch1 and Dll1, which are essential for somite segmentation and maintenance of somite borders.

In DeStrooper *et al.* (1999). the link between Notch-1 and PS1 is examined in cells from the PS1 knockout mice. Previous work from this lab (DeStrooper *et al.* 1998) using neuronal cultures derived from PS1 knockout mouse embryos showed α- and β-secretase cleavage of APP was unaffected whereas cleavage by γ-secretase was inhibited. This resulted in accumulation of carboxyl-terminal fragments of APP and a reduction in Aβ peptide. In this latest paper they show evidence that supports the theory that a PS1-dependent γ-secretase-like protease mediates release of NICD since PS1 deficiency reduces the proteolytic release of NICD from a truncated Notch construct. Moreover, several known APP γ-secretase inhibitors block this step in Notch processing indicating that similar protease activities are responsible for cleavage of Notch and APP.

The papers by Struhl and Greenwald (1999) and Ye *et al.* (1999) look at the *PS* gene in *Drosophila*. They show that PS is required for the proteolytic release of NICD from the membrane following ligand-induced activation of Notch. Null mutations in the *Drosophila PS* gene abolish Notch signal transduction and prevent NICD from entering the nucleus. PS is shown to be required for the normal proteolytic production of C-terminal Notch fragments, and to act upstream of both the membrane-bound form and the activated nuclear form of Notch.

Wolfe and colleagues (Wolfe *et al.* 1999*b*) show that mutation of either of two conserved transmembrane aspartate residues in PS1, Asp 257 (in TM6), and Asp 385 (in TM7) to alanines, substantially reduces Aβ production and increases the amounts of the C-terminal fragments of APP (see Appendix II for schematic of PS1). This is seen in three different cell lines and in cell-free microsomes. Mutation of either aspartate also prevents the normal endoproteolysis of PS1. The two transmembrane aspartate residues appear to be critical for both PS1 endoproteolysis and γ-secretase activity. But in the ΔE9 PS1 variant, which does not undergo cleavage, the Asp385Ala mutation is still able to inhibit γ-secretase activity. The authors suggest that PS1 is either a diaspartyl cofactor for γ- secretase or is itself γ-secretase, an autoactivated intramembranous aspartyl protease.

The same group (Wolfe *et al.* 1999*a*) recently described a difluoro ketone peptidomimetic that blocks Aβ production at the γ-secretase level, able to block both Aβ1–40 and Aβ1–42 formation. Various amino acid changes still resulted in inhibition of Aβ1–40 and Aβ1–42, suggesting relatively loose specificity by γ-secretase. Alcohol counterparts of selected difluoro ketones also lowered Aβ levels, indicating that the ketone carbonyl is not essential for activity and suggesting that these compounds inhibit an aspartyl protease.

3-α-**secretase activity**

Two recent papers provide evidence that α-secretase is a member of the ADAMs (a disintegrin and metalloprotease-like) family of membrane-associated zinc metalloproteinases. In the first paper (Lammich *et al.* 1999), overexpression of ADAM10 in HEK 293 cells resulted in a large increase in α-secretase activity. The proteolytically activated form was localized in the plasma membrane, the majority of the proenzyme was found in the Golgi implying that APP may be cleaved both at the cell surface and along the secretory pathway. Futhermore, endogenous α-secretase activity was inhibited by ADAM 10 with a point mutation in the zinc binding site. The authors suggest that increasing expression and activity might be beneficial for the treatment of AD.

In the second paper (Buxbaum *et al.* 1998), using a knockout of TACE (tumour necrosis factor alpha converting enzyme, also a member of the ADAMs family) the authors show that this enzyme plays a central role in regulated α-cleavage of APP. The data suggests that TACE may be the α-secretase responsible for the majority of regulated α- cleavage in cultured cells. Inhibiting this enzyme affected both APP secretion and Aβ formation in cultured cells.

References

Buxbaum, J. D., Liu, K. N., Luo, Y. X., *et al.* (1998). Evidence that tumor necrosis factor alpha converting enzyme is involved in regulated alpha-secretase cleavage of the Alzheimer amyloid protein precursor. *Journal of Biological Chemistry*, **273**, 27765–7.

DeStrooper, B., Saftig, P., Craessaerts, K., *et al.* (1998). Deficiency of presenilin-1 inhibits the normal cleavage of amyloid precursor protein. *Nature*, **391**, 387–90.

DeStrooper, B., Annaert, W., Cupers, P., *et al.* (1999). A presenilin-1-dependent gamma-secretase-like protease mediates release of Notch intracellular domain. *Nature*, **398**, 518–22.

Hussain, I., Powell, D., Howlett, D. R., *et al.* (1999). Identification of a novel aspartic protease (Asp 2) as β–secretase. *Molecular and Cellular Neuroscience*, **14**, 419–27.

Lammich, S., Kojro, E., Postina, R., *et al.* (1999). Constitutive and regulated alpha-secretase cleavage of Alzheimer's amyloid precursor protein by a disintegrin metalloprotease. *Proceedings of the National Academy of Sciences USA*, **96**, 3922–7.

Vassar, R., Bennett, B. D., BabuKhan, S., *et al.* (1999). Beta-secretase cleavage of Alzheimer's amyloid precursor protein by the transmembrane aspartic protease BACE. *Science*, **286**, 735–41.

Shen, J., Bronson, R. T., Chen, D. F., *et al.* (1997). Skeletal and CNS defects in presenilin-1-deficient mice. *Cell*, **89**, 629–39.

Sinha, S., Anderson, J. P., Barbour, R., *et al.* (1999). Purification and cloning of amyloid precursor protein β-secretase from human brain. *Nature*, **402**, 537–40.

Struhl, G. and Greenwald, I. (1999). Presenilin is required for activity and nuclear access of Notch in *Drosophila*. *Nature*, **398**, 522–5.

Wolfe, M. S., Xia, W. M., Moore, C. L., *et al.* (1999*a*). Peptidomimetic probes and molecular modeling suggest that Alzheimer's gamma-secretase is an intramembrane-cleaving aspartyl protease. *Biochemistry*, **38**, 4720–7.

Wolfe, M. S., Xia, W. M., Ostaszewski, B. L., *et al.* (1999*b*). Two transmembrane aspartates in presenilin-1 required for presenilin endoproteolysis and gamma-secretase activity. *Nature*, **398**, 513–17.

Wong, P. C., Zheng, H., Chen, H., *et al.* (1997). Presenilin 1 is required for Notch1 and DII1 expression in the paraxial mesoderm. *Nature*, **387**, 288–92.

Yan, R., Bienkowsi, M. J., Shuck, M. E., *et al.* (1999). Membrane-anchored aspartyl protease with Alzheimer's disease β-secretase activity. *Nature*, **402**, 533–7.

Ye, Y. H., Lukinova, N., and Fortini, M. E. (1999). Neurogenic phenotypes and altered Notch processing in *Drosophila* presenilin mutants. *Nature*, **398**, 525–9.

BACE

Protein Name Beta-secretase; Synonym(s) beta-site APP cleaving enzyme, beta-site amyloid precursor protein cleaving enzyme; aspartyl protease 2, ASP2
Gene name(s) *BACE*

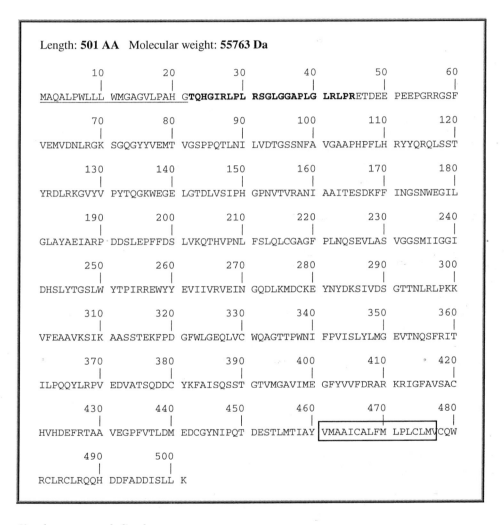

Length: **501 AA**   Molecular weight: **55763 Da**

```
          10         20         30         40         50         60
          |          |          |          |          |          |
MAQALPWLLL WMGAGVLPAH GTQHGIRLPL RSGLGGAPLG LRLPRETDEE PEEPGRRGSF

          70         80         90        100        110        120
          |          |          |          |          |          |
VEMVDNLRGK SGQGYYVEMT VGSPPQTLNI LVDTGSSNFA VGAAPHPFLH RYYQRQLSST

         130        140        150        160        170        180
          |          |          |          |          |          |
YRDLRKGVYV PYTQGKWEGE LGTDLVSIPH GPNVTVRANI AAITESDKFF INGSNWEGIL

         190        200        210        220        230        240
          |          |          |          |          |          |
GLAYAEIARP DDSLEPFFDS LVKQTHVPNL FSLQLCGAGF PLNQSEVLAS VGGSMIIGGI

         250        260        270        280        290        300
          |          |          |          |          |          |
DHSLYTGSLW YTPIRREWYY EVIIVRVEIN GQDLKMDCKE YNYDKSIVDS GTTNLRLPKK

         310        320        330        340        350        360
          |          |          |          |          |          |
VFEAAVKSIK AASSTEKFPD GFWLGEQLVC WQAGTTPWNI FPVISLYLMG EVTNQSFRIT

         370        380        390        400        410        420
          |          |          |          |          |          |
ILPQQYLRPV EDVATSQDDC YKFAISQSST GTVMGAVIME GFYVVFDRAR KRIGFAVSAC

         430        440        450        460        470        480
          |          |          |          |          |          |
HVHDEFRTAA VEGPFVTLDM EDCGYNIPQT DESTLMTIAY VMAAICALFM LPLCLMVCQW

         490        500
          |          |
RCLRCLRQQH DDFADDISLL K
```

Signal sequence underlined
Pro-domain in bold
Putative transmembrane domain boxed

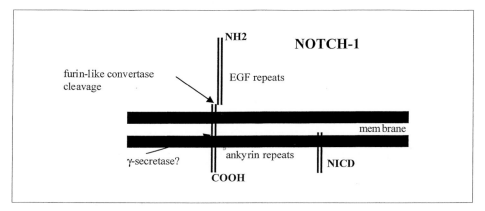

Fig. AVI.1 Schematic of notch-1 receptor at the plasma membrane showing positions of cleavage by furin and possibly γ-secretase. Notch is first cleaved by furin in the transgolgi network; the two resulting fragments remain associated at the plasma membrane. A putative ligand induced second cleavage is indicated. This cleavage releases the intracellular domain of the receptor which translocates to the nucleus to activate transcription. EGF Epidermal growth factor. NICD Notch intracellular domain

Index